D1327788

THE REQUISITES

Breast Imaging

The Requisites Series

SERIES EDITOR

James H. Thrall, MD
Radiologist-in-Chief Emeritus
Massachusetts General Hospital
Distinguished Juan M. Taveras Professor of Radiology
Harvard Medical School
Boston, Massachusetts

TITLES IN THE SERIES

Breast Imaging
Cardiac Imaging
Emergency Imaging
Gastrointestinal Imaging
Genitourinary Imaging
Musculoskeletal Imaging
Neuroradiology Imaging
Nuclear Medicine
Pediatric Imaging
Thoracic Imaging
Ultrasound
Vascular and Interventional Imaging

THE REQUISITES

Breast Imaging

THIRD EDITION

Debra M. Ikeda, MD, FACR, FSBI
Professor
Department of Radiology
Stanford University School of Medicine
Stanford, California

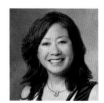

Kanae K. Miyake, MD, PhD
Program-Specific Assistant Professor
Department of Diagnostic Imaging and Nuclear Medicine
Kyoto University Graduate School of Medicine
Kyoto, Japan
Visiting Assistant Professor
Department of Radiology
Stanford University School of Medicine
Stanford, California

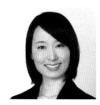

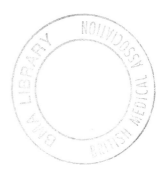

ELSEVIER

ELSEVIER

3251 Riverport Lane
St. Louis, Missouri 63043

THE REQUISITES: BREAST IMAGING, THIRD EDITION

ISBN: 978-0-323-32904-0

Notices

Knowledge and best practice in this field are constantly changing. As new research and experience broaden our understanding, changes in research methods, professional practices, or medical treatment may become necessary.

Practitioners and researchers must always rely on their own experience and knowledge in evaluating and using any information, methods, compounds, or experiments described herein. In using such information or methods they should be mindful of their own safety and the safety of others, including parties for whom they have a professional responsibility.

With respect to any drug or pharmaceutical products identified, readers are advised to check the most current information provided (i) on procedures featured or (ii) by the manufacturer of each product to be administered, to verify the recommended dose or formula, the method and duration of administration, and contraindications. It is the responsibility of practitioners, relying on their own experience and knowledge of their patients, to make diagnoses, to determine dosages and the best treatment for each individual patient, and to take all appropriate safety precautions.

To the fullest extent of the law, neither the Publisher nor the authors, contributors, or editors assume any liability for any injury and/or damage to persons or property as a matter of products liability, negligence or otherwise, or from any use or operation of any methods, products, instructions, or ideas contained in the material herein.

Library of Congress Cataloging-in-Publication Data

Names: Ikeda, Debra M., author. | Miyake, Kanae K., author.
Title: Breast imaging / Debra M. Ikeda, Kanae K. Miyake.
Other titles: Requisites series.
Description: Third edition. | St. Louis, Missouri : Elsevier, [2017] |
Series: Requisites | Includes bibliographical references and index.
Identifiers: LCCN 2016032302 | ISBN 9780323329040 (hardcover : alk. paper)
Subjects: | MESH: Mammography | Breast Diseases–diagnosis | Ultrasonography,
Mammary | Magnetic Resonance Imaging–methods
Classification: LCC RG493.5.R33 | NLM WP 815 | DDC 618.1/907572–dc23 LC record available at
    https://lccn.loc.gov/2016032302

Executive Content Strategist: Robin Carter
Content Development Specialist: Angie Breckon
Publishing Services Manager: Julie Eddy
Book Production Specialist: Clay S. Broeker
Design Direction: Amy Buxton

Printed in China

Working together
to grow libraries in
developing countries

www.elsevier.com • www.bookaid.org

Last digit is the print number: 9   8   7   6   5   4   3   2   1

For my mother, Dorothy Yoshie Kishi Ikeda
Pearl City, Hawaii
and
For my father, Otto Masaru Ikeda, and brother
Clyde Seiji Ikeda
Puowaina (Punchbowl), Honolulu, Hawaii
Debra M. Ikeda

For my mother, Chikako Miyake
Gifu, Japan
and
For my father, Akihide Miyake
Tokiwacho, Kyoto, Japan
Kanae K. Miyake

Contributors

Bruce L. Daniel, MD
Professor of Radiology
Stanford University School of Medicine
Stanford, California

Frederick M. Dirbas, MD
Associate Professor of Surgery
Stanford University School of Medicine
Leader, Breast Disease Management Group
Stanford Cancer Center
Stanford, California

Dipti Gupta, MD
Assistant Professor
Section of Breast Imaging
Northwestern Memorial Hospital
Chicago, Illinois

R. Edward Hendrick, PhD, FACR, FSBI, FAAPM, FISMRM
Clinical Professor of Radiology
University of Colorado-Denver School of Medicine
Aurora, Colorado

Kathleen C. Horst, MD
Assistant Professor
Department of Radiation Oncology
Stanford University School of Medicine
Stanford, California

Debra M. Ikeda, MD, FACR, FSBI
Professor
Department of Radiology
Stanford University School of Medicine
Stanford, California

Ellen B. Mendelson, MD, FACR, FSBI, FSRU
Lee F. Rogers Professor of Medical Education in Radiology
Professor of Radiology
Department of Radiology
Feinberg School of Medicine, Northwestern University
Chicago, Illinois

Kanae K. Miyake, MD, PhD
Program-Specific Assistant Professor
Diagnostic Imaging and Nuclear Medicine
Kyoto University Graduate School of Medicine
Kyoto, Japan
Visiting Assistant Professor
Department of Radiology
Stanford University School of Medicine
Stanford, California

Camila Mosci, MD, MSc
Professor of Nuclear Medicine
Department of Radiology
University of Campinas
Campinas, Sao Paulo, Brazil

Dung H. Nguyen, MD, PharmD
Clinical Assistant Professor
Stanford University
Stanford, California
Director of Breast Reconstruction
Stanford Cancer Center
Palo Alto, California

Andrew Quon, MD
Medical Director, Clinical PET-CT
Associate Professor of Radiology
Stanford University School of Medicine
Stanford, California

Foreword

The first two editions of *Breast Imaging: The Requisites* were both outstanding texts and captured the philosophy of the *Requisites in Radiology* series by presenting complex material in a concise, logical, and straightforward way, making the material very accessible to the reader. Drs. Ikeda and Miyake and their contributors have again succeeded in achieving these attributes for the third edition of their book. Important new material has been added, and material on all enduring methods has been updated.

In light of the trend toward standardized reporting in radiology, it is noteworthy that breast imaging has been an exemplar within the specialty for the use of standardized reporting through the use of BI-RADS®. Indeed, understanding the use of this reporting system is crucial to successful clinical practice in breast imaging. To this end, Drs. Ikeda and Miyake have systematically incorporated the revised BI-RADS® 2013 system that encompasses ultrasound and MRI reporting as well as mammography, and they explain how to use the BI-RADS® 2013 lexicon correctly. Readers will find this material of daily practical use.

Screening and diagnostic applications of x-ray mammography remain the most commonly performed procedures in breast imaging, but the technology for performing these studies has changed dramatically over the last decade, with widespread use of digital imaging and increasing use of tomosynthesis. These advances in technology are comprehensively described in the third edition of *Breast Imaging: The Requisites.* Many positive consequences related to the use of digital mammography and tomosynthesis have been more firmly established since the previous edition, such as improved cancer detection and reduced callback rates.

Beyond x-ray–based mammography, no area of specialization in radiology has seen more expansion of scope or complexity than breast imaging. The specialty now encompasses the use of all medical imaging methods—x-ray, ultrasound, MRI, nuclear medicine—and addresses a spectrum of applications that includes screening, diagnosis, surveillance, interventions, and assessment of therapeutic efficacy. Functional and molecular information is now incorporated into the practice of breast imaging. Separate chapters of *Breast Imaging: The Requisites* are devoted to each of these topics. The chapters are laid out in a logical fashion, with a succinct summary statement of key elements at the end.

New material in the third edition incorporates substantial advances in our understanding of the challenges of diagnosing breast cancer and therewith development of optimal strategies for employing different imaging methods. For example, strategies for enhanced surveillance using ultrasound and MRI have been informed by advances in our understanding of the genetics of breast cancer and genotype-related risks. Likewise, strategies incorporating nuclear medicine, ultrasound, and MRI methods have been developed to help better detect disease in women with dense breast tissue.

High-quality images are a fundamental basis for successful radiology practice. Presentation of high-quality images is even more important in textbooks in order to provide the reader with clear, easily comprehended examples of image findings. Drs. Ikeda and Miyake and their contributors have achieved a high standard in this regard. Readers will again find that this edition of *Breast Imaging: The Requisites* is generously illustrated with very high-quality material.

While the technology and scientific understanding of breast imaging continue to advance, the special relationship of breast imaging specialists and their patients has not changed. Breast imaging radiologists have a special responsibility as stewards of patient care in going from screening to diagnosis, to assessment of surgical specimens, to clinical staging, and finally to assessment of therapeutic outcome and long-term follow-up. The intimate relationship between radiologists and their patients with breast disease is unique in radiology practice. As in the previous editions of *Breast Imaging: The Requisites,* Drs. Ikeda and Miyake have captured the importance of this relationship and especially the philosophy that the fundamental goal is to save women's lives.

The *Requisites in Radiology* series is well into its third decade and is now an old friend to a large number of radiologists around the world. The intent of the series has always been to provide residents, fellows, and clinical practitioners with reliable, factual material, uncluttered with conjecture or speculation, that can serve as a durable basis for daily practice. As series editor, I have always asked writers to include what they use in their own practices and what they teach their own trainees and to not include extraneous material just for the sake of "completeness." Reference books are also valuable but serve a different purpose.

I would like to congratulate Drs. Ikeda and Miyake for sustaining the goals of the *Requisites* series and for producing another outstanding book. Readers will benefit from the authors' knowledge and also from their experience and wisdom in one of the most challenging areas of medical practice.

James H. Thrall, MD
Radiologist-in-Chief Emeritus
Massachusetts General Hospital
Distinguished Taveras Professor of Radiology
Harvard Medical School
Boston, Massachusetts

Preface

The specialty of breast imaging is a uniquely challenging and personal combination of imaging, biopsy procedures, clinical correlation, advances in technology, and compassion. A breast cancer diagnosis is intensely personal and potentially devastating for the patient. The radiologist's job is to detect and diagnose the cancer and gently support the patient through discovery, diagnosis, treatment, and follow-up. The radiologist's role has changed from simply identifying cancers to being deeply involved in diagnosis, biopsy, and follow-up. Instead of sitting alone in a dark room, the radiologist is truly part of a team of oncologic surgeons, pathologists, radiation oncologists, medical oncologists, plastic surgeons, geneticists, and, most importantly, the patient.

This is a very simple book. Its purpose is to help the first-year resident understand why the mammogram, the ultrasound, and the MRI look the way they do in benign disease or in cancer. The other purpose is to help senior residents/fellows pass their boards. With careful scrutiny of each chapter, residents will know clinical scenarios in which cancers occur; develop a systematic method of analyzing images; be able to generate a differential diagnoses for masses, calcifications, and enhancement; and know how manage patients.

Even though the book is simple, the pictures and tools in the book can be adapted to your general clinical practice. Thus, when you come upon a tough case out in the "real world," look to the skills that you learned in this book to solve problems. Use all the tricks you learned on each tough case, because there *will* be tough cases. Adversity is inevitable. If you welcome adversity as your personal challenge and opportunity, and if you use *common sense*, you will most certainly succeed. Remember, the goal of imaging is for the good of the patient—to diagnose and treat breast cancer so that the patient will live. Therefore, with each challenging case, view the adversity of the difficult diagnosis as your responsibility, your challenge, and your opportunity. Keep using the tools in this book until you overcome your problem. As Bruce Daniel told me when I was flailing around in the most difficult of MRI-guided procedures, *within the realm of common sense, "Never give up!"*

Two days before Christmas in 1986, in my junior year as a resident, my 62-year-old mother's mammogram showed a 7-mm suspicious spiculated nonpalpable breast mass. The mass was detected because the University of Michigan had hired Visiting Professor Dr. Ingvar Andersson from Malmo, Sweden (principal investigator of the randomized, controlled, population-based Malmo Mammographic Screening Project), who updated our equipment, started a QA program, and taught faculty/trainees state-of-the-art breast imaging interpretation. Because of him, my mother underwent a brand-new diagnostic technique brought from Sweden: fine-needle aspiration under x-ray guidance using a grid coordinate plate. The aspirate showed cancer. We were devastated. My mom had a second opinion for surgery on Christmas Eve and underwent mastectomy 2 days after Christmas. On New Year's Eve, we got the good news that it was a very small invasive tumor, that there were negative axillary lymph nodes, and that she had a good prognosis.

Naturally, I wanted to learn everything about breast imaging because of my experience of what happens within families when a loved one is diagnosed with breast cancer. I knew that diagnosis and treatment of early-stage breast cancers can result in a long, healthy life for the woman. I knew that we, as radiologists, could train to find and diagnose early breast cancer, profoundly affecting women and their families for the better. So I learned breast imaging from excellent teachers. Dr. Miyake and I want you to learn breast imaging, find the little cancer like my mother's tumor, and save her life again.

My mom is now 92 years old and living in Hawaii. Remember our story. I want everyone who reads this book to have the opportunity to perceive and diagnose small cancers, intervene, and have this outcome. When this outcome is not possible, I want everyone who reads this book to use their knowledge to help their patient through her journey. Someday we may not need this book because there will be further advances in science. Until that happy day comes, we ask those who read this book to use your knowledge to help women.

Debra M. Ikeda, MD, FACR, FSBI

Acknowledgments

I would like to thank my mentors, Dr. Edward A. Sickles and Dr. Ingvar Andersson, who inspired me, taught me breast cancer imaging, and have always supported my career. I especially thank my wonderful husband, Glenn C. Carpenter, who is so generously supportive, giving me the "gift of time" to work on the book. Most of all, I wish to thank my awesome co-editor, Dr. Kanae Kawai Miyake, who wrote, reviewed, and cropped images; trained assistants; provided an incredible database for our project; and has been so wonderful to work with as a meticulous, organized scientist, making sure every image, reference, and statement had appropriate scientific or clinical relevance. I was truly blessed when Dr. Kaori Togashi supported Dr. Miyake's sabbatical from Kyoto University to work at Stanford. I have rarely seen anyone so dedicated and devoted to making complex ideas so very simple that even I can understand them! Dr. Miyake has done outstanding work to improve and update this book, and it could not have been done without her tenacity and generous nature. Our collaboration and friendship is an experience I will never forget.

Dr. Debra M. Ikeda

It was a great pleasure for me to be a part of this book, having the opportunity to share these educational cases with readers worldwide. I have been working with Dr. Ikeda as a Visiting Assistant Professor at Stanford since October 2013, since which time we have been working on *Breast Imaging* together. I still remember that I read a previous edition of this book when I was a young radiologist and used to keep it on my desk so that I could refer to it when I met difficult cases. It was an indescribable honor for me to be able to contribute to the new edition.

The previous edition was an excellent book, providing fundamental knowledge and useful tips to diagnose breast cancer, written in a reader-friendly manner. I was moved to tears when I read Dr. Ikeda's preface, filled with her sense of responsibility for patients, her strong fighting spirit to battle against breast cancer, and her consideration for all breast radiologists. Through editing the new edition, I have realized that she is truly such a person. She is a wonderful expert, an enthusiastic teacher, and an affectionate woman. Her noble intention and tenacious efforts inspired me, and her dedication and leading ideas made the book evolve. I hope that our book will provide practical help to patients and doctors fighting against breast cancer as they face the difficulties that lay ahead of them. I greatly thank Dr. Debra M. Ikeda for including me in this work.

I thank Dr. Kaori Togashi, the current chair of Department of Radiology at Kyoto University, Japan, who has always supported me and encouraged me as a radiologist and a nuclear medicine physiologist. I thank Dr. Junji Konishi, a former chair of Department of Radiology at Kyoto University, who helped me have the wonderful opportunity to work at Stanford. I thank my mentors, Dr. Yuji Nakamoto and Dr. Shotaro Kanao, who taught me PET and breast imaging while I was at Kyoto University. I thank my beloved little son, Toma Kawai, who brings happiness into my life, and my husband and best friend, Toshiyuki Kawai, who always supports my work and walks the path of joyful life together with me. I thank my dad, Akihide Miyake, who has affectionately looked over our family from the sky since the age of 36, and my mom, Chikako Miyake, who bravely raised three kids and always wishes happiness and good health to all.

Dr. Kanae K. Miyake

No book is completed without tremendous efforts on the part of many people. We wish to acknowledge our co-authors, Dr. R. Edward Hendrick, Dr. Ellen B. Mendelson, Dr. Dipti Gupta, Dr. Bruce L. Daniel, Dr. Kathleen C. Horst, Dr. Frederick M. Dirbas, Dr. Dung Hoang Nguyen, Dr. Andrew Quon, and Dr. Camila Mosci for their invaluable scientific and educational contributions in their book chapters. We wish to thank our assistants Adrian C. Carpenter, Catherine M. Carpenter, and John Chitouras for their dogged, painstaking, but cheerful help with the massive files of images, references, tables, and text. We thank Mark Riesenberger for his fabulous HIPAA compliant, web-based IT support, without which we would have been frozen 2 years ago. We thank our Elsevier editors Robin Carter, Angie Breckon, and Julia Roberts for their support and (sometimes) gentle prodding to complete the book.

We thank Dr. Jafi Lipson, Dr. Sunita Pal, and Dr. Jennifer Kao for sharing ideas of what might be good tools or illustrations for teaching residents and providing images. We thank our physician contributors at Kyoto University, Japan, Dr. Shotaro Kanao and Dr. Yuji Nakamoto for their beautiful images and written contributions to the book to increase our knowledge of MRI and PET.

We thank Dr. Kaori Togashi, Radiology Chairman at Kyoto University, who generously supported Dr. Kanae Kawai Miyake in writing this book and in her research. We both wish to emulate her superb example as a chairman, scientist, physician, and compassionate mentor to radiologists and women. We thank Dr. S. Sanjiv (Sam) Gambhir, Radiology Chairman at Stanford University, and the late Dr. Gary M. Glazer for their vision and support of Stanford Breast Imaging, who were always and constantly seeking ways to provide the best technology and the earliest detection and keenly pursuing newest research for our women to save them from breast cancer.

We thank all the scientists, doctors, engineers, and physicists who support our breast cancer patients and women and who battle breast cancer on their behalf. We especially wish to recognize the struggle of our many breast cancer patients and women undergoing screening; this book was written for them, directed to all who wish to help them by learning about breast imaging. Thank you.

Dr. Debra M. Ikeda and Dr. Kanae K. Miyake

Contents

Video Contents

Chapter 1

Mammography Acquisition

Screen-Film, Digital Mammography and Tomosynthesis, the Mammography Quality Standards Act, and Computer-Aided Detection

R. Edward Hendrick, Debra M. Ikeda, and Kanae K. Miyake

Mammography is one of the most technically challenging areas of radiography, requiring high spatial resolution, excellent soft-tissue contrast, and low radiation dose. It is particularly challenging in denser breasts because of the similar attenuation coefficients of breast cancers and fibroglandular tissues. The Digital Mammographic Imaging Study Trial (DMIST) and other recent studies have shown that digital mammography offers improved cancer detection compared with screen-film mammography (SFM) in women with dense breasts (Pisano et al., 2005b). As of March 2015, 96% of the mammography units in the United States are digital units, and some sites are using digital breast tomosynthesis (DBT) systems for screening and diagnostic mammography. Computer-aided detection (CAD) systems specific to mammography are also in common use.

Randomized controlled trials (RCTs) of women invited to mammography screening conducted between 1963 and 2000 based on SFM have shown that early detection and treatment of breast cancer have reduced the proportion of late-stage breast cancers and led to a 20% to 30% decrease in breast cancer mortality among these women. More recent observational studies of screening programs in Europe have shown that screening mammography reduces breast cancer mortality by 38% to 48% among women screened compared with unscreened women (Broeders et al., 2012). A similar observational study in Canada showed breast cancer mortality reduced by 44% among screened women aged 40 to 49, 40% in screened women aged 50 to 59, 42% in screened women aged 60 to 69, and 35% in screened women aged 70 to 79 compared with unscreened women (Coldman et al., 2007). The different mammography screening recommendations of several major organizations are shown in Box 1.1 (Lee et al., 2010; Oeffinger et al., 2015; Siu, 2016).

In all of these studies, image quality was demonstrated to be a critical component of early detection of breast cancer.

To standardize and improve the quality of mammography, in 1987 the American College of Radiology (ACR) started a voluntary ACR Mammography Accreditation Program. In 1992, the U.S. Congress passed the Mammography Quality Standards Act (MQSA; P.L. 102-539), which went into effect in 1994 and remains in effect with reauthorizations in 1998, 2004, and 2007. The MQSA mandates requirements for facilities performing mammography, including equipment and quality assurance requirements, as well as personnel qualifications for physicians, radiologic technologists, and medical physicists involved in the performance of mammography in the United States (Box 1.2).

This chapter outlines the basics of image acquisition using SFM, digital mammography, and DBT. It reviews the quality assurance requirements for mammography stipulated by the MQSA and also describes the essentials of CAD in mammography.

BOX 1.1 Mammography Screening Recommendations for Normal Risk Women from Several Major Organizations

American College of Radiology and Society of Breast Imaging: Annual screening starting at age 40 and continuing until a woman's life expectancy is less than 5-7 years
American Cancer Society: Annual screening ages 45-54, then biennial screening until a woman's life expectancy is less than 10 years, with the option to begin annual screening at age 40 and to continue annual screening beyond age 54.
United States Preventive Services Task Force: Biennial screening ages 50-74.

Congressional act to regulate mammography
Regulations enforced by the Food and Drug Administration (FDA) require yearly inspections of all U.S. mammography facilities
All mammography centers must comply; noncompliance results in corrective action or closure
Falsifying information submitted to the FDA can result in fines and jail terms
Regulations regarding equipment, personnel credentialing and continuing education, quality control, quality assurance, and day-to-day operations

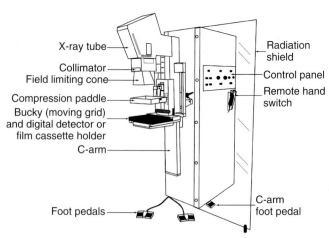

FIG. 1.1 Components of an x-ray mammography unit.

BOX 1.3 **Mammography Generators**

Provide 24–32 kVp, 5–300 mA
Half-value layer between kVp/100 + 0.03 and kVp/100 + 0.12 (in millimeters of aluminum) for Mo/Mo anode/filter material
Average breast exposure is 26–28 kVp (lower kVp for thinner or fattier breasts, higher kVp for thicker or denser breasts)
Screen-film systems deliver an average absorbed dose to the glandular tissue of the breast of 2 mGy (0.2 rad) per exposure

Mo, molybdenum.

TECHNICAL ASPECTS OF MAMMOGRAPHY IMAGE ACQUISITION

Mammography is performed on specially designed, dedicated x-ray machines using either x-ray film and paired fluorescent screens (SFM) or digital detectors to capture the image. All mammography units are comprised of a rotating anode x-ray tube with matched filtration for soft-tissue imaging, a breast compression plate, a moving grid, an x-ray image receptor, and an automatic exposure control (AEC) device that can be placed under or detect the densest portion of the breast, all mounted on a rotating C-arm (Fig. 1.1). A technologist compresses the patient's breast between the image receptor and compression plate for a few seconds during each exposure. Breast compression is important because it spreads normal fibroglandular tissues so that cancers can be better seen on the superimposed structured noise pattern of normal breast tissues. It also decreases breast thickness, decreasing exposure time, radiation dose to the breast, and the potential for image blurring as a result of patient motion and unsharpness.

Women worry about breast pain from breast compression and about the radiation dose from mammography. Breast pain during compression varies among individuals and may be decreased by obtaining mammograms 7 to 10 days after the onset of menses when the breasts are least painful. Breast pain is also minimized by taking oral analgesics, such as acetaminophen, before the mammogram or by using appropriately designed foam pads that cushion the breast without adversely affecting image quality or increasing breast dose.

Current mammography delivers a low dose of radiation to the breast. The most radiosensitive breast tissues are the epithelial cells, which, along with connective tissues, make up fibroglandular elements. The best measure of breast dose is mean glandular dose, or the average absorbed dose of ionizing radiation to the radiosensitive fibroglandular tissues. The mean glandular dose received by the average woman is approximately 2 mGy (0.2 rad) per exposure or 4 mGy (0.4 rad) for a typical two-view examination. Radiation doses from digital mammography exposures tend to be 20% to 30% lower than those from SFM. Radiation doses to thinner compressed breasts are substantially lower than doses to thicker breasts.

The main patient risk from mammographic radiation is the possible induction of breast cancer 5 to 30 years after exposure. The estimated risk of inducing breast cancer is linearly proportional to the radiation dose and inversely related to age at exposure. The lifetime risk of inducing a fatal breast cancer as a result of two-view mammography in women aged 45 years old at exposure is estimated to be about 1 in 100,000 (Hendrick, 2010). For a woman aged 65 at exposure, the *risk* is less than 0.3 in 100,000. The *benefit* of screening mammography is the detection of breast cancer before it is clinically apparent. The likelihood of an invasive or in situ cancer present in a woman screened at age 45 is about 1 in 500. The likelihood that the cancer would be fatal in the absence of mammography screening is about 1 in 4, and the likelihood that screening mammography will convey a mortality benefit is 15% (RCT estimate for women aged 40–49) to about 45% (observational study estimate). Hence, the likelihood of screening mammography saving a woman's life at this age is about 1 in 4400 to 1 in 13,000, yielding a benefit-to-risk ratio of 8:1 to 23:1. For a woman aged 65 at screening, the likelihood of a mortality benefit from mammography is about 1 in 2000 to 1 in 4000 (assuming a 25% to 50% mortality benefit), yielding a benefit-to-risk ratio of approximately 90:1 to 180:1. Screening mammography is only effective when regular periodic exams are performed.

The generator for a mammography system provides power to the x-ray tube. The peak kilovoltage (kVp) of mammography systems is lower than that of conventional x-ray systems, because it is desirable to use softer x-ray beams to increase both soft-tissue contrast and the absorption of x-rays in the image receptor. Low kVp is especially important for SFM, in which screen phosphor thickness is limited to minimize image blur. Typical kVp values for mammography are 24 to 32 kVp for molybdenum (Mo) targets and 26 to 35 kVp for rhodium (Rh) or tungsten (W) targets. A key feature of mammography generators is the electron beam current (milliampere [mA]) rating of the system. The higher the mA rating, the shorter is the exposure time for total tube output (milliampere second [mAs]). A compressed breast of average thickness (5 cm) requires about 150 mAs at 26 kVp to achieve proper film densities in SFM. If the tube rating is 100 mA (typical of the larger focal spots used for nonmagnification mammography), the exposure time would be 1.5 seconds. A higher output system with 150-mA output would cut the exposure time to 1 second for the same compressed breast thickness and kVp setting. Because of the wide range of breast thicknesses, exposures require mAs values ranging from 10 to several hundred mAs. Specifications for generators are listed in Box 1.3.

BOX 1.4 Anode-Filter Combinations for Mammography

Mo/Mo
Mo/Rh
Rh/Rh
W/Rh, W/Ag, or W/Al

Ag, silver; *Al*, aluminum; *Mo*, molybdenum; *Rh*, rhodium; *W*, tungsten.

The most commonly used anode/filter combination is Mo/Mo consisting of an Mo anode (or target) and an Mo filter (25–30 μm thick). This is used for thinner compressed breasts (<5 cm thick). Most current manufacturers also offer an Rh filter to be used with the Mo target (Mo/Rh), which produces a slightly more penetrating (harder) x-ray beam for use with thicker breasts. Some manufacturers offer other target materials, such as Rh/Rh, which is an Rh target paired with an Rh filter, and a W target paired with a Rh filter (W/Rh or with an aluminum [Al] filter [W/Al]). These alternative anode/filter combinations are designed for thicker (>5 cm) and denser breasts. Typically, higher kVp settings are used with these alternative target/filter combinations to create a harder x-ray beam for thicker breasts, because fewer x-rays are attenuated with a harder x-ray beam (Box 1.4). One of the best parameters to measure the hardness or penetrating capability of an x-ray beam is the half-value layer (HVL), which represents the thickness of Al that reduces the x-ray exposure by one-half. The harder the x-ray beam, the higher is the HVL. The typical HVL for mammography is 0.3 to 0.5 mm of Al. The Food and Drug Administration (FDA) requires that the HVL for mammography cannot be less than kVp/100 ± 0.03 (in millimeters of Al), so that the x-ray beam is not too soft (ie, does not contain too many low-energy x-rays that contribute to breast radiation dose but not to image contrast because they are all absorbed in breast tissue). For example, at 28 kVp the HVL cannot be less than 0.31 mm of Al. There is also an upper limit on the HVL that depends on the target–filter combination. For Mo/Mo, the HVL must be less than kVp/100 +0.12 (in mm of Al); thus, for 28 kVp, the HVL must be less than 0.4 mm of Al.

The usual mammography focal spot size for standard contact (ie, nonmagnification) mammography is typically 0.3 mm. Magnification mammography requires a smaller focal spot, (about 0.1 mm) to reduce penumbra (geometric blurring of structures in the breast produced because the breast is closer to the x-ray source and farther from the image receptor to produce greater "geometric" magnification). The effect of focal spot size on resolution in the breast is tested by placing a line pair (lp) pattern in the location of the breast at a specific distance (4.5 cm) from the breast support surface. For SFM, the larger 0.3-mm mammography focal spot used for standard, contact mammography should produce an image that resolves at least 11 lp/mm when the lines of the test pattern run in the direction perpendicular to the length of the focal spot (this measures the blurring effect of the length of the focal spot) and at least 13 lp/mm when the lines run parallel to the focal spot (measuring the blurring effect of the width of the focal spot). Thus, although the SFM image receptor can resolve 18 to 21 lp/mm, the geometry of the breast in contact mammography and the finite-sized larger focal spot reduce the limiting spatial resolution of the system to 11 to 15 lp/mm *in the breast*. The limiting spatial resolution of digital mammography systems is less (5–10 lp/mm), caused by pixelization of the image by the digital image receptor. In digital, a *line* is 1 pixel width, and a line pair is 2 pixels. For example, for a digital detector with 100-micron (0.1-mm) pixel size or pitch (the center-to-center distance between adjacent pixels), a line pair consists of 2 pixels or 200 microns (0.2 mm). Therefore, one can fit five line pairs (at 0.2 mm each) into a 1-mm length, or the

detector has a limiting spatial resolution of 5 lp/mm. By similar reasoning, a digital detector with 50-micron pixels has a limiting spatial resolution of 10 lp/mm.

The x-ray tube and image receptor are mounted on opposite ends of a rotating C-arm to obtain mammograms in almost any projection. The source-to-image receptor distance (SID) for mammography units must be *at least* 55 cm for contact mammography. Most systems have SIDs of 65 to 70 cm.

Geometric magnification is achieved by moving the breast farther from the image receptor (closer to the x-ray tube) and switching to a small focal spot, about 0.1 mm in size (Fig. 1.2). Placing the breast halfway between the focal spot and the image receptor (see Fig. 1.2B) would magnify the breast by a factor of 2.0 from its actual size to the image size because of the divergence of the x-ray beam. The MQSA requires that mammography units with magnification capabilities must provide at least one fixed magnification factor of between 1.4 and 2.0 (Table 1.1). Geometric magnification makes small, high-contrast structures such as microcalcifications more visible by making them larger relative to the noise pattern in the image (increasing their signal-to-noise ratio [SNR]). Optically or electronically magnifying a contact image, as is done with a magnifier on SFM or using a zoom factor greater than 1 on a digital mammogram, does not increase the SNR of the object relative to the background, because both object and background are increased in size equally. To avoid excess blurring of the image with geometric magnification, it is important to use a sufficiently small focal spot (usually 0.1 mm nominal size) and not too large a magnification factor (2.0 or less). When the small focal spot is selected for geometric magnification, the x-ray tube output is decreased by a factor of 3 to 4 (to 25–40 mA) compared with that from a large focal spot (80–150 mA). This can extend imaging times for magnification mammography, even though the grid is removed in magnification mammography. The air gap between the breast and image receptor provides adequate scatter rejection in magnification mammography without the use of an antiscatter grid.

Collimators near the x-ray tube control the size and shape of the x-ray beam to decrease patient exposure to tissues beyond the compressed breast and image receptor. In mammography, the x-ray beam is collimated to a rectangular field to match the image receptor rather than the breast contour, because x-rays striking the image receptor outside the breast do not contribute to breast dose. By federal regulation, the x-ray field cannot extend beyond the chest wall of the image receptor by more than 2% of the SID. Thus for a 60-cm SID unit, the x-ray beam can extend beyond the chest wall edge of the image receptor by no more than 1.2 cm.

The compression plate and image receptor assembly hold the breast motionless during the exposure, decreasing the breast thickness and providing tight compression, better separating fibroglandular tissues in the breast (Fig. 1.3). The compression plate has a posterior lip that is more than 3 cm high and usually is oriented at 90 degrees to the plane of the compression plate at the chest wall. This lip keeps chest wall structures from superimposing and obscuring posterior breast tissue in the image. The compression plate must be able to compress the breast for up to 1 minute with a compression force of 25 to 45 lb. The compression plate can be advanced by a foot-controlled motorized device and adjusted more finely with hand controls. Because the radiation dose to the breast is decreased in thinner breasts, breast compression, which thins the breast, also decreases radiation dose.

Screen-Film Mammography Image Acquisition

In SFM, the image receptor assembly holds a screen-film cassette in a carbon-fiber support with a moving antiscatter grid in front of the cassette and an AEC detector behind it (see Fig. 1.3A).

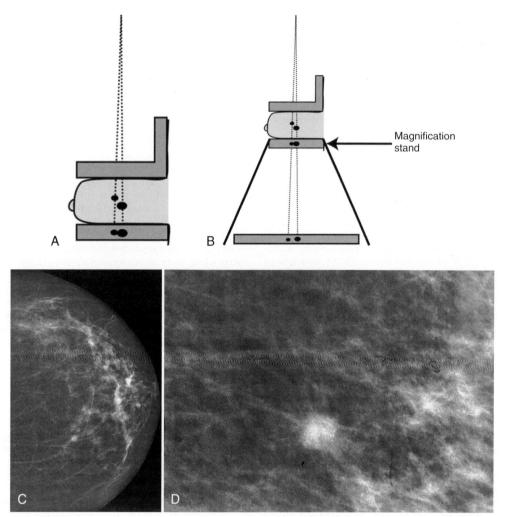

FIG. 1.2 Magnification mammography improves resolution. Nonmagnified, or contact, mammography (A) and geometrically magnified mammography (B). Using a small or microfocal (0.1-mm) focal spot with the configuration shown in (B), higher spatial resolution can be obtained in the breast compared with (A) in which a larger (0.3-mm) focal spot is used. (C) Craniocaudal mammogram shows a possible benign mass in the inner breast. (D) Microfocal magnification shows irregular borders not seen on the standard view.

TABLE 1.1   Mammography Focal Spot Sizes and Source-to-Image Distances

Mammography Type	Nominal Focal Spot Size (mm)	Source-to-Image Distance (cm)
Contact film screen	0.3	≥55
Magnification	0.1	≥55

The Mammography Quality Standards Act requires magnification factors between 1.4 and 2.0 for systems designed to perform magnification mammography.

Screen-film image receptors are required to be 18 × 24 cm and 24 × 30 cm in size to accommodate both smaller and larger breasts (Box 1.5). Each size image receptor must have a moving antiscatter grid composed of lead strips with a grid ratio (defined as the ratio of the lead strip height to the distance between strips) between 3.5:1 and 5:1. The reciprocating grid moves back and forth in the direction perpendicular to the grid lines during the radiographic exposure to eliminate grid lines in the image by blurring them out. One manufacturer uses a hexagonal-shaped grid pattern to improve scatter rejection; this grid is also blurred by reciprocation during exposure. Use of

a grid improves image contrast by decreasing the fraction of scattered radiation reaching the image receptor. Grids increase the required exposure to the breast by approximately a factor of 2 (the Bucky factor), because of the attenuation of primary, as well as scattered, radiation. Grids are not used with magnification mammography. Instead, in magnification mammography, scatter is reduced by collimation and by rejection of scattered x-rays due to a significant air gap between the breast and image receptor.

The AEC system, also known as the *phototimer*, is calibrated to produce a consistent film optical density (OD) by sampling the x-ray beam after it has passed through the breast support, grid, and cassette. The AEC detector is usually a D-shaped sensor that lies along the midline of the breast support and can be positioned by the technologist closer to or farther from the chest wall. If the breast is extremely thick or inappropriate technique factors are selected, the AEC will terminate exposure at a specific backup time (usually 4–6 seconds or 300–750 mAs) to prevent tube overload or melting of the x-ray track on the anode.

Screen-film cassettes used in mammography have an inherent spatial resolution of 18 to 21 lp/mm. Such resolution is achieved typically by using a single-emulsion film placed emulsion side

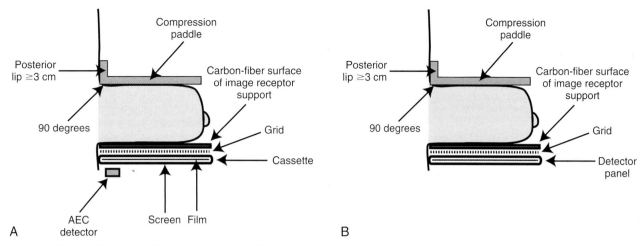

FIG. 1.3 Schematic of a compression paddle and image receptor of screen-film mammography (A) and of digital mammography (B), showing the components of the cassette holder, the compression plate, and the breast. The film emulsion faces the screen. AEC, automatic exposure control. (Adapted from Farria DM, Kimme-Smith C, Bassett LW: Equipment, processing, and image receptor. In Bassett LW, editor: *Diagnosis of diseases of the breast*, Philadelphia, 1997, WB Saunders, pp 32 and 34.)

BOX 1.5   Compression Plate and Imaging Receptor

Both 18 × 24-cm and 24 × 30-cm sizes are required
A moving grid is required for each image receptor size
The compression plate has a posterior lip >3 cm and is oriented 90 degrees to the plane of the plate
Compression force of 25–45 lb
Paddle advanced by a foot motor with hand-compression adjustments
Collimation to the image receptor and not the breast contour

---

down against a single intensifying screen that faces upward toward the breast in the film cassette. The single-emulsion film with a single intensifying screen is used to prevent the parallax unsharpness and crossover exposure that occur with double-emulsion films and double-screen systems. One manufacturer has introduced a double-emulsion film with double-sided screens (EV System, Carestream Health, formerly Eastman Kodak Health Group) with a thinner film emulsion and screen on top to minimize parallax unsharpness. Most screen-film processing combinations have relative speeds of 150 to 200, with speed defined as the reciprocal of the x-ray exposure (in units of Roentgen) required to produce an OD of 1.0 above base plus fog (1.15–1.2, because base plus fog OD is 0.15–0.2).

Film processing involves development of the latent image on the exposed film emulsion. The film is placed in an automatic processor that takes the exposed film and rolls it through liquid developer to amplify the latent image on the film, reducing the silver ions in the x-ray film emulsion to metallic silver, resulting in film darkening in exposed areas. The developer temperature ranges from 92°F to 96°F. The film is then run through a fixer solution containing thiosulfate (or *hypo*) to remove any unused silver and preserve the film. The film is then washed with water to remove residual fixer, which if not removed can cause the film to turn brown over time. The film is then dried with heated air.

Film processing is affected by many variables, and the most important is developer chemistry (weak or oxidized chemistry makes films lighter and lower contrast), developer temperature (too hot may make films darker, and too cool may make films lighter), developer replenishment (too little results in lighter,

TABLE 1.2   Variables Affecting Image Quality of Screen-Film Mammograms

Film too dark	Developer temperature too high Wrong mammographic technique (excessive kVp or mAs) Excessive plus-density control
Film too light	Inadequate chemistry or replenishment Developer temperature too low Wrong mammographic technique
Lost contrast	Inadequate chemistry or replenishment Water to processor turned off Changed film
Film turns brown	Inadequate rinsing of fixer
Motion artifact	Movement by patient Inadequate compression applied Inappropriate mammographic technique (long exposure times)

lower contrast films), inadequate agitation of developer, and uneven application of developer to films (causing film mottling; Table 1.2).

Film viewing conditions must be appropriate (Fig. 1.4). Because mammography viewboxes have high luminance levels (>3000 cd/m² [3000 nit]), mammograms should be masked so that no light strikes the radiologist's eye without passing through the exposed film. Because of high luminance levels film collimation of x-ray exposure should be rectangular and extend slightly beyond the edge of the image receptor so that film is darkened to its edges. Viewbox luminance should be reasonably uniform across all viewbox panels. In addition, the ambient room illumination should be low (<50 lux, and preferably less) to minimize "dazzle glare" from film surfaces. Both viewbox luminance and room illumination should be checked annually by the medical physicist as part of the site quality control program, as specified in the *ACR Mammography Quality Control Manual*.

Digital Mammography Image Acquisition

In digital mammography, the image is obtained in the same manner as in screen-film mammography, using a compression plate and an x-ray tube, with the screen-film cassette replaced by a digital detector (see Fig. 1.3B). Digital image acquisition has several potential advantages in terms of image availability, image processing, making annotations (Fig. 1.5), and CAD. One advantage is elimination of the film processor, which eliminates artifacts and image noise added during film processing. The image contrast of digital mammography is different among vendors depending on the digital look-up curve, which governs how digital signals are translated into pixel gray scale values. Figure 1.6 shows digital mammograms that were obtained with two machines from different vendors demonstrating how the image contrast varies.

Digital mammography uses indirect or direct digital detectors. Indirect digital detectors use a fluorescent screen made of materials such as cesium iodide (CsI) to convert each absorbed x-ray to hundreds of visible light photons. Behind the fluorescent material, light-sensitive detector arrays made of materials such as amorphous silicon diodes or charge-coupled devices measure the produced light pixel by pixel. The weak electronic signal measured in each pixel is amplified and sent through an analog-to-digital converter, enabling computer storage of each pixel's measured detector signal.

Direct digital detectors use detector elements that capture and count x-rays directly, although amplification and analog-to-digital conversion are still applied. Another method to produce digital mammograms involves amorphous selenium. An amorphous selenium plate is an excellent absorber of x-rays and an excellent capacitor, storing the charge created by ionization when x-rays are absorbed. After exposure, an electronic device is used to read out the charge distribution on the selenium plate, which is in proportion to local exposure. This can be done by scanning the selenium plate with a laser beam or by placing a silicon diode array in contact with one side of the plate, with bias voltage applied, to read out the stored charge. Each of these methods allows production of high-resolution digital images.

Another approach to full-field digital mammography (FFDM) is computed radiography (CR), which uses a photostimulable phosphor composed of barium fluorobromide doped with europium (BaFBr:Eu). Computed radiography uses the same dedicated mammography units as SFM, replacing the screen-film cassettes and film processor with CR cassettes (in sizes of 18 × 24 cm and 24 × 30 cm) and a CR processor. The phosphor plate within the CR cassette is used to absorb x-rays just as the screen in a screen-film cassette. Rather than emitting light immediately after exposure (through fluorescence), x-ray absorption in the phosphor causes electrons within the phosphor crystals to be promoted to higher energy levels (through photostimulation).

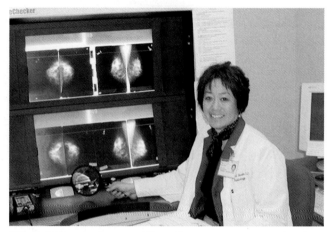

FIG. 1.4 Film-viewing conditions. Because mammography viewboxes have high luminance levels (>3000 cd/m² [3000 nit]), mammograms should be masked so that no light strikes the radiologist's eye without passing through the exposed film. Because of the high luminance, film collimation should be rectangular and extend slightly beyond the edge of the image receptor so that film is darkened to its edges. Viewbox luminance should be reasonably uniform across all viewbox panels. In addition, the ambient room illumination should be low (<50 lux, and preferably less) to minimize "dazzle glare" from film surfaces. Both viewbox luminance and room illumination should be checked annually by the medical physicist as part of the site quality control program (see the *ACR Mammography Quality Control Manual*, 1999 edition).

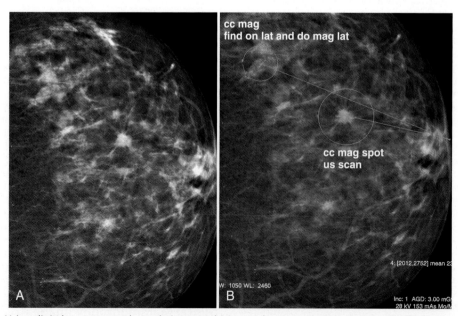

FIG. 1.5 Using digital mammography and picture archiving and communication systems (PACS) for screening recall, two spiculated masses representing infiltrating ductal carcinoma on the craniocaudal view (A) were marked by computer-aided detection and were recalled. The radiologist annotates the images and sends them to PACS for the technologist to retrieve when the patient returns for workup (B).

The plate is removed from the cassette in the CR processor and a red laser light scans the phosphor plate point by point, releasing electrons and stimulating emission of a higher energy (blue) light in proportion to x-ray exposure. In conventional x-ray systems, CR phosphor plates have an opaque backing and are read from only one side. In at least one FDA-approved CR system for mammography (Fuji 5000D CR, Fujifilm Medical Systems), the CR cassette base is transparent and light emitted from the plate during laser scanning is read from both sides to increase reading efficiency.

No matter which digital detector is used, its job is to measure the quantity of x-rays passing through the breast, compression plate, grid (in contact mammography), and breast holder. The signal measured in each pixel is determined by the total attenuation in the breast along a given ray.

The choice of an analog-to-digital converter determines how many bits of memory will be used to store the signal for each pixel; the more bits per pixel, the more dynamic range there is for the image, but at a higher digital data storage cost. Specifically, if 12 bits per pixel are used, 2^{12} or 4096 signal values can be stored. If 14 bits per pixel are used, 2^{14} or 16,384 signal values can be stored. Usually 12- to 14-bit storage per pixel is used. In either case, 2 bytes per pixel are required (8 bits = 1 byte) to store the image. For example, the GE Senographe 2000D and DS digital detectors have 1920 × 2304 pixel arrays, or 4.4 million pixels, requiring 8.8 million bytes (8.8 megabytes; MB) of storage per image. Other FFDM systems require up to 52 MB of storage per image.

Screen-film image receptors used for mammography have a line pair resolution of 18 to 21 lp/mm. To equal this spatial resolution, a digital detector would require 25-micron pixels, which would yield noisier images and pose a storage issue caused by the large data sets required to store those images. FFDM systems have spatial resolutions ranging from 5 lp/mm (for 100-micron pixels) to 10 lp/mm (for 50-micron pixels). In digital mammography systems, it is the size of the pixels, or more correctly their center-to-center distance (pitch), that determines (and limits) the spatial resolution of the imaging chain.

The lower limiting spatial resolution of FFDM systems compared with film is offset by the increased contrast resolution of FFDM systems. Unlike SFM, in which the image cannot be manipulated after exposure and processing, FFDM images can be optimized after image capture by image postprocessing and adjustment of image display. For fixed digital detectors, such as CsI and silicon diode arrays (used by GE) and selenium and amorphous silicon diode arrays (used by Hologic and Siemens), one image-processing step that can minimize image noise and structured artifacts is flat-field correction, or *gain correction* of each acquired digital image. This is done by making and storing a sensitivity map of the digital detector and using that map to correct all exposures. Typically, slot-scanning devices (such as the older SenoScan digital system, Fischer Medical Systems) and CR systems do not perform flat-field correction of digital images. Beyond this, all digital systems have the ability to process the acquired digital image to minimize or eliminate the signal difference that results from the roll-off in thickness of the breast toward the skin line (thickness equalization); some devices add processing to help enhance the appearance of microcalcifications (eg, GE Premium View and FineView). The window width and window level for all digital images viewed with soft copy display on review workstations can be adjusted, changing the contrast and brightness of the images, respectively, as well as digitally magnifying images.

Another important difference between SFM and FFDM is that screen-film images have a linear relationship between the logarithm of x-ray exposure and film OD only in the central portion of the characteristic curve. In FFDM, there is a linear relationship between x-ray exposure and signal over the entire dynamic range of the detector. Thus digital images (at least their "raw" or "for processing" presentation) do not suffer contrast loss in underexposed or overexposed areas of the mammogram (as long as detector saturation does not occur); instead, they show similar contrast over the full dynamic range of signals. Different manufacturers apply different look-up tables to digital images in transforming them from initially acquired raw or for processing images to *processed* or *for presentation* images. These different

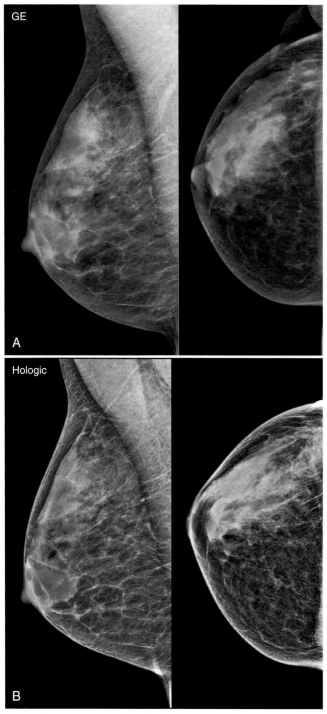

FIG. 1.6 Image contrast of digital mammography differs among vendors because of differences in image acquisition and postprocessing. Full-field digital mammogram obtained with a GE machine (GE Healthcare, Milwaukee, WI) (A) and with Hologic machine (Hologic, Bedford, MA) (B) in the same patient. Mediolateral oblique (*left*) and craniocaudal views (*right*) are shown. The skin line and the Cooper's ligaments are emphasized in B compared with A.

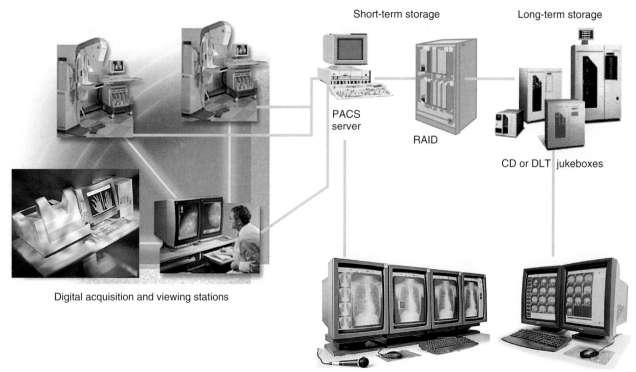

Short-term storage

Long-term storage

PACS server

RAID

CD or DLT jukeboxes

Digital acquisition and viewing stations

Hi-resolution multimodality workstations

FIG. 1.7 Schematic of a full-field digital mammography unit, workstation, picture archiving and communication system (PACS), or long-term storage and workstation displays. CD, compact disc; DLT, digital linear tape; RAID, redundant array of independent disks. (Adapted from figures provided by GE Healthcare, Waukesha, WI.)

look-up tables affect the contrast of final presentation digital images. Some, such as Hologic's linear look-up table, yield higher contrast images, whereas others, such as GE's sigmoidal look-up table, yield images presented with less contrast and more like screen-film images. In either case, thickness equalization is used to equalize signal differences from the center of the breast to the skin line. FFDM also has the advantage of eliminating the variability and noise added by film processing that is inherent to SFM.

In terms of breast dose, FFDM has a mean glandular dose lower than, or comparable with, the radiation dose of SFM. Results from the American College of Radiology Imaging Network (ACRIN) DMIST found the average single-view mean glandular dose for FFDM to be 1.86 mGy, 22% lower than the average SFM mean glandular dose of 2.37 mGy (Hendrick et al., 2010). Specific manufacturers, especially those using slot-scanning techniques, produce lower doses than SFM. Slot-scanning systems have a narrow slot of detector elements that are scanned under the breast in synchronization with a narrow fan beam of x-rays swept across the breast. This design, although more technically difficult to implement, has the advantage of eliminating the need for a grid to reduce scattered radiation. Scatter is partially eliminated by the narrow slot itself. The absence of a grid reduces the amount of radiation to the breast needed to get the same SNR in the detector. Most full area digital detectors also have demonstrated lower breast doses compared with SFM, especially for thicker breasts.

Once captured and processed, the image data are transferred to a reading station for interpretation on high-resolution (2048 × 2560 or 5-Mpixel) monitors or printed on film by laser imagers (with approximately 40-micron spot sizes, so that film printing does not reduce the inherent spatial resolution of digital mammograms) for interpretation of hardcopy images on film

viewboxes or alternators (Fig. 1.7). Digital data can be stored on optical disks, magnetic tapes, picture archiving and communication systems (PACS), or CDs for later retrieval.

The MQSA states that FFDM images must be made available to patients as hardcopy films, as needed, which means the facility must have access to an FDA-approved laser printer for mammography that can reproduce the gray scale and spatial resolution of FFDM images. The images may also be given to the patient on a CD with an image viewer, if this is acceptable to the patient.

A number of studies have evaluated the performance of FFDM compared with SFM for screening asymptomatic women for breast cancer. Early studies showed comparable or slightly worse results (but not statistically significant differences) for receiver operating characteristic (ROC) curve area and sensitivity (Lewin et al., 2001, 2002) or cancer detection rate (Skaane and Skjennald, 2004) of FFDM compared with SFM. Larger studies, however, showed some benefits of FFDM compared with SFM. The ACRIN DMIST paired study (Pisano et al., 2005b) showed no difference overall, but found that FFDM had statistically significantly higher ROC curve areas than SFM for women under age 50, for premenopausal and perimenopausal women, and for women with denser breasts (Breast Imaging Reporting and Data System [BI-RADS] density categories C and D). These findings are supported by Kerlikowske et al. (2011) who showed in clinical practice in the United States that FFDM had higher, but not necessarily significantly higher, sensitivity than SFM in most age groups, including women 40 to 49, premenopausal and perimenopausal women, and women with extremely dense breasts. The sensitivity of FFDM was significantly higher than for SFM among women aged 40 to 79 who had estrogen receptor–negative cancers, and especially so among women aged 40 to 49 (95% versus 55%; $p = 0.007$) The Oslo II trial

- GE Senographe 2000D Full Field Digital Mammography (FFDM) System: 1/28/00
- Fischer Imaging SenoScan Full Field Digital Mammography (FFDM) System: 9/25/01
- Lorad Digital Breast Imager Full Field Digital Mammography (FFDM) System: 3/15/02
- Lorad/Hologic Selenia Full Field Digital Mammography (FFDM) System: 10/2/02
- GE Senographe DS Full Field Digital Mammography (FFDM) System: 2/19/04
  - Siemens Mammomat Novation DR Full Field Digital Mammography (FFDM) System: 8/20/04
  - GE Senographe Essential Full Field Digital Mammography (FFDM) System: 4/11/06
  - Fuji Computed Radiography Mammography Suite (FCRMS): 7/10/06
  - Hologic Selenia Full Field Digital Mammography (FFDM) System with a Tungsten target: 11/2007
- Siemens Mammomat Novation S Full Field Digital Mammography (FFDM) System: 2/11/09
- Hologic Selenia S Full Field Digital Mammography (FFDM) System: 2/11/09
- Hologic Selenia Dimensions 2D Full Field Digital Mammography (FFDM) System: 2/11/09
- Carestream Directview Computed Radiography (CR) Mammography System: 11/3/10
- Siemens Mammomat Inspiration Full Field Digital Mammography (FFDM) System: 2/11/11
- Hologic Selenia Dimensions Digital Breast Tomosynthesis (DBT) System: 2/11/11
- Philips (Sectra) MicroDose L30 Full-Field Digital Mammography (FFDM) System: 4/28/11
- Hologic Selenia Encore Full-Field Digital Mammography (FFDM) System: 6/15/11
- Siemens Mammomat Inspiration Pure Full-Field Digital Mammography (FFDM) System: 8/16/11
- Planmed Nuance Full-Field Digital Mammography (FFDM) System: 9/23/11
- Planmed Nuance Excel Full-Field Digital Mammography (FFDM) System: 9/23/11
- GE Senographe Care Full-Field Digital Mammography (FFDM) System: 10/7/11
- Fuji Aspire HD Full-Field Digital Mammography (FFDM) System: 9/1/11
- Giotto Image 3D-3DL Full-Field Digital Mammography (FFDM) System: 10/27/11
- Fuji Aspire Computed Radiography for Mammography (CRM) System: 12/8/11
- Agfa Computed Radiography (CR) Mammography System: 12/22/11
- Konica Minolta Xpress Digital Mammography Computed Radiography (CR) System: 12/23/11
- Fuji Aspire HD-s Full-Field Digital Mammography (FFDM) System: 9/21/12
- Fuji Aspire HD Plus Full-Field Digital Mammography (FFDM) System: 9/21/12
- Philips MicroDose SI Model L50 Full-Field Digital Mammography (FFDM) System: 2/01/13
- iCRco 3600M Mammography Computed Radiography (CR) System: 4/26/13
- Siemens Mammomat Inspiration Prime Full-Field Digital Mammography (FFDM) System: 6/11/13
- Fuji Aspire Cristalle Full-Field Digital Mammography (FFDM) System: 3/25/14
- GE SenoClaire Digital Breast Tomosynthesis (DBT) System: 8/26/14
- Siemens Mammomat Inspiration with Tomosynthesis Option (DBT) System: 4/21/15
- Siemens Mammomat Fusion: 9/14/15

showed that digital mammography had a significantly higher cancer detection rate (5.9 cancers per 1000 women screened) than SFM (3.8 cancers per 1000 women screened) (Skaane et al., 2007).

Interpretation times for screening exams using FFDM tend to take 1.5 to 2 times longer than screening exams on SFM (Berns et al., 2006; Haygood et al., 2009). As of May 2016, 98% of the mammography units in the United States are digital mammography systems. The FDA-approved manufacturers for digital mammography units and their approval dates are listed in Box 1.6.

Tomosynthesis Acquisition

Digital breast tomosynthesis obtains a set of rapidly acquired low-dose digital projections taken at multiple angles through the compressed breast to reconstruct a stack of high-resolution, mammographic-quality planar images through the entire breast (Fig. 1.8). The reconstructed planes are parallel to the plane of the breast support (perpendicular to the central ray of the x-ray unit) and are spaced every 0.5 mm or 1 mm apart. The technique is similar to the previous technique of linear film tomography, but with one major difference. In film tomography, a full sweep of the x-ray tube resulted in a single planar image through the patient, with tissues in the selected plane in focus

while tissues outside that single plane were blurred. In digital tomosynthesis, a single sweep of the x-ray tube and reconstruction of the stored digital data results in a stack of dozens of parallel images through the breast, each image with a single in-focus plane, with blurring of the tissues above and below each focal plane.

The stack of reconstructed in-focus planar images from DBT permits improved visualization of lesion margins and can reveal suspicious lesions with greater clarity than conventional mammography (Fig. 1.9) (Video 1.1). This is possible because DBT minimizes structured noise caused by overlapping tissues, which is a significant limitation of conventional two-dimensional (2D) screen-film or digital mammography. DBT images also reduce callbacks for additional imaging by eliminating or reducing the complication of superimposed fibroglandular tissues that can appear suspicious in conventional 2D projection mammography.

Different manufacturers have taken different approaches to DBT in terms of the number of acquired low-dose projections, angular range of the projections, detector types, and scan time. Table 1.3 presents DBT design parameters for four different DBT manufacturers. As of May 2016, three manufacturers (Hologic, GE Healthcare, and Siemens Healthcare) have received FDA approval for clinical use of DBT for screening and diagnostic breast imaging in the United States.

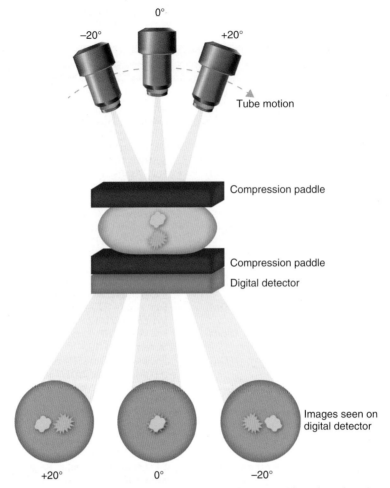

FIG. 1.8 Digital breast tomosynthesis (DBT) obtains a set of rapidly acquired low-dose digital projections taken at multiple angles through the compressed breast. A stack of reconstructed in-focus high-resolution, mammographic-quality planar images through the entire breast is reconstructed with the image data.

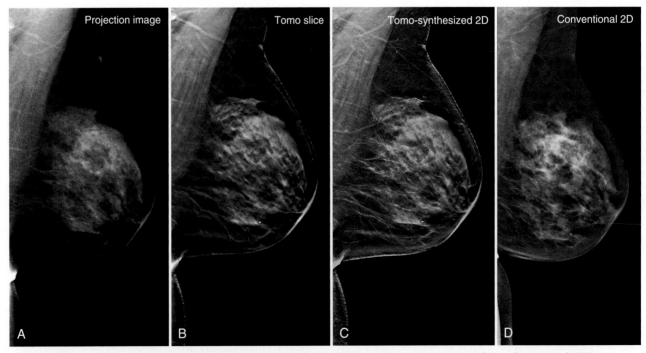

FIG. 1.9 Three-dimensional digital breast tomosynthesis (DBT) images and conventional two-dimensional (2D) digital mammogram. (A) A DBT projection image at the +7.53-degree position (Video 1.1A). First, low-dose digital projection images are taken at multiple angles. In this system (Hologic), 15 projection images (one image per degree of angle) are obtained. (B) DBT slice (Video 1.1B). By using the projection image data, a stack of high-resolution, mammographic-quality planar images through the entire breast is reconstructed for diagnostic use. These images are parallel to the plane of breast support. (C) DBT-synthesized 2D image. A reconstructed 2D image is synthesized from tomosynthesis data using software. The advantage of the synthesized 2D image over conventional 2D images is that additional radiation exposure is not required. (D) Conventional 2D mammogram of the same breast.

TABLE 1.3   Digital Breast Tomosynthesis Design Parameters for Four Different Manufacturers

Manufacturer Parameter	GE Healthcare	Hologic	IMS Giotto	Siemens
Tube motion	Step-and-shoot	Continuous	Step-and-shoot	Continuous
Angular range	25 degrees	15 degrees	40 degrees	50 degrees
Number of projections	9	15	13	25
Scan time (s)	7	4	12	25
Detector pixel size for digital breast tomosynthesis	100 μm	140 μm[a]	85 μm	85 μm
Grid	Yes	No	No	No
Reconstruction algorithm	Iterative	Back-projection	Iterative	Iterative

[a]As a result of binning two 70-μm pixels in each direction

A multireader FDA approval study of Hologic DBT by Rafferty et al. (2013, 2014) found significantly higher ROC curve areas for two-view DBT added to two-view FFDM compared with FFDM alone. Most clinical studies of DBT have reported similar results, with higher breast cancer detection rates and/or higher sensitivity with two-view DBT added to two-view FFDM, than with FFDM alone. They have also shown significantly lower recall rates with DBT plus FFDM compared with DBT alone. For example, Rose et al. (2013) compared the performance of 13,856 screening FFDM studies finding 56 cancers in 2010 to 9499 studies with FFDM plus DBT finding 51 cancers from May 2011 to early 2012. They found that cancer detection rates increased from 4.0 to 5.4 per 1000 screenings ($p = 0.18$, not significant), whereas recall rates dropped from 8.7% to 5.5% ($p < 0.001$, highly significant), and positive predictive value for recalls increased from 4.7% to 10.1% ($p < 0.001$). Similar results were found by Skaane et al. (2013) in Oslo and by Ciatto et al. (2013) in Italy: significantly higher cancer detection rates and significantly lower false-positive rates with DBT plus FFDM compared with FFDM alone.

Breast radiation doses with DBT added to FFDM are approximately double that of FFDM alone (Rafferty et al., 2013). Recently, however, Hologic has received FDA approval to replace DBT plus FFDM acquisitions with DBT acquisitions in which 2D FFDM (C view) images are synthesized from DBT data, reducing breast radiation doses from two-view DBT with C view images to approximately the same as two-view FFDM. GE's approach to DBT approved by the FDA was to acquire a DBT mediolateral oblique (MLO) view and 2D craniocaudal (CC) FFDM view of each breast at the same dose as two-view FFDM. GE systems also have the capability to acquire DBT CC views at approximately the same dose as 2D FFDM CC views.

Interpretation times for screening exams using DBT plus FFDM tend to be longer than for FFDM alone by 47% to 102% (Dang et al., 2014; Skaane et al., 2013).

Views and Positioning

The two views obtained for screening mammography are the CC and MLO projections. The names for the mammographic views and abbreviations are based on the ACR BI-RADS, a lexicon system developed by experts for standard mammographic terminology. The first word in the mammographic view indicates the location of the x-ray tube, and the second word indicates the location of the image receptor. Thus a CC view would be taken with the x-ray tube pointing at the breast from the head (cranial) down through the breast to the image receptor in a more caudal (toward the feet) position.

For positioning, the technologist tailors the mammogram to the individual woman's body habitus to get the best image. The breast is relatively fixed in its medial borders near the sternum and the upper breast, whereas the lower and outer portions of the breast are more mobile. The technologist takes advantage of the mobile lower outer breast to obtain as much breast tissue on the mammogram as possible. One component of ACR Mammography Accreditation is clinical image review in which clinical images are submitted for peer review of one patient with dense breasts and one patient with fatty breasts acquired on each mammography unit every 3 years. To pass ACR accreditation clinical image review, the MLO mammogram must show most of the breast tissue in one projection, with portions of the upper inner and lower inner quadrants partially excluded (Figs. 1.10 and 1.11). Clinical evaluation of the MLO view should show fat posterior to the fibroglandular tissue and a large portion of the pectoralis muscle, which should be convex and extend inferior to the posterior nipple line (PNL; Figs. 1.12 and 1.13). The nipple must be in profile on at least one of the two images. The PNL describes an imaginary line drawn from the nipple to the pectoralis muscle or chest wall image edge and perpendicular to the pectoralis muscle. The PNL should intersect the pectoralis muscle in the MLO view in more than 80% of women. The MLO view should show adequate compression, exposure, contrast, and an open inframammary fold (Fig. 1.14), in which both the lower portion of the breast and a portion of the upper abdominal wall should be seen.

To pass ACR clinical image review, the CC view should include the medial posterior portions of the breast without sacrificing the outer portions (Fig. 1.15; see Fig. 1.10). With proper positioning technique, the technologist should be able to include the medial portion of the breast without rotating the patient medially by lifting the lower medial breast tissue onto the image receptor. The pectoralis muscle should be seen when possible on the CC view. On the CC view, the PNL extends from the nipple to the pectoralis muscle or the chest wall edge of the image and perpendicular to the pectoralis muscle or image edge. For a given breast, the length of the PNL on the CC view should be within 1 cm of its length on the MLO view.

Although the technologist tries to avoid producing skin folds on the image when possible, they are seen occasionally and sometimes the image needs to be repeated, and other times they may not cause problems for the radiologist reading the image (Fig. 1.16).

Bassett et al. (2000a) described reasons why 1034 mammographic clinical images failed ACR accreditation, which included positioning in 20%, contrast in 13%, labeling in 8%, and noise in

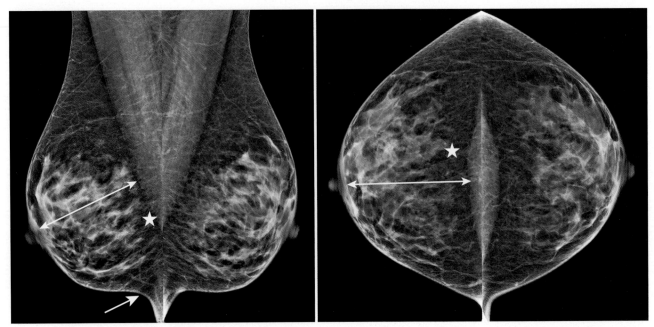

FIG. 1.10 Example of good positioning. Mediolateral oblique (MLO) views (*left*) and craniocaudal views (*right*). The posterior nipple lines (*double-sided arrows*), and the retroglandular fat (*stars*) are ideally visualized. The open inframammary fold (*arrow*) and abdomen are displayed with the breast pulled up and away from the chest on MLO views.

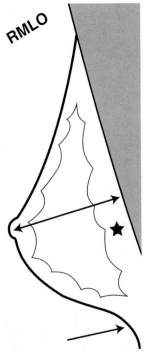

FIG. 1.11 Positioning for a normal mediolateral oblique (MLO) mammogram. By convention, the view type and side (*R*, right; *L*, left) labels are placed near the axilla. On a properly positioned MLO view, the inferior aspect of the pectoralis muscle should extend down to the posterior nipple line, which is an imaginary line drawn from the nipple back to and perpendicular to the pectoral muscle (*double-sided arrow*). The anterior margin of the pectoralis muscle should be convex in a properly positioned MLO view. Ideally, the image shows fat posterior to the glandular tissue (*star*). The open inframammary fold (*arrow*) and abdomen are displayed with the breast pulled up and away from the chest.

5% at a time when only film-screen mammography was available. They included the deficiencies mentioned previously as reasons for failure and also included these reasons: sagging breast tissue, portions of the breast not visualized, other body parts included on the mammogram, breast positioned too high on the image receptor, motion artifact, poor compression resulting in poor separation of breast tissues, poor contrast or exposure, and unsharpness.

Image Labeling in Mammography

Image labeling is important (Box 1.7) because proper labeling ensures accurate facility, patient, laterality, and projection identification. Guidelines from the ACR Mammography Accreditation Program for image labeling state that an identification label on the mammogram should specify the patient's first and last name, unique identification number, facility name and address, date, view and laterality, an Arabic number indicating the cassette used (for SFM and CR), and the technologist's initials. The laterality and projection marker should be placed near the axilla on all screen-film and digital mammograms.

BOX 1.7 Film Labeling

Patient's first and last names
Unique patient identification number
Name and address of the facility
Mammography unit
Date
View and laterality placed near the axilla
Arabic number indicating the cassette
Technologist's initials

From Hendrick et al: *Mammography quality control manual*, Reston, VA, 1999, American College of Radiology, p 27.

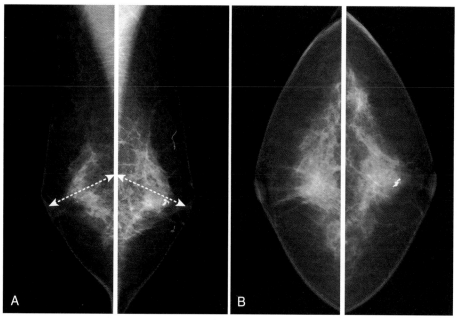

FIG. 1.12 Improper positioning. (A) Inadequate pectoralis muscle and sagging breast tissue on this full-field digital mediolateral oblique view shows that the posterior nipple line (*dashed double-sided arrows*) requirements are not met. (B) The craniocaudal view is rotated laterally. Note the calcifying fibroadenoma on the left.

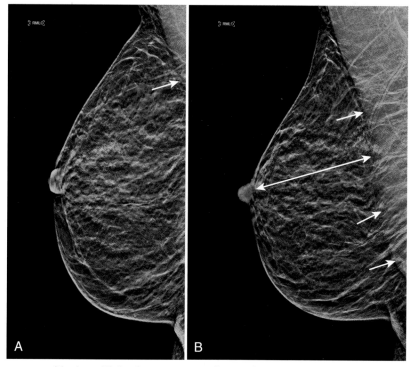

FIG. 1.13 Improper positioning. (A) Inadequate pectoralis muscle (*arrow*) on the full-field digital mediolateral oblique (MLO) view shows that the posterior nipple line (PNL) requirements are not met. (B) After the breast was pulled out, the pectoralis muscle (*arrows*) became convex. This MLO meets PNL requirements (*double-sided arrow*).

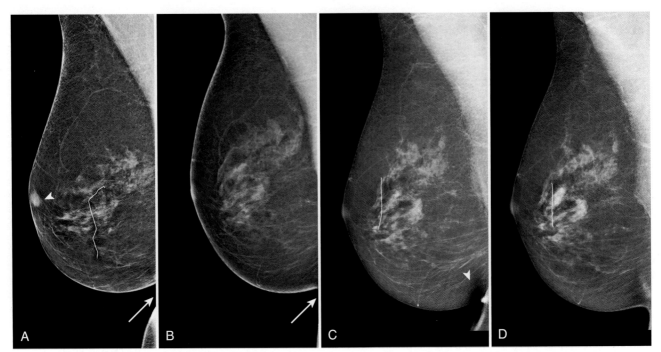

FIG. 1.14 Right mediolateral oblique (MLO) screening mammograms showing various positioning problems in a 73-year-old woman. (A) Right MLO mammogram shows that the inframammary fold is not included (*arrow*), the nipple is not in profile (*arrowhead*), and the posterior nipple line (PNL) is inadequate because a 90-degree line from the nipple to the chest wall does not reach the pectoralis muscle. Note the linear skin scar marker showing the location of a prior biopsy. (B) Right MLO mammogram now shows the nipple in profile and adequate PNL, but it does not include the inframammary fold (*arrow*). (C) Right MLO mammogram shows nipple in profile, adequate PNL, and inclusion of the inframammary fold, but now there is skin fold and air obscuring the lower breast (*arrowhead*). Note the linear skin scar marker showing the location of a prior biopsy. (D) Right MLO shows good positioning with the nipple in profile, open inframammary fold, no skin folds, and pectoralis muscle in correct PNL position. Note the linear skin scar marker showing the location of a prior biopsy.

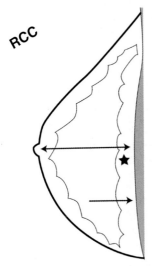

FIG. 1.15 Normal craniocaudal (CC) mammogram. The posterior nipple line (PNL) on the CC view is the distance between the nipple and the posterior aspect of the image. The PNL on the CC view (*double-sided arrow*) should be within 1 cm of the PNL on the mediolateral oblique (MLO) view. The goal is to include posterior medial tissue (excluded on the MLO view) (*arrow*) and as much retroglandular fat (*star*) as possible.

IMAGE EVALUATION AND ARTIFACTS

Clinical images are evaluated based on positioning, compression, contrast, proper exposure, random noise (radiographic mottle or quantum mottle produced by varying numbers of x-rays contributing to the image in different locations, even with a uniform object), sharpness, and artifacts (structured noise). Imaging on a phantom is helpful in evaluating most of these factors, except for positioning and compression (Fig. 1.17) (Video 1.2).

In SFM, adequate exposure (to achieve adequate film OD) and adequate contrast (OD difference) are important to ensure detection of subtle abnormalities (Fig. 1.18). Artifacts seen on SFM images include processing artifacts (roller marks, wet pressure marks, and guide shoe marks), white specklike artifacts from dust or lint between the fluorescent screen and film emulsion, grid lines from incomplete grid motion, motion artifacts from patient movement (made more likely by longer exposure times), skin folds from positioning, tree static caused by static electricity from low humidity in the dark room, or film handling artifacts (fingerprints, crimp marks, or pressure marks; Figs. 1.19–1.22).

Commonly encountered artifacts on digital mammography include patient-related artifacts (motion, antiperspirant, and thin breast artifacts; Fig. 1.23), hardware-related artifacts (signal nonuniformity caused by poor detector calibration and

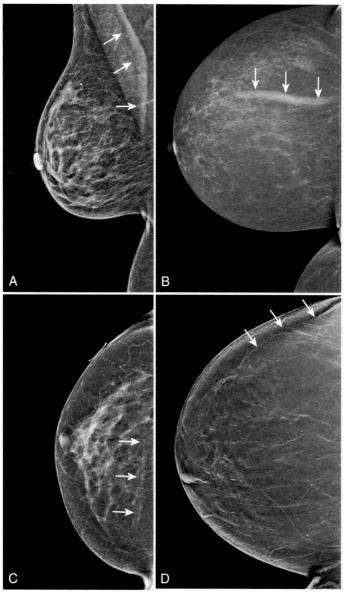

FIG. 1.16 Skin folds (A–D; *arrows*). Skin folds in compressed breasts are shown as linear white lines on mammograms in A and B. In C and D the minimal skin fold has caused a dark line in which air occurs adjacent to the skin.

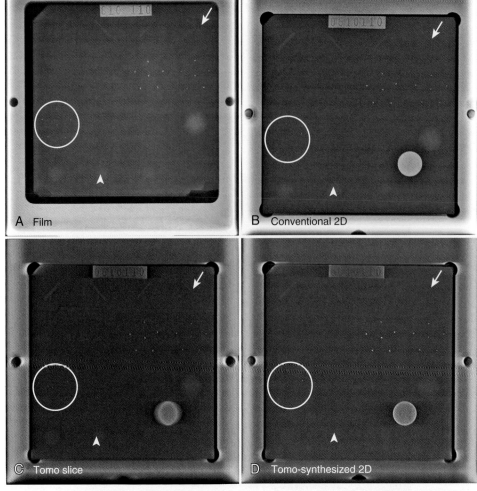

FIG. 1.17 Images of the American College of Radiology mammography phantom. (A) Film-screen mammography image. (B) Two-dimensional (2D) full-field digital mammography image obtained on mammographic unit capable of tomosynthesis. (C) Tomosynthesis slice (see Video 1.2). (D) Tomosynthesis-synthesized 2D view. Note that images B–D were obtained with the same phantom on a mammographic unit capable of tomosynthesis on the same day, but A was separately obtained with another phantom on a film-screen mammography unit. Fibers, speck groups, and masses in graduated sizes are embedded in a 4.5-cm thick phantom. All images shown here reach to the minimum requirements: four fibers (*arrows*), three speck groups (*circles*), and three masses (*arrowheads*).

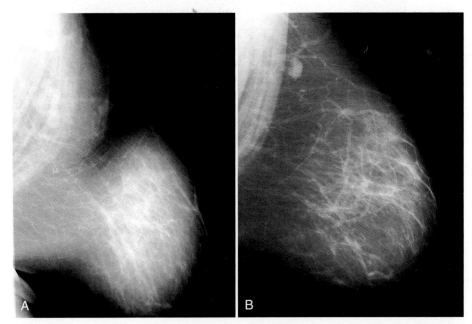

FIG. 1.18 Inadequately and adequately exposed and compressed breasts. (A) Underpenetration and an inadequately exposed and compressed breast produce a light film and poor separation of breast tissue; even though the pectoralis muscle is adequately included, skin folds are apparent in the upper portion of the image. (B) A mammogram of a properly exposed and compressed breast shows normal glandular tissue.

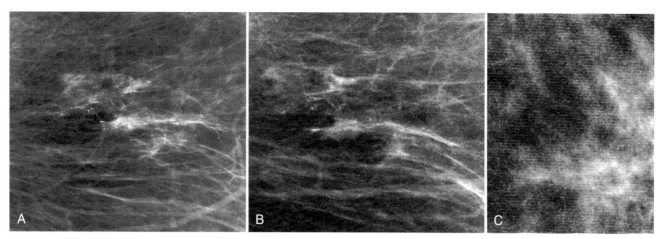

FIG. 1.19 Grid lines on screen-film mammography. (A and B) Cancer without (A) and with (B) grid lines as a result of cessation of grid motion during exposure. (C) Magnified view of grid lines from a moving grid that has stopped because of malfunction.

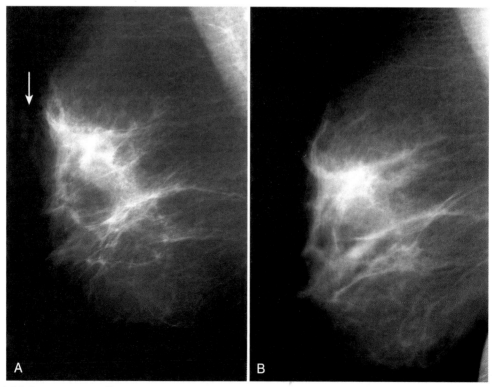

FIG. 1.20 Dust on screen-film mammography. (A) Blurring is caused by a large dust particle (*arrow*) shown as a white dot in the upper part of the breast and is caused by poor film-screen contact as the dust lifts the film off the screen. (B) After the large dust particle is removed, the dust artifact and blur are gone.

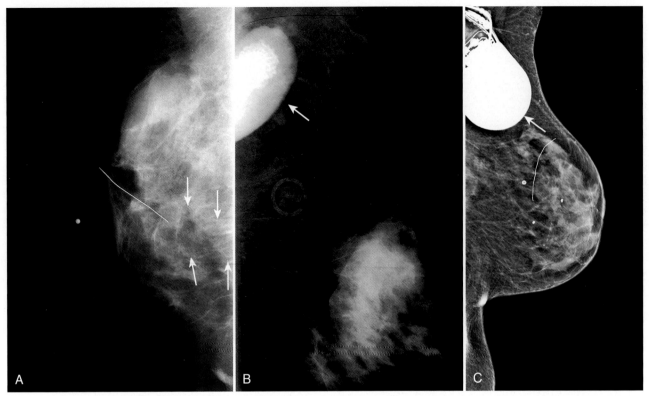

FIG. 1.21 Interposed objects at x-ray exposure. (A) A mediolateral oblique (MLO) view after biopsy and radiation therapy shows tiny bright white specks (*arrows*) over the biopsy scar compatible with dust on the film. Dust can interfere with a search for microcalcifications. Note the nipple marker and linear scar marker showing the previous biopsy site. (B) Patient's fingertip (*arrow*) is visible in the film. (C) Pacemaker (*arrow*) is seen in the upper left breast in left MLO view. Note the linear scar marker showing the previous biopsy site.

detector-associated artifacts such as bad pixels, bad lines, or detector element failures; collimator misalignment; underexposure; grid lines; grid misplacement; vibration artifact; and edge of small breast paddle; Figs. 1.24 and 1.25), and software processing artifacts (*breast-within-a-breast* or improper thickness equalization artifacts, vertical processing bars, loss of edge, and high-density artifacts). Although some of these artifacts, such as patient-related artifacts and hardware-related artifacts, are similar to those seen with SFM, some are unique to digital mammography—specifically, those caused by software processing errors or digital detector deficiencies. In addition, digital mammography artifacts depend on detector technology and therefore can be vendor specific.

Unique artifacts on DBT include dark edge or shadow artifacts beside metallic markers or dense calcifications in the plane of focus (Fig. 1.26), and out-of-plane artifacts caused by clips, markers, or other high-attenuation objects causing artifacts in out-of-focus planes (Fig. 1.27).

QUALITY ASSURANCE IN MAMMOGRAPHY AND THE MAMMOGRAPHY QUALITY STANDARDS ACT

The MQSA, a federal law regarding mammography enforced by the FDA, stipulates that all institutions performing mammography must be certified by the FDA. A prerequisite to FDA certification is accreditation to perform mammography by an FDA-approved accrediting body, such as the ACR or an FDA-approved state accrediting body. Arkansas, Iowa, and Texas are approved to accredit mammography facilities in their own states. The

MQSA final regulations are listed in the *Federal Register*. To update facilities on the latest regulation changes and updates, the FDA maintains an MQSA website (http://www.fda.gov), which includes a section to guide users who have questions on MQSA compliance.

The MQSA certification involves an initial application to the FDA and FDA approval to perform mammography, continuous documentation of compliance, and annual facility inspection by an MQSA or state inspector. Noncompliance with regulations may result in FDA citations, with time limits on deficiency corrections. Serious noncompliance issues may result in facility closure. Falsification of data submitted to the FDA can result in monetary fines and jail terms.

The MQSA equipment requirements for mammography are summarized in Box 1.8, and the MQSA qualification requirements for radiologists, technologists, and medical physicists are outlined in Boxes 1.9 to 1.11.

One radiologist at each facility must be designated as the *Lead Interpreting Physician* to oversee the facility's quality assurance (QA) program (Boxes 1.12 and 1.13). The *Audit Interpreting Physician* oversees assessment of mammography outcomes to evaluate the accuracy of interpretation. The facility must have a method for recording outcomes on interpretation of all abnormal mammographic findings and tallying these interpretations for each individual physician and for the group as a whole, providing feedback to each radiologist on a yearly basis (Box 1.14). A portion of the medical audit includes review of the pathology in cases recommended for biopsy.

One radiologic technologist, designated as the *QC technologist*, oversees the quality control (QC) tasks outlined in Table 1.4,

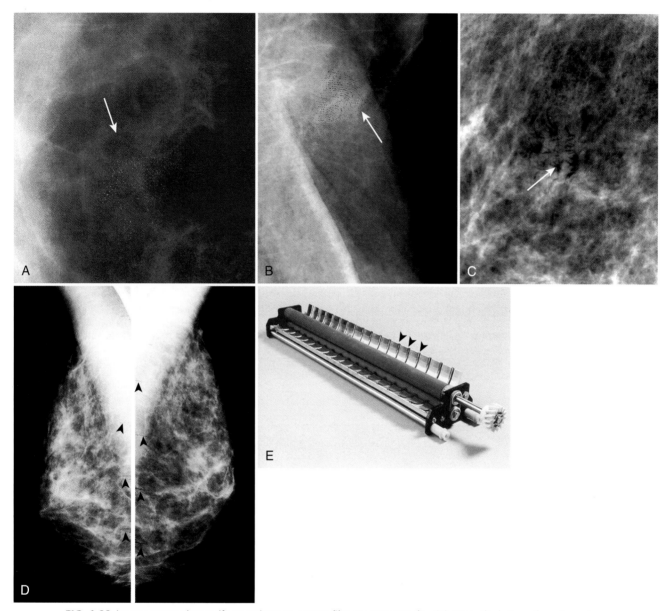

FIG. 1.22 Image-processing artifacts unique to screen-film mammography. (A) Magnified view of a minus-density (*white*) fingerprint artifact (*arrow*), usually caused by contact with the film before exposure. (B) Magnified view of a plus-density (*dark*) fingerprint artifact (*arrow*), usually caused by contact with the film after exposure but before processing. (C) Subtle plus-density tree static artifacts (*arrow*) caused by static discharge in a limited region of the film. The light emitted from the static discharge causes localized film exposure before processing. (D and E) Guide shoe marks. Dark lines (D, *arrowheads*) at the edge of the film in the direction of film travel that are evenly spaced are caused by excessive pressure on the film emulsion from guide shoes as the film travels through the processor. Guide shoe marks can sometimes result in minus-density linear artifacts in the direction of film travel as well. A film guide turns the film as it passes through the processor. Such guides (E, *arrowheads*) are located at the top and bottom of each tank. Improperly adjusted film guides can lead to excessive pressure on the film emulsion and result in guide shoe artifacts.

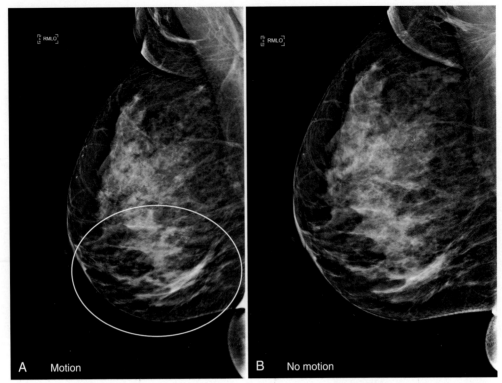

FIG. 1.23 Motion artifact on digital mammography. (A) Right mediolateral oblique (RMLO) view shows blurred breast tissue most evident in lower breast (*circle*). (B) On a corrected RMLO, the breast tissue and Cooper's ligaments appears more distinct against a fatty background. Longer exposure times can lead to patient motion.

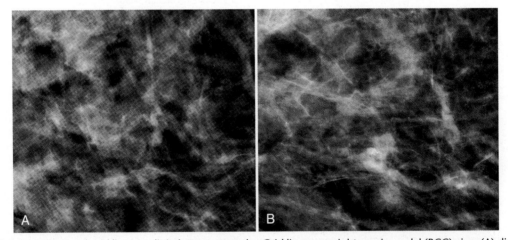

FIG. 1.24 Hexagonal grid lines on digital mammography. Grid lines on a right craniocaudal (RCC) view (A) disappeared in a corrected RCC view (B). This artifact may be attributed to the stopping or slowing down of grid oscillation in the Bucky, causing the grid lines to be superimposed on the image. To correct this artifact, the technologist should repeat the exposure and, if the artifact persists, a call should be made for servicing the equipment.

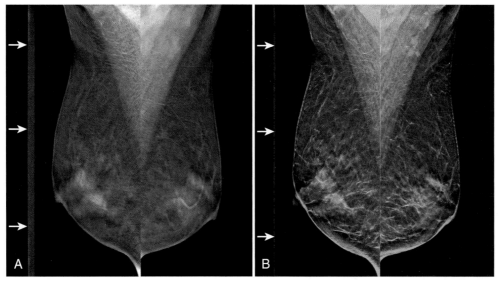

FIG. 1.25 Edge of small breast paddle. A unilateral vertical linear artifact (*arrows*) is seen outside the right breast on a tomosynthesis slice (A) as a tomosynthesis-synthesized 2D image (B). These vertical linear artifacts are the edge of the small breast paddle used to compress small breasts. Usually, the paddle edge is not included on the images.

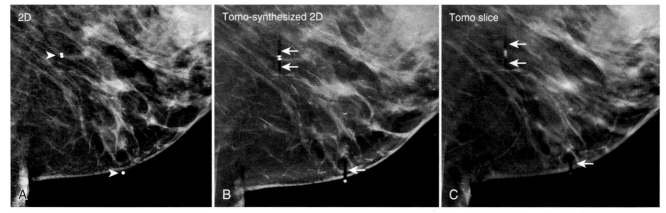

FIG. 1.26 Shadow artifacts on tomosynthesis. (A) Conventional digital 2D. (B) Tomosynthesis-synthesized 2D. (C) Tomosynthesis slice. There are two small metal BBs and an external skin marker (A). Tomosynthesis images (B and C) show artifactual black lines (*arrows*) above and below high-attenuation objects such as metal markers or macrocalcifications caused by the tomosynthesis reconstruction. The *shadow* artifacts shown in this image are a result of reconstruction of limited angle projections. They occur on relatively small-size extremely bright objects such as clips, pins, BBs, large calcifications, etc. Software is being developed to reduce these artifacts.

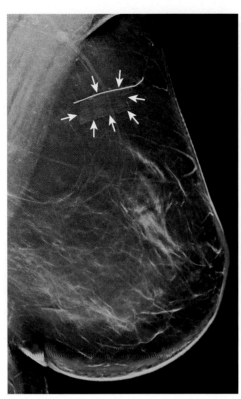

FIG. 1.27 Out-of-plane artifacts on tomosynthesis. Tomosynthesis-synthesized two-dimensional (2D) image shows multiple lines (*arrows*) under the linear scar marker that were caused by ghost artifacts from the metallic marker in out-of-focus planes.

BOX 1.8   Mammography Quality Standards Act Equipment Requirements for Mammography

Be specifically designed for mammography

Have a breast compression device and have additional hand-operated compression to augment motor-driven compression

Have image receptors, moving grids, and compression paddles for both 18 × 24-cm and 24 × 30-cm image receptors (screen-film only)

The mean glandular dose to a 4.5-cm thick breast is less than 3 mGy (0.3 rad) when the site's clinical technique is used

Can angulate 180 degrees from craniocaudal orientation in at least one direction

X-ray system must have a functioning postexposure display of the actual x-ray focal spot and the target material used during each exposure.

Other minimum standards for beam limitation and light field, magnification capability, automatic exposure control, and, for screen-film mammography, requirements for x-ray film, intensifying screens, film processing solutions, lighting and hot lights, film masking devices

Modified from the *Federal Register.* Available at http://www.fda.gov

---

BOX 1.9   Mammography Quality Standards Act Qualifications for Interpreting Physicians

Be licensed to practice medicine in a state,
and

Be certified by a body approved by the Food and Drug Administration to certify interpreting physicians or have 3 months' full-time training in mammography interpretation, radiation physics, radiation effects, and radiation protection,
and

Have earned 60 hours of documented mammography continuing medical education (CME) (time in residency will be accepted if documented in writing) and 8 hours of training in each modality (such as screen-film or digital mammography),
and

Have read at least 240 examinations in the preceding 6 months under supervision or have read mammograms under the supervision of a fully qualified interpreting physician (see the *Federal Register* for exact requirements),
and

Have read 960 mammograms over a period of 24 months,
and

Have earned at least 15 Category 1 CME credits in mammography over a 36-month period, with 6 credits in each modality used,
and

To perform a new imaging modality (eg, digital mammography, digital breast tomosynthesis), the interpreting physician must have 8 CME credits specific to that modality before starting the modality.

To reestablish qualifications, either interpret or double read 240 mammograms under direct supervision or bring the total to 960 over a period of 24 months and accomplish these tasks within the 6 months immediately before resuming independent interpretation. Regarding CME, if the requirement of 15 hours per 36 months is not met, the total number of CME hours must be brought up to 15 per 36 months before resuming independent interpretation.

Modified from the *Federal Register.* Available at http://www.fda.gov

---

BOX 1.10   Mammography Quality Standards Act Qualifications for Radiologic Technologists

Have a license to perform radiographic procedures in their state or be certified by one of the bodies (such as the American Registry of Radiologic Technologists) approved by the Food and Drug Administration,
and

Have undergone 40 hours of documented mammography training, with 8 hours of instruction in each modality used, and have completed at least 25 mammography examinations,
and

Complete 200 examinations in the previous 24 months and complete (or teach) at least 15 continuing education units (CEUs) in the past 36 months, including 6 in each modality used.

Modified from the *Federal Register.* Available at http://www.fda.gov

Note: To reestablish qualifications, must complete 25 examinations under direct supervision and complete 15 CEUs per 36 months.

BOX 1.11 Mammography Quality Standards Act Qualifications for Medical Physicists

Have a license or approval by a state to conduct evaluations of mammography equipment under the Public Health Services Act or have certification in an accepted area by one of the accrediting bodies approved by the Food and Drug Administration, *and*

Have at least a master's degree or higher in a physical science with at least 20 semester hours (30 quarter hours) of graduate or undergraduate physics, *and*

Have at least 20 contact hours of mammography facility survey training, *and*

Have the experience of conducting surveys of at least 1 mammography facility and at least 10 mammography units, *and*

Before independently performing surveys or mammography equipment evaluations on any new mammographic modality, have at least 8 hours of training in the modality, *and*

Have conducted a minimum of two mammography facility surveys and a total of six mammography unit surveys during the 24 months immediately preceding the date of the facility's annual MQSA inspection, *and*

Have taught or completed at least 15 continuing education units (CEUs) in medical physics or mammography during the 36 months immediately preceding the date of the facility's annual MQSA inspection.

Modified from the *Federal Register.*Available at http://www.fda.gov

BOX 1.12 Quality Assurance Program for Equipment

All facilities must establish and maintain a quality assurance (QA) program with written designation of a lead interpreting physician, medical physicist, and quality control technologist.

For screen-film systems, the QA program is the same as described in Hendrick et al. (1999); for digital and digital breast tomosynthesis units, a QA program as described by the image receptor manufacturer's QC manual.

Maintenance of log books documenting compliance and corrective actions for each unit.

Establish and maintain radiographic images of phantoms to assess performance of the mammography system for each unit.

Major changes from the interim regulations include weekly phantom image quality testing and mammography unit performance tests after each relocation of a mobile unit.

Modified from the *Federal Register.*Available at http://www.fda.gov

BOX 1.13 Quality Assurance for Clinical Images

Monitoring of repeat rate for repeated clinical images and their causes

Record keeping, analysis of results, and remedial actions taken on the basis of this monitoring

Modified from the *Federal Register.*Available at http://www.fda.gov

BOX 1.14 Quality Assurance for Interpretation of Clinical Images

Establishment of systems for reviewing outcome data from mammograms, including

Disposition of all positive mammograms

Correlation of surgical biopsy results with mammogram reports

Designation of a specific physician to ensure data collection and analysis and show that the analysis is shared with the facility and individual physicians

Modified from the *Federal Register.*Available at http://www.fda.gov

TABLE 1.4 Technologist Quality Control Tests for Screen-Film Mammography

Periodicity	Quality Control Test	Desired Result
Daily	Darkroom cleanliness	No dust artifacts
Daily	Processor quality control	Density difference and mid-density changes not to exceed control limits of ±0.15
Weekly	Screen cleanliness	No dust artifacts on films
Weekly	Viewbox cleanliness	No marks on panels, uniform lighting
Weekly	Phantom image evaluation	Film density >1.4 with control limits of ±0.20 Densities do not vary over time or between units Minimum test objects seen: four largest fibers, three largest speck groups, three largest masses
Monthly	Visual checklist	Each item on checklist present and functioning properly
Quarterly	Repeat analysis	Overall repeat rate of <5% Percent repeats similar for each category
Quarterly	Analysis of fixer retention	Residual sodium thiosulfate (hypo) ≤0.05 μg/cm³
Semiannually	Darkroom fog	Fog ≤0.05 optical density difference for 2-minute exposure in darkroom
Semiannually	Screen-film contact	Large areas (>1 cm) of poor contact unacceptable
Semiannually	Compression	Power mode: 25–45 lb Manual mode: >25 lb

From Hendrick et al: *Mammography quality control manual*, Reston, VA, 1999, American College of Radiology, p. 119.

which specifies the minimum frequency of each QC test and action limits for test performance. One important test performed by the QC technologist and reviewed by the interpreting physician is acquisition and evaluation of the mammography phantom image; this test is performed at least weekly and evaluates the entire imaging system. The phantom consists of fibers, speck clusters, and masses of various sizes imbedded in a uniform phantom material. The technologist takes a phantom radiograph using the site's clinical technique for a 4.5-cm thick compressed breast, the radiograph is processed on the site's film

---

BOX 1.15   Phantom Image

Evaluates the entire mammographic imaging chain (other than technologist positioning)
Performed at least weekly
Must see four fibers, three speck groups, three masses
Must be free of significant artifacts

From Hendrick et al: *Mammography quality control manual*, Reston, VA, 1999, American College of Radiology, p 119.

BOX 1.16   Medical Physicist's Screen-Film Mammography Quality Control Tests (Annually and after Major Equipment Changes)

1. Unit assembly evaluation
2. Assessment of collimation
3. Evaluation of system resolution
4. Automatic exposure control (AEC) assessment of performance
5. Uniformity of screen speed
6. Artifact evaluation
7. Evaluation of image quality
8. kVp accuracy and reproducibility
9. Assessment of beam quality (half-value layer measurement)
10. Breast entrance exposure, AEC reproducibility, average glandular dose, and radiation output rate
11. Viewbox luminance and room luminance

From Hendrick et al: *Mammography quality control manual*, Reston, VA, 1999, American College of Radiology.

---

processor or produced by the digital system, and the image is evaluated for the number of objects seen in each category. To pass accreditation and meet MQSA requirements, the phantom should show a minimum of four fibers, three speck groups, and three masses (Box 1.15). The phantom image should also be free of significant artifacts. These and other tests are used to evaluate the entire imaging system.

The medical physicist surveys the equipment just after installation, after important major equipment repairs or upgrades, and at least annually, performing the QC tests outlined in Box 1.16. The medical physicist's survey report is an important component of the QA program and is reviewed by the supervising physician to ensure high-quality mammography. The facility is responsible for correcting deficiencies pointed out by the site medical physicist and documenting corrective actions.

Each year, the mammography facility is inspected by state or federal inspectors who evaluate compliance with MQSA regulations. Site QA records and site personnel qualifications are routinely checked by the MQSA inspector. Correction of deficiencies specified in the medical physicist's report is an important item checked by MQSA inspectors. Noncompliance with MQSA requirements may result in warnings requiring corrective actions or, in extreme cases, facility closure.

Screen-Film Mammography Quality Control

For SFM, MQSA specifies the QA/QC tests to be performed by the QC technologist and the site medical physicist, as well as how frequently these tests must be performed. Technologist test frequencies range from daily to semiannually, as specified in Table 1.4. Medical physicist tests are required annually, on acceptance of new equipment, or after major equipment changes and before its use on patients or volunteers (see Box 1.16). The technologist and medical physicist tests for SFM are described in detail in the 1999 edition of the ACR *Mammography Quality Control Manual* (Hendrick, 1999).

BOX 1.17   Educational Requirements for New Personnel Using Digital Mammography

Eight hours of training specific to digital mammography before its use
Six hours of Category 1 continuing medical education or continuing education unit credits in this new modality every 3 years; the 6 hours can be part of the required 15 hours of continuing education in mammography required by the Mammography Quality Standards Act

---

Full-Field Digital Mammography Quality Assurance and Quality Control

To comply with MQSA requirements, all personnel must have 8 hours of training specific to digital mammography, and that training must be documented in writing before clinical use of FFDM units in that facility (Box 1.17). Specifically, the radiologist must receive 8 hours of training in interpretation of digital mammography, with the strong recommendation from the FDA that training includes instruction from a radiologist experienced in digital mammography interpretation on the specific system used. Technologists and medical physicists also must have documented training by appropriately qualified individuals; for example, the manufacturer's application specialists or other qualified individuals should train technologists, and medical physicists qualified in digital mammography should provide hands-on training for medical physicists. After meeting initial education requirements, all personnel involved in digital mammography should receive 6 hours of Category 1 continuing medical education (CME) or continuing educational units (CEU) specifically in digital mammography every 3 years, which may be part of the required 15 hours of continuing education required for all personnel in mammography. The completion of the required 15 hours of Category 1 CME in mammography every 3 years must be documented in writing.

The MQSA requires that QC testing for FFDM is performed by the facility "according to the image receptor manufacturer's specification." Each digital manufacturer has a detailed QC manual specifying tests, test frequencies, and pass–fail criteria. All manufacturers' QC manuals differ in the specific tests, frequencies, and criteria.

For some tests, such as mean glandular dose for the ACR phantom being less than 3 mGy, the FDA specifies that failures must be corrected immediately before that component of the FFDM system (eg, the digital mammography unit, review workstation, laser imager) can be used. Test failures that must be corrected immediately include phantom image quality, contrast-to-noise ratio, radiation dose, and review workstation calibration. For other test failures, such as repeat analysis, collimation assessment, and other physics tests, 30 days are permitted for correction after problem identification. Typical digital mammography QC tests are listed in Box 1.18, although these vary somewhat by digital manufacturer.

Digital Breast Tomosynthesis Quality Assurance and Quality Control

As with digital mammography, DBT is considered a *new modality*. To add DBT capability to an existing mammography unit, the facility must apply to the FDA to have its certificate extended to include the DBT portion of the unit. The certification extension applies only to the DBT portion of the unit. The facility must have the 2D portion of the unit accredited by one of the accreditation bodies already approved to accredit digital mammography systems. In addition, the MQSA requires that all personnel involved in the performance of DBT (radiologists, technologists,

---

BOX 1.18 Medical Physicist's Digital Mammography Quality Control Tests (Annually and after Major Equipment Changes)

1. Full-field digital mammography (FFDM) unit assembly evaluation
2. Flat-field uniformity test[a]
3. Artifact evaluation
4. Automatic exposure control mode and signal-to-noise ratio check[a]
5. Phantom image quality test[a]
6. Contrast-to-noise ratio test[a]
7. Modulation transfer function measurement[a]
8. Assessment of collimation
9. Evaluation of focal spot size
10. kVp accuracy and reproducibility
11. Assessment of beam quality (half-value layer measurement)
12. Breast entrance exposure, mean glandular dose,[a] and radiation output rate
13. Image quality of the display monitor

---

[a]Indicates immediate correction required before using the FFDM unit.

---

and medical physicists) must have 8 hours of training specific to DBT, either including or supplemented by training in the unique features of the specific manufacturer's DBT system(s) used. New modality training must be documented in writing before clinical use of DBT in that facility. After meeting initial DBT educational requirements, all personnel involved in DBT should receive 6 hours of Category 1 CME or CEU in DBT every 3 years, which may be part of the required 15 hours of continuing education every 3 years required for all personnel in mammography.

The MQSA requires that QC testing for DBT, like digital mammography, is performed by the facility according to the DBT manufacturer's specifications. Each DBT manufacturer has a QC manual specifying DBT QC tests, test frequencies, and pass–fail criteria. Most tests are identical to those performed for 2D digital mammography, but may include additional tests unique to DBT. Both 2D and DBT-specific QC tests should be performed on the equipment used for DBT. A list of QC tests appropriate for a DBT system is given in Box 1.19, although these differ somewhat by manufacturer. These tests should be performed in addition to conventional FFDM QC tests with any DBT-specific hardware or software installed.

COMPUTER-AIDED DETECTION

Radiologists are trained to detect early, subtle signs of breast cancer, such as pleomorphic calcifications and spiculated masses on mammograms. The CAD systems use algorithms to review mammograms for bright clustered specks and converging lines, which represent pleomorphic calcifications and spiculated masses, respectively. These programs were developed to help radiologists search for signs of cancer against the complex background of fat and fibroglandular breast tissues.

Some facilities use CAD as a *second reader. Double reading* in screening mammography involves two observers reviewing the same mammograms to increase detection of cancer, decrease the false-negative rate or, in some facilities, decrease the false-positive recall rate by using a consensus. Studies have shown that double reading, depending on its implementation, increases the rate of detection of cancer by 5% to 15%. However, the expense and logistical problems of a second interpretation limit double reading of mammography in clinical practice in the United States.

Mammographic data are sent to CAD systems directly from FFDM/tomosynthesis units or from digitized screen-film mammograms. The digital or digitized mammograms undergo

---

BOX 1.19 Typical Digital Breast Tomosynthesis Quality Control Tests and Intervals for Radiologic Technologists and Medical Physicists

RADIOLOGIC TECHNOLOGIST DBT QC TESTS AND INTERVALS

Flat-field test: DBT acquisition	Weekly
Phantom image quality test: 2D and DBT	Weekly
Artifact evaluation	Weekly
SNR test: 2D	Weekly
CNR test: 2D	Weekly
MTF test: 2D	Weekly
SNR test: 2D	Weekly
Grid texture test: 2D (GE only)	Monthly
Automatic exposure control test: 2D and DBT	Monthly
Visual checklist	Monthly
Geometry calibration: DBT	Semiannually
Compression force test	Semiannually

MEDICAL PHYSICIST DBT QC TESTS (ANNUALLY OF AFTER MAJOR DBT EQUIPMENT CHANGE)

Flat-field test: DBT acquisition
Phantom image quality test: 2D and DBT
Artifact evaluation
SNR test: 2D
CNR test: 2D
MTF test: 2D
System resolution test: 2D
Grid texture test: 2D (GE only)
Automatic exposure control test: 2D and DBT
Collimation assessment and compression paddle to chest-wall alignment test
Breast entrance exposure and average glandular dose: 2D and DBT
Flat-field uniformity test: 2D
Volume coverage test: DBT

CNR, contrast-to-noise ratio; DBT, digital breast tomosynthesis; MTF, modulation transfer function; QC, quality control; SNR, signal-to-noise ratio.

---

analysis by computer algorithms that mark potential abnormal findings. For film-screen mammography, the CAD marks are printed on a low-resolution paper print or displayed on a monitor below the film-screen mammograms on an alternator (Figs. 1.28 and 1.29). For FFDM, CAD highlights potential abnormalities on the workstation monitor. The FDA requires that images are displayed first without CAD markings; a single toggle button may show or hide CAD marks highlighting potential lesions. The radiologist first interprets the mammogram and then pushes the CAD button and analyzes the marked CAD findings, either dismissing them as insignificant or recalling them for further workup (Fig. 1.30).

The CAD detects and marks microcalcifications, masses, and parenchymal distortions on mammograms. Its computer algorithms were developed from training sets comprised of large numbers of mammograms with biopsy-proven findings, resulting in *true-positive* and *false-positive* in known cases. The optimized algorithms were then tested on both known subtle and obvious cancers. Using the optimized schemes, commercial CAD systems mark abnormalities that represent cancers (true-positive marks and a measure of CAD sensitivity) and findings that do *not* represent cancer or where no known cancer has occurred. Because mass or calcification detection by the CAD scheme is directly affected by image quality, good-quality mammograms are required to obtain good CAD output. Mammograms of suboptimal quality will result in poor CAD output. CAD output also can be affected by the type and reproducibility of the digitizer if CAD data are from digitized SFM. Thus it is essential to have high-quality mammograms with SFM or FFDM,

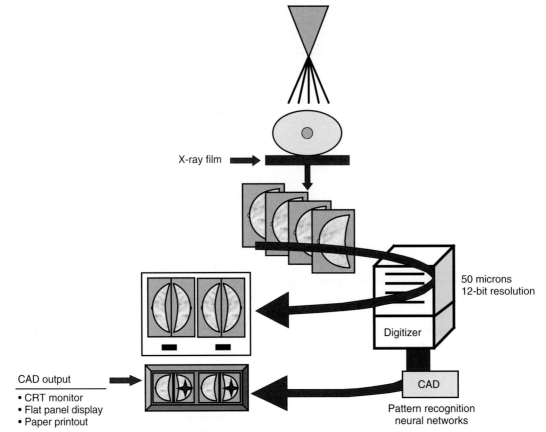

X-ray film

50 microns
12-bit resolution

Digitizer

CAD output

- CRT monitor
- Flat panel display
- Paper printout

CAD

Pattern recognition
neural networks

FIG. 1.28 Computer-aided detection (CAD) schematic for screen-film and full-field digital mammograms. Film digitizers typically operate at 50-micron pixel (or 10 lp/mm) spatial resolution. Digital spatial resolution is set by the digital detector (see Table 1.3). CRT, cathode ray tube. (Courtesy of R. Castellino, R2 Technology, San Jose, CA.)

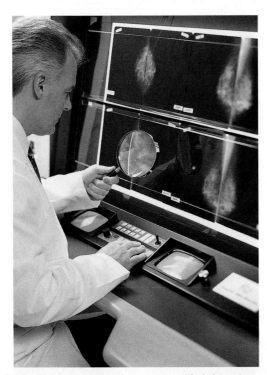

FIG. 1.29 Mammograms and computer-aided detection output. For screen-film mammography, the technologist digitizes the mammograms and then mounts the images on an alternator for the radiologist to interpret. A computer marks potential findings on the mammogram and displays the findings on low-resolution images on the monitor below the films. (Courtesy of R. Castellino, R2 Technology, San Jose, CA.)

because CAD cannot overcome poor image quality. The FDA has approved CAD systems for breast cancer detection in both screening and diagnostic mammography using both screen-film and digital mammography.

A retrospective study by Warren-Burhenne et al. (2000) of breast cancers found on mammography determined that a CAD program marked 77% (89/115) of screening-detected breast cancers. Birdwell et al. (2001) reviewed "negative" mammograms obtained the year before the diagnosis of 115 screen-detected cancers in 110 patients. They reported that a CAD program marked reader-missed findings in 77% (88/115) of false-negative mammograms. Specifically, CAD marked 86% (30/35) of missed calcifications and 73% (58/80) of missed masses.

Freer and Ulissey (2001) reported that in a prospective community breast center study of 12,860 women undergoing screening mammography, CAD increased their cancer detection rate by 19.5%. Radiologists detected 41 of 49 cancers and missed 8 cancers found by the CAD system (7 of 8 were calcifications). The CAD detected 40 of the 49 cancers, but it did not mark 9 radiologist-detected masses that were proven to be cancers.

The CAD system does not diagnose all cancers, and it should not be used as the only evaluator of screening mammograms. As in the study by Freer and Ulissey (2001), radiologists initially made a decision about the mammogram, used CAD, and then re-reviewed the marked mammogram. The radiologist's decision to recall a potential abnormality could not be changed by failure of the CAD system to mark the potential finding. Findings marked by CAD could be recalled even if the finding was not initially detected by the radiologist but was judged to be abnormal in retrospect. This means that radiologists should read the mammogram first so they are not influenced by CAD marks initially, because not all cancers are marked by CAD.

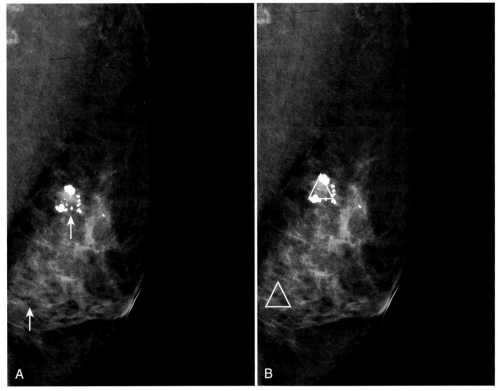

FIG. 1.30 Computer-aided detection (CAD). (A) Left digital mediolateral oblique mammogram before CAD shows calcifications (*arrows*). (B) The CAD scheme puts a triangular mark on the calcification clusters in the upper and lower breast.

The CAD marks have low specificity. Freer and Ulissey (2001) showed that 97.6% of CAD marks were dismissed by the interpreting radiologists. Furthermore, the radiologists had identified almost all of the 2.4% of CAD-marked findings that were selected for recall, which means that high-sensitivity CAD systems will mark significant potential findings as well as numerous insignificant findings. Accordingly, many insignificant findings will be marked by the CAD system, most of which can be dismissed readily, and yet the radiologists' attention will still be drawn to overlooked suspicious areas.

Other CAD studies have shown somewhat less positive results. Gur et al. (2004) assessed changes in screening mammography recall rate and cancer detection rate after the introduction of a CAD system into a single academic radiology practice. Based on 56,432 cases interpreted without CAD and 59,139 cases interpreted with CAD by 24 radiologists, recall rates were identical without and with CAD (11.39% versus 11.40%, respectively; $p = 0.96$), as were breast cancer detection rates without and with CAD (3.49 versus 3.55 per 1000 women screened, respectively; $p = 0.68$). Feig et al. (2004) used Gur's data to point out that lower volume readers benefited from CAD by having a 19.7% higher cancer detection rate, but at the price of a 14% increase in recall rate, from 10.5% to 12%.

Fenton et al. (2007) conducted a retrospective study comparing SFM without and with CAD in early implementation (2–25 months). They showed that adding CAD led to a nonsignificant increase in sensitivity (from 80.4% without CAD to 84% with CAD; $p = 0.32$), a significant decrease in specificity (from 90.2% without CAD to 87.2% with CAD; $p < 0.001$), and a significant decrease in accuracy (area under the ROC curve decreased from 0.919 without CAD to 0.871 with CAD; $p = 0.005$).

A study by Gromet (2008) compared CAD-aided readings of screening mammograms with double reading without CAD. The study found that CAD-aided readings had a nonsignificantly higher sensitivity than double reading (90.4% versus 88.0%), with a significantly lower recall rate (10.6% versus 11.9%, respectively; $p > 0.0001$).

The CAD programs have the potential to increase detection of cancer, particularly for readers with less experience or lower reading volumes, at the price of somewhat lower specificity and slightly longer interpretation times. In the end, however, it is the radiologist's knowledge and interpretive skills that have an impact on cancer detection, whether CAD is used or not.

CONCLUSION

Mammography acquisition is determined by a number of variables, including factors affecting image quality, such as the x-ray equipment, processing technique, technologist positioning, breast compression, and patient differences, such as breast density, lesion type, and the skills of the interpreting radiologist. It is important for radiologists to understand equipment requirements and the effect of imaging parameters on image quality; in addition, practitioners should be able to solve imaging problems that occur in everyday clinical practice. The MQSA regulations were put into effect to mandate many of the technical factors that are known to affect image quality and to improve the quality of mammography. Every radiologist who performs breast imaging should understand MQSA requirements and be able to supervise a high-quality mammography practice, working toward improved technical quality and interpretive skills based on follow-up and feedback from sound quality assurance practices.

Key Elements

American College of Radiology and Society of Breast Imaging guidelines for breast cancer screening of asymptomatic women include annual mammography starting at age 40.

The Mammography Quality Standard Act of 1992 is a congressional act enforced by the Food and Drug Administration (FDA) under which, since October 1994, mammography facilities in the United States are regulated.

Continued

The usual exposure for a mammogram is 24–32 kVp at 25–200 mAs.

Screen-film and digital systems deliver a mean glandular breast dose of about 2 mGy per exposure (4 mGy per two-view examination) to a woman of average breast thickness and glandularity; mean glandular dose is lower for thin breasts and higher for thick breasts.

Anode/filter combinations for mammography are Mo/Mo, Mo/Rh, Rh/Rh, W/Rh, W/Ag, or W/Al.

Screen-film image receptors are 18 × 24 cm and 24 × 30 cm in size.

Focal spot sizes for contact mammography and magnification mammography are nominally 0.3 and 0.1 mm, respectively.

Magnification mammography is achieved by moving the breast farther from the image receptor and closer to the x-ray source; FDA requires that magnification mammography have a magnification factor of 1.4× to 2.0×.

Moving grids with grid ratios between 3.5:1 and 5:1 are used to reduced scattered radiation for contact mammography; grids are not used for magnification mammography; instead the air gap between the breast and image receptor is used to reduce scatter.

The phantom image using the American College of Radiology mammography phantom evaluates the entire mammography imaging chain, is performed weekly, and at a minimum should detect four fibers, three speck groups, and three masses.

Film labeling includes the patient's first and last names and unique identification number, the name and address of the facility, the date, the view and laterality positioned near the axilla, numbers indicating the cassette and the mammography unit, and the technologist's initials.

The mediolateral oblique view should show good compression, contrast, exposure, sharpness, little noise, a posterior nipple line that intersects a convex pectoralis muscle, and an open inframammary fold.

The craniocaudal view should show good compression, contrast, exposure, sharpness, little noise, and a PNL that has a distance within 1 cm of the mediolateral oblique PNL length, and it should include medial breast tissue without sacrificing lateral breast tissue.

The MQSA requires specific training, experience, and continuing education for technologists, radiologists, and medical physicists.

To use a new modality, such as digital mammography or DBT, technologists, radiologists, and medical physicists are all required to have an initial 8 hours of training on that new modality prior to use.

Digital mammography detectors are composed of cesium iodide plus amorphous silicon diodes, cesium iodide plus arrayed charge-coupled devices, charged selenium plate read by silicon diodes, or computed radiography plates consisting of a barium fluorobromide plate read by a computed radiography laser scanner.

Digital mammograms may be interpreted on printed films or on high-resolution 2 × 2.5K (5 Mpixel) or higher monitors.

Studies indicate that the addition of DBT to 2D mammography increases sensitivity and cancer detection rate while decreasing recall rate when compared with 2D alone.

Computer-aided detection programs can detect subtle but suspicious mammographic findings in dense or complex breast tissue.

Computer-aided detection programs do not detect every breast cancer.

When computer-aided detection is used to aid interpretation of mammograms, the decision to recall a finding on a mammogram rests solely on the radiologist's experience and judgment.

Ag, silver; *Al*, aluminum; *Mo*, molybdenum; *Rh*, rhodium; *W*, tungsten.

SUGGESTED READINGS

Alonzo-Proulx O, Mawdsley GE, Patrie JT, et al.: Reliability of automated breast density measurements, *Radiology* 275:366-376, 2015.

American College of Radiology: *ACR BI-RADS®—mammography*, ed 4, Reston, VA, 2003, American College of Radiology.

Ayyala RS, Chorlton M, Behrman RH, et al.: Digital mammographic artifacts on full-field systems: what are they and how do I fix them? *Radiographics* 28:1999-2008, 2008.

Baker JA, Rosen EL, Lo JY, et al.: Computer-aided detection (CAD) in screening mammography: sensitivity of commercial CAD systems for detecting architectural distortion, *AJR Am J Roentgenol* 181:1083-1088, 2003.

Bassett LW, Farria DM, Bansal S, et al.: Reasons for failure of a mammography unit at clinical image review in the American College of Radiology Mammography Accreditation Program, *Radiology* 215:698-702, 2000a.

Bassett LW, Feig SA, Hendrick RE, et al.: *Breast disease (third series) test and syllabus*, Reston, VA, 2000b, American College of Radiology.

Berns EA, Hendrick RE, Cutter GR: Performance comparison of full-field digital mammography to screen-film mammography in clinical practice, *Med Phys* 29:830-834, 2002.

Berns EA, Hendrick RE, Solari M, et al.: Digital and screen-film mammography: comparison of image acquisition and interpretation times, *AJR Am J Roentgenol* 187:38-41, 2006.

Birdwell RL, Ikeda DM, O'Shaughnessy KF, et al.: Mammographic characteristics of 115 missed cancers later detected with screening mammography and the potential utility of computer-aided detection, *Radiology* 219:192-202, 2001.

Broeders M, Moss S, Nyström L, et al.: The impact of mammographic screening on breast cancer mortality in Europe: a review of observational studies, *J Med Screen* 19(Suppl 1):14-25, 2012.

Choi YJ, Cha JH, Kim JH, et al.: Analysis of prior mammography with negative result in women with interval breast cancer, *Breast Cancer*, published online March 29, 2015.

Ciatto S, Del Turco MR, Risso G, et al.: Comparison of standard reading and computer aided detection (CAD) on a national proficiency test of screening mammography, *Eur J Radiol* 45:135-138, 2003.

Ciatto S, Houssami N, Bernardi D, et al.: Integration of 3D digital mammography with tomosynthesis for population breast-cancer screening (STORM): a prospective comparison study, *Lancet Oncol* 14:583-589, 2013.

Coldman A, Phillips N, Warren L, et al.: Breast cancer mortality after screening mammography in British Columbia women, *Int J Cancer* 120:1076-1080, 2007.

Curry TS, Dowdy JE, Murray RC: *Christensen's Physics of diagnostic radiology*, ed 4, Malvern, PA, 1990, Lea & Febiger.

Dang PA, Freer PE, Humphrey KL, et al.: Addition of tomosynthesis to conventional digital mammography: effect on image interpretation time of screening examinations, *Radiology* 270:49-56, 2014.

Duffy SW, Tabar L, Chen THH, et al.: for The Swedish Organized Service Screening Evaluation Group: reduction in breast cancer mortality from organized service screening with mammography: 1. Further confirmation with extended data, *Cancer Epidemiol Biomarkers Prev* 15:45-51, 2006.

Durand MA, Haas BM, Yao X: Early clinical experience with digital breast tomosynthesis for screening mammography, *Radiology* 274:85-92, 2015.

Feig SA, Sickles EA, Evans WP, Linver NM: Re: Changes in breast cancer detection and mammography recall rates after the introduction of a computer-aided detection system, *J Natl Cancer Inst* 96:1260-1261, 2004.

Fenton JJ, Taplin SH, Carney PA, et al.: Influence of computer-aided detection on performance of screening mammography, *N Engl J Med* 356:1399-1409, 2007.

Freer PE, Niell B, Rafferty EA: Preoperative tomosynthesis-guided needle localization of mammographically and sonographically occult breast lesions, *Radiology* 140515, 2015.

Freer TW, Ulissey MJ: Screening mammography with computer-aided detection: prospective study of 12,860 patients in a community breast center, *Radiology* 220:781-786, 2001.

Friedewald SM, Rafferty EA, Conant EF: Breast cancer screening with tomosynthesis and digital mammography—reply, *JAMA* 312:1695-1696, 2014.

Galen B, Staab E, Sullivan DC, et al.: Congressional update: Report from the Biomedical Imaging Program of the National Cancer Institute. American College of Radiology Imaging Network: the digital Mammographic Imaging Screening Trial—An Update, *Acad Radiol* 9:374-375, 2002.

Greenberg JS, Javitt MC, Katzen J, et al.: Clinical performance metrics of 3D digital breast tomosynthesis compared with 2D digital mammography for breast cancer screening in community practice, *AJR Am J Roentgenol* 203:687-693, 2014.

Gromet M: Comparison of computer-aided detection to double reading of screening mammograms: review of 231,221 mammograms, *AJR Am J Roentgenol* 190:854-859, 2008.

Gur D, Sumkin JH, Rockette HE: Changes in breast cancer detection and mammography recall rates after the introduction of a computer-aided detection system, *J Natl Cancer Inst* 96:185-190, 2004.

Hakim CM, Catullo VJ, Chough DM, et al.: Effect of the availability of prior full-field digital mammography and digital breast tomosynthesis images on the interpretation of mammograms, *Radiology* 142009, 2015.

Hardesty LA: Issues to consider before implementing digital breast tomosynthesis into a breast imaging practice, *AJR Am J Roentgenol* 204(3):681-684, 2015.

Haygood TM, Wang J, Atkinson EN, et al.: Timed efficiency of interpretation of digital and film-screen screening mammograms, *AJR Am J Roentgenol* 192:216-220, 2009.

Hemminger BM, Dillon AW, Johnston RE, et al.: Effect of display luminance on the feature detection rates of masses in mammograms, *Med Phys* 26:2266-2272, 1999.

Hendrick RE: Radiation doses and cancer risks from breast imaging studies, *Radiology* 257:246-253, 2010.

Hendrick RE, Bassett LW, Botsco MA, et al.: *Mammography quality control manual*, Reston, VA, 1999, American College of Radiology.

Hendrick RE, Botsco M, Plott CM: Quality control in mammography, *Radiol Clin North Am* 33:1041–1057, 1995.

Hendrick RE, Cole E, Pisano ED, et al.: ACRIN DMIST retrospective multi-reader study comparing the accuracy of softcopy digital and screen-film mammography by digital manufacturer, *Radiology* 247:38–48, 2008.

Hendrick RE, Cutter G, Berns EA, et al.: Community-based screening mammography practice: services, charges and interpretation methods, *AJR Am J Roentgenol* 84:433–438, 2005.

Hendrick RE, Pisano ED, Averbukh A, et al.: Comparison of acquisition parameters and breast dose in digital mammography and screen-film mammography in the American College of Radiology Imaging Network Digital Mammographic Screening Trial, *AJR Am J Roentgenol* 194:362–369, 2010.

Houssami N, Macaskill P, Bernardi D, et al.: Breast screening using 2D-mammography or integrating digital breast tomosynthesis (3D-mammography) for single-reading or double-reading—evidence to guide future screening strategies, *Eur J Cancer* 50:1799–1807, 2014.

Keller BM, McCarthy AM, Chen J, et al.: Associations between breast density and a panel of single nucleotide polymorphisms linked to breast cancer risk: a cohort study with digital mammography, *BMC Cancer* 15:143, 2015.

Kerlikowske K, Hubbard RA, Miglioretti DL, et al.: Comparative effectiveness of digital versus film-screen mammography in community practice in the United States, *Ann Intern Med* 155:493–502, 2011.

Kim MY, Choi N, Yang JH, et al.: Background parenchymal enhancement on breast MRI and mammographic breast density: correlation with tumour characteristics, *Clin Radiol* 70:706–710, 2015.

Lacson R, Harris K, Brawarsky P, et al.: Evaluation of an automated information extraction tool for imaging data elements to populate a breast cancer screening registry, *J Digit Imaging* 28:567–576, 2015.

Lee CI, Cevik M, Alagoz O, et al.: Comparative effectiveness of combined digital mammography and tomosynthesis screening for women with dense breasts, *Radiology* 274:772–780, 2015.

Lei J, Yang P, Zhang L, et al.: Diagnostic accuracy of digital breast tomosynthesis versus digital mammography for benign and malignant lesions in breasts: a meta-analysis, *Eur Radiol* 24:595–602, 2014.

Lewin JM, D'Orsi CJ, Hendrick RE, et al.: Clinical comparison of full-field digital mammography and screen-film mammography for detection of breast cancer, *AJR Am J Roentgenol* 179:671–677, 2002.

Lewin JM, Hendrick RE, D'Orsi CJ, et al.: Comparison of full-field digital mammography with screen-film mammography for cancer detection: results of 4,945 paired examinations, *Radiology* 218:873–880, 2001.

Linver MN, Osuch JR, Brenner RJ, et al.: The mammography audit: a primer for the Mammography Quality Standards Act (MQSA), *AJR Am J Roentgenol* 165:19–25, 1995.

Lourenco AP, Barry-Brooks M, Baird GL, et al.: Changes in recall type and patient treatment following implementation of screening digital breast tomosynthesis, *Radiology* 274:337–342, 2015.

Mariscotti G, Houssami N, Durando M, et al.: Digital breast tomosynthesis (DBT) to characterize MRI-detected additional lesions unidentified at targeted ultrasound in newly diagnosed breast cancer patients, *Eur Radiol* 25:2673–2681, 2015.

Markey MK, Lo JY, Floyd Jr CE: Differences between computer-aided diagnosis of breast masses and that of calcifications, *Radiology* 223:489–493, 2002.

McCarthy AM, Kontos D, Synnestvedt M: Screening outcomes following implementation of digital breast tomosynthesis in a general-population screening program, *J Natl Cancer Inst* 106, 2014.

Monsees BS: The Mammography Quality Standards Act. An overview of the regulations and guidance, *Radiol Clin North Am* 38:759–772, 2000.

Morrish OW, Tucker L, Black R, et al.: Mammographic breast density: comparison of methods for quantitative evaluation, *Radiology* 275:356–365, 2015.

MQSA (Mammography Quality Standards Act) final rule released. American College of Radiology, *Radiol Manage* 20:51–55, 1998.

Nass SJ, Henderson IC, Lashof IJ, editors: *Mammography and beyond: developing technologies for the early detection of breast cancer*, Washington, DC, 2001a, National Academy Press.

Nass SJ, Henderson IC, Lashof JC: *Institute of Medicine (U.S.). Committee on Technologies for the Early Detection of Breast Cancer and National Cancer Policy Board (U.S.). Committee on the Early Detection of Breast Cancer: Mammography and beyond: developing technologies for the early detection of breast cancer*, Washington, DC, 2001b, National Academy Press.

Pisano E, Cabras T, Montaldo C, et al.: Peptides of human gingival crevicular fluid determined by HPLC-ESI-MS, *Eur J Oral Sci* 113:462–468, 2005a.

Pisano ED, Cole EB, Kistner EO, et al.: Interpretation of digital mammograms: comparison of speed and accuracy of soft-copy versus printed-film display, *Radiology* 223:483–488, 2002.

Pisano ED, Cole EB, Major S, et al.: For the International Digital Mammography Development Group: radiologists' preferences for digital mammographic display, *Radiology* 216:820–830, 2000a.

Pisano ED, Cole EB, Major S, et al.: Radiologists' preferences for digital mammographic display. The International Digital Mammography Development Group, *Radiology* 216:820–830, 2000b.

Pisano ED, Gatsonis C, Hendrick E, et al.: Diagnostic performance of digital versus film mammography for breast-cancer screening, *N Engl J Med* 353:1773–1783, 2005b.

Pisano ED, Gatsonis CA, Yaffe MJ, et al.: American College of Radiology Imaging Network digital mammographic imaging screening trial: objectives and methodology, *Radiology* 236:404–412, 2005c.

Pisano ED, Hendrick RE, Yaffe MJ, et al.: Diagnostic accuracy of digital versus film mammography: exploratory analysis of selected population subgroups in DMIST, *Radiology* 246:376–383, 2008.

Pisano ED, Yaffe MJ: Digital mammography, *Radiology* 234:353–361, 2005d.

Quek ST, Thng CH, Khoo JB, et al.: Radiologists' detection of mammographic abnormalities with and without a computer-aided detection system, *Australas Radiol* 47:257–260, 2003.

Rafferty EA, Park JM, Philpotts LE: Diagnostic accuracy and recall rates for digital mammography and digital mammography combined with one-view and two-view tomosynthesis: results of an enriched reader study, *AJR Am J Roentgenol* 202:273–281, 2014.

Rafferty EA, Park JM, Philpotts LE, et al.: Assessing radiologist performance using combined digital mammography and breast tomosynthesis compared with digital mammography alone: results of a multicenter, multireader trial, *Radiology* 266:104–113, 2013.

Rong XJ, Shaw CC, Johnston DA, et al.: Microcalcification detectability for four mammographic detectors: flat-panel, CCD, CR, and screen/film, *Med Phys* 29:2052–2061, 2002.

Rose SL, Tidwell AL, Bujnoch LJ, et al.: Implementation of breast tomosynthesis in a routine screening practice: an observational study, *AJR Am J Roentgenol* 200:1401–1408, 2013.

Rothenberg LN, Feig SA, Hendrick RE, et al.: *A Guide to mammography and other breast imaging procedures*, Bethesda, MD, December 31, 2004, National Council of Radiation Protection and Measurements. NCRP Report #149.

Saslow D, Boetes C, Burke W, for the American Cancer Society Breast Cancer Advisory Group, et al.: American Cancer Society guidelines for breast screening with MRI as an adjunct to mammography, *CA Cancer J Clin* 57:75–89, 2007.

Schrading S, Distelmaier M, Dirrichs T: Digital breast tomosynthesis-guided vacuum-assisted breast biopsy: initial experiences and comparison with prone stereotactic vacuum-assisted biopsy, *Radiology* 274(3):654–662, 2015.

Seidenwurm D, Rosenberg R: Breast cancer screening with tomosynthesis and digital mammography, *JAMA* 312:1695, 2014.

Shin SU, Chang JM, Bae MS, et al.: Comparative evaluation of average glandular dose and breast cancer detection between single-view digital breast tomosynthesis (DBT) plus single-view digital mammography (DM) and two-view DM: correlation with breast thickness and density, *Eur Radiol* 25:1–8, 2015.

Skaane P, Bandos AI, Eben EB, et al.: Two-view digital breast tomosynthesis screening with synthetically reconstructed projection images: comparison with digital breast tomosynthesis with full-field digital mammographic images, *Radiology* 271:655–663, 2014.

Skaane P, Bandos AI, Gullien R, et al.: Comparison of digital mammography alone and digital mammography plus tomosynthesis in a population-based screening program, *Radiology* 267:47–56, 2013.

Skaane P, Hofvind S, Skjennald A: Randomized trial of screen-film versus full-field digital mammography with soft-copy reading in population-based screening program: follow-up and final results of Oslo II study, *Radiology* 244:708–717, 2007.

Skaane P, Skjennald A: Screen-film mammography versus full-field digital mammography with soft-copy reading: randomized trial in a population-based screening program—the Oslo II study, *Radiology* 232:197–204, 2004.

Smith RA, Saslow D, Sawyer KA, et al.: American Cancer Society guidelines for breast cancer screening: update 2003, *CA Cancer J Clin* 53:141–169, 2003.

Swedish Organised Service Screening Evaluation, G: Reduction in breast cancer mortality from organized service screening with mammography: 1. Further confirmation with extended data, *Cancer Epidemiol Biomarkers Prev* 15:45–51, 2006.

Tabar L, Yen MF, Vitak B, et al.: Mammography service screening and mortality in breast cancer patients: 20-year follow-up before and after introduction of screening, *Lancet* 361:1405–1410, 2003.

Tagliafico A, Mariscotti G, Durando M, et al.: Characterisation of microcalcification clusters on 2D digital mammography (FFDM) and digital breast tomosynthesis (DBT): does DBT underestimate microcalcification clusters? Results of a multicentre study, *Eur Radiol* 25:9–14, 2015.

Trubo R: Recent findings may inform breast density notification laws, *JAMA* 313:452–453, 2015.

U.S. Department of Health and Human Services: Food and Drug Administration: Compliance guidance: the mammography quality standards act final regulations document #1; Availability. Notice, *Fed Reg* 64:13590–13591, 1999.

U.S. Department of Health and Human Services: Food and Drug Administration: State certification of mammography facilities. Final rule, *Fed Reg* 67:5446–5469, 2002.

U.S. Department of Health and Human Services: Public Health Service. Food and Drug Administration: quality mammography standards. Direct final rule, *Fed Reg* 64(116):32404–32407, 1999.

Vedantham S, Karellas A, Suryanarayanan S, et al.: Breast imaging using an amorphous silicon-based full-field digital mammographic system: stability of a clinical prototype, *J Digit Imaging* 13:191–199, 2000a.

Vedantham S, Karellas A, Suryanarayanan S, et al.: Full breast digital mammography with an amorphous silicon-based flat panel detector: physical characteristics of a clinical prototype, *Med Phys* 27:558–567, 2000b.

Venta LA, Hendrick RE, Adler YT, et al.: Rates and causes of disagreement in interpretation of full-field digital mammography and film-screen mammography in a diagnostic setting, *AJR Am J Roentgenol* 176:1241–1248, 2001.

Warren Burhenne LJ, Wood SA, D'Orsi CJ, et al.: Potential contribution of computer-aided detection to the sensitivity of screening mammography, *Radiology* 215:554–562, 2000.

Zheng B, Shah R, Wallace L, et al.: Computer-aided detection in mammography: an assessment of performance on current and prior images, *Acad Radiol* 9(1):245–1250, 2002.

Zhou XQ, Huang HK, Lou SL: Authenticity and integrity of digital mammography images, *IEEE Trans Med Imaging* 20:784–791, 2001.

Chapter 2

Mammogram Analysis and Interpretation

Debra M. Ikeda and Kanae K. Miyake

CHAPTER OUTLINE

In the United States, statistics indicate that one in eight American women will develop breast cancer if women live a 90-year life span. The incidence of breast cancer in women in the United States is rising, and although the rate of increase has slowed recently, the rate of in situ breast cancer continues to increase. The United States breast cancer death rates have decreased since the early 1990s, with decreases of 2.5% per year among white women. These decreased breast cancer deaths are attributed to both improved breast cancer treatments and mammography screening. Randomized, controlled population trials of women invited to breast cancer screening using x-ray mammography showed an approximate 30% reduction in breast cancer deaths in the invited group compared with women the control group. The National Comprehensive Cancer Network (NCCN) recommends annual screening mammography for women aged 40 years and older (V1.2015). Societies such as the American Cancer Society (ACS) and the U.S. Preventive Services Task Force recommend annual screening after ages 45 and 50, respectively, whereas other societies differ widely from every other year to no screening mammography at all.

This chapter reviews breast cancer risk factors, signs, and symptoms of breast cancer; the normal mammogram; mammographic findings of breast cancer; basic interpretation of screening mammograms; and workup of findings detected at screening with additional mammographic views and tomosynthesis.

BREAST CANCER RISK FACTORS

Risk factors for breast cancer are important to consider when reading mammograms because they indicate a pretest probability of breast cancer. Compiling risk information on a breast history sheet or compiled by the technologist on a computerized form provides interpreting radiologists quick access to this important information (Fig. 2.1). Breast cancer risk factors are listed in Box 2.1. The most important risk factors are personal or family history of breast cancer/ovarian cancer, genetic mutations predisposing to breast cancer such as *BRCA 1/2*, older age, and female gender. Men also develop breast cancer, but only 1% of all breast cancers occur in men in the United States.

Breast cancer risk increases with increasing age and drops off at 80 years old. Women with a personal history of breast cancer have a higher risk of developing breast cancer in the ipsilateral or contralateral breast than does the general population. After breast cancer surgery, the conservatively treated breast has a 1% per year risk of developing recurrent or new cancer.

Breast cancer risk assessment uses breast cancer risk assessment models based on a detailed family history of breast or ovarian cancer looking for genetic predispositions for breast cancer, and calculates lifetime risks for breast cancer. The BRCAPRO, BOADICEA, modified Gail model, and Tyrer–Cuzick model take into account the age, number, and cancer types in affected relatives, as well as other risk factors, to estimate a lifetime risk for breast cancer. Both the NCCN and ACS consider a >20% to 25% lifetime risk to be high risk. Women with a first-degree relative (mother, daughter, or sister) with breast cancer have approximately double the risk of the general population and are at particularly high risk if the cancer was premenopausal or bilateral. If many relatives had breast or ovarian cancer, the woman may be a carrier of *BRCA1* or *BRCA2*, the autosomal dominant breast cancer susceptibility genes. Genetic testing is most appropriately performed by genetic counseling professionals who evaluate, counsel, and support women because of untoward social effects of either positive or negative results. Carriers of the breast cancer susceptibility gene *BRCA1* on chromosome 17 have a breast cancer risk of 85% and an ovarian cancer risk of 63% by age 70. Women with *BRCA2* on chromosome 15 have a high risk

LABEL

Patient Phone #:_____

Is this your first mammogram?   Yes   No

I am having the following **PROBLEM(S)**: (Circle **R** for Right, or **L** for Left); or **NO PROBLEMS** ____

R L ___ Bloody discharge   R L ___ Implant problem

R L ___ Cancer elsewhere   R L ___ Difficult physical exam

R L ___ Image detected calcifications   R L ___ Image detected mass

R L ___ Large nodes under my arm   R L ___ Other lump or thickening

R L ___ Nipple problem   R L ___ Non-bloody discharge

R L ___ Pain in the breast   R L ___ Palpable abnormality or lump

R L ___ Other skin changes to breast

R L ___ Skin thickening or retraction on clinical examination

Check all of the following **RISK FACTORS** that you have had (if any); or **NONE** ____

___ I do not know my personal breast cancer history   ___ Been through menopause

___ Breast cancer   ___ Never had children

___ Endometrial cancer   ___ First child after age 30

___ Ovarian caner   ___ BRCA1 gene mutation

___ Chest/Breast radiation therapy   ___ BRCA2 gene mutation

___ Breast biopsy that showed a high-risk lesion

FMILY BREAST CANCER AND OVARIAN CANCER History: (Circle)

Relationship: Maternal/Paternal: Age cancer developed:

Sister   Brother   Aunt (M or P)   Grandmother (M or P)   _____

Daughter   Son   Uncle (M or P)   Grandfather (M or P)   _____

Mother   Father   Cousin (M or P)   Half-sister (M or P)   Breast or Ovarian: ___

                                 Half-brother (M or P)   _____

                                                                             _____

HORMONE History: Please check all hormones you have used; or NEVER USED ____

	Age when last used:	Currently using? (**Y** or **N**)
Hormonal contraceptives	_____	_____
Estrogen	_____	_____
Progesterone	_____	_____
Tamoxifen	_____	_____
Raloxifene	_____	_____
Arimidex	_____	_____
Other hormones	_____	_____

MENSTRUAL History:

Age when periods started   _____   Currently pregnant?   Yes   No

Age at menopause   _____   Age at first full-term pregnancy _____

Age at right ovary removal _____   Age at hysterectomy   _____

Age at left ovary removal   _____   Parity (number of live births)   _____

FIG. 2.1 Breast history form. It includes a diagrammatic breast template and places to record the patient's history and current problems or complaints.

Menstrual cycle phase, if applicable:

___ 1st week after   ___ 2nd week after   ___ 3rd week after   ___ Presently menstruating

Menopausal status:

___ Pre-menopausal   ___ Peri-menopausal   ___ Post-menopausal

BREAST PROCEDURE History

Procedure	Side	Date Performed	Benign	Malignant	High-risk
Breast reduction	R ___ L ___	_____	_____	_____	_____
Core needle biopsy	R ___ L ___	_____	_____	_____	_____
Cyst aspiration	R ___ L ___	_____	_____	_____	_____
Surgical biopsy	R ___ L ___	_____	_____	_____	_____
Implant removal	R ___ L ___	_____	_____	_____	_____
Breast reconstruction	R ___ L ___	_____	_____	_____	_____
Cancer lumpectomy	R ___ L ___	_____	_____	_____	_____
Mastectomy	R ___ L ___	_____	_____	_____	_____
Radiation therapy	R ___ L ___	_____	_____	_____	_____
Unknown biopsy	R ___ L ___	_____	_____	_____	_____

If you have IMPLANTS, indicate the type (for example; Silicone gel, Saline, Combination) **and/or location** (for example; Pre-pectoral, Sub-pectoral, Retro-pectoral); or **NONE** ____

Type   **Location**

RIGHT: Implant type: _____   (Circle): Pre-pectoral, Sub-pectoral, Retro-pectoral, Unknown

LEFT: Implant type: _____   (Circle): Pre-pectoral, Sub-pectoral, Retro-pectoral, Unknown

Have you ever received chemotherapy for any type of cancer?   ____ Yes ____ No ____ Unknown

Comments: (Please mark on the diagram any **NEW** symptoms)

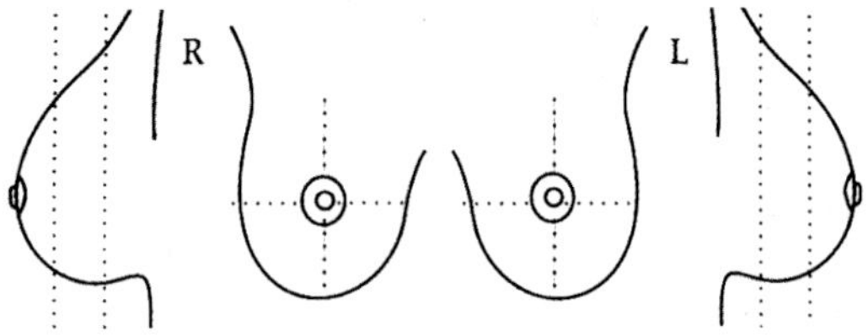

	Right	Left		Right	Left
Nipple inversion or retraction:	____	____	Pain:	____	____
Nipple discharge:	____	____	Moles:	____	____
Skin thickening or retraction:	____	____	Scars:	____	____
Tissue thickening:	____	____	Lump or Mass:	____	____

Other: _____   ____ ____

Patient Signature: _____   Date: _____

Technologist Signature: _____   Date: _____

FIG. 2.1, cont'd

of breast cancer and a low risk of ovarian cancer. These genes account for 5% of all breast cancers in the United States and for 25% of breast cancers in women younger than age 30 years old. Women of Ashkenazi (Eastern European) Jewish heritage have a slightly higher risk of breast cancer than does the general population (Box 2.2), but additional work is being done to determine whether this population has a higher rate of breast and ovarian cancer related to *BRCA1* and *BRCA2* mutations. Other genetic syndromes that have a higher risk of breast cancer include the Li-Fraumeni, Cowden, and ataxia-telangiectasia syndromes.

Factors such as early menarche (before age 12), late menopause (after age 55), nulliparity, and first live birth after age 30 bestow a slightly higher risk for breast cancer, as a result of having more menstrual cycles and longer exposure to estrogen and progesterone. Data from a 2003 study, part of the Women's Health Initiative, which is a randomized, controlled trial of the effects of estrogen plus progestin (combination hormone replacement therapy [CHRT]) versus placebo, showed a 24% greater incidence of breast cancer in women receiving CHRT compared with the control group. Whereas previous data showed an adjusted relative risk of 1.46 for the development of breast cancer in women receiving CHRT for more than 5 years, the 2003 analysis showed the risk for breast cancer rising within 5 years of starting CHRT; in addition, it showed more difficulty in detecting cancers by mammography.

A breast biopsy showing atypical ductal hyperplasia (ADH) histology increases the risk for breast cancer to four to five times that of the general population. The presence of lobular carcinoma in situ (LCIS) also increases the risk for breast cancer, but at a much higher rate than ADH (about 10 times that of the normal population). The acronym LCIS is a misnomer and not a cancer at all; rather, LCIS is a high-risk marker for developing breast cancer. A woman with LCIS has a 27% to 30% chance of developing

invasive ductal or lobular cancer in the ipsilateral or contralateral breast over a 10-year period. Thus a biopsy showing LCIS results in patient management of either "watchful waiting" with increased surveillance by frequent imaging and physical examination, or bilateral mastectomy.

Women who had an early exposure to radiation also have an increased risk for breast cancer. A medical history of radiation therapy to the mediastinum for Hodgkin disease, multiple fluoroscopic examinations for tuberculosis, ablation of the thymus, or treatment of acne with radiation infers scattered radiation to the breasts at an early age, which may induce breast cancer. The risk for developing breast cancer is so high in women treated for Hodgkin disease that in 2007 the ACS recommended magnetic resonance breast cancer screening for Hodgkin disease survivors as well as *BRCA1/2* genetic mutation carriers or women with a high lifetime risk of breast cancer >20% to 25% lifetime risk.

Extensive mammographic breast density, defined as a large amount of fibroglandular tissue within the breast by volume as measured on the mammogram, is associated with the risk of breast cancer. However, the association and the reasons for this finding, as well as its relative association among different ethnicities, are still being studied.

Other lifestyle choices also affect breast cancer risk. One of these is drinking alcohol. One drink per day bestows a very small risk, but two to five drinks per day increases the risk to 15 times that of women who do not drink. Being overweight or obese also increases the risk of cancer, especially if the weight gain happens after menopause and the fat is around the abdomen. A woman with an "apple-shaped" body is at higher risk than one with a "pear-shaped" body. Exercise has been shown to reduce breast cancer risk after menopause, with one study suggesting that cancer risk was reduced at least in part via hormonal pathways. However, more study of these changeable risk factors is needed.

Despite all that is known about breast cancer risk factors, 70% of all women with breast cancer have none of these risk factors other than older age and female gender. What can women do to prevent breast cancer? The ACS recommends adopting a healthy lifestyle including exercise, maintenance of an appropriate body mass index, and decreased alcohol consumption. Women at very high risk also may take antiestrogen medications to prevent breast cancer.

SIGNS AND SYMPTOMS OF BREAST CANCER

A breast lump is one of the most common symptoms for which women seek advice (Box 2.3), but most lumps are benign, often found by the woman herself or her partner, and most commonly caused by breast cysts or solid fibroadenomas (the most common solid benign breast masses in women). Breast lumps are worrisome for cancer if they are new, growing, hard, stuck to the skin or chest wall, causing skin dimpling or nipple retraction, or are associated with bloody nipple discharge.

Nipple discharge is another finding for which women often seek advice. Nipple discharge is usually benign, especially if it is whitish, green, or yellow or produced from several ducts, and it is usually caused by fibrocystic change. Nipple discharge is

---

BOX 2.1   Breast Cancer Risk Factors

Female
Older age
Personal history of breast cancer
First-degree relative with breast cancer (see also models for breast cancer risk based on family history of breast and ovarian cancer, such as Tyrer–Cuzick and modified Gail model)
Early menarche
Late menopause
Nulliparity
First birth after age 30
Atypical ductal or lobular hyperplasia
BRCA1, BRCA2, and other genetic predispositions
Radiation exposure
Lobular carcinoma in situ

BOX 2.2   Family History Suggesting an Increased Risk of Breast Cancer

>2 relatives with breast or ovarian cancer
Breast cancer in relative age <50 years
Relatives with breast and ovarian cancer
Relatives with two independent breast cancers or breast plus ovarian cancer
Male relative with breast cancer
Family history of breast or ovarian cancer and Ashkenazi Jewish heritage
Li-Fraumeni syndrome
Cowden syndrome
Ataxia-telangiectasia

BOX 2.3   Signs and Symptoms of Breast Cancer

Breast lump
Nipple discharge (new and spontaneous, bloody, serosanguineous or serous but copious)
New nipple inversion
Skin retraction or skin tethering
Peau d'orange
Nothing (cancer detected on screening mammography)

suspicious for cancer if it is new, expressed from only one duct, bloody or serosanguineous, spontaneous, copious, or serous. An example of a suspicious clinical history is a woman describing new bloody or serous nipple discharge on her nightgown or undergarments. Other causes of bloody nipple discharge are benign intraductal papilloma, pregnancy, or trauma.

Nipple change may be caused by benign etiologies or to Paget disease of the nipple. Nipple irritation caused by nursing is common, and nipple irritation with associated mastitis is not uncommon but is benign. However, Paget disease of the nipple is a malignancy, and may present with a bright red nipple initially, can proceed to an eczema-like flakiness simulating infection, and later, frank tumor invasion and tissue destruction. Patients with Paget disease of the nipple are often treated for months with antibiotics until the true diagnosis of malignancy is made by nipple tissue punch biopsy.

Long-standing nipple inversion is not uncommon and is benign if it is present at birth. On the other hand, new nipple inversion is worrisome because retroareolar breast cancers can pull in the nipple by productive fibrosis or invasion, causing the nipple retraction.

Skin retraction or skin dimpling is a sign of breast cancer and is caused by superficial cancers tethering or invading the skin and pulling the skin in toward the breast. On physical examination, skin retraction or tethering might become evident when the woman raises her arms as she inspects her breasts in the mirror. Raising her arms or placing her hands on her hips pulls in the pectoralis muscle, which pulls on the cancer, which pulls on the skin, and dimples the skin in toward the cancer.

Peau d'orange is a French word for "orange peel" skin or pitting of the skin caused by breast edema. The pitting is caused by fluid accumulating in the skin and rising around the bases of tethered hair follicles, resulting in skin pitting. Breast edema is a nonspecific finding and can be caused by mastitis, trauma, inflammatory cancer, edema from radiation therapy, or axillary lymph node obstruction.

Lymphadenopathy can cause large or painful axillary lymph nodes in the armpits for which women seek advice. Bilateral lymphadenopathy may be caused by systemic illnesses such as widespread infection, lymphoma, leukemia, collagen vascular disease, and widespread malignancy, to name a few etiologies. Causes of unilateral lymphadenopathy are infection, tumors that include breast cancer, and granulomatous disease, whereas other causes are rarer. In the breast, the radiologist looks at the ipsilateral breast tissue to exclude breast cancer as the cause for the patient's complaint of unilateral lymphadenopathy.

Despite all these signs and symptoms of breast cancer, some women have no physical findings or symptoms at all despite having breast cancer. Their breast cancers are detected on screening mammography and are asymptomatic.

Breast pain is not generally caused by cancer, but it deserves special mention because breast pain is very common. If cyclic, breast pain is usually endocrine in nature. Although breast pain is usually caused by benign etiologies, unfortunately, both breast pain and breast cancer are common. Thus the physician's goals are to reassure patients with breast pain, search for treatable causes of breast pain such as cysts, and exclude coexistent malignancy.

THE NORMAL MAMMOGRAM

Anatomy and Image Contrast

A normal breast has glandular breast elements surrounded by fat and breast stroma, which is surrounded by a honeycomb fibrous structure of thin strandlike Cooper's ligaments. The glandular elements are composed of lactiferous ducts leading from the nipple and branch into excretory ducts, interlobular ducts, and terminal ducts that lead to acini that produce milk (Fig. 2.2). The ducts are lined by epithelium composed of an outer cellular myoepithelial

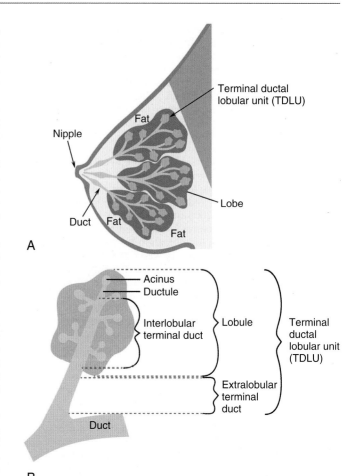

FIG. 2.2 Schematic of a normal breast. (A) Schematic of a normal breast showing the nipple, ducts, and lobes that contain terminal ductal lobular units (TDLUs). (B) A TDLU consists of acini, ductules, and terminal ducts. Breast milk is produced in TDLUs.

layer and an inner secretory cellular layer. The ducts and glandular tissue extend posteriorly in a fanlike distribution consisting of 15 to 20 lobes draining each of the lactiferous ducts, with most of the glandular tissue found in the upper outer breast near the axilla. Fatty tissue surrounds the glandular tissue. Posterior to the glandular tissue is retroglandular fat, described by Dr. Laszlo Tabar as a "no man's land," in which no glandular tissue should be seen. The pectoralis muscle lies behind the fat on top of the chest wall.

Mammography provides image contrast by using the differences in the x-ray attenuation among the different breast tissue types, such as fat, fibroglandular tissue, and carcinoma. With lower energy x-rays used by mammography (approximately 25–28 keV), the attenuation difference between the fibroglandular tissue and carcinoma is more pronounced than on standard radiographs, which use a 50-keV x-ray. Fatty tissue is the least dense and most translucent to x-rays and appears dark on mammography. Fibroglandular tissue, muscle, and lymph nodes are more dense and radiopaque (whiter) than fatty tissue, and are white on mammography. Cancers and fluid-filled cysts may be denser and whiter than normal surrounding fibroglandular tissue. Calcifications and metals are the brightest and whitest of all structures on mammography.

On the normal mediolateral oblique (MLO) mammogram, the pectoralis muscle is a concave white structure posterior to the retroglandular fat near the chest wall (Fig. 2.3). Normal lymph nodes high in the axilla overlie the pectoralis muscle. Normal lymph nodes are sharply marginated, oval, or lobulated dense

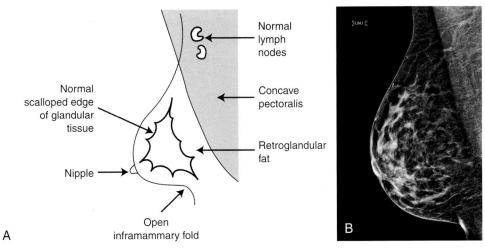

FIG. 2.3 Normal breast anatomy and correlative mammograms. (A) Schematic of a normal mediolateral oblique (MLO) mammogram. Note the normal scalloped edge of glandular tissue, retromammary fat, concave pectoralis muscle, and normal lymph nodes. (B) Normal MLO mammogram.

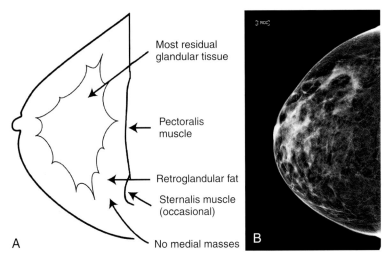

FIG. 2.4 (A) Schematic of a normal craniocaudal (CC) mammogram. Note the normal fat in the medial and retroglandular regions and the location of the pectoralis muscles. Most of the residual glandular tissue and the sternalis muscle remain in the upper outer quadrants. (B) Normal CC mammogram.

white masses with a radiolucent fatty hilum. They are commonly found in the axilla and in the upper outer quadrant of the breast along blood vessels. Lymph nodes can also occur normally but less commonly in any quadrant of the breast and are called normal *intramammary* lymph nodes. A normal lymph node has a typical, sharply marginated kidney bean shape; a white outer cortex; and a dark, fatty hilum on the mammogram and should be left alone. If one is uncertain about whether a mass represents an intramammary lymph node, a tomosynthesis slice or mammographic magnification views may help display the fatty hilum, or an ultrasound may show the typical hypoechoic appearance of the lymph node and the echogenic fatty hilum.

On the normal craniocaudal (CC) projection, the pectoralis muscle produces a half-moon–shaped or bandlike density near the chest wall (Fig. 2.4). Fat lies anterior to the muscle, and the white glandular tissue lies anterior to the fat. In older women, most of the glandular tissue in the medial breast undergoes fatty involution, and most of the residual dense glandular tissue persists in the upper outer breast.

There should be only fatty tissue in the medial breast near the chest wall on the CC view. The only normal exception is the sternalis muscle, which is a white slip of muscle hugging the medial chest wall on the CC view that should not be mistaken for a

mass (Fig. 2.5). If there is a question that a density in the medial breast is a mass instead of the sternalis muscle, a tomosynthesis slice should show that it is sternalis muscle. If there is no tomosynthesis, a cleavage view (CV) mammogram or ultrasound can prove that the density is a just a sternalis muscle, is normal, and can be ignored.

Breast Density, Breast Density Notification Legislation, and Breast Density Classification Based on the Breast Imaging Reporting and Data System

Breast *density* is an important feature of the mammogram that describes how much of the breast volume is filled with white glandular tissue. Breast fibroglandular tissue is white on the mammogram, and fat is black on the mammogram. Women have varying ratios of glandular and fatty tissue in their breasts genetically. The definition of a *dense* breast is one that contains a lot of glandular breast tissue and looks mostly white on the mammogram. The opposite of a dense breast is a *fatty* breast, which looks mostly black on the mammogram. A dense breast does not mean the breast is hard to the touch. Breast density on the mammogram has little correlation to how hard or soft the breast feels

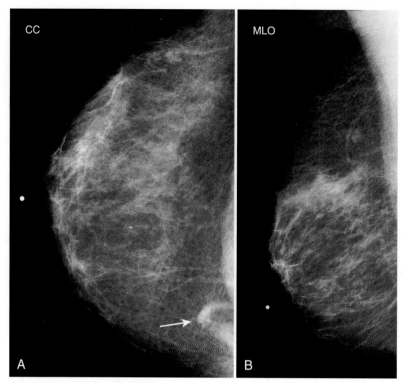

FIG. 2.5 Sternalis muscle. (A) The breast is composed of scattered fibroglandular density. A muscle-like density seen in the right breast medial to the half-moon or triangular shape of the pectoralis muscle (*arrow*) near the chest wall on the craniocaudal (CC) view represents the sternalis muscle. (B) The sternalis muscle is not seen on the mediolateral oblique (MLO) view.

on physical examination; that is, you cannot predict how soft a breast will feel to the touch by looking at the mammogram density. Conversely, there is no correlation of how white the mammogram will be based on how hard, lumpy, or soft the breast feels on physical examination.

The American College of Radiology's (ACR) Breast Imaging Reporting and Data System (BI-RADS) lexicon classifies breast density on mammograms into four groups: extremely dense, heterogeneously dense, scattered areas of fibroglandular density, and almost entirely fatty (Fig. 2.6; Box 2.4). From 2004 to 2013, extremely dense, heterogeneous dense, scattered areas of fibroglandular density, and almost entirely fatty defined, in quartiles, how dense or how white the breast looked on the mammogram. Dense was defined as >75% to 100% dense tissue by volume, heterogeneously dense was 51% to 75% dense, scattered 26% to 75% dense, and fatty was <25% dense by volume. Dense and heterogeneously dense glandular tissue lowered the sensitivity of mammography, because breast cancer is also white on the mammogram, and the white dense normal background of glandular tissue can hide a cancer, just like a polar bear can hide in a snowstorm.

The fifth edition of BI-RADS, published in 2013, no longer defines breast density in the quartile system (Fig. 2.7). Instead, dense and heterogeneously dense describe whether there is enough breast tissue on the mammogram to obscure a cancer. Thus a heterogeneously dense normal background of glandular tissue may have less than 50% dense breast tissue by volume on the mammogram but contains enough dense tissue to obscure a cancer. In the mammographic report, radiologists describe breast density so that referring doctors will know how white the breast looks and how confident the radiologist is in excluding cancer.

Breast density notification legislation in the United States began in 2009 in the state of Connecticut, where the law mandated that women with dense and heterogeneously dense breast tissue on mammograms receive a letter informing them that they have dense breast tissue, that dense breast tissue is normal, that

dense breast tissue carries a higher risk of breast cancer, that dense breast tissue may hide breast cancer, and that they may wish to discuss supplemental screening tests with their doctor. BI-RADS 2013 shows that in the United States about 50% of all women have heterogeneously dense or dense breast tissue on mammograms. As of May 2016, 27 states have proposed or enacted dense breast notification federal legislation.

It is important to know that the breast is normally dense at a young age and decreases in density with time as glandular tissue normally involutes into fat. Young women have mostly glandular breasts, and their mammograms are usually dense or white on mammograms (see Fig. 2.6A). As women age, their fibroglandular tissue involutes into fat, which is black. Therefore the natural progression of the mammogram is mostly white (dense) at a young age when the breasts are filled with glandular tissue and it becomes progressively darker (fatty) as the woman ages. The amount of remaining glandular tissue varies from woman to woman and depends on genetics, parity, and exogenous hormone replacement therapy. Some older women have surprisingly large amounts of dense white tissue on the mammogram, but generally as women age there are greater amounts of fat and less dense glandular tissue, which usually remains in the upper outer quadrants of the breast (see Fig. 2.6D), producing a darker mammogram. Normal increases in breast density occur only in pregnant and lactating women, or in women starting exogenous hormone replacement therapy, because of the increase in fibroglandular tissue in response to female hormones. The breast density does not increase normally otherwise. Any unexplained increases in breast density should be viewed with suspicion and worked up.

MAMMOGRAPHIC FINDINGS OF BREAST CANCER

Radiologists detect breast cancers when the tumor produces findings that are different from the normal fibroglandular/fatty

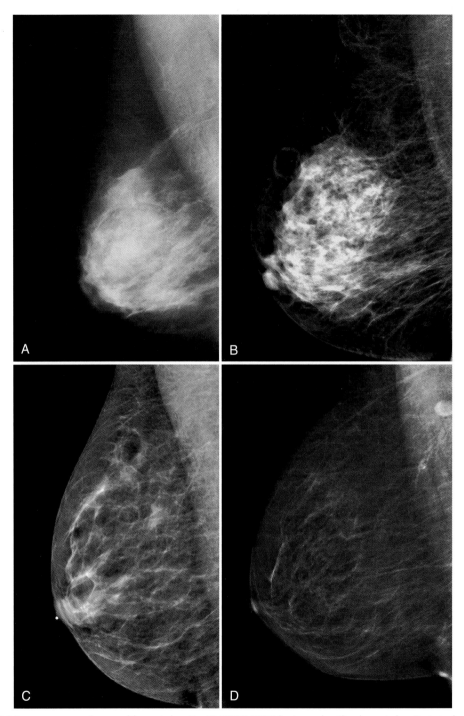

FIG. 2.6 Mammograms of normal breast density. BI-RADS 2013 lexicon classifies breast density into four types. (A) "Dense" glandular tissue, which lowers the sensitivity of mammography. A mammogram of a young woman is shown. (B) "Heterogeneously dense" breast tissue, which may obscure small masses. (C) "Scattered" densities with scattered areas of fibroglandular tissue. (D) A "fatty" breast composed of almost entirely fatty tissue. A mammogram of an older women is presented.

BOX 2.4 ACR BI-RADS Terms for Breast Density

Breast is almost entirely fat
There are scattered fibroglandular densities
Breast tissue is heterogeneously dense, which could obscure detection of small masses
Breast tissue is extremely dense

From ACR BI-RADS Mammography, In *ACR BI-RADS atlas, breast imaging reporting and data system*, Reston, VA, 2013, American College of Radiology.

background. Common mammographic findings of breast cancer include pleomorphic calcifications, spiculated masses, masses containing calcifications, round masses, or architectural distortion. Less common mammographic signs of cancer include a focal asymmetry, a developing asymmetry, breast edema, lymphadenopathy, a single dilated duct, or the cancer can be mammographically occult (nothing is seen; Table 2.1). The radiologist has to perceive the finding, recognize it as abnormal, and correctly interpret it as "actionable" (something to be acted upon; Box 2.5). Calcifications are discussed in detail in Chapter 3,

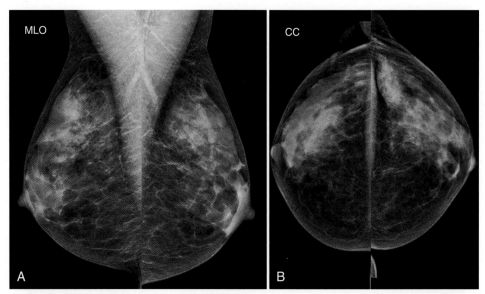

FIG. 2.7 The fifth edition of BI-RADS no longer indicates the ranges of percentage dense tissue of the four density categories. In this case, the breast density is classified as *heterogeneously dense* based on BI-RADS 2013 because the fibroglandular tissue could mask small cancers, even though far less than 50% of volume of the breast contains fibroglandular-density tissue. Mediolateral oblique (MLO) view (A) and craniocaudal (CC) view (B).

TABLE 2.1   Mammographic Findings of Breast Cancer

Finding	Differential Diagnosis
Pleomorphic calcifications	Cancer (most common), benign disease, fat necrosis
Spiculated mass	Cancer, postsurgical scar, radial scar, fat necrosis
Mass with calcifications	Cancer, fibroadenoma, papilloma; exclude calcifying oil cyst
Round mass	Cyst, fibroadenoma, cancer, papilloma, metastasis
Architectural distortion	Postsurgical scarring, cancer
A focal asymmetry	Normal asymmetric tissue (3%), cancer (suspicious: new, palpable, a mass containing suspicious calcifications or spiculation)
Developing asymmetry	Cancer, hormone effect, focal fibrosis
Breast edema	Unilateral: mastitis, postradiation therapy, inflammatory cancer Bilateral: systemic disease (liver disease, renal failure, and congestive heart failure)
Lymphadenopathy	Unilateral: mastitis, cancer Bilateral: systemic disease (collagen vascular disease, lymphoma, leukemia, infection, and adenocarcinoma of unknown primary)
Single dilated duct	Normal variant, papilloma, cancer
Nothing	10% of all cancers are false-negative on mammography

BOX 2.5   Steps in Radiologists Recognizing Cancer on Mammograms

Radiologist sees the finding
Radiologist recognizes the finding is different from normal tissue
Radiologist correctly interprets the finding as abnormal/possibly abnormal
Radiologist acts on the finding (recall/biopsy)

mammogram is negative, the decision for biopsy should be based on clinical grounds alone.

Next is described an approach to the mammogram using a consistent, reproducible viewing display, a systematic search pattern, a list of "danger zones" in which cancers are commonly missed, and detailed methods to find these cancers.

DISPLAY OF MAMMOGRAMS

Optimization of Reading Room and Image Display

If the mammograms are screen-film studies, the images are viewed on high-intensity viewboxes with the light parts of the films masked to block extraneous light. For full-field digital mammograms (FFDMs) and tomosynthesis images viewed on soft copy, the images are displayed on high-resolution bright monitors in a dark room with little to no ambient light, comparing old studies with new ones in the display protocol. Additionally, an ergonomic setup for the radiologist as described in our article on repetitive stress injury in breast radiologists will help the radiologist avoid injury (Thompson et al., 2014).

First Look at Two-Dimensional Views and Older Studies

The standard set of mammograms consists of paired MLO views and paired CC views. Normal breast tissue is usually symmetric, or "mirror image." To evaluate for mammographic symmetry, the MLO and CC views are displayed back to back, and asymmetries

breast masses in Chapter 4, and findings associated with clinical problems in Chapter 10.

Between 10% and 15% of breast cancers are mammographically occult, which means that breast cancer is present but the mammogram is normal. Dense fibroglandular background tissue can hide up to 30% to 50% of cancers. Accordingly, if there are suspicious clinical symptoms or physical findings and the are easily identified using the comparison of the right and left breasts (Fig. 2.8). Look at the whitest part of the mammograms for normal fibroglandular symmetry to see if there is more white tissue on one side than on the other (an asymmetry) or if there are any abnormal spots focally whiter than background (a focal asymmetry).

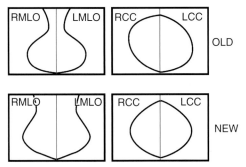

FIG. 2.8 Schematic of viewing normal mammograms to judge the symmetry and change over time. The mediolateral oblique (MLO) and craniocaudal (CC) mammograms are viewed with the right and left sides placed back to back. Older mammograms are placed above to check for change from year to year. *R*, right; *L*, left.

Asymmetries can be normal. For example, normal asymmetric glandular tissue is defined as a larger volume of normal fibroglandular tissue in one breast than the other, but with one breast not necessarily being larger than the other; this occurs in about 3% of women. A normal asymmetry should be stable over time.

To detect changes over time, good quality older mammograms are placed above the new ones. Because subtle changes may take longer than a year to become evident, one compares new mammograms with last year's mammogram, one more than 2 years old, and the oldest images of comparable quality.

Unexplained increases in breast density may indicate breast cancer. An unexplained generalized increase in breast density associated with skin thickening may represent breast edema, which has many etiologies, including inflammatory cancer. An unexplained *new* asymmetric focal density is called a "developing asymmetry" and should prompt investigation because developing asymmetries represent cancer in 15% of cases.

Comparing old studies with current studies makes it easier to see new or developing changes. A normal mammogram does not usually change from year to year after taking into account the normal involution of glandular tissue (Fig. 2.9). Contrastingly, malignant lesions increase in size and can change the mammographic appearance over time. However, the changes on mammography caused by tumors can be very subtle. Some tumors may infiltrate into the breast tissue without producing an apparent contrast against fat (Fig. 2.10). The doubling time of breast

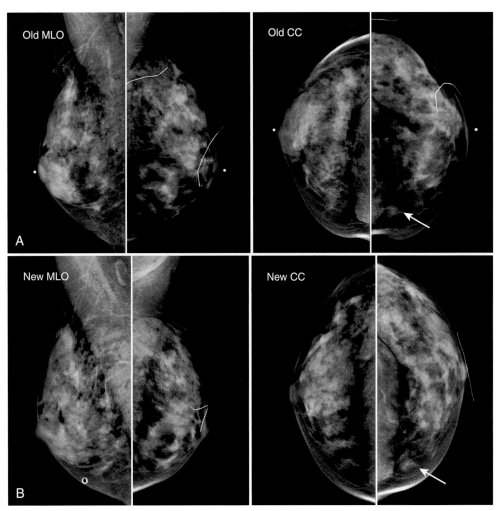

FIG. 2.9 Example of normal stable mammograms in viewing scheme. (A) Normal old mediolateral oblique (MLO) and craniocaudal (CC) views are placed back to back above the new views. (B) Normal new MLO and CC views, also placed back to back. Comparing the new and old studies shows no change in dense tissue and a stable benign nodule (*arrow* in A and B) in the medial left CC view over a 4-year period.

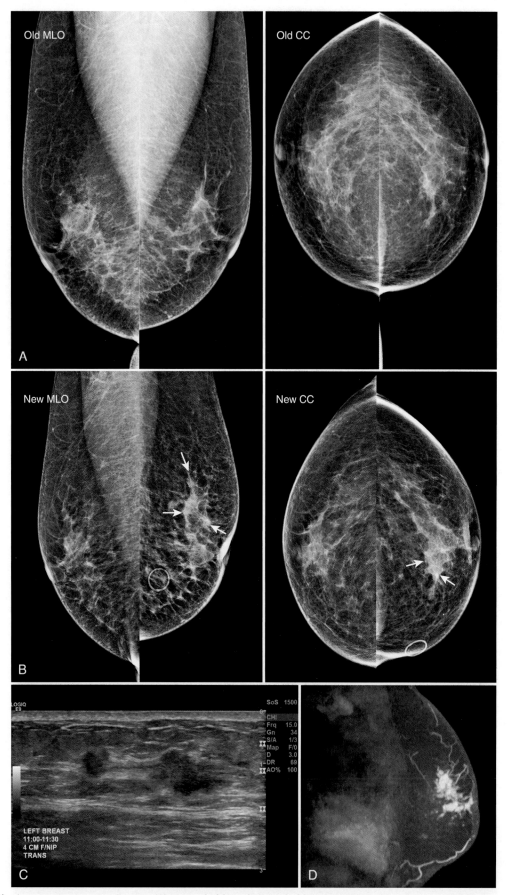

FIG. 2.10 Developing asymmetry over 3 years. (A) Normal old mediolateral oblique (MLO) and craniocaudal (CC) views are placed back to back above the new views. (B) New MLO and CC views, also placed back to back, showing developing asymmetry (*arrows*) in the medial upper left breast. Although the asymmetry looks subtle, comparison of the new study with the older study performed 3 years before (A) helps to identify this abnormality. (C) Ultrasonography shows two masses in the 11:00 to 11:30 position. (D) A sagittal plane of contrast enhanced magnetic resonance imaging shows masses and nonmass enhancement involving the nipple in the upper left breast. This patient was proven to have invasive ductal cancer.

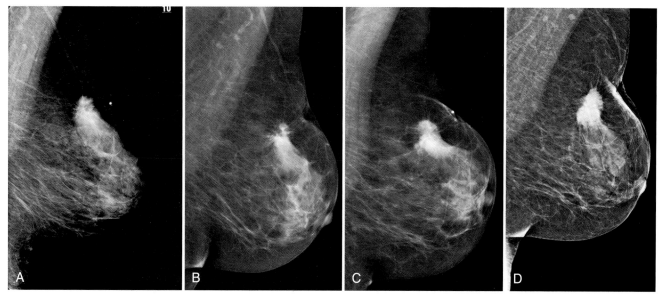

FIG. 2.11 Natural course of slow-growing breast cancer. Mediolateral oblique (MLO) views obtained 4 years prior (A), 2 years prior (B), and 1 year prior (C) to the current mammogram (D). This patient has an infiltrating carcinoma, but refused treatment. Annual follow-up mammograms show a spiculated mass with skin retraction in the left upper breast. This tumor has been growing over 4 years, but is rather stable. Even invasive cancer can have slow-growing nature over time like this case, although others may grow rapidly. Note the BB skin marker on the palpable mass in A and C.

cancer is typically approximately 50 to 200 days, but some can grow more slowly (Fig. 2.11).

Systematic Search on Each Mammographic Two-Dimensional View and Tomosynthesis

Once the radiologist judges the mammographic density and asymmetries, they search for masses, calcifications, and distortions on the mammograms. A common search pattern uses zigzags or strips of each image, like mowing a lawn with a lawnmower or searching for a lost boat at sea with a rescue helicopter. For two-dimensional (2D) digital mammography, the radiologist electronically magnifies the mammograms in quartiles, the upper half and the lower half of the 2D MLO views and the inner and outer 2D CC views (Fig. 2.12).

On tomosynthesis, the radiologist first reviews the 2D or synthesized 2D mammogram initially using the zigzag/strip method, then proceeds to magnify the 2D/synthesized 2D mammogram in quartiles because it is harder to see the overall breast in tomosynthesis slices or slabs alone. Then the radiologist scrolls through tomosynthesis slices or slabs. Some radiologists synchronize the tomosynthesis slabs or slices together, back to back, similar to the 2D display, to look for symmetry and auto scroll the tomosynthesis as a movie to get an overall view of the breast. For detailed tomosynthesis analysis, similar to reading a computed tomography (CT) scan or magnetic resonance imaging (MRI), it is important for the radiologist to keep his or her eyes in one place as the movie is scrolled/played to analyze a specific area. Otherwise, the eye is moving and the images are moving, and a finding could be missed. For example, the radiologist scrolls through all the tomosynthesis slices/slabs keeping his or her eye on the upper right breast MLO throughout the series, the lower right MLO, the upper left MLO, and then the lower left MLO. The radiologist then repeats the procedure for the CC studies. The method to review the tomosynthesis is described in Fig. 2.13. If the radiologist is reviewing the tomosynthesis on slabs, and there is a suspicious finding seen on a slab, then the findings are reviewed on the tomosynthesis slices.

LOCATION OF A FINDING

This section defines BI-RADS location terminologies, shows how to track findings on mammograms on different projections, how to predict ultrasound locations from the mammograms, how to know the three-dimensional (3D) position of a finding before surgical resection, and how to correlate palpable findings to the mammogram.

Location Description Based on BI-RADS 2013

Finding locations are described by laterality (right or left breast), quadrant and clock face, depth, and distance from the nipple. The breast quadrants describe the breast as the breast was divided into four areas with the nipple at the crosshairs of quadrants and as if the patient is facing the examiner (Fig. 2.14). The *upper outer quadrant* is the upper breast quadrant closest to the axilla, the *upper inner quadrant* is the upper breast near the sternum, the *lower inner quadrant* is the lower inner breast near the sternum, and the *lower outer quadrant* is the lower breast not near the sternum nor the axilla. The "clock face" description of a breast finding location imagines a clock superimposed on each breast as the woman faces the examiner (see Fig. 2.14). This means that the upper outer quadrant in the right breast is between the 9-o'clock and 12-o'clock positions, but the upper outer quadrant in the left breast is between the 12-o'clock and 3-o'clock positions. Although it is simple to see how clock-face lesion location can be easily mixed up (right upper outer quadrant versus left upper outer quadrant), the clock face allows the radiologist and surgeon to describe lesions that fall between quadrants, for example, a lesion located at the 12 o'clock or the 6 o'clock position of the breast. The breast depth includes the anterior, middle, and posterior third (Fig. 2.15) of the breast. Distance from the nipple for a specific lesion is measured as the distance between the root of the nipple and the anterior edge of the lesion on one of the projections that provide the best visualization of the lesion.

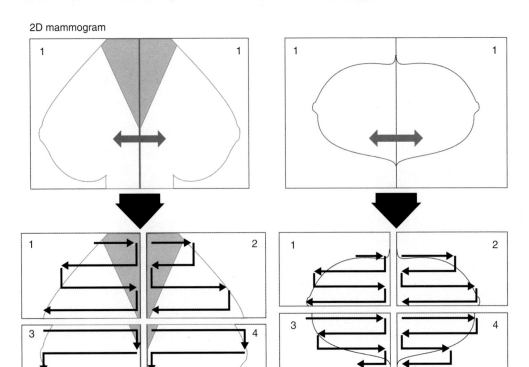

FIG. 2.12 Systemic search on digital mammography. First, display the paired mediolateral oblique (MLO) views and the paired craniocaudal (CC) views with the right and left breasts back to back and do the overall search by comparing the breasts. Look though the entire breast using the zigzag approach. Second, display the paired views of the upper half of the electronically magnified breasts. Focus on the right-side view and search for abnormalities very carefully using the zigzag approach to not miss subtle findings. Then do the zigzag search on the left-side view. Repeat the same process for the lower half of the magnified breasts.

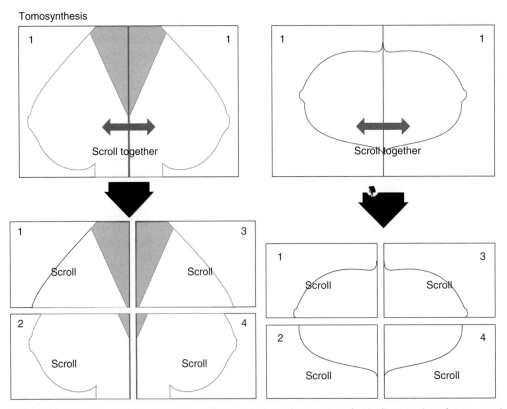

FIG. 2.13 Systemic search on tomosynthesis. Before evaluating the tomosynthesis slices, review the conventional two-dimensional (2D) mammograms or the tomosynthesis-synthesized 2D view using the method described in Fig. 2.12. Then display the paired mediolateral oblique and the craniocaudal projections of tomosynthesis images with the right and left breasts back to back. Scroll the linked right- and left-side images together, and look through the entire breast comparing both breasts. Next, display the upper half of the electronically magnified right breast, and scroll tomosynthesis images of this series, looking very carefully for abnormalities. Then display the tomosynthesis slices of the lower half of the magnified right breast and check for the abnormality. Repeat the same process for the left breast using the electronically magnified views.

Keys to Identify the Location of a Finding
Distance from the Nipple

Basically, the distance from the nipple to a breast lesion is consistent among many projections to within about a centimeter. When a radiologist finds a suspicious finding on one projection and wants to look for the corresponding finding on another projection, the radiologist measures the distance from the nipple to the finding and then searches the other view for the finding at this distance (Fig. 2.16). This process determines if finding is included on two projections and gives an estimate of where the finding might lie on the other view. This process also indicates if the finding might be excluded from the second projection if the finding is expected to project outside of the field of view.

Two-Dimensional Triangulation

Triangulation is an important process of localizing a finding on two orthogonal views on 2D mammograms, providing a clear 3D

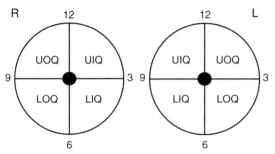

FIG. 2.14 Schematic for breast quadrant and clock face. Breast quadrants are divided by cross lines that have the center at the nipple. The clock face location of breast findings is described by imaging a clock on both the left and the right breast as the woman faces the examiner. Note that the outer portion of the breast on the right is at the 9 o'clock position and the outer portion on the left is at the 3 o'clock position. *UIQ,* upper inner quadrant; *LIQ,* lower inner quadrant; *UOQ,* upper outer quadrant; *LOQ,* lower outer quadrant.

position of a finding for subsequent imaging or biopsy. Triangulation predicts a lesion's position on a true mediolateral mammogram from the CC and MLO views. Triangulation is commonly used when a finding is seen on only two of the three (CC, MLO, or lateral) mammographic views.

To predict a finding's location from the CC and MLO screening views, place the CC, MLO, and lateral views so that the breasts face the same direction and the nipple is at the same level, but always with the MLO view in the middle of the CC and lateral views. Draw an imaginary line through the finding on the CC and MLO views. This line will predict the lesion's location on the lateral view (Fig. 2.17). In practice, if any two of the three (CC, MLO, and lateral) views are available, place the MLO between the CC and lateral views, with the nipple at the same level on each view, and an imaginary line will connect the target on the three views (Fig. 2.18). An imaginary line drawn through the lesion on any two of the three views will predict where the lesion will be on the third view.

Medial (inner) findings on the CC view will rise or project higher on the MLO projection and even higher on the MLO projection using triangulation. Lateral (outer) findings on the CC view will fall or project lower on the MLO view and even lower on the mediolateral projection. Remember the pneumonic LEAD FALLS for "**Lateral** breast lesions **Falling** from the CC projection to the MLO, to the lateral view, like lead falling when dropped." If you remember the pneumonic MUFFINS RISE for "**Medial** breast lesions **Rise** from the CC projection to the MLO to the lateral view, just like a muffin dough rises in the oven when baked," then you can remember which way lesions should move using triangulation. I did not make up this pneumonic, it has been around for a very long time, so I cannot give credit to whomever originally made it up, but they must have been a baker.

Tomosynthesis Triangulation Using Slice Locators

On tomosynthesis, the slice locator bar indicates the location of the slice within the breast volume and, similar to a CT or MRI scans, can be used to predict the actual location of a target within the breast volume. If a radiologist finds a suspicious lesion on a CC slice, the side bar of the CC tomosynthesis view series will indicate if the finding is near the upper or lower breast, just like the slice locators on CT or MRI show the location of findings

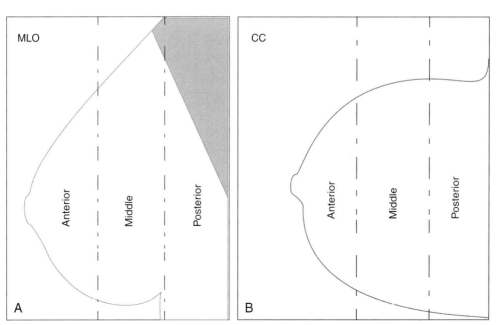

FIG. 2.15 Schematic for breast depth. (A) Schematic of mediolateral oblique (MLO) views. (B) Schematic of craniocaudal (CC) view. Breast depth is classified as the anterior, middle, and posterior third.

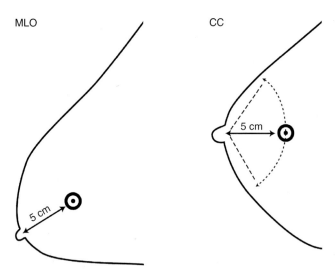

FIG. 2.16 Schematic for locating a lesion on two different mammographic projections. The radiologist measures the distance from the finding to the nipple (*left*) and then inspects the second view at the same distance from the nipple (*right*) for the finding.

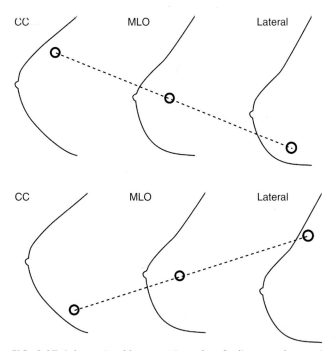

FIG. 2.17 Schematic of how to triangulate findings on the craniocaudal (CC), mediolateral oblique (MLO), and lateral views. Each view area is oriented with the nipples at the same level and the breasts pointing the same way. An imaginary line drawn through the lesions will predict its location on the third view. (Modified from Sickles EA: Practical solutions to common mammographic problems: tailoring the examination, *AJR Am J Roentgenol* 151:31–39, 1988.)

within the body. Similarly, the side bar of the MLO tomosynthesis views series will indicate if the finding is near the outer or inner breast. Although the obliquity of the breast and compression may not allow perfect triangulation of the lesion, radiologists should be able to estimate the lesion location, or they can do a mediolateral tomosynthesis series for further triangulation. If the suspicious finding is not identified in the expected quadrant, the finding may either be hidden and need ultrasound or may represent a summation artifact (Fig. 2.19).

Two-Dimensional Rolled Views

Sometimes only the CC view shows a suspicious finding not displayed on the lateral or MLO views. Rolled 2D CC views can show if true masses are located in the upper or lower breast. The technologist does a rolled CC view called a "rolled" CC lateral (RL) view (top-rolled laterally) by rolling the top of the breast toward the axilla and the bottom of the breast medially (Fig. 2.20). The radiologist compares the laterally rolled view with the standard CC view because a true mass will roll to the side with the breast tissue it is located within. An upper breast mass should roll laterally with the rolled upper breast tissue. A lower breast mass should roll medially with the lower breast tissue. The radiologist looks at the "regular" CC view and sees how the finding moves on the RL view. If the mass moves toward the axilla, the mass must be in the upper portion of the breast. If the mass moves medially on the RL view, the mass must be in the lower portion of the breast (Fig. 2.21).

SYSTEMATIC APPROACH TO MAMMOGRAPHY INTERPRETATION

Before Reading Mammogram

Many tools help the radiologist correctly interpret mammograms (Table 2.2). The first is the breast history and physical findings form, alerting the radiologist to the patient's risk factors, pretest probability of cancer, and any important lumps or patient complaints (see Fig. 2.1). The history sheet includes the patient's clinical history of breast biopsies and a schematic diagram of their location so that old scars are not misinterpreted as cancer.

A technologist or aide usually interviews the patient and marks the location of any palpable findings on a diagram on the history sheet. Positions of findings in the breast are described in breast quadrants and in the "clock face" (see Fig. 2.14).

The radiologist then reviews the breast history sheet and the technologist's marks (indicating masses, skin moles, biopsies, scars, or implants). The technologist may place special skin markers on moles or palpable masses before taking the mammogram to draw the radiologist's attention for a specific purpose, and should write down why the skin markers were placed to clarify the reason for their placement for the radiologist.

Systematic Approach to Interpretation of Mammogram

The radiologist then starts a targeted systematic review of each film (Table 2.3). The radiologist first evaluates the images for good positioning, contrast, and compression. Next, the radiologist looks at the dense breast tissue for symmetry between the left and right breasts, which should be symmetric. The radiologist then looks at the whitest, or densest, part of the mammogram to see whether there is a mass or distortion there.

The radiologist inspects all edges of the glandular tissue where it interfaces with fat. Abnormal findings along the glandular tissue edge include a "pulling in" or tethering of tissue (the *tent sign*) or masses that pop out along the glandular tissue edge. The radiologist looks at the skin/nipple/areolar complex for thickening or retraction, which may indicate a mass. Next, the radiologist inspects the retroareolar region, the axilla, retroglandular fat, breast tissue at the film edge, and the skin as normal. The radiologist then completes his or her search of the mammogram for calcifications by using a magnifying lens (on screen-film mammograms) or an electronic magnifier (digital mammograms) using the zigzag/strip method described earlier. The radiologist then compares the new films with older films of the same quality to evaluate for changes. The radiologist last uses computer-aided detection (CAD) to do a "second look" of findings marked on the mammograms by the CAD system.

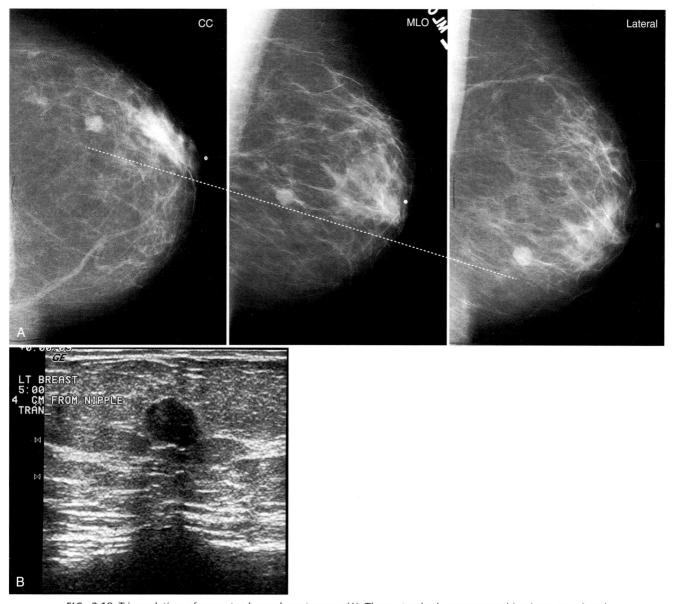

FIG. 2.18 Triangulation of an outer lower breast mass. (A) Three standard mammographic views are placed with the mediolateral oblique (MLO) view at the middle. An imaginary line (*dashed line*) connecting an outer lower mass can be drawn in a linear fashion. When drawn though the craniocaudal (CC; *left*) and MLO views, the imaginary line (*dashed line*) points at an even lower position of the breast on the lateral view (*right*). Note that even though the mass is at nipple level on the MLO view, its actual location on the lateral view is at the 5 o'clock position and not the 3 o'clock position. Triangulation is helpful for predicting the lateral position from CC and MLO. (B) Ultrasound shows a round microlobulated mass at the 5 o'clock position of the left breast that was diagnosed as invasive ductal cancer.

The following section details the individual components of the systematic approach to the mammogram (see Table 2.3).

Step 1. Overall Search: Quality of Images and Balance of Breast Tissue Density

The first step is the overall search of the whole set of mammograms, including bilateral MLO views, bilateral CC views, and additional views if available. Initially, the radiologist looks at the mammographic technique for good quality and then evaluates the balance of the breast tissue density between the breasts and within a breast, ie, the symmetry of breast density and the white parts, respectively.

Checking symmetry between the breasts is essential to detect an abnormal finding on mammography. The normal breast tissue is usually symmetric between the breasts, and an abnormal lesion can produce an asymmetry. However, the normal breast tissue sometimes is asymmetric, meaning that there is more normal glandular tissue in one breast than the other; this is a normal variant, like having one foot bigger than the other. Normal asymmetry consists of a normal asymmetric volume of breast tissue with more in one side than the other. On the CC and MLO views, the glandular asymmetry should "spread out" and not look like a mass (Fig. 2.22). Normal asymmetry can also be caused by removal of fibroglandular tissue from one breast by biopsy, making the other breast look like it has more tissue.

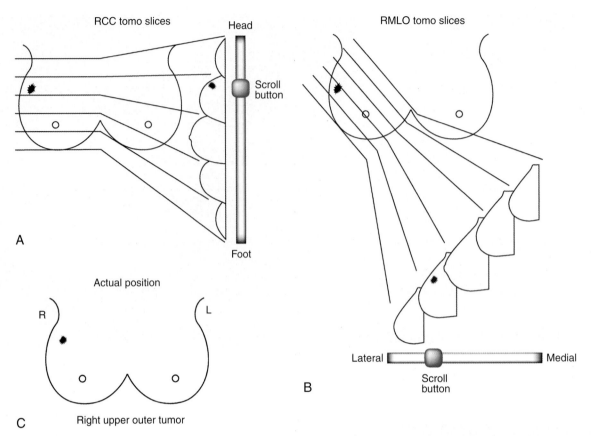

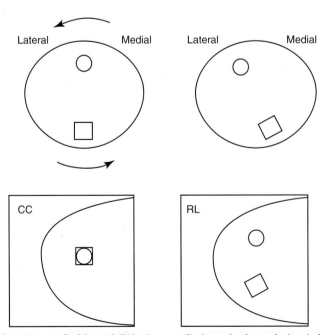

FIG. 2.19 Schematic of use of scroll button to identify the location for breast tumors on tomosynthesis. The example is in the upper outer quadrant. (A) Right craniocaudal (RCC) tomosynthesis slice shows a mass in the outer breast; the slice with the mass is second from the top or in the upper part of the breast. Thus the mass must be in the upper outer quadrant. (B) Right mediolateral oblique (RMLO) slice shows a mass in the upper breast; the slice with the mass is second from the lateral or outer part of the breast. Thus the mass must be in the upper outer quadrant. (C) Actual location of the mass in the upper outer right breast.

FIG. 2.20 Schematic showing a rolled lateral (RL) view predicting whether a lesion is located in the upper or lower part of the right breast. The initial craniocaudal (CC) view superimposes two lesions on each other (*left*). When the top of the breast is rolled laterally (*right*), the superior lesion rolls laterally with the top of the breast tissue. The inferior lesion moves medially with the lower part of the breast tissue. Comparing whether the lesion moves laterally on the rolled CC lateral (RL) view with respect to the standard CC view will help predict whether the lesion is in the upper or lower part of the breast. (Modified from Sickles EA: Practical solutions to common mammographic problems: tailoring the examination, *AJR Am J Roentgenol* 151:31–39, 1988.)

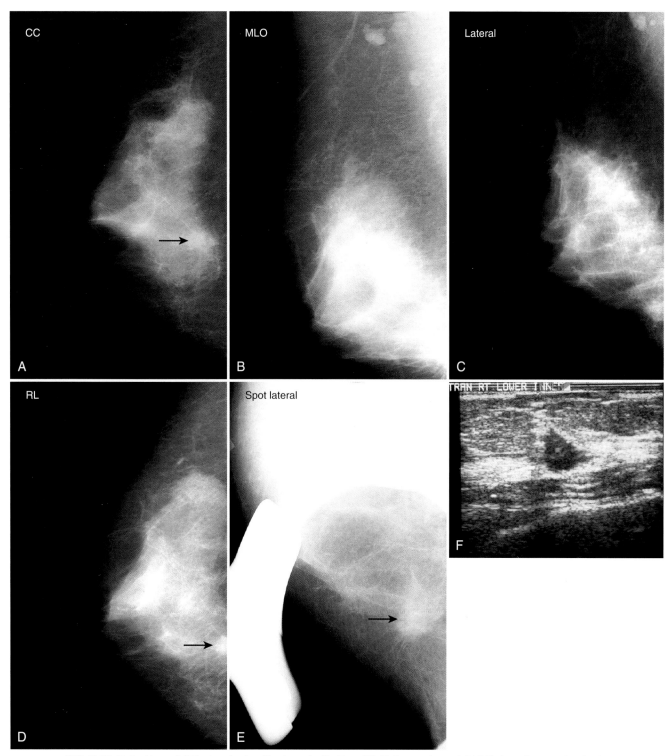

FIG. 2.21 Rolled lateral (RL) view for localization of a finding. (A) Right craniocaudal (CC) view shows a density in the posterior medial aspect of the breast (*arrow*). (B) On the mediolateral oblique (MLO) view the mass was not seen at the time of interpretation. In retrospect, spiculation is seen extending into the lower part of the breast from outside the field of view at the edge of the film. (C) The lateral view does not show a definite mass at the time of interpretation. (D) A CC view with the top of the breast rolled laterally, ie, the rolled CC lateral (RL) view shows that the mass (*arrow*) is medial in comparison with that seen on the original CC view, indicating that it rolled medially with the lower part of the breast. (E) Spot compression in the lower portion of the breast reveals a spiculated mass (*arrow*). (F) Ultrasound directed to the lower portion of the breast shows a hypoechoic irregular mass that was diagnosed as invasive ductal cancer.

Normal asymmetries should have no suspicious calcifications, spiculations, or palpable masses, are stable when compared with older studies, and are composed of fibroglandular tissue. An asymmetry may be abnormal or indicate cancer if it is palpable, has suspicious calcifications or spiculations, is new, or is a mass and not an asymmetry at all; if the patient has any of these findings with an asymmetry they should undergo a workup with ultrasound or biopsy.

The white parts of mammograms can hide masses. Radiologists can see masses if they are whiter than the surrounding tissue or if there is a round or spiculated mass edge projected against dark fat. If the radiologist sees a mass on one projection, the radiologist looks for the mass on the orthogonal view. To do this, the radiologist measures the distance from the nipple to the mass and searches the orthogonal view for the mass at this distance

(see Fig. 2.16). If the finding is seen on two views, it is considered a *mass* or *focal asymmetry*. If the "mass" is seen on only one view, it is called an *asymmetry* or a *density* and represents either a summation artifact (Fig. 2.23) or a mass that is obscured on the second view (Fig. 2.24). The decision to recall this type of finding and prompt a workup is based on the radiologist's experience and the degree of suspicion of the one-view finding.

Step 2. Targeted Search: Anatomical Structures

If there was no mass on the initial study and the overall mammogram was normal on the initial impression, the radiologist would look closer at each mammogram individually. Specifically, the next step is to focus in on one view of one of the breasts breast and perform the zigzag systemic search over the breast as described earlier (see Fig. 2.14). During this process, the radiologist pays attention to the morphology of anatomical structures, the presence of abnormal density, and the presence of calcifications. The first targets are the anatomical structures to be checked, which include the edge of the glandular tissue, the nipple and areolar complex, the retroareolar region, the skin, and the axilla.

The normal glandular tissue edges interface with fat. A layer of fat typically surrounds the cone of normal fibroglandular tissue and should contain no masses. As part of the systematic review, the radiologist checks the fat all around the glandular tissue to make sure that no masses are present. These edges should be gently curving, scalloped, and without tethering. Masses at the glandular edge or in breast tissue can "pull in" the fat, producing a tent sign caused by productive fibrosis from cancer retracting Cooper's ligaments and breast ducts. In other cases, tumor spiculation produces straight lines extending into the glandular tissue that draw attention to a mass at the center of the radius of spicules (Fig. 2.25). Subtle equal-density cancers can be difficult to detect, but looking for secondary signs of straightened lines in glandular tissue or tethering of the glandular tissue edge guides the radiologist to the cancer.

TABLE 2.2   Tools Used for Interpretation of Mammograms

Tool	Use
Breast history, risk factors	Evaluate patient's complaint and risks
Technologist's marks	Show skin lesions, scars, problem areas
Putting images back to back	Detection of asymmetry Look for whitest part of study
Bright light (SFM)	View skin, dark parts of film
Window/level (FFDM)	Contrast for masses, calcifications
Magnifying lens or magnifier	Visualize mass borders, calcifications
Old films	Compare for changes
CAD (if available)	Look for CAD marks *after* initial interpretation

CAD, computer-aided detection; *FFDM*, full-field digital mammogram; *SFM*, screen-film mammogram.

TABLE 2.3   Systematic Approach to Interpretation of Mammograms

Search Pattern/Objects	Normal Findings
OVERALL SEARCH	
Evaluation of technique	Good technique
Fibroglandular symmetry	Breast tissue usually symmetric Asymmetric tissue in 3%; be alert for new, palpable, three-dimensional masses or suspicious calcifications/distortions
White areas in glandular tissue	No mass or distortion; white areas look like normal tissue on the orthogonal views
TARGETED SEARCH	
Edge of glandular tissue	No pulling in or tent sign, no concave masses
Nipple/areolar complex	Nipple everted, no skin thickening
Retroareolar region	Normal ducts, vessels, nipple in profile on at least one view
Skin	2–3 mm in thickness, no edema
Axilla	Normal lymph nodes, normal variant axillary breast tissue
Medial breast	Mostly fat, normal variant medial sternalis muscle
Retroglandular fat	All fat, no masses between glandular tissue and chest wall
Film edge	No mass or spiculation from findings lying outside the field of view
Use magnifying lens or magnifier	No pleomorphic calcifications, subtle distortion, or masses
Use bright light (SFM) or adjust window/level (FFDM)	Evaluate dark areas as needed
FURTHER EVALUATION	
Tomosynthesis	Do a detailed evaluation using thin image sections
Compare with old films	No change; be alert for a developing asymmetry, new or changing calcifications or masses
CAD	Do a second look of the marked areas; CAD comes last because it does not pick up all cancers

CAD, computer-aided detection; *FFDM*, full-field digital mammogram; *SFM*, screen-film mammogram.

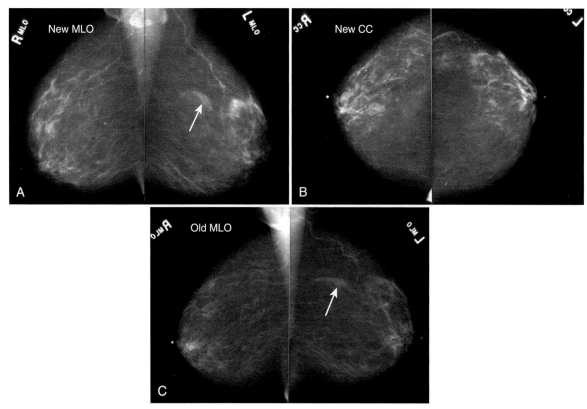

FIG. 2.22 Normal asymmetry. (A and B) Mediolateral (MLO) view (A) shows an asymmetry in the upper left breast, which is not as apparent on the craniocaudal (CC) view (B), representing normal overlapping tissue. (C) An older MLO mammogram shows that the asymmetry is stable.

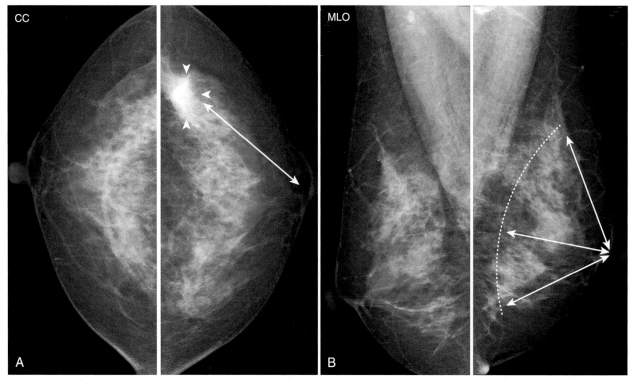

FIG. 2.23 Asymmetry on one view caused by a summation artifact. (A) On the craniocaudal (CC) view an asymmetric density (*arrowheads*) is seen in the outer left breast. (B) Review of the mediolateral oblique (MLO) view shows no mass of the same shape or density at the same distance from the nipple (*double arrows*), suggesting a confluence of shadows. In addition, the asymmetry has no spiculations or calcifications, was not associated with a palpable finding, and did not appear to be a mass. Workup showed that the density represented a summation artifact.

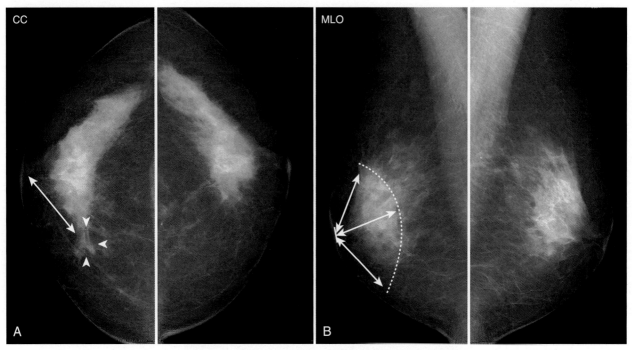

FIG. 2.24 Asymmetry on one view caused by cancer. (A) More breast tissue is seen in the medial aspect of the right breast on the craniocaudal (CC) view (*arrowheads*) than in the medial aspect of the left breast. Closer examination shows the density to have a slightly round shape and possible spiculations, unlike the asymmetric density seen in Fig. 2.9. (B) The abnormal density is not identified at the same distance from the nipple as in A (*double arrows*) on the mediolateral oblique (MLO) view. Follow-up examination confirmed the density to be a true mass and invasive ductal cancer.

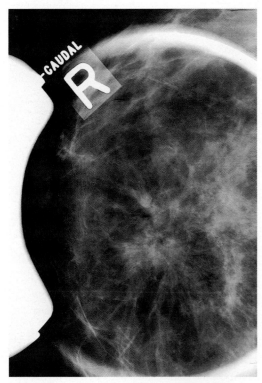

FIG. 2.25 Use of the surrounding architecture to detect masses. A craniocaudal spot magnification view shows an equal-density spiculated mass (radial scar at biopsy) producing subtle distortion of the tissue with straightening of Cooper's ligaments.

The radiologist sees if the nipple is everted and reviews the complex structures of ducts and vessels in the retroareolar region. The nipple should be seen in profile on at least one mammographic view. If the nipple is not in profile on at least one view, it may overlie the retroareolar region and obscure a mass, or it might be retracted by cancer. If the nipple is not seen in profile on any view, the mammogram should be repeated with the nipple in profile. If the nipple is truly inverted on the mammogram, the radiologist should check the breast history form to see if it was inverted at birth (normal variant) or if the nipple inversion is new. New nipple inversion is of concern for a retroareolar cancer and prompts a workup.

Normal breast skin is approximately 2-mm to 3-mm thick on the mammogram, and normal subcutaneous fat is dark. The skin should be smooth all around the breast and not pulled in (Fig. 2.26). Skin thickening greater than 2 mm to 3 mm that is asymmetric to the contralateral side is abnormal and is especially worrisome if the subcutaneous tissue has become gray and the thin tethering lymphatics and ligaments become thick and trabeculated. This is worrisome for breast edema. Generally, skin thickening from cancer should be investigated.

The axilla normally contains lymph nodes, which are smooth oval-shaped or kidney bean–shaped masses containing fatty hila on the mammogram (Fig. 2.27A). Lymph nodes that grow larger become dense, round, and lose their fatty hila; they represent lymphadenopathy and are abnormal (Fig. 2.27B).

Axillary breast tissue is a normal variant and consists of breast tissue in the axilla (Fig. 2.28). It develops along the normal nipple line that extends (in animals) from the axilla along the chest to the abdomen. Axillary breast tissue can be, but is rarely, attached to an extra nipple. Spiculated masses in the axilla can mimic normal lymph nodes or axillary breast tissue. Any masses in the axilla should be scrutinized carefully to make sure they are normal lymph nodes or axillary tissue and not cancer (Fig. 2.29).

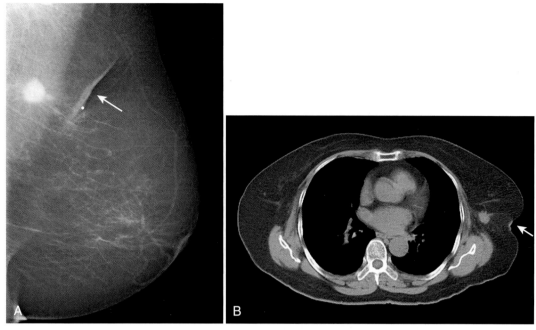

FIG. 2.26 Skin retraction and skin thickening. (A) An axillary spiculated mass, proven to be invasive ductal cancer, is accompanied with a secondary sign of indrawing of the skin (*arrow*), marked by a metallic BB skin marker. The dark air is seen adjacent to the skinfold. (B) An axial plane of computed tomography shows the skin thickening (*arrow*) at the site of skin retraction caused by the spiculated mass.

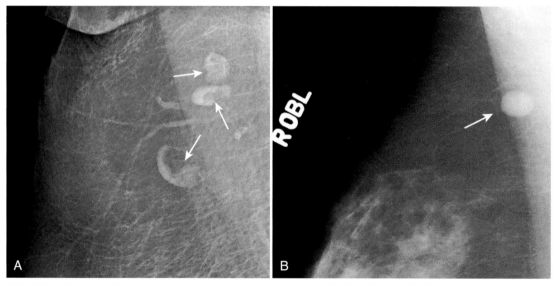

FIG. 2.27 Normal axillary and abnormal lymph nodes. (A) A magnified mediolateral oblique view shows multiple normal lymph nodes that have kidney bean shapes with the fatty hilum well visualized (*arrows*) suggesting they are "normal." The large fatty hilum with thin cortex causes the lymph node to have a C shape. (B) Abnormal axillary lymph node without a fatty hilum (*arrow*), characteristic of lymphadenopathy, and representing lymphoma. If the axilla had not been reviewed, this finding would have been missed.

Step 3. Targeted Search: Abnormal Density in Danger Zones

The second target is abnormal densities in so-called danger zones. These include a few locations in the breast in which any density can be abnormal and deserves both special mention and a second look. The danger zones include the medial breast, the retroglandular fat, and the film edge.

The medial portion of the breast usually becomes fattier over time (Fig. 2.30). Masses or densities in the medial part of the breast should be scrutinized carefully because usually only fat is present here. The only exception is the normal sternalis muscle seen on the CC view near the chest wall (see Fig. 2.5). A second danger zone is the retroglandular fat, or fat between the cone of normal fibroglandular tissue and the chest wall (Fig. 2.31). The area between the glandular tissue and pectoralis muscle should include only fat, with the only exception again being the sternalis muscle. This retroglandular fat is the no man's land mentioned earlier. Any masses here are abnormal and should be worked up. The third danger zone is the film edge at the chest wall (Fig. 2.32;

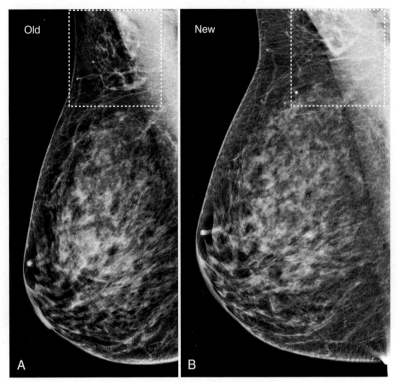

FIG. 2.28 Normal axillary breast tissue. (A) A right screening mediolateral oblique (MLO) view shows glandular tissue (*box*) high in the axilla over the pectoralis muscle, representing normal axillary breast tissue. (B) The axillary breast tissue (*box*) is unchanged on the 1-year follow-up screening study.

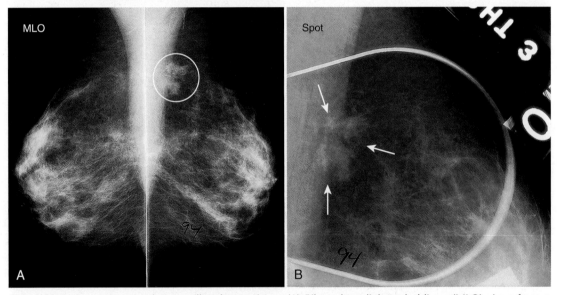

FIG. 2.29 Breast cancer simulating axillary breast tissue. (A) Bilateral mediolateral oblique (MLO) views from a screening study show dense tissue in the axilla (*circle*). (B) Spot view shows that the density (*arrows*) retains its shape, does not separate into fibroglandular components, and represents a mass—specifically, invasive ductal cancer.

Video 2.1). Here, the hint of a mass edge or spiculations may barely stick out into the field of view and suggest that a tumor is not fully imaged on the mammogram. In these cases, only special mammographic views will display the mass.

Step 4. Targeted Search: Calcifications

The last and the most challenging targets are calcifications. Because calcifications can be too small to be identified on the standard views, the radiologist needs a magnifying lens (for screen-film studies) or an electronic magnifier (for FFDMs and tomosynthesis; see Figs. 3.9 and 3.10). Radiologists should look at screen-film mammograms with the magnifying lens until they see dust, which ensures that they have looked hard enough to find the calcifications that form in breast cancer. For screen-film mammography, the radiologist uses a hot light to illuminate dark portions of the mammogram as needed. For FFDMs and tomosynthesis images, the images are viewed at optimal windowing and

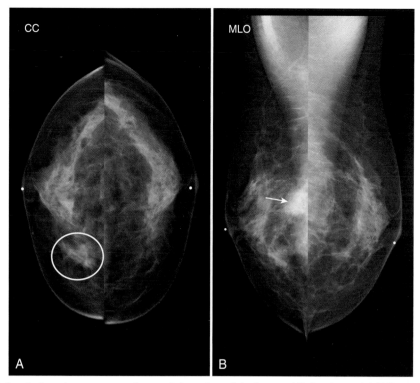

FIG. 2.30 A density in a danger zone—the medial portion of the breast. (A) Craniocaudal (CC) views show a focal asymmetry (*circle*) in the medial portion of right breast, suggestive of breast cancer. (B) Mediolateral oblique (MLO) views show a focal density (*arrow*) in the upper left breast that is more dense than the surrounding breast tissue. This was proven to be an invasive ductal cancer with ductal carcinoma in situ. Please note BB skin markers at the nipples.

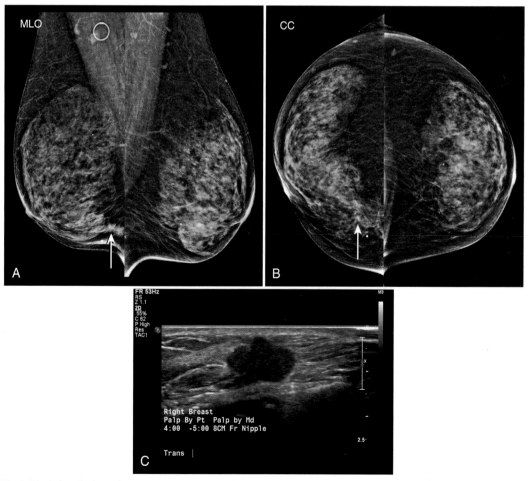

FIG. 2.31 A density in a danger zone—retroglandular fat. (A and B) Mediolateral oblique (MLO; A) and craniocaudal (CC; B) views show a focal asymmetry (*arrows*) in the retroglandular fat at the medial lower right breast. Note BB was placed on the palpable mass. (C) An irregular mass is clearly depicted on ultrasonography. This was proven to be invasive ductal cancer.

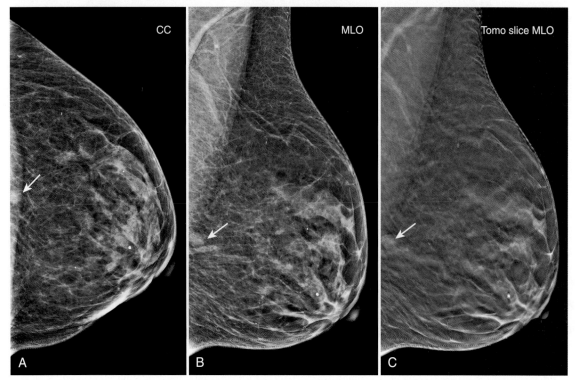

FIG. 2.32 A density in a danger zone—the film edge at the chest wall. (A) Left craniocaudal (CC) view shows a small mass (*arrow*) overlapped by the chest wall at the film edge. (B) Left mediolateral oblique (MLO) view shows the mass (*arrow*) deep in the middle breast. (C) A tomosynthesis slice of MLO projection shows the mass (*arrow*) apart from the normal fibroglandular tissue (see Video 2.1). This was proven to be invasive ductal cancer.

leveling to see calcifications, and the radiologist views all portions of the images under electronic magnification that shows skin pores to make sure the films are displayed at a high enough magnification to display tiny calcifications in cancer. To make sure no areas are missed for calcifications, the systemic zigzag search over the breast is important.

Step 5. Tomosynthesis

Tomosynthesis provides reconstructed image sections as thin as 1 mm. It can help provide greater detail about the internal structure of the breast tissue and overcomes mammography's limitation caused by the overlaying tissue that confounds the clear depiction of lesion margin and shape analysis. To detect and analyze abnormal findings using tomosynthesis, the radiologist starts by reviewing the tomosynthesis-synthesized 2D mammograms or conventional 2D mammograms. The radiologist then scrolls the tomosynthesis images of the entire breast, the upper half and the lower half of the magnified breast, using the process described earlier (see Fig. 2.13).

Step 6. Compare Current and Older Films

The radiologist then compares the current mammogram with older films of the same quality to check for developing densities and to look for new or progressive changes.

Step 7. Use Computer-Aided Detection

If CAD devices are used, it is done so only after the initial review of the mammogram. Computer-provided marks should function as a second look, because CAD misses some breast cancers that are only detected by the radiologist. In a prospective study of CAD on more than 9000 mammograms in an academic center, CAD and the radiologist found 13 of 19

cancers, CAD found 2 cancers undetected by the radiologist, but the radiologist found 4 cancers not marked by CAD. Because CAD does not find all the cancers, it should not be used alone to read mammograms. The radiologist should read the mammogram and then use CAD as a second look. If the radiologist sees a suspicious finding that he or she truly thinks needs to be recalled, that finding should be worked up no matter what CAD says because CAD misses some cancers that the radiologist sees.

REPORTING OF MAMMOGRAPHIC FINDINGS BASED ON BI-RADS 2013

The BI-RADS (5th edition, published in 2013) developed by the ACR provides standardized breast imaging terminology in a "breast imaging lexicon." This lexicon provides a standard report organization, assessment structure, and a classification system for mammography, ultrasound, and MRI. The BI-RADS enables radiologists to provide a succinct review of breast imaging findings to communicate the results to the referring physician in a clear and consistent fashion with a final assessment and a specific course of action. In the mammography report, radiologists describe mammographic findings using BI-RADS terminology and write their final impression, which should be coded based on BI-RADS categories.

The BI-RADS 2013 terminology for mammography is shown in Table 2.4. Further details of this BI-RADS mammography terminology are discussed in Chapters 3 and 4, as well as later in this chapter.

The radiologists' final impressions of the study are sorted into categories numbered BI-RADS category 0 through 6 (Table 2.5). The first BI-RADS category, category 0, is used for screening recalls or when more studies are needed at the end of a case to make a final assessment. Categories 1 and 2 are used for normal mammograms or for findings requiring no action.

Category 3 is used for findings thought to have a 2% or less chance of malignancy and for which a short-term, 6-month follow-up mammogram and yearly follow-up for 2 to 3 years may be implemented, with the expectation that the finding will be stable. Specifically, this category is often used for a solitary group of round or punctate benign-appearing calcifications, a noncalcified circumscribed solitary solid mass, or an asymmetry without other associated mammographic abnormality. Category 4 encompasses a wide variety of findings for which biopsy is recommended. It can be further subcategorized into 4A, 4B, and 4C for lesions that require biopsy but with a low, intermediate, or moderate suspicion for cancer, respectively. Category 5 is reserved for mammographic findings highly suggestive of cancer, with a 95% or greater likelihood of cancer. Category 6 is intended for cancers for which a known diagnosis has been established before definite therapy such as surgery or chemotherapy. For example, women with large breast cancers diagnosed by percutaneous core biopsy who will be undergoing subsequent neoadjuvant chemotherapy would be designated as category 6.

By United Stated federal law (Mammography Quality Standards Act [MQSA]; P.L. 102-539), all mammograms must have a summary BI-RADS code. Both the BI-RADS number and the words must be spelled out in the report. Yearly, federal inspectors read mammographic reports at all U.S. facilities and check them for BI-RADS summary codes and words. It is against U.S. federal law to exclude the BI-RADS codes and words on mammogram repeats. Both monetary fines and jail sentences can be imposed on facilities that do not comply with MQSA.

DIAGNOSTIC MAMMOGRAPHY

Diagnostic versus Screening Mammography

There is a crucial difference between *diagnostic* and *screening* mammography. Diagnostic mammography is used for symptomatic women or for women with findings detected on screening mammography (Table 2.6). A radiologist is on-site for diagnostic mammograms to personally guide the workup by using special mammographic views or ultrasound.

Screening mammography is performed without a radiologist on-site and is meant for asymptomatic women. The usual scenario for a screening mammogram is that an asymptomatic woman has her mammogram and goes home, and a radiologist reads the mammogram later. In the United States, mammographic screening includes two views of each breast: CC and MLO projections of the left and right breasts.

Women with lumps or symptoms need diagnostic mammograms, not screening mammograms. From 10% to 15% of all cancers are not seen at screening mammography; this usually happens in women with palpable breast lumps that are cancer. Screening studies can result in false-negative findings even when

TABLE 2.4 American College of Radiology BI-RADS Mammography Lexicon Terms and Classification Scheme

BREAST COMPOSITION
The breast is almost entirely fatty
There are scattered areas of fibroglandular density
The breast is heterogeneously dense, which may obscure small masses
The breast is extremely dense, which lowers the sensitivity of mammography

MASSES
Shape
  Oval
  Round
  Irregular
Margin
  Circumscribed
  Obscured
  Microlobulated
  Indistinct
  Spiculated
Density
  High density
  Equal density
  Low density
  Fat containing

CALCIFICATIONS
Typically benign
  Skin
  Vascular
  Coarse or "popcorn like"
  Large rod like
  Round
  Rim
  Dystrophic
  Milk of calcium
  Suture

Suspicious morphology
  Amorphous
  Coarse heterogeneous
  Fine pleomorphic
  Fine linear or fine-linear branching
Distribution
  Diffuse
  Regional
  Grouped
  Linear
  Segmental

ARCHITECTURAL DISTORTION
ASYMMETRIES
  Asymmetry
  Global asymmetry
  Focal asymmetry
  Developing asymmetry

INTRAMAMMARY LYMPH NODE
SKIN LESION
SOLITARY DILATED DUCT
ASSOCIATED FEATURES
  Skin retraction
  Nipple retraction
  Skin thickening
  Trabecular thickening
  Axillary adenopathy
  Architectural distortion
  Calcifications

LOCATION OF LESION
  Laterality
  Quadrant and clock face
  Depth
  Distance from the nipple

From ACR BI-RADS Mammography, In *ACR BI-RADS atlas, breast imaging reporting and data system,* Reston, VA, 2013, American College of Radiology.

TABLE 2.5 ACR BI-RADS Code Assessment Categories

BI-RADS Category	Definition	Likelihood of Malignancy	Management Recommendation
0	Incomplete	N/A	Recall for additional imaging and/or comparison with prior examination(s)
1	Negative	0%	Routine mammography screening
2	Benign	0%	Routine mammography screening
3	Probably benign[a]	>0% but ≤2%	Short-interval (6-month) follow-up or continued surveillance mammography
4A	Low suspicion for malignancy	>2% to ≤10%	Tissue diagnosis
4B	Moderate suspicion for malignancy	>10% to ≤50%	Tissue diagnosis
4C	High suspicious for malignancy	>50% to <95%	Tissue diagnosis
5	Highly suggestive of malignancy	≥95%	Tissue diagnosis
6	Known biopsy-proven malignancy	N/A	Surgical excision when clinically appropriate

[a]Noncalcified circumscribed solid mass, focal asymmetry, and solitary group of punctate calcifications are placed in category 3.
From ACR BI-RADS Mammography, In *ACR BI-RADS atlas, breast imaging reporting and data system*, Reston, VA, 2013, American College of Radiology.

the woman has felt her own lump. The false-negative screening mammogram may delay diagnosis. Some cancers that are felt as a lump may need tangential views, spot views, or ultrasound to reveal their presence. These supplemental studies are only done with a diagnostic mammogram, in which the radiologist recognizes the danger of the palpable mass and gets the other views or an ultrasound. Therefore women with lumps or symptoms need to undergo a diagnostic rather than a screening mammogram because the on-site radiologist can recognize the woman's problem and target a dedicated workup to that problem to find the cancer.

Additional Two-Dimensional Mammographic Views and Tomosynthesis

In 2D diagnostic mammography, radiologists use additional mammographic views in three common scenarios: to differentiate between a real lesion and a summation artifact, to visualize findings in "hard to see" locations, and to characterize a true lesion (Box 2.6). Tomosynthesis is also helpful in these scenarios. A large study from England (a comparison of TOMosynthesis with digital MammographY or the TOMMY Trial) demonstrated a tendency for higher specificity for 2D plus tomosynthesis compared with 2D alone for distortion/asymmetry because tomosynthesis showed either overlapping tissue or an underlying mass. In another study by Nam et al. (2015), lesions on tomosynthesis were seen as a more specific and localized pattern (eg, mass or focal asymmetry rather than asymmetry) than those on 2D mammogram; cancers were more often classified as *constantly visible* on tomosynthesis than on 2D mammography, and asymmetries were more often classified as *focal asymmetry* on tomosynthesis. Decreased recalls from screening in our own practice were often caused by tomosynthesis showing overlapping tissue that could be dismissed as benign versus true distortion/mass that might be cancer.

To Differentiate between a Real Lesion and a Summation Artifact

A common reason to use additional views is in the setting of a "one-view-only" finding. Specifically, the radiologist sees a finding on one view that is not confirmed on the orthogonal view. Additional special mammographic views determine whether the finding is real. The first step is to estimate the finding's location on the orthogonal view by measuring the distance from the nipple to the finding. The breast tissue is scrutinized along a radius of the same distance on the orthogonal view to identify the finding (see Figs. 2.16, 2.23, and 2.24). If the finding shows up on the

second view, it is considered a true finding and the radiologist then uses additional views to characterize the lesion. If the finding is invisible on the second view, it may represent a true finding hidden on the second view or a fortuitous summation of normal breast tissue. In either case, an ultrasound at the distance from the nipple may reveal the lesion subsequently.

Other supplemental mammographic views can be used to determine whether a one-view finding is a true lesion or a summation artifact (Box 2.7; Tables 2.7 and 2.8).

BOX 2.7 Views Used to Confirm or Exclude a Lesion (Commonly a One-View-Only Finding)

Lateral view
Spot compression
Spot compression magnification
Rolled views (with or without spot compression or magnification)
Repeat the same view
Step oblique views
Ultrasound
Tomosynthesis

TABLE 2.7 Mammographic Views and Techniques Used to Visualize and Characterize Findings

Mammographic Problem	Mammographic View
True finding versus summation	Rolled views, spot view, step oblique views; repeat the same view; tomosynthesis
Triangulation	Line up CC, MLO, and ML views and draw an imaginary line through the lesion. Use rolled views to determine whether the mass is upper or lower tomosynthesis
Outer breast finding	XCCL, Cleopatra
Inner breast finding	XCCM, CV, spot view
Upper breast finding	Compression from below (or CC view), upper-breast-only view
Retroareolar finding	Spot compression with the nipple in profile
Lower inner finding	Superior–inferior oblique
Palpable finding	Spot compression over the mass or a tangential view; tomosynthesis
Characterization of a mass	Magnification, spot magnification, or calcification views; tomosynthesis

CC, craniocaudal; *CV*, cleavage view; *ML*, mediolateral; *MLO*, mediolateral oblique; *XCCL*, laterally exaggerated craniocaudal; *XCCM*, medially exaggerated craniocaudal.

TABLE 2.6 Screening versus Diagnostic Studies

Screening	Asymptomatic women CC and MLO mammograms Films taken and patient released Films batch interpreted after patient is gone
Diagnostic	Symptomatic women or mammographic finding CC and MLO mammograms Additional mammograms tailored to the problem With or without breast ultrasound Radiologist on-site to guide workup with patient present

CC, craniocaudal; *MLO*, mediolateral oblique.

BOX 2.6 Use of Additional Mammographic Views

To differentiate between a real lesion and a summation artifact
To visualize findings in hard to see locations
To characterize a true lesion

TABLE 2.8 Mammographic Views and Abbreviations

View	Abbreviation
Craniocaudal	CC
Mediolateral oblique	MLO
Mediolateral	ML
Lateromedial	LM
Laterally exaggerated craniocaudal	XCCL
Medially exaggerated craniocaudal	XCCM
Cleavage view	CV
Rolled lateral view	RL
Rolled medial view	RM
From-below	FB

By convention, the side (left or right) precedes the view abbreviation.
From *Mammography quality control manual*, Reston, VA, 1999, American College of Radiology.

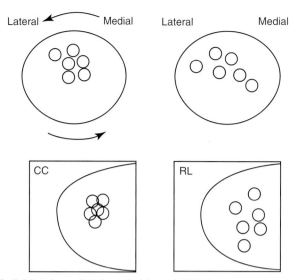

FIG. 2.33 Schematic of a rolled lateral (RL) view separating summation artifacts into their fibroglandular components. The initial craniocaudal (CC) view of the right breast on the lower left shows a "mass" composed of overlapping glandular tissue. The rolled CC lateral (RL) view on the lower right shows the fibroglandular components separated into normal structures. In contradistinction, a mass should retain shape, form, and density, as seen on the original mammogram. (Modified from Sickles EA: Practical solutions to common mammographic problems: tailoring the examination, *AJR Am J Roentgenol* 151:31–39, 1988.)

A one-view finding often prompts requests for rolled views. Rolled CC views separate fake masses from summation artifacts of normal fibroglandular elements into their individual components (see Table 2.7). To obtain the RL CC view, the technologist positions the breast as if he or she is going to take a CC mammogram, rolls the breast tissue so that the top of the breast is rolled toward the axilla, and then recompresses the breast and takes the picture (Fig. 2.33; see also Fig. 2.20). The bottom of the breast is now directed toward the sternum. This action rolls the fibroglandular components that formed the "fake mass" away from each other. On the rolled view, a summation artifact is separated into its normal fibroglandular components and the mass goes away (Fig. 2.34). On the other hand, true masses retain their shape and size on the rolled view (see Fig. 2.21).

Another way to separate true masses from fake ones is to use *spot compression*. A small spot compression paddle is used to compress tightly and directly over a finding. This provides greater compression on the area of interest. If used to determine whether a finding is a real mass or a superimposition, spot compression separates fake summation artifacts into normal fibroglandular components (Figs. 2.34 and 2.35). If the finding is a real mass, the mass should persist within the spot compression field of view (Fig. 2.36). A true mass will retain its shape, size, and density, whereas a summation artifact will disperse into its fibroglandular components. It is important to perform the spot view in the projection in which the finding is best seen or displayed against fat to increase the chance of discovering if it is real (Fig. 2.37).

Step oblique views are mammograms obtained at slightly different oblique angles (ie, 45, 50, 60 degrees) that throw fibroglandular elements into slight variations of obliquity. As with rolled views, true lesions should persist on multistep oblique views. Summation artifacts, on the other hand, will separate into their fibroglandular components.

Tomosynthesis provides tomographic images and sometimes helps to identify a true mass. Unlike 2D images that may suffer from overlapping tissue, including fibroglandular tissues, Cooper's ligaments and vessels, tomosynthesis can provide thin-slice images focusing the target. Spiculation with a center or architectural distortion caused by a tumor may be more clearly visualized on tomosynthesis slices, without the interference of overlapping structures (Figs. 2.38 and 2.39; Videos 2.2A–B). The differentiation of a summation artifact from a true mass may be easier to differentiate with tomosynthesis than with 2D mammograms (Fig. 2.40; Video 2.3B). The decrease in screening mammogram recalls is often caused by a decrease in the number of 2D asymmetries and fake summation artifacts in published series. In some cases, the use of the spot compression on tomosynthesis may be helpful to differentiate between a summation artifact and a true mass (Fig. 2.41; see Video 2.3A).

In all cases in which a mass is suspected, ultrasound provides indispensable information. The negative ultrasound confirms findings on "negative" mammograms. If the ultrasound is positive, a mass is confirmed. A repeat mammogram with a marker over the ultrasound-detected mass may show ultrasound findings that correspond to the mammographic findings and show a mass (Fig. 2.42). If they do not correspond, more workup is needed.

To Visualize Findings in Hard to See Locations

The following section details mammographic projections modified to visualize findings in specific hard-to-see locations that are commonly missed by standard CC, MLO, and lateral views. It is not uncommon to see a suspicious lesion on one view and not see it on the orthogonal projection. This can be because of the patient's body configuration or because the location of the finding makes it hard to see on the mammogram.

Some lesions are located in the extreme outer part of the breast not included on the standard CC view. A view that sees more of the outer breast is the CC view exaggerated laterally (XCCL; Figs. 2.43 and 2.44 and Figs. e2.1 and e2.2). The technologist obtains an XCCL by modifying a standard CC view. The patient's body is rotated to display more outer breast tissue than is seen on a standard CC view and excludes the medial portion of the breast. This projection sees more outer breast but does not see the inner breast.

The Cleopatra view also includes more outer breast tissue. In this view, the patient rotates laterally, as in the XCCL, but also leans obliquely like Cleopatra reclining on a bed of pillows (Fig. 2.45). The Cleopatra view includes much more of the outer part of the breast while excluding inner breast tissue, but unlike the XCCL, which is taken with the patient standing straight up, the Cleopatra view is taken with the patient leaning slightly backward and obliquely.

For inner breast lesions, CC views exaggerated medially (XCCM) image the medial portion of the breast while excluding the outer breast tissue (see Fig. 2.43, Fig. 2.46, and Fig. e2.3). Another view that visualizes the inner breast is the CV (see Fig. 2.43), or valley view, which includes the medial portions of both breasts on the image receptor in a modified CC projection. Such views allow visualization of even more of the inner part of the breast than is seen on standard CC views, but also images some of the opposite inner breast (Fig. 2.47).

Some lesions are so close to the chest wall they are hard to image with normal-sized compression paddles. The small spot compression paddles can get closer to the chest wall. The technologist can use the small spot compression paddles to image extremely inner or deep lesions because they are smaller than the bulky normal compression paddles (see Fig. 2.43).

Some lesions in the upper part of the breast are so far back against the chest wall that they can be pushed out of the field of view by the compression paddle (Fig. 2.48A–B). This problem can be solved by the from-below (FB) or CC view (Fig. 2.48C). For this view, the image receptor is placed on the

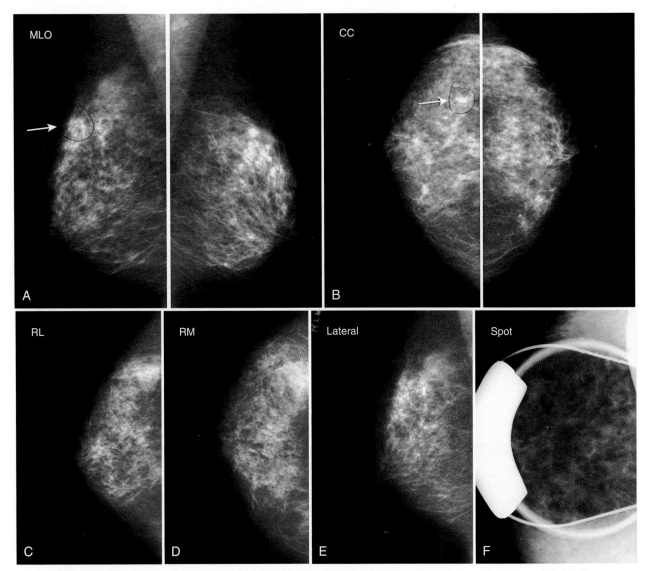

FIG. 2.34 The use of rolled views for a possible mass. Final diagnosis: a summation artifact. (A and B) Medio-lateral oblique (MLO; A) and craniocaudal (CC; B) screening mammograms show a possible mass (*circles with arrows*) in the upper outer right breast. (C and D) Rolled CC lateral (RL) view (C) and rolled CC medial (RM) view (D) show no focal density. (E) The lateral view shows no mass. (F) The double spot compression view shows no mass. This possible mass actually represents overlapping tissue. (Modified from Sickles EA: Practical solutions to common mammographic problems: tailoring the examination, *AJR Am J Roentgenol* 151:31–39, 1988.)

upper part of the breast. The breast is then compressed from below, excluding the lower part of the breast but including tissue high on the chest wall. In another approach for imaging lesions high on the chest wall, the image receptor is placed on the midportion of the breast with the lower portion excluded; this approach, first described by Sickles et al. (1988), incorporates more of the upper portion of the breast because the compression paddle does not have to include lower breast tissue in the field of view.

Another area that is hard to see is the region immediately behind the nipple, which can be hidden by adjacent blood vessels and ducts. Spot compression compresses normal ducts, blood vessels, and tissue while pulling the nipple into profile (Fig. 2.49). The nipple should be in profile on at least one view to see the retroareolar region; otherwise, the nipple may hide a cancer.

Lesions in the lower inner part of the breast are very hard to see. A superior–inferior oblique (SIO), or reverse oblique, view visualizes the lower inner breast. In this view, the technologist

places the imaging receptor on the medial part of the breast and the compression plate on the superior breast while the patient leans over the imaging receptor (Fig. 2.50). The compression paddle approaches the breast from the superior axillary side, allowing more of the inner breast tissue to be visualized.

Palpable findings imaged near the periphery of the breast are seen better with spot compression. This type of spot compression tangential to the palpable finding can push the mass against subcutaneous fat, allowing it to be seen. Spot compression directly over the palpable mass, previously known as a *lumpogram*, also can show masses by compressing the surrounding glandular tissue away from the suspicious finding (Fig. 2.51).

To Characterize True Findings

After the radiologist determines that a mass or cluster of calcifications is a true finding and triangulates its position within the breast, additional mammographic views are used to characterize the finding (Box 2.8). Microfocal spot air-gap magnification views

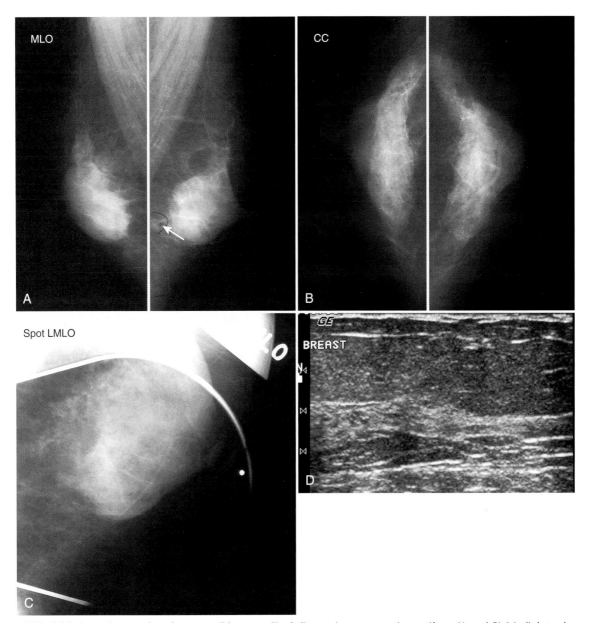

FIG. 2.35 Spot view workup for a possible mass. Final diagnosis: a summation artifact. (A and B) Mediolateral oblique (MLO; A) and craniocaudal (CC; B) screening mammograms; a possible mass is seen in the lower part of the left breast on the MLO view near the chest wall (*circle with arrow*) but not on the CC view. (C) A spot compression film shows no mass. (D) Ultrasound in this region shows fatty and scant fibroglandular tissue. This possible mass is overlapping tissue.

of clustered calcifications sharpen and separate calcification forms and display calcifications not detected on nonmagnified studies. Magnification can also depict mass shapes and margins to greater advantage, showing spiculated or irregular margins not discernible at lower resolutions.

Spot compression magnification views not only provide greater visualization of the region of interest by pushing fibroglandular tissue away from the finding, but also produce higher resolution of mass margins and calcification shapes (Fig. 2.52). Thus spot compression magnification mammograms are a mainstay of the radiologist's diagnostic tools to characterize both masses and calcifications.

Another option to characterize true findings is tomosynthesis. Thin slices obtained by tomosynthesis may increase the chance to read the margin of a mass or to detect subtle calcifications compared with 2D images. Tomosynthesis may be helpful particularly in characterizing true findings in women with dense breasts (Fig. 2.53;Video 2.4A).

DIAGNOSTIC LIMITATIONS

Breast Cancer Missed by Mammography

Nondetection of breast cancer on mammography is of concern to the patient, the referring physician, and the radiologist. Nondetection of cancer on mammography is the result of a variety of factors, including the mammographic technique, experience of the radiologist, morphology of the breast tumor, and the background on which it is displayed. Errors can occur at any levels, ie, in technique, in detection, and in interpretation (Table 2.9). Cancers can best be displayed by good mammographic technique, optimal positioning, and a tumor

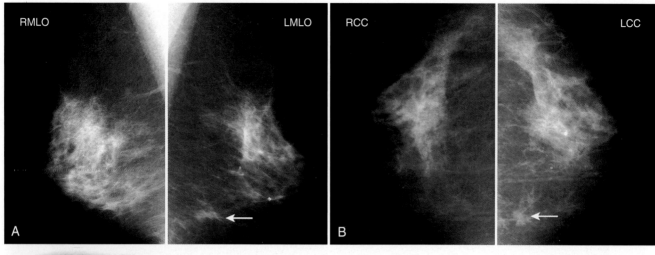

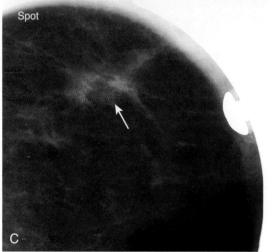

FIG. 2.36 Spot view workup for a possible mass. Final diagnosis: cancer. (A and B) A mass (*arrows*) is seen on mediolateral oblique (MLO; A) craniocaudal (CC; B) screening mammograms in the lower inner portion of the left breast. (C) A spot compression view shows that the density persists and is suggestive of spiculation, representing a mass (*arrow*). Invasive ductal cancer was diagnosed. *R*, right; *L*, left.

location that can be displayed on the film. Approximately 10% to 15% of breast cancers are mammographically occult, even on good images, and will not be detected on mammography in the best of hands.

Missed cancers on mammography can be categorized into several types (Box 2.9). First, the tumor may have a morphology that is undetectable on the mammographic background on which it is displayed and is therefore mammographically occult. Second, the tumor may display findings that are visible, but below the threshold of any radiologist for consideration as cancer. Such findings have been termed *nonspecific*, examples of which include mammographic findings suggesting normal islands of fibroglandular tissue, a few benign-appearing calcifications, or a benign-appearing mass among many other benign-appearing masses that do not represent cancer. Third, the tumor may show subtle findings that represent cancer but are atypical, such as a single dilated duct, a developing asymmetry, or other less common features of breast cancer that are perceptible but may have been unrecognized. Fourth, signs that are classic for breast cancer may have been present on the mammogram but either were not perceived or were misinterpreted at the time of diagnosis.

Box 2.10 shows mammographic features of missed cancer, according to the review of previous studies. Birdwell et al. (2001)

reviewed possible reasons why cancers were not identified on previous mammograms. They postulated that findings were hidden among many other findings ("busy breasts") or that distracting findings other than the cancer were present on the film. Other contributing factors included dense breast tissue, small calcifications or masses that may have been overlooked, cancers hiding in the axilla and simulating lymph nodes, linear microcalcifications simulating vascular calcifications, findings seen on only one mammographic view, and findings at the edge of the film or at the edge of the glandular tissue producing either a tent sign or concavity that was missed at the time of screening. Of note, most of these cancers were located in the upper outer quadrant, where 50% of all cancers occur. Also, not all the cancers that were missed were small; at least half of the tumors were 1 cm or larger at the time they were missed.

To decrease the number of missed breast cancers, the radiologist should use a systematic approach to reviewing the mammogram that minimizes distractions, paper shuffling, or other busy work in the reading room at the time of interpretation. Next, comparison with older films may reveal subtle changes not apparent on only the current examination. Finally, the radiologist should be aware of subtle or nonspecific findings of breast cancer.

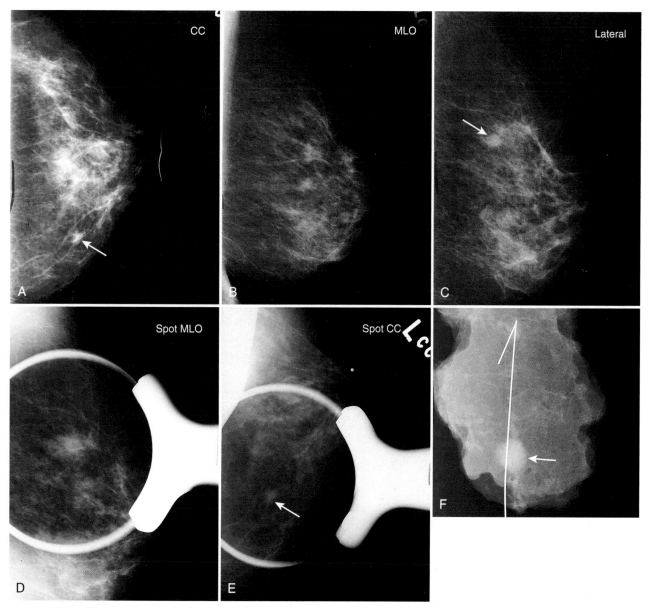

FIG. 2.37 Importance of using a spot view over an area of fat. (A and B) Craniocaudal (CC; A) and mediolateral oblique (MLO; B) screening mammograms; a possible mass is seen at the inner portion of the left breast on the CC view (*arrow*) but is not apparent on the MLO view. Incidentally, note the linear metallic scar marker over a skin scar in A. (C) On the lateral view, the mass (*arrow*) is seen in the upper part of the breast. (D) A spot compression film in the mediolateral view is taken over glandular tissue but shows no mass. (E) When the spot view is repeated over the fatty area on the CC view, it shows a spiculated mass (*arrow*) in the medial breast against the dark fat that was hidden against the glandular tissue on the mediolateral spot view (D). (F) The specimen shows the hookwire used for preoperative localization and the mass (*arrow*), which was invasive ductal cancer.

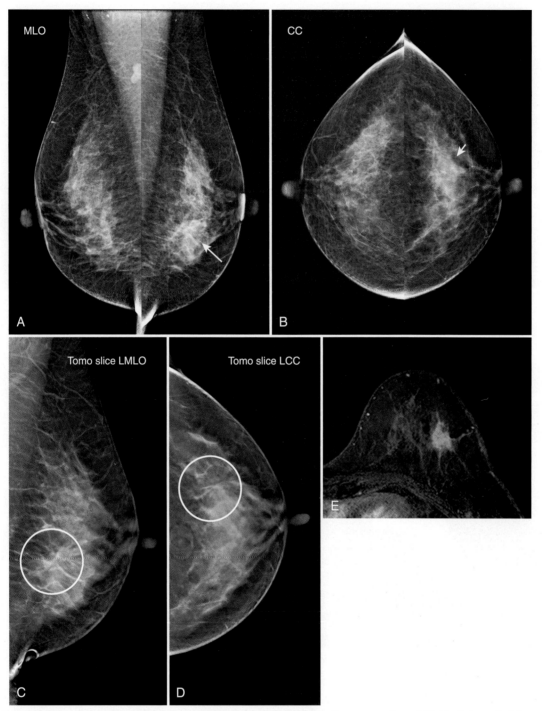

FIG. 2.38 Tomosynthesis workup for a possible mass. Final diagnosis: cancer. (A and B) Mediolateral oblique (MLO; A) and craniocaudal (CC; B) screening mammograms; a focal asymmetry with possible architectural distortion is seen in the lower outer portion of the left breast (*arrows*), but the finding is not apparent because of the overlapping fibroglandular tissue. (C and D) Tomosynthesis MLO (C; see Video 2.2A) and CC (D; see Video 2.2B) projections depict the architectural distortion or spiculated mass (*circles*) clearly, suggesting a malignancy. (E) Contrast enhanced magnetic resonance image of the left breast shows a spiculated mass, which is proven to be invasive ductal cancer. *L*, left.

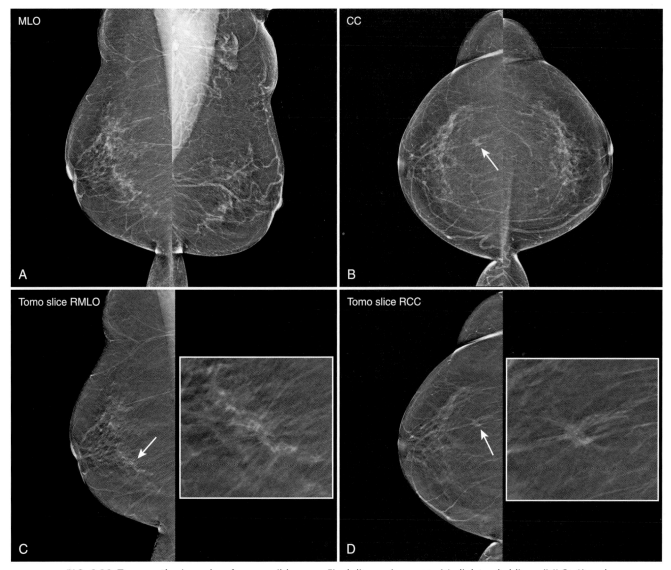

FIG. 2.39 Tomosynthesis workup for a possible mass. Final diagnosis: cancer. Mediolateral oblique (MLO; A) and craniocaudal (CC; B) screening mammograms; a one-view asymmetry is seen in the outer portion of the right breast (*arrow*) on CC, but is not seen on MLO. Tomosynthesis MLO (C; *see* Video 2.3A) and CC (D; *see* Video 2.3B) projections with photography magnified views on the right depict a spiculated mass (*arrows*), suggesting a malignancy. This was proven to be invasive ductal cancer. *R,* right.

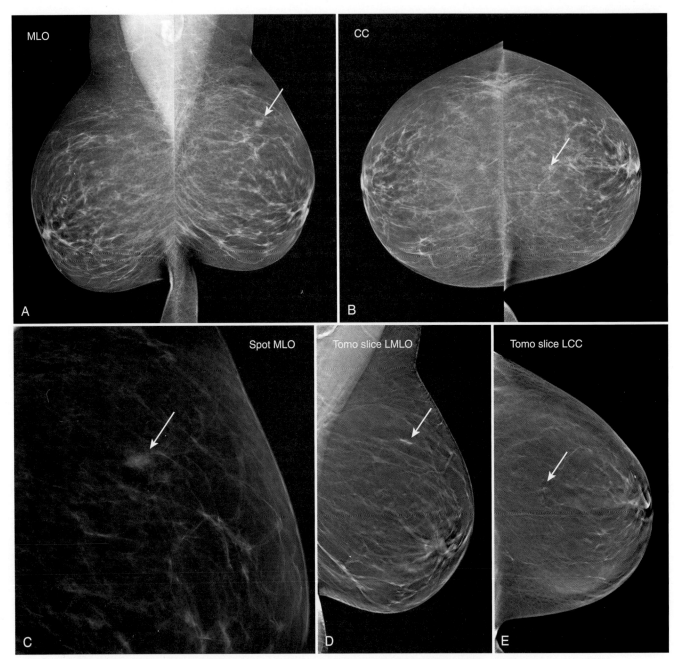

FIG. 2.40 Tomosynthesis workup for a possible mass. Final diagnosis: a summation artifact. (A and B) Mediolateral oblique (MLO; A) and craniocaudal (CC; B) screening mammograms show a two-view focal asymmetry (*arrows*) in the upper middle left breast. (C) A possible mass shadow (*circle*) persists on the spot magnified MLO view. (D and E) Tomosynthesis MLO (D) (see Video 2.4) and CC projections show no mass, but just a breast tissue without a convex margin (*arrows*). The focal asymmetry was diagnosed as a summation artifact. *L*, left.

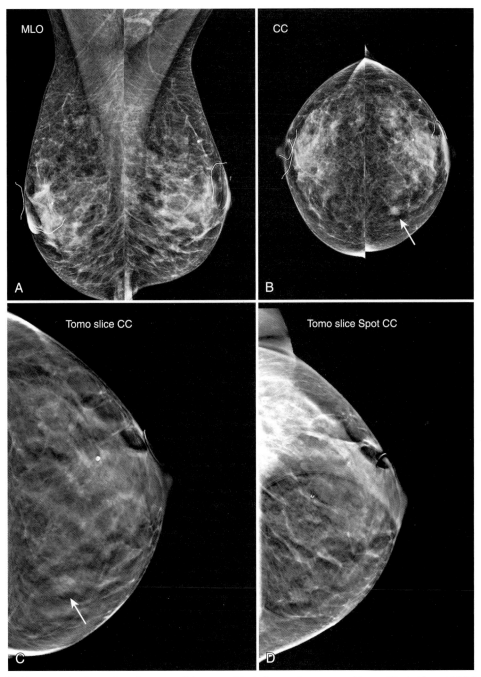

FIG. 2.41 Tomosynthesis workup for a possible mass. Final diagnosis: a summation artifact. (A and B) Mediolateral oblique (MLO; A) and craniocaudal (CC; B) screening mammograms. A one-view asymmetry (*arrows*) is seen in the inner left breast on the CC view that is not visualized on the MLO view. Because this density has a relatively convex-outward border, further workup was performed to exclude the possibility of malignancy. Please note scar markers on the skin in the bilateral breasts. (C) On tomosynthesis CC (see Video 2.5A) projection, the asymmetry persists (*arrow*). (D) However, with the use of spot compression, this asymmetry disappeared on the tomosynthesis CC projection (see Video 2.5B–C). The asymmetry was diagnosed as a summation artifact.

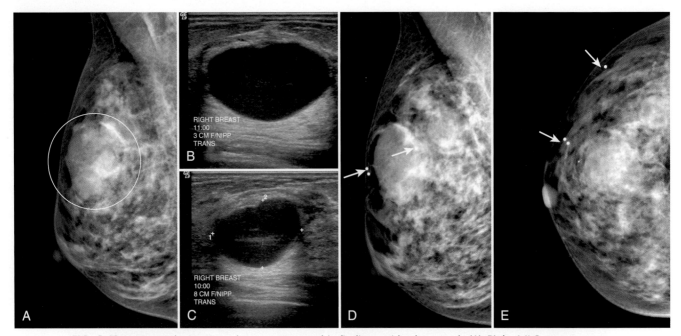

FIG. 2.42 Using markers to correlate mammographic findings with ultrasound. (A) Right MLO mammogram showed a large equal density mass (*circle*) in the upper right breast. (B and C) Ultrasound showed two large cysts. (D and E) A right MLO (D) and CC view (E) with BBs (*arrows*) placed over the cysts seen at ultrasound show that the masses correlate with the cysts.

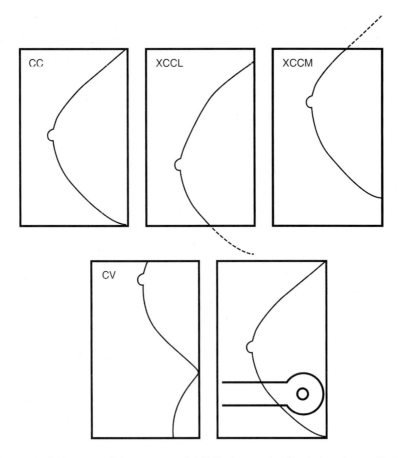

FIG. 2.43 Schematic of variations of the craniocaudal (CC) view to visualize lesions in specific locations. The CC view exaggerated laterally (XCCL) includes outer breast tissue but excludes medial breast tissue. The CC view exaggerated medially (XCCM) includes medial breast tissue while excluding outer breast tissue. The cleavage view (CV) includes the medial portions of both breasts on the mammogram. Spot compression may visualize findings close to the chest wall that are excluded by a larger compression paddle.

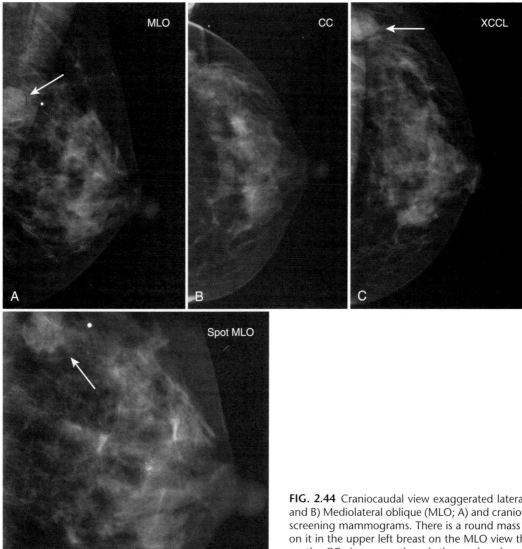

FIG. 2.44 Craniocaudal view exaggerated laterally (XCCL). (A and B) Mediolateral oblique (MLO; A) and craniocaudal (CC; B) screening mammograms. There is a round mass with a marker on it in the upper left breast on the MLO view that is not seen on the CC view, even though the marker shows the palpable mass. (C) An XCCL now shows the mass by including it in the field of view. (D) A spot compression MLO view shows the mass, and it is invasive ductal cancer.

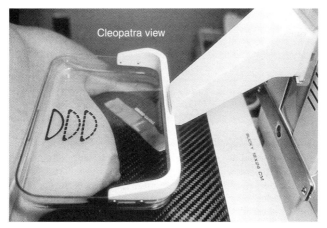

FIG. 2.45 Cleopatra view. For this view the patient leans outward and back, essentially performing an outer craniocaudal view exaggerated laterally with a degree of obliquity to image more outer tissue.

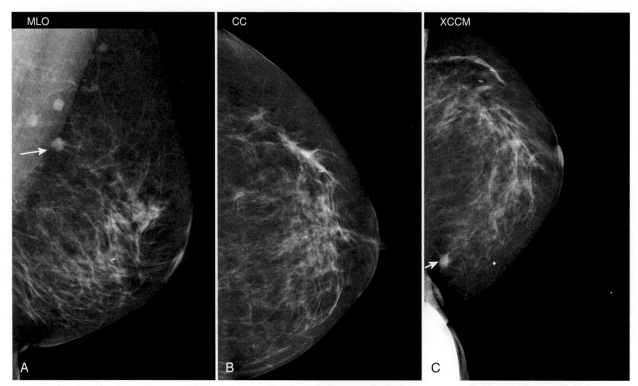

FIG. 2.46 Craniocaudal view exaggerated medially (XCCM). (A) A left mediolateral oblique (MLO) view shows the mass (*arrow*) deep in the upper breast at the chest wall. (B) However, the left craniocaudal (CC) view shows no mass. (C) XCCM successfully shows a small mass (*arrow*) in the medial portion of the breast. This was proven to be invasive ductal cancer. Note that there are two ribbon markers in the outer right breast tissue.

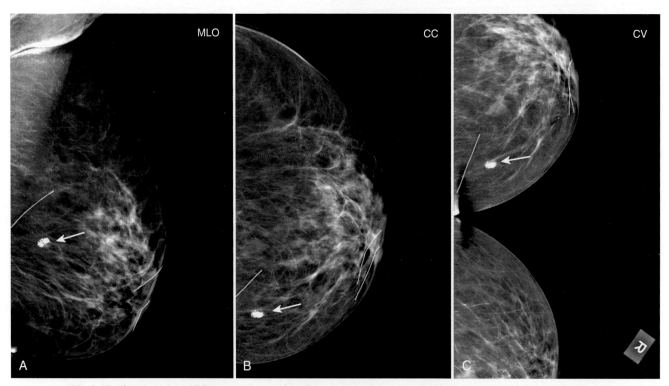

FIG. 2.47 Cleavage view (CV) mammogram that shows more of the inner breast. (A and B) Mediolateral oblique (MLO; A) and craniocaudal (CC; B) screening mammograms show a calcified degenerating fibroadenoma (*arrows*) in the middle inner left breast. (C) The CV mammogram shows the fibroadenoma in the inner breast to the best advantage and also includes some of the inner portion of the contralateral breast. Incidentally, note the linear metallic scar marker over skin scars in A–C.

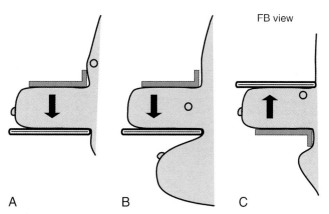

FIG. 2.48 Methods to visualize high breast lesions. (A) The compression paddle may exclude high breast masses by compressing them out of the field of view. (B) A view with the cassette holder above the nipple to allow compression of only the upper breast tissue. (C) The right image shows a from-below (FB) view in which the image receptor is placed over the upper part of the breast and the compression paddle approaches the receptor from the lower part of the breast. (Modified from Sickles EA: Practical solutions to common mammographic problems: tailoring the examination, *AJR Am J Roentgenol* 151:31–39, 1988.)

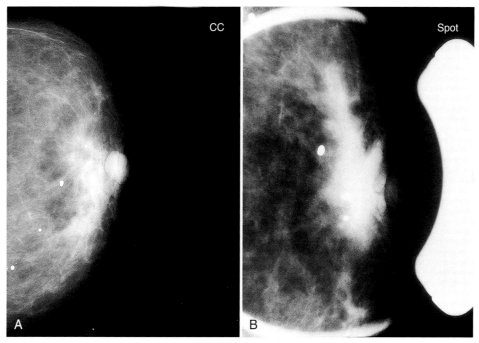

FIG. 2.49 Spot view showing a mass in the retroareolar region. (A) A craniocaudal (CC) view shows a vague density behind the nipple, but the nipple is not in profile. (B) A spot view with the nipple in profile shows a spiculated mass that was diagnosed as invasive lobular cancer.

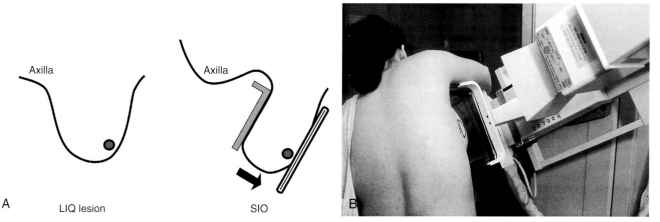

FIG. 2.50 Superior–inferior oblique (SIO) view. (A) Schematic shows a lower inner quadrant (LIQ) lesion in the left image. The SIO view is obtained with the image receptor next to the inner breast lesion and the compression plate compressing from the superior axillary side. (B) Model demonstrating positioning for the SIO view.

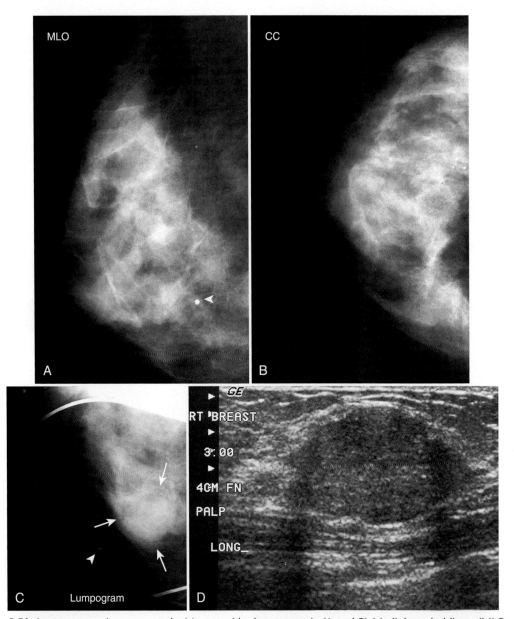

FIG. 2.51 Spot compression over a palpable mass (the lumpogram). (A and B) Mediolateral oblique (MLO; A) and craniocaudal (CC; B) views show no defined mass at the 3 o'clock position on the right breast with the palpable abnormality. Note a BB skin marker (A; *arrowhead*) placed at the palpable portion. (C) Spot tangential view over the lump with the BB marker (*arrowhead*) in the CC projection shows a possible round mass (*arrows*) against the dense tissue. (D) Ultrasound shows an oval smooth mass, representing a fibroadenoma on biopsy.

BOX 2.8   Mammographic Views to Characterize a True Lesion

Magnification
Spot compression magnification
Tomosynthesis

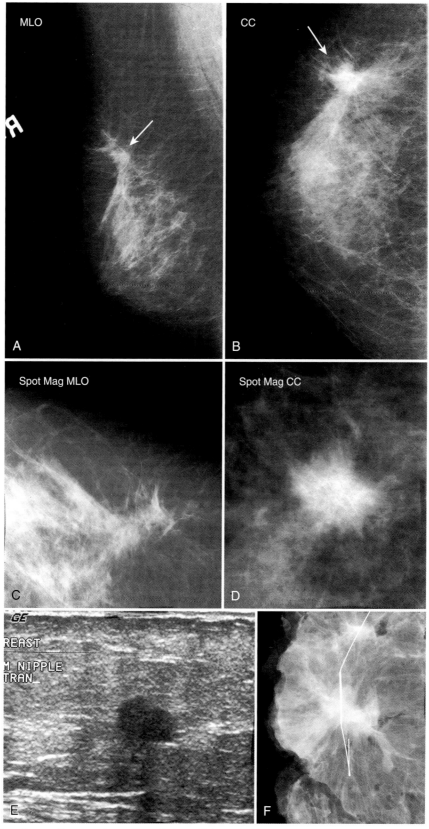

FIG. 2.52 Use of magnification views. (A and B) Mediolateral oblique (MLO; A) and craniocaudal (CC; B) mammograms show a spiculated mass (*arrows*), which is seen better on the CC view than on the MLO view. Distortion and the tent sign are evident in the upper part of the breast. (C and D) Spot magnification views show the spiculated mass to better advantage on both the MLO (C) and CC (D) views. (E) Ultrasound shows an oval (a very hypoechoic mass that has no acoustic spiculation or shadowing) corresponding to the mass on the mammogram. (F) The mass was localized by ultrasound and was removed, as shown by the specimen. Note the localizing hookwire. Invasive ductal cancer was the diagnosis.

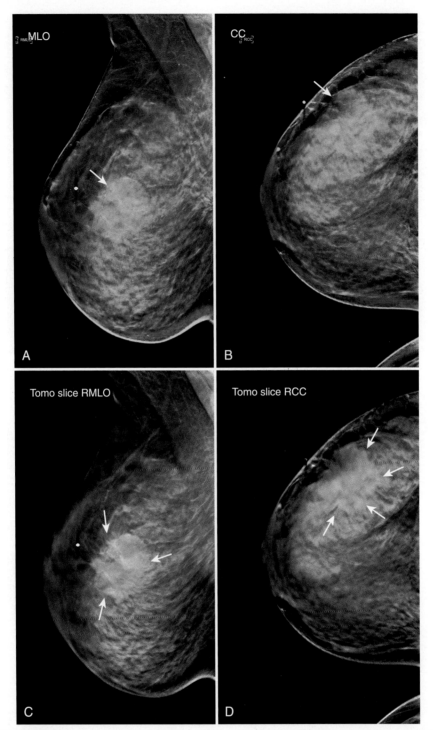

FIG. 2.53 Tomosynthesis to characterize a true finding in extremely dense breasts. (A and B) Mediolateral oblique (MLO; A) and craniocaudal (CC; B) projections of tomosynthesis-synthesized 2D mammograms show a possible mass (*arrows*) below the BB skin marker in the right upper outer breast. However, its margin is largely obscured by the overlapped dense fibroglandular tissue. (C and D) Tomosynthesis slices depict the spiculated margin better on both MLO (C; see also Video 2.6A) and CC (D) (see also Video 2.6B) projections. On tomosynthesis slices, the mass appears more dense and more homogenous compared with the surrounding fibroglandular tissue that has heterogeneous density caused by marbled fat tissue. Invasive ductal cancer was the diagnosis. *R*, right.

TABLE 2.9 Reasons for Missed Cancers

Errors in technique	Poor technique Poor positioning Cancer in location not included in standard field of view
Errors in detection	"Overlooked, missed": characteristic cancer findings, present in retrospect; this commonly occurs particularly in tumors with morphology that is similar to background fibroglandular tissue displayed on mammography "Unrecognized sign": atypical finding perceived but not acted on, such as round mass or developing focal asymmetry "Nonspecific findings" that look normal (not actionable, not an error)
Errors in interpretation	Radiologist sees and perceives finding, incorrectly interprets finding as nonactionable
True negative study	Tumor cannot be seen even in retrospect

From Ikeda DM, Andersson I, Wattsgard C, et al: Interval carcinomas in the Malmö Mammographic Screening Trial: Radiographic appearance and prognostic considerations, *AJR Am J Roentgenol* 159:287–294, 1992.

BOX 2.9 Types of Findings on Mammograms in Patients with Missed Breast Cancer

Occult on mammography (negative)
Nonspecific findings (normal or benign findings)
Atypical findings (subtle)
Classic cancer findings overlooked or misinterpreted

From: Ikeda DM, Andersson I, Wattsgard C, et al: Interval carcinomas in the Malmö Mammographic Screening Trial: Radiographic appearance and prognostic considerations, *AJR Am J Roentgenol* 159:287–294, 1992.

BOX 2.10 Features of Cancer Missed on Previous Mammography

Lesion seen on only one view
Distracting lesions
Radiolucent lines of fat through the lesion
Too few calcifications
Small masses
Calcifications look like calcifying blood vessel
Lesion in dense breast tissue
Lesion at the edge of glandular tissue
Lesion at the edge of the film
Lesion in the axilla that looks like a lymph node
Benign-appearing lesion
Lesion in large breast
Lesion obscured by a blood vessel
Lesion on mammography with suboptimal technique
Lesion outside the image

From: Birdwell RL, Ikeda DM, O'Shaughnessy KF, Sickles EA: Mammographic characteristics of 115 missed cancers later detected with screening mammography and the potential utility of computer-aided detection, *Radiology* 219:192–202, 2001.

Key Elements

Breast cancer screening in women invited to undergo mammography decreases breast cancer mortality by about 30%.
Risk factors for breast cancer include age older than 50 years, personal history of or first-degree relative with breast cancer, nulliparous status, early menarche, late menopause, first birth after age 30, radiation treatment, atypical ductal hyperplasia, lobular carcinoma in situ, and presence of *BRCA1* or *BRCA2* breast cancer susceptibility genes.

Seventy percent of women who have breast cancer have no risk factors other than being female and being older than age 50.
Signs and symptoms of breast cancer include a breast lump, bloody or new spontaneous nipple discharge, new nipple or skin retraction, *peau d'orange*, and symptoms from metastasis.
Signs of breast cancer on mammography include a spiculated mass, pleomorphic calcifications, a round mass, architectural distortion, a developing density, an asymmetric density, a single dilated duct, lymphadenopathy, and breast edema; in some patients, no mammographic signs are present (occult cancer).
A normal mammogram is dense in young women and becomes darker over time as the dense tissue is replaced by fat.
Increasing breast density may be caused by pregnancy or hormone replacement therapy.
Unexplained increasing breast density should prompt a work-up to exclude breast edema or cancer.
Evaluation of a normal mammogram includes routine inspection for fibroglandular symmetry and examination of the periglandular edges, the skin, retroareolar region and nipple, retroglandular fat, medial part of the breast, chest wall, and axilla.
Normal asymmetric glandular tissue occurs in 3% of women and looks like an asymmetry of normal glandular tissue without a palpable mass, suspicious calcifications or spiculations, a three-dimensional mass, or new findings.
Be alert for findings in the medial part of the breast; the normal sternalis muscle variant is the one normal finding in the medial breast.
To detect developing densities, change, or asymmetries, view films back to back and compare them with old films.
Review both the breast history and the technologist's physical sheet before interpretation of the mammogram to know where previous biopsies were, the meaning of skin markers, and to be aware of patient complaints.
Women with breast cancer have normal mammograms 10% to 15% of the time.
The skin should normally be 2 to 3 mm thick. Skin thicker than 2 to 3 mm might be breast edema or scarring.
Special mammographic views confirm or exclude questionable findings seen on screening mammography, characterize true lesions, and triangulate the location of a lesion.
Rolled views, compression views, and step oblique views distinguish true lesions from summation artifacts.
Magnification spot compression views characterize mass margins and shapes and see calcification numbers, shapes, and forms better.
Air-gap magnification views resolve the shape and number of calcifications better than standard mammograms.
Laterally exaggerated craniocaudal (CC) and Cleopatra views display the outer part of the breast.
Medially exaggerated CC and cleavage views display the inner portion of the breast.
From-below and upper breast views display the upper part of the breast.
Spot compression and nipple-in-profile images view the nipple and retroareolar region.
Superior–inferior oblique views (reverse oblique) display the lower inner portion of the breast.
The breast location most often excluded by screening mammograms is the upper inner quadrant.
Lesions displayed at the nipple level on the mediolateral oblique (MLO) view may be in the upper, lower, or mid-portion of the breast on the ML view.
Triangulation with the CC and MLO views can be used to predict the location of the lesion on the lateral view.

SUGGESTED READINGS

Andersson I, Janzon L: Reduced breast cancer mortality in women under age 50: updated results from the Malmö Mammographic Screening Program, *J Natl Cancer Inst Monogr* 22:63-67, 1997.

Bent CK, Bassett LW, D'Orsi CJ, Sayre JW: The positive predictive value of BI-RADS microcalcification descriptors and final assessment categories, *AJR Am J Roentgenol* 194:1378-1383, 2010.

Berg WA, Arnoldus CL, Teferra E, et al.: Biopsy of amorphous breast calcifications: pathologic outcome and yield at stereotactic biopsy, *Radiology* 221:495-503, 2001.

Beyer T, Moonka R: Normal mammography and ultrasonography in the setting of palpable breast cancer, *Am J Surg* 185:416-419, 2003.

Birdwell RL, Bandodkar P, Ikeda DM: Computer-aided detection with screening mammography in a university hospital setting, *Radiology* 236(2):451-457, 2005.

Birdwell RL, Ikeda DM, O'Shaughnessy KF, et al.: Mammographic characteristics of 115 missed cancers later detected with screening mammography and the potential utility of computer-aided detection, *Radiology* 219:192-202, 2001.

Bjurstam N, Bjorneld L, Duffy SW, et al.: The Gothenburg breast screening trial: first results on mortality, incidence, and mode of detection for women ages 39-49 years at randomization, *Cancer* 80:2091-2099, 1997.

Boyd NF, Guo H, Martin LJ, et al.: Mammographic density and the risk and detection of breast cancer, *NEJM* 356(3):227-238, 2007.

Boyd NF, Martin LJ, Rommens JM, et al.: Mammographic density: a heritable risk factor for breast cancer, *Methods Mol Biol* 472:343-360, 2009.

Bradley FM, Hoover Jr HC, Hulka CA, et al.: The sternalis muscle: an unusual normal finding seen on mammography, *AJR Am J Roentgenol* 166:33-36, 1996.

Brenner RJ, Sickles EA: Acceptability of periodic follow-up as an alternative to biopsy for mammographically detected lesions interpreted as probably benign, *Radiology* 171:645-646, 1989.

Burnside ES, Ochsner JE, Fowler KJ, et al.: Use of microcalcification descriptors in BI-RADS 4th edition to stratify risk of malignancy, *Radiology* 242:388-395, 2007.

Claus EB, Risch N, Thompson WD: Autosomal dominant inheritance of early-onset breast cancer. Implications for risk prediction, *Cancer* 73:643-651, 1994.

Claus EB, Risch N, Thompson WD: Genetic analysis of breast cancer in the cancer and steroid hormone study, *Am J Hum Genet* 48:232-242, 1991.

Colditz GA, Egan KM, Stampfer MJ: Hormone replacement therapy and risk of breast cancer: results from epidemiologic studies, *Am J Obstet Gynecol* 168:1473-1480, 1993.

Colditz GA, Willett WC, Hunter DJ, et al.: Family history, age, and risk of breast cancer. Prospective data from the Nurses' Health Study, *JAMA* 270:338-343, 1993.

Cook KL, Adler DD, Lichter AS, et al.: Breast carcinoma in young women previously treated for Hodgkin disease, *AJR Am J Roentgenol* 155:39-42, 1990.

Faulk RM, Sickles EA: Efficacy of spot compression-magnification and tangential views in mammographic evaluation of palpable breast masses, *Radiology* 185:87-90, 1992.

Gail MH, Brinton LA, Byar DP, et al.: Projecting individualized probabilities of developing breast cancer for white females who are being examined annually, *J Natl Cancer Inst* 81:1879-1886, 1989.

Gilbert FJ, Tucker L, Gillan MG, et al.: Accuracy of digital breast tomosynthesis for depicting breast cancer subgroups in a UK Retrospective Reading Study (TOMMY Trial), *Radiology* 277:697-706, 2015.

Gilbert FJ, Tucker L, Gillan MG, et al.: The TOMMY trial: a comparison of TOMosynthesis with digital MammographY in the UK NHS Breast Screening Programme–a multicentre retrospective reading study comparing the diagnostic performance of digital breast tomosynthesis and digital mammography with digital mammography alone, *Health Technol Assess* 19(i-xxv):1-136, 2015.

Goergen SK, Evans J, Cohen GP, MacMillan JH: Characteristics of breast carcinomas missed by screening radiologists, *Radiology* 204:131-135, 1997.

Gunhan-Bilgen I, Bozkaya H, Ustun EE, Memis A: Male breast disease: clinical, mammographic, and ultrasonographic features, *Eur J Radiol* 43:246-255, 2002.

Hartge P, Struewing JP, Wacholder S, et al.: The prevalence of common BRCA1 and BRCA2 mutations among Ashkenazi Jews, *Am J Hum Genet* 64:963-970, 1999.

Helvie MA, Pennes DR, Rebner M, et al.: Mammographic follow-up of low-suspicion lesions: compliance rate and diagnostic yield, *Radiology* 178:155-158, 1991.

Homer MJ: Proper placement of a metallic marker on an area of concern in the breast, *AJR Am J Roentgenol* 167:390-391, 1996.

Homer MJ, Smith TJ: Asymmetric breast tissue, *Radiology* 173:577-578, 1989.

Ikeda DM, Andersson I, Wattsgard C, et al.: Interval carcinomas in the Malmö Mammographic Screening Trial: radiographic appearance and prognostic considerations, *AJR Am J Roentgenol* 159:287-294, 1992.

Ikeda DM, Birdwell RL, O'Shaughnessy KF, et al.: Analysis of 172 subtle findings on prior normal mammograms in women with breast cancer detected at follow-up screening, *Radiology* 226(2):494-503, 2003.

Jonsson H, Bordas P, Wallin H, et al.: Service screening with mammography in Northern Sweden: effects on breast cancer mortality—an update, *J Med Screen* 14(2):87-93, 2007.

Kopans DB: Negative mammographic and US findings do not help exclude breast cancer, *Radiology* 222:857-859, 2002.

Kopans DB, Swann CA, White G, et al.: Asymmetric breast tissue, *Radiology* 171:639-643, 1989.

Larsson LG, Andersson I, Bjurstam N, et al.: Updated overview of the Swedish Randomized Trials on Breast Cancer Screening with Mammography: age group 40-49 at randomization, *J Natl Cancer Inst Monogr* 22:57-61, 1997.

Leung JW, Sickles EA: Developing asymmetry identified on mammography: correlation with imaging outcome and pathologic findings, *AJR Am J Roentgenol* 188:667-675, 2007.

Li Y, Baer D, Friedman GD, et al.: Wine, liquor, beer and risk of breast cancer in a large population, *Eur J Cancer* 45(5):843-850, 2009.

Liberman L, Abramson AF, Squires FB, et al.: The breast imaging reporting and data system: positive predictive value of mammographic features and final assessment categories, *AJR Am J Roentgenol* 171:35-40, 1998.

Logan WW, Janus J: Use of special mammographic views to maximize radiographic information, *Radiol Clin North Am* 25:953-959, 1987.

Lynch HT, Watson P, Conway T, et al.: Breast cancer family history as a risk factor for early onset breast cancer, *Breast Cancer Res Treat* 11:263-267, 1988.

Miki Y, Swensen J, Shattuck-Eidens D, et al.: A strong candidate for the breast and ovarian cancer susceptibility gene BRCA1, *Science* 266:66-71, 1994.

Nam KJ, Han BK, Ko ES, et al.: Comparison of full-field digital mammography and digital breast tomosynthesis in ultrasonography-detected breast cancers, *Breast* 24:649-655, 2015.

National Comprehensive Cancer Network (NCCN): NCCN Clinical Practice Guidelines in Oncology (NCCN Guidelines) Breast Cancer Screening and Diagnosis, *Version 1*, 2015.

Nystrom L, Andersson I, Bjurstam N, et al.: Long-term effects of mammography screening: updated overview of the Swedish randomised trials, *Lancet* 359:909-919, 2002.

Oeffinger KC, Fontham ETH, Etzioni R, et al.: Breast cancer screening for women at average risk 2015 guideline update from the American Cancer Society, *JAMA* 314(15):1599-1614, 2015.

Park JM, Franken Jr EA: Triangulation of breast lesions: review and clinical applications, *Curr Probl Diagn Radiol* 37(1):1-14, 2008.

Pearson KL, Sickles EA, Frankel SD, et al.: Efficacy of step-oblique mammography for confirmation and localization of densities seen on only one standard mammographic view, *AJR Am J Roentgenol* 174:745-752, 2000.

Ries LAG, Melbert D, Krapcho M, et al.: *SEER Cancer Statistics Review 1975-2005*, Bethesda, MD, 2008, National Cancer Institute. www.seer.cancer.gov/csr/1975_2005/. (based on November 2007 SEER data submission, posted to the SEER Web site. Accessed April 12, 2010.

Rosen EL, Sickles E, Keating D: Ability of mammography to reveal nonpalpable breast cancer in women with palpable breast masses, *AJR Am J Roentgenol* 172:309-312, 1999.

Saslow D, Boetes C, Berke W, et al.: American Cancer Society guidelines for breast screening with MRI as an adjunct to mammography, *CA Cancer J Clin* 57(2):75-89, 2007.

Schmidt ME, Steindorf K, Mutschelknauss E, et al.: Physical activity and postmenopausal breast cancer: effect modification by breast cancer subtypes and effective periods in life, *Cancer Epidemiol Biomarkers Prev* 17(12):3402-3410, 2008.

Schubert EL, Mefford HC, Dann JL, et al.: BRCA1 and BRCA2 mutations in Ashkenazi Jewish families with breast and ovarian cancer, *Genet Test* 1:41-46, 1997.

Shapiro S, Venet W, Strax P, et al.: Ten- to fourteen-year effect of screening on breast cancer mortality, *J Natl Cancer Inst* 69:349-355, 1982.

Sickles EA: Mammographic features of 300 consecutive nonpalpable breast cancers, *AJR Am J Roentgenol* 146:661-663, 1986.

Sickles EA: Periodic mammographic follow-up of probably benign lesions: results in 3,184 consecutive cases, *Radiology* 179:463-468, 1991.

Sickles EA: Practical solutions to common mammographic problems: tailoring the examination, *AJR Am J Roentgenol* 151:31-39, 1988.

Sickles EA, D'Orsi CJ, Bassett LW, et al.: ACR BI-RADS® Mammography. In *ACR BI-RADS® atlas, breast imaging reporting and data system*. Reston, VA, 2013, American College of Radiology.

Siegel RL, Miller KD, Jemal A: Cancer statistics, 2015, *CA Cancer J Clin* 65:5-29, 2015.

Silvera SA, Jain M, Howe GR, et al.: Energy balance and breast cancer risk: a prospective cohort study, *Breast Cancer Treat* 97(1):97-106, 2006.

Smith RA, Cokkinides V, Eyre HJ: American Cancer Society guidelines for the early detection of cancer, 2003, *CA Cancer J Clin* 53:27-43, 2003.

Smith RA, Saslow D, Sawyer KA, et al.: American Cancer Society guidelines for breast cancer screening: update 2003, *CA Cancer J Clin* 53:141-169, 2003.

Tabar L, Vitak B, Chen HH, et al.: The Swedish Two-County Trial 20 years later. Updated mortality results and new insights from long-term follow-up, *Radiol Clin North Am* 38:625-651, 2000.

Tabar L, Yen MF, Vitak B, et al.: Mammography service screening and mortality in breast cancer patients: 20-year follow-up before and after introduction of screening, *Lancet* 361:1405-1410, 2003.

Thompson AC, Kremer Prill MJ, Biswal S, et al.: Factors associated with repetitive strain, and strategies to reduce injury among breast-imaging radiologists, *J Am Coll Radiol* 11:1074-1079, 2014.

Varas X, Leborgne F, Leborgne JH: Nonpalpable, probably benign lesions: role of follow-up mammography, *Radiology* 184:409-414, 1992.

Varas X, Leborgne JH, Leborgne F, et al.: Revisiting the mammographic follow-up of BI-RADS category 3 lesions, *AJR Am J Roentgenol* 179:691-695, 2002.

Vizcaíno I, Gadea L, Andreo L, et al.: Short-term follow-up results in 795 nonpalpable probably benign lesions detected at screening mammography, *Radiology* 219:475-483, 2001.

Warren Burhenne LJ, Wood SA, D'Orsi CJ, et al.: Potential contribution of computer-aided detection to the sensitivity of screening mammography, *Radiology* 215:554-562, 2000.

Wolverton DE, Sickles EA: Clinical outcome of doubtful mammographic findings, *AJR Am J Roentgenol* 167:1041-1045, 1996.

Wooster R, Neuhausen SL, Mangion J, et al.: Localization of a breast cancer susceptibility gene, BRCA2, to chromosome 13q12-13, *Science* 265:2088-2090, 1994.

Chapter 3

Mammographic Analysis of Breast Calcifications

Debra M. Ikeda and Kanae K. Miyake

CHAPTER OUTLINE

Breast calcifications are commonly seen on mammograms, are usually composed of calcium carbonate, and are mostly seen in benign entities. However, breast calcifications also form in breast cancer and are sometimes the only sign that something is wrong on the mammogram. Fifty percent to eighty percent of breast cancers contain calcifications at pathology, but fewer cancers actually display calcifications on mammograms. This chapter will review a systematic method of analyzing breast calcifications using the 2013 Breast Imaging Reporting and Data System (BI-RADS) terms for typically benign calcifications, suspicious calcification morphology, and calcification distributions.

NORMAL BREAST ANATOMY AND CALCIFICATIONS

Breast anatomy explains why calcific shapes or distributions suggest benign or malignant disease. The structures in which calcifications form influence calcification morphology and distribution appearances on mammograms.

The breast is composed of approximately 15 to 20 breast lobes extending from 7 to 9 breast ducts (Fig. 3.1). Each lobe has 20 to 40 lobules and branches over a quarter of the breast. In each lobe, a collecting duct starts in the nipple and branches to smaller ducts, each ending in a terminal ductal-lobular unit (TDLU), which is the basic functional unit that produces milk and contains terminal ducts and a cluster of ductules and acini. A normal TDLU size ranges from 1 to 4 mm. The TDLUs and ducts are surrounded by interlobular stroma, extralobular stroma, and fat.

Calcifications forming within the breast ducts and acini/ductules include benign and malignant entities. For example, both large rodlike calcifications from benign secretory disease and fine-linear or fine linear–branching calcifications from ductal carcinoma in situ (DCIS) have pathognomonic morphologies reflecting the shape of ducts or ductules. Their shapes are very different from each other, even though they both form in ducts. The benign secretory disease calcifications are large and rodlike, as shown in Fig. 3.2, because they form in larger ducts (Fig. 3.2A). Cancer calcifications are tiny and irregular because they generally start in smaller peripheral ducts and form in the interstices of cancers within pathologic ducts (Fig. 3.2B).

Calcifications forming in the location of interlobular stroma; in periductal locations; or in blood vessels, fat, or skin are usually benign. By understanding the pathologies in which calcifications form and how they interact with structures in which they develop, one can understand why calcification shapes and distributions suggest either cancer or benign entities.

BREAST DUCTS, TERMINAL DUCTAL LOBULAR UNITS, PATHOLOGY, AND CALCIFICATIONS

Benign round punctate calcifications often form in normal terminal breast acini or lobules. Benign round (BI-RADS size <1 mm for round) or punctate calcifications (<0.5 mm for punctate) are densely calcified and sharply marginated. These calcifications take on the round shape of the acini in which they form (Figs. 3.3 and 3.4).

Calcifications forming in DCIS are not as dense or sharply marginated as benign round or punctate calcifications because they form within central tumor necrosis or secretions. DCIS is a noninvasive cancer, grows within mammary ducts, and is classified into high-grade, intermediate-grade, and low-grade types. The histologic architecture of DCIS includes the *comedocarcinoma*, which describes the appearance of the comedos of thick tenacious material extruding from the ducts on its cut surface at pathology, resembling pimples (Fig. 3.5). The terms *micropapillary, solid,* and *cribriform* reflect the DCIS architecture showing small DCIS papillary extensions into the duct, a solid tumor, or a tumor with little cribriform holes, respectively.

Because DCIS grows within ducts, and because the comedo and micropapillary DCIS calcifications form in the center of the tumor, these calcifications may take on a ductal or linear shape. In cribriform DCIS, calcifications form in tiny tumor holes and take on a round, irregular shape, and are much smaller, less sharp, and more numerous than the benign

FIG. 3.1 Schematic of a normal breast duct. The breast has approximately 15 to 20 breast lobes extending from 7 to 9 breast ducts. Each duct branches into smaller ducts, with the ducts terminating in a terminal ductal lobular unit (TDLU). Note that the branching duct extends over almost an entire breast quadrant and form one lobe (*left*). The ducts branch into smaller ducts, similar to bronchioles and alveoli in the lung, and end in TDLUs. A TDLU consists of a terminal duct, ductules, and acini (*right*). A lobule contains intralobular terminal ducts, ductules, and acini. Each duct and lobule are lined by breast epithelium, which is where breast cancer starts.

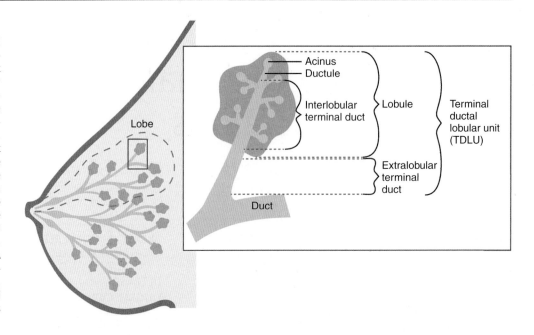

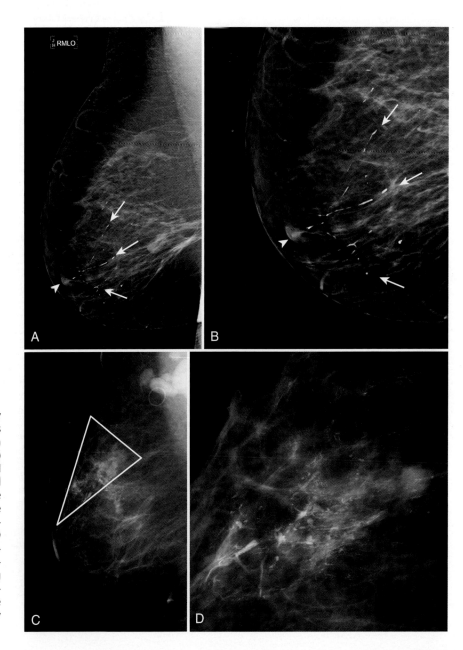

FIG. 3.2 Calcifications along mammary ducts. (A and B) Large rodlike calcifications from benign secretory disease are shown on the mediolateral oblique view (MLO) (A) and the photographically magnified view (B). Large rodlike calcifications (A and B; *arrows*) formed in ducts radiate from the nipple (A and B; *arrowhead*). (C and D) Fine pleomorphic calcifications from ductal carcinoma in situ (DCIS) are shown on MLO (C) and the magnified lateral view (D). Intraductal cancer spread results in calcifications within ducts in linear and branching distributions, and if extensive, forms a segmental distribution (C; *triangle*). Note the axillary lymph node metastases marked by a ring-shaped marker in the axilla in C.

round or punctate calcifications. The DCIS calcifications can be as small as 50 to 100 μm, which is equal to or smaller than the width of a human hair (approximately 100 μm). The classic appearance of DCIS calcification is the fine-linear or fine linear–branching individual calcifications, which have a 70% chance of malignancy (Fig. 3.6A–B). Also, DCIS is typically suggested by calcifications in linear or segmental distributions, in which individual calcifications can have any morphology, including amorphous, fine pleomorphic, coarse heterogeneous, or fine linear/fine-linear branching (Fig. 3.6C–D). Linear and segmental distributions have a 60% to 62% chance of malignancy. Figure 3.7 shows four example cases of DCIS with the correlation of mammographic features and pathologic findings. Not all calcifications seen on pathology can be seen on the mammogram.

Benign milk of calcium forms in enlarged cystic acini or ductules. Large rodlike calcifications representing benign duct ectasia, secretory disease, or plasma cell mastitis form in proximal ducts. Both milk of calcium and ductal ectasia have unique pathognomonic calcification shapes caused by their morphology and distribution, which allows them to be left alone.

Thus individual calcification morphologies and distributions are clues as to whether calcifications are associated with benign or malignant disease based on the anatomic structures in which they form (Fig. 3.8).

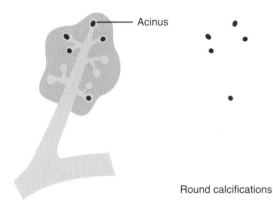

FIG. 3.3 Schematic of round calcifications in benign disease. Calcifications in benign disease form in the acini or lobules, so they look round (*left*). On the mammogram, these calcifications are sharply marginated, dense, round, or punctate (*right*) because they form in round structures.

TECHNIQUE FOR FINDING CALCIFICATIONS

Calcifications are bright white specks, like grains of sand, to be detected against dense white glandular tissue. To find calcifications on two-dimensional (2D) screen-film mammography (SFM), radiologists use a bright light to illuminate the darker parts of the film. They view the mammogram with a handheld magnifying glass, enlarging the image and making calcifications easier to see. On 2D digital mammography, the radiologist adjusts the viewing monitor window and level to optimize the whiteness of the calcifications against the glandular tissues and then views the entire breast in magnified sections. The radiologist uses a systematic search pattern for calcifications to make sure no areas are missed. It is common to search the entire breast in a zigzag pattern or in strips, like mowing a lawn with a lawnmower or searching for a lost boat at sea in a rescue helicopter (Fig. 3.9).

To find calcifications on tomosynthesis studies, the radiologist first reviews the conventional 2D mammogram or tomosynthesis-synthesized 2D mammogram to detect calcifications initially using the method described earlier. The 2D mammograms show a better overall view of calcifications compared with tomosynthesis slices alone. After finding calcifications on one 2D image, the radiologist looks for the calcifications on the orthogonal view to figure out the calcifications' location within the breast and to determine whether the calcifications are grouped or scattered. The radiologist then knows where to search for the calcifications on individual tomosynthesis slices and confirms their location and grouping. Then he or she analyzes the targeted calcifications on the individual tomosynthesis slides in detail and looks for additional findings (Fig. 3.10; Video 3.1). Optical magnification and the systemic search of images using zigzag reading on the tomosynthesis slices are keys to detecting and evaluating tiny calcifications appropriately. Sometimes calcifications are detected initially on tomosynthesis slices because they are shown better than when obscured by overlapping breast tissue.

However, tomosynthesis may not be as effective as conventional 2D mammography in detecting microcalcifications. Tomosynthesis microcalcification detection varies in the literature, partly because of variations in image reconstruction techniques, and placing individual slice combinations into slabs to optimize calcification visualization. A subgroup analysis from a large study in England (Comparison of Tomosynthesis with Digital Mammography [TOMMY] Trial) showed that synthetic 2D plus tomosynthesis was less optimal than conventional 2D or 2D plus tomosynthesis in calcification detection or in detecting 11- to 20-mm DCIS (mostly detected by microcalcifications). Because of this, a 2D mammogram could possibly

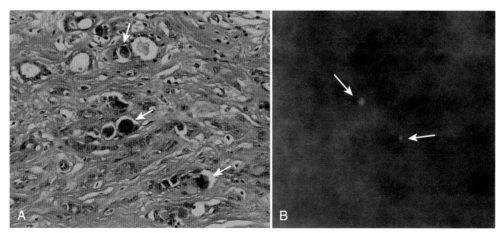

FIG. 3.4 Typically benign round calcifications: microscopic and radiologic correlation. (A) A specimen (H&E stain) shows multiple primary round calcifications (*arrows*) in acini or ductules, seen in sclerosing adenosis. (B) Mammogram shows round benign white calcifications (*arrows*), corresponding to the microscopic findings. (Courtesy Shotaro Kanao, M.D., Ph.D. and Tatsuki R. Kataoka, M.D., Ph.D., Kyoto University, Kyoto, Japan.)

be required for optimal microcalcification detection when using tomosynthesis. Adding 2D mammography to tomosynthesis would increase radiation dose. However, other groups have suggested that the decreased dose from not using 2D mammograms may be worth the trade-off in not detecting a small numbers of DCIS cases (shown by calcifications). Tomosynthesis imaging improvements will continue to evolve, and no doubt there will be continuing changes in viewpoints on the use of synthesized 2D plus tomosynthesis views as the only imaging modality for calcification detection.

After detecting calcifications on conventional mammograms or tomosynthesis, 0.1-mm focal spot air-gap magnification mammography should be performed on all calcifications requiring further analysis (see Fig. 1.2). Air-gap magnification mammography increases the resolution power of the imaging system by about 1.8 times, separates closely grouped calcifications into their individual forms, sharpens individual

Comedo   Micropapillary   Cribriform   Solid

FIG. 3.5 Schematic of architectural pattern of ductal carcinoma in situ (DCIS) in cross section. Note the spaces (*white*) in the DCIS tumors, in which the calcifications form. These calcifications may be amorphous, coarse heterogeneous, fine pleomorphic, fine-linear, or fine linear–branching shapes.

calcification shapes for analysis, and displays faint calcifications not detected on standard mammography (Fig. 3.11). Magnifying screen-film mammograms with a magnifying glass or electronically magnifying digital mammograms makes the original image bigger but does not sharpen the calcification shapes or show faint calcifications displayed only on true magnification mammography.

CALCIFICATION CLASSIFICATIONS BASED ON BREAST IMAGING REPORTING AND DATA SYSTEM 2013

The American College of Radiology (ACR) BI-RADS provides terminology to describe benign and suspicious calcification morphology and distributions on mammography (Box 3.1) as well as associated findings (Box 3.2). The BI-RADS report of calcifications includes size of calcific group, location, morphology/distribution, associated findings, change from previous studies, BI-RADS Final Assessment category, and management recommendations (Box 3.3). The BI-RADS helps radiologists classify calcifications into benign or malignant entities, prompting patient management, and provides powerful descriptors that help clinicians understand the seriousness of a finding. For example, the suspicious BI-RADS calcification term *fine pleomorphic* prompts the radiologist to classify the calcifications into BI-RADS Final Assessment category 4 Suspicious and prompts biopsy. The BI-RADS term *large rodlike* indicates benign ductal ectasia and prompts classification to

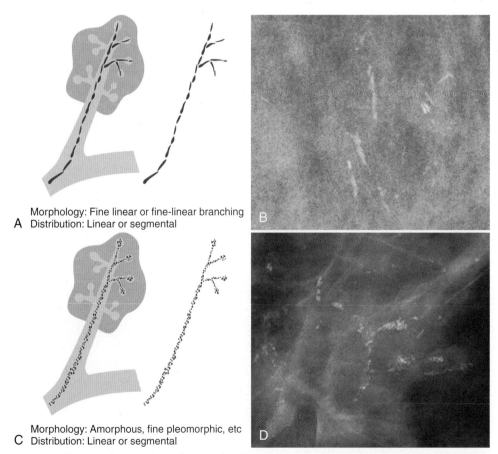

Morphology: Fine linear or fine-linear branching
A Distribution: Linear or segmental

Morphology: Amorphous, fine pleomorphic, etc
C Distribution: Linear or segmental

FIG. 3.6 Classical morphology and distribution of calcifications in ductal carcinoma in situ (DCIS). (A and B) Intraductal spread can result in fine-linear or fine linear–branching individual calcification morphologies when the DCIS calcified necrotic center extends along the duct. This morphology of calcifications is typical for comedo-type DCIS. Schematic (A) and representative case (B). (C and D) However, DCIS does not always produce fine-linear or fine linear–branching calcifications. For example, when calcifications form in lumens or small pockets of DCIS, the morphology of individual calcification particles may be amorphous or fine pleomorphic. If the duct is packed with tiny calcifications, the mammography can show linear (including linear branches) or segmental calcification distributions. This distribution pattern is also suggestive of DCIS components.

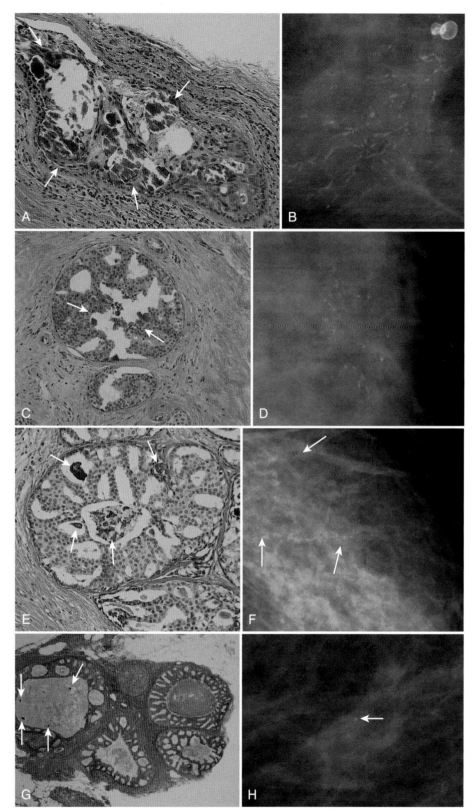

FIG. 3.7 Variety of calcifications in ductal carcinoma in situ (DCIS). Pathologic–radiologic correlation. (A and B) High-grade DCIS with comedo necrosis. Large central calcifications (A; *arrows*) developing in comedo necrosis results in fine-linear and fine linear–branching calcifications on mammography highly suggestive of DCIS (B). (C and D) Intermediate-grade DCIS showing cribriform architecture. Microcalcifications (C; *arrows*) within ducts produces fine pleomorphic calcifications in linear distributions on mammography (D). The linear distribution is typical for DCIS. (E and F) Low-grade DCIS with cribriform and papillary architecture. Microcalcifications in small pockets and central lumens of cribriform DCIS (E; *arrows*) are shown as amorphous calcifications (F; *arrows*) on mammography. This case has no unique findings for DCIS, and it is difficult to differentiate amorphous calcifications in DCIS from amorphous calcifications in benign disease. (G and H) Intermediate-grade DCIS with cribriform architecture. Multiple small microcalcifications (G; *arrows*) are likely caused by the secretions within ducts. On mammography, there is only one calcification seen (H; *arrow*). Note that not all calcifications seen on pathology can be seen on the mammogram. (Courtesy Shotaro Kanao, M.D., Ph.D. and Tatsuki R. Kataoka, M.D., Ph.D., Kyoto University, Kyoto, Japan.)

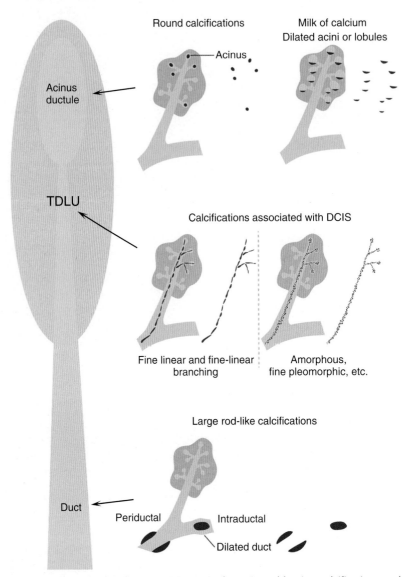

FIG. 3.8 Calcification location correlated to BI-RADS terminology. Round benign calcifications and milk of calcium form in acini or ductules. The ductal carcinoma in situ (DCIS) starts in the terminal ductal and lobular unit (TDLU) epithelium and can extend into ducts. Benign large rodlike calcifications from secretory disease or duct ectasia also forms in or around ducts but are larger, sharper, and coarser than DCIS calcifications. To distinguish benign-appearing from malignant-appearing calcifications, analyze *both* the individual calcification morphology and their distribution.

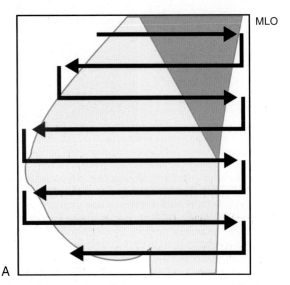

FIG. 3.9 Systemic search to find calcifications on digital mammography. (A) First, do a systemic search in stripes over the entire breast.

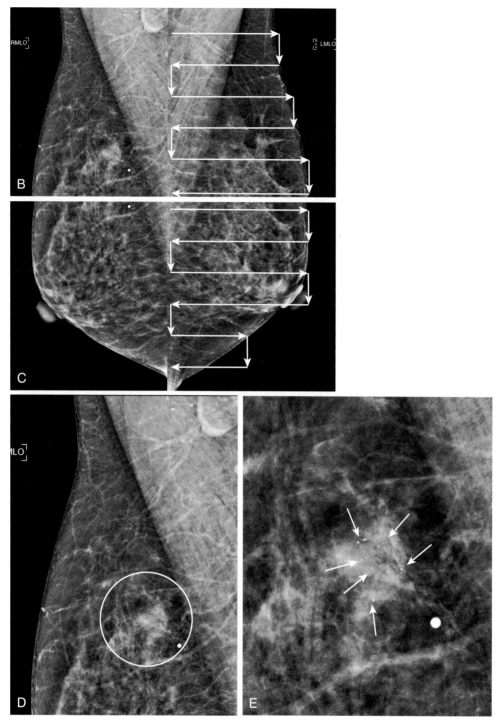

FIG. 3.9 cont'd (B) Second, on electronically magnified views, systematically search the upper half of the magnified breast. (C) Third, systematically search for the lower half of the magnified breast. (D) Then, you can find the calcifications associated with a mass (*circle*). (E) A photographically magnified view of D shows bright white calcifications (*arrows*) within the mass shadow. Biopsy showed invasive ductal cancer. Note that a BB marker is placed at the palpable portion on the skin.

BI-RADS Final Assessment category 2 Benign, return to screening. This chapter will illustrate and classify breast calcifications in benign or malignant categories using BI-RADS terminology.

Typically Benign Calcifications

Recognizing typically benign calcifications as "don't touch" lesions allows the radiologist to leave them alone (Box 3.4).

Generally, benign calcifications are dense and have a unique morphology or location. Classic benign calcifications require no further workup and should prompt no further action. However, some benign calcifications mimic malignant calcifications (Box 3.5), and tiny, subtle calcifications may be difficult to classify as benign or malignant in particular. However, recognizing clues for classification into appropriate BI-RADS lexicon terms may help the radiologist make the correct diagnosis. Box 3.6 shows

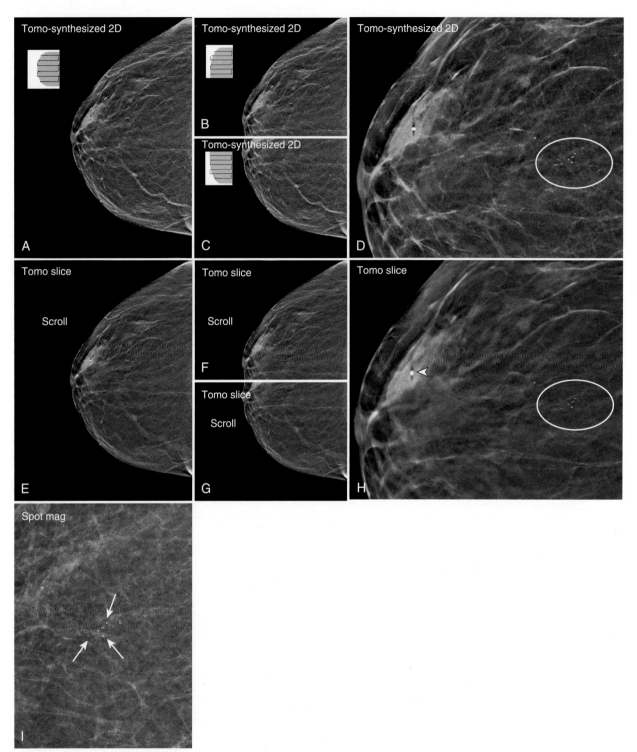

FIG. 3.10 Systemic search to find calcifications on tomosynthesis. (A–D) Tomosynthesis synthesized 2D mammograms of right craniocaudal (CC) views. To detect and analyze calcifications using tomosynthesis, start by reviewing the synthesized 2D mammograms (or conventional 2D). Do a systemic search in a zigzag pattern or in stripes over the entire breast (A), the upper half (B), and the lower half (C) of the magnified breast, using the same process described in Fig. 3.9. The photographic magnification view (D) shows grouped microcalcifications (*circle*) in the middle right breast. (E–H) Key slices of tomosynthesis right CC projection views at the level of calcifications. Try to find microcalcifications in a movie showing all tomosynthesis slices in Video 3.1A (standard view) and B (electronically magnified). First, review the entire breast in slices with scrolling slices (E). Place your attention on the upper half (F) and the lower half (G) of the breast with scrolling slices. Finally, pay attention to the retroareolar and axillary regions with scrolling slices. Then scroll through any suspicious areas with electronic magnification and correlate to the area on the orthogonal view, just like you would with a 2D mammogram. Then direct your attention to the location of the detected calcifications on the appropriate tomosynthesis slices and carefully analyze the calcifications (*circle*) with electronic magnification to determine whether they need further analysis (H; Video 3.1B). Try to find microcalcifications in a movie showing all tomosynthesis slices in Video 3.1A (standard view) and B (electronically magnified view). In this case you would detect and recall grouped microcalcifications initially spotted on the synthesized 2D mammogram. Note a benign round calcification with a linear shadow artifact (*arrowhead*). (I) Spot magnification CC view of the conventional 2D mammogram shows grouped fine pleomorphic calcifications.

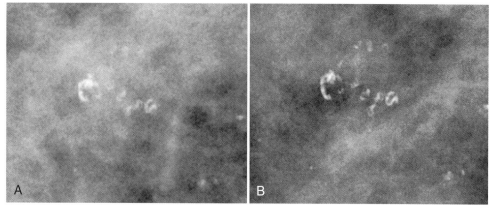

FIG. 3.11 Air-gap spot magnification view using a 0.1-mm focal spot: a technique to visualize calcifications better. (A) Photographically magnified view of conventional 2D craniocaudal (CC) view of calcifications taken with a 0.3-mm focal spot. (B) Photographically magnified view of air-gap spot magnification mammogram of the calcifications with a 0.1-mm focal spot showing the calcifications sharper than the conventional mammogram (A).

BOX 3.1 Breast Imaging Reporting and Data System Terms for Calcifications

TYPICALLY BENIGN

Skin
Vascular
Coarse or "popcorn-like"
Large rodlike
Round
Rim
Dystrophic
Milk of calcium
Suture

SUSPICIOUS MORPHOLOGY

Amorphous
Coarse heterogeneous
Fine pleomorphic
Fine linear or fine-linear branching

DISTRIBUTION

Diffuse
Regional
Grouped
Linear
Segmental

From ACR BI-RADS Mammography, In *ACR BI-RADS atlas, breast imaging reporting and data system*, Reston, VA, 2013, American College of Radiology.

BOX 3.2 Associated Findings with Calcifications

Mass
Architectural distortion
Axillary adenopathy
Skin retraction
Nipple retraction
Skin thickening
Trabecular thickening (breast edema)

From ACR BI-RADS Mammography, In *ACR BI-RADS atlas, breast imaging reporting and data system*, Reston, VA, 2013, American College of Radiology.

BOX 3.3 Calcification Report

Size of the calcific group
Location (right or left breast, quadrant or clock position, centimeters from the nipple)
Calcification descriptors, including characteristics of the worst-looking individual calcifications in the group
Distribution of the calcifications
Associated findings
Change, if previous films are compared
BI-RADS code
Management recommendation

BI-RADS, Breast Imaging Reporting and Data System.
From ACR BI-RADS Mammography, In *ACR BI-RADS atlas, breast imaging reporting and data system*, Reston, VA, 2013, American College of Radiology.

BOX 3.4 Typically Benign Calcifications (American College of Radiology Breast Imaging Reporting and Data System Terminology): Don't Touch Calcifications

Skin calcifications
Vascular calcifications (tram-track appearance)
Coarse or "popcorn-like"
    Fibroadenoma (mass with round, coarse peripheral calcifications)
Large rodlike
    Plasma cell mastitis or secretory disease (needle-like or sausage-shaped calcifications pointing toward the nipple; found in middle-aged women; benign entity, usually asymptomatic)
Round calcifications
Rim calcifications (with radiolucent centers)
    Calcifying oil cysts
Intraparenchymal calcifications
Skin calcifications (obtain tangential views)
Fat necrosis (postbiopsy, posttrauma)
Dystrophic calcifications (be alert for such calcifications in women after biopsy for cancer)
Milk of calcium (linear on the mediolateral view, smudgy on the craniocaudal view)
Suture calcifications (cat gut, postradiation)

BOX 3.5 Benign Calcifications that Simulate Ductal Carcinoma in Situ

SKIN CALCIFICATIONS

Scattered calcifications projecting as a group in one projection
Sclerosing adenosis
Fibrocystic change

INDIVIDUAL CALCIFICATION FORM
Round
Punctate

CALCIFICATION DISTRIBUTION (IF INDIVIDUAL SHAPES ARE BENIGN, STABLE)
Grouped
Regional
Diffuse

BOX 3.7 **Other Typically Benign Calcifications (Non-American College of Radiology Breast Imaging Reporting and Data System Terminology)**

Artifacts (deodorant, hair, fingerprints)
Skin artifacts: antiperspirant, material in moles
Calcifications in the fibrous implant capsule
Calcifications in polyurethane-type implant coverings
Silicon/paraffin injections
Dermatomyositis

characteristics of benign calcifications according to individual morphologies and distributions that distinguish them from malignancy. Artifacts mimicking calcifications are not included in the BI-RADS lexicon, but these fake "calcifications" will also be illustrated in this chapter (Box 3.7).

Skin Calcifications

Skin calcifications are tiny, the size of skin pores, are single or clustered, and often (but not always) have a calcific rim surrounding a radiolucent center. On mammograms, they look like little calcified eggshells within the white line of the skin (Fig. 3.12). Skin calcifications deserve special attention because sometimes they have no lucent center and simulate grouped intraparenchymal calcifications that need biopsy (Fig. 3.13). Attempts to needle localize skin calcifications will result in dismal failures because the hookwire tip will never project onto the calcifications (because the calcifications are in the skin and not in the breast).

Skin calcifications may be diffuse and bilateral, scattered, or occasionally grouped (Fig. 3.14). The radiologist suspects skin calcifications if calcifications are in the breast periphery; if there are other skin calcifications on the mammogram; if they occur at sites where skin touches skin, such as in the axilla, the inframammary fold, in the cleavage areas; or if the calcifications show up on the first or last tomosynthesis slice (that displays the skin; Fig. e3.1; Video 3.2; Box 3.8).

To prove that calcifications are in the skin, one does a "skin calcification study." This is a mammographic procedure in which a

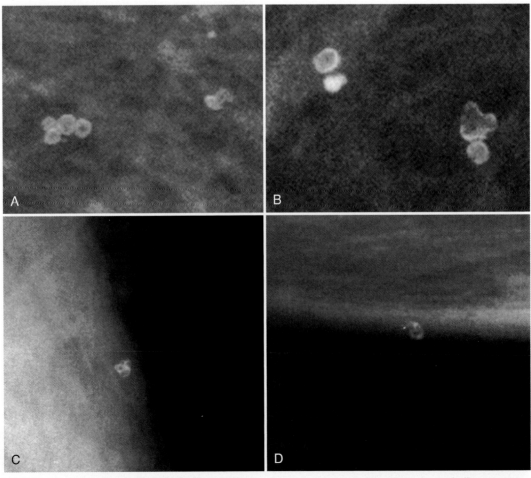

FIG. 3.12 Typically benign: skin calcifications with rim appearances. (A–C) Rim (former eggshell) appearances of skin calcifications show the typically benign appearance of clustered or a single round rim calcified structure with lucent centers. (D) A view tangential to the calcification in C shows the calcifications are in the skin and can be dismissed as benign.

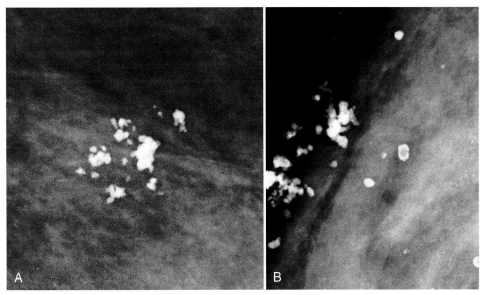

FIG. 3.13 Typically benign: skin calcifications with no lucent center (not rim). (A) Grouped coarse skin calcifications sometimes have no lucent center, no rim, and can simulate intraparenchymal calcifications. (B) A view tangential to the calcifications confirms their dermal origin.

metallic marker, usually a BB, is placed directly on top of the skin containing the calcifications. A technologist takes a mammogram tangential to the BB to show the calcifications in the skin, virtually excluding malignancy.

To do a skin calcification study, the technologist uses a mammographic compression plate containing a rectangular hole that has letters and numbers around the edge of the hole (a "localizing grid"). The technologist places the grid directly over the skin containing the calcifications and takes a mammogram (Fig. 3.15). With the patient still in compression, the technologist looks at the mammogram to find the coordinates of the calcifications. A metallic BB is placed on the patient's skin at the calcification grid coordinates, superimposing the marker on the calcifications. The mammogram is repeated to make sure that the marker superimposes on the calcifications. The technologist then takes a mammogram tangential to the skin marker. Skin calcifications will be directly under the BB in the skin. Intraparenchymal calcifications will be in breast tissue under the marker away from the skin (Fig. 3.16). This process can take from 10 to 30 minutes, depending on whether the facility performs digital (10 minutes) or analog mammography (30 minutes).

It is a common mistake to put the localizing grid on the breast opposite from where the calcifications lie, particularly if the calcifications are in the lower breast. For example, calcifications at the 6 o'clock position (lower breast) will project in the midbreast on a craniocaudal (CC) view. One could mistakenly place the grid on the upper breast, thinking the calcifications are at the 12 o'clock position. A BB placed here will superimpose over the calcifications on the CC view. A tangential view to the 12 o'clock position BB will show no skin calcifications and mislead the radiologist (because the skin calcifications actually lie in the lower breast at the 6 o'clock position). Therefore it is important to look at both CC and lateral views to determine which part of the breast contains the calcifications so that the localizing grid can be placed on the skin containing the calcifications.

Vascular Calcifications

Arterial calcifications have a characteristic appearance of two parallel calcified lines, representing calcification in the arterial wall on edge, with sheetlike calcifications between the lines representing calcifications in the arterial wall en face (Fig. 3.17). Early

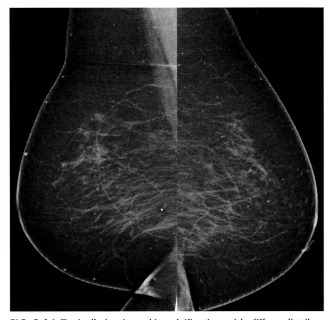

FIG. 3.14 Typically benign: skin calcification with diffuse distribution. Paired mediolateral oblique views show bilateral diffuse skin calcifications that spread toward the axilla regions.

BOX 3.8 Reasons to Suspect Skin Calcifications[a]

Peripheral location in the breast
Location close to the skin surface on one view
Location in the axilla, inframammary fold, or medial part of the breast
Size similar to skin pores
Other skin calcifications present
Location on the first or last tomosynthesis slice

[a]A skin calcification study should be performed to exclude calcifications (see text).

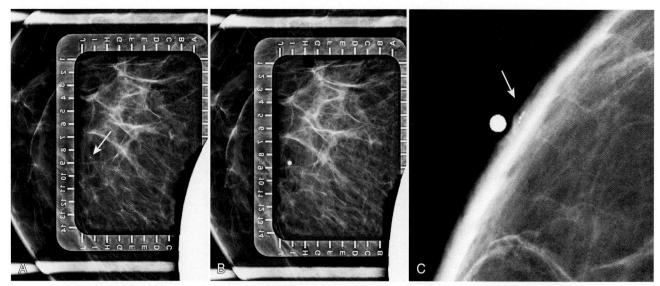

FIG. 3.15 Mammographic skin calcification study proves calcifications are in the skin. (A) For the skin calcification study the technologist places a grid coordinate plate over the skin suspected to contain the calcifications (*arrow*) and takes a mammogram. (B) The technologist places a BB at the coordinates identifying the calcifications, superimposing the BB on the calcifications. (C) A mammogram is taken tangential to the BB, which shows the BB over calcifications within the skin (*arrow*).

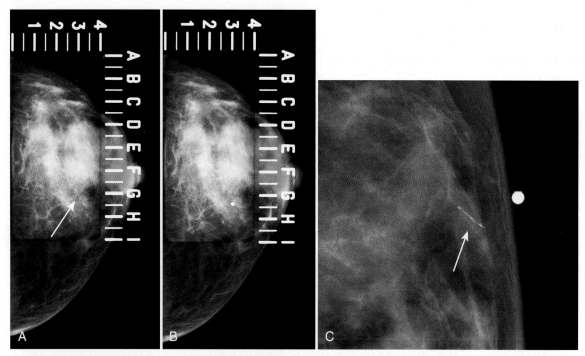

FIG. 3.16 Skin calcification study proving calcifications in breast tissue. (A) Craniocaudal (CC) view shows a grid coordinate plate on the skin over suspicious calcifications (*arrow*). (B) A BB is superimposed over the calcifications by its placement at the coordinates identifying the calcifications. (C) A mammogram tangential to the BB shows the calcification is located in the breast tissue, not in the skin. The calcifications were caused by fat necrosis after trauma.

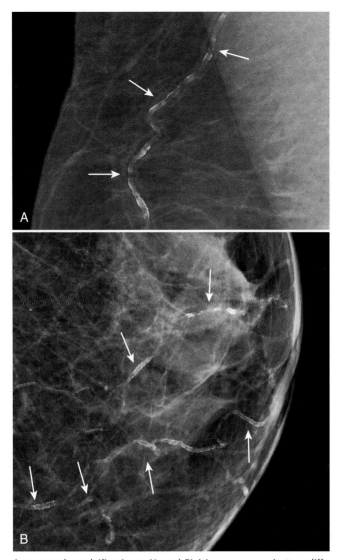

FIG. 3.17 Typically benign: vascular calcifications. (A and B) Mammograms in two different cases show a characteristic appearance of vascular calcifications (*arrows*). Two parallel calcified lines represent calcification in the arterial wall on edge, whereas calcifications between the two lines are vascular calcifications en face.

arterial calcification along vascular walls may simulate suspicious linear calcifications in DCIS. Seeing a noncalcified vessel leading to the calcifications may establish that the calcifications are in a calcified part of the blood vessel. Tomosynthesis may be helpful to visualize the noncalcified portion of blood vessels adjoining the calcified part, which resolves if the calcifications are arterial or not (Fig. 3.18; Video 3.3). Magnification views of vascular calcifications will show arterial tram-track calcifications in two parallel lines, with coarse calcifications en face in the vessel wall between them, and also magnify and separate any grouped suspicious calcifications mimicking vascular calcifications from them (Fig. 3.19).

Coarse or "Popcorn-Like" Calcifications (Calcifying Fibroadenomas)

Fibroadenomas are common solid benign breast tumors that usually form between puberty and 30 years of age. They are benign oval well-circumscribed solid masses equal in density to breast tissue on the mammogram and may have a lobulated border containing up to three to four gentle lobulations. If they do not calcify they are impossible to distinguish from

cysts on the mammogram. Classic coarse or popcorn-like calcifications occurring in involuting fibroadenomas are large, dense, sharply marginated, >2 to 3 mm in size, and usually start at the mass periphery (Fig. 3.20A–B). The calcifications can enlarge and occasionally completely replace the fibroadenoma (Fig. 3.20C).

Fibroadenomas have intracanalicular and pericanalicular forms, are multiple in approximately 10% to 20% of cases (Fig. 3.20D), and result from epithelial and intraductal proliferation of breast elements. Although classic popcorn-like fibroadenoma calcifications are easy to identify as benign, some fibroadenoma calcifications have small, coarse heterogeneous shapes in their early stages and prompt biopsy. Periodic mammography may show slow progression of the calcifications from the coarse heterogeneous forms to the more classic, dense popcorn-like appearance (Fig. 3.21). If the calcifications are not typical for fibroadenomas or if the mass shape or other features are suspicious, consideration should be given to needle biopsy to establish a histologic diagnosis. Otherwise, the classic, characteristic benign mass shape and typical coarse popcorn-like calcifications of involuting fibroadenomas should be recognized and left alone.

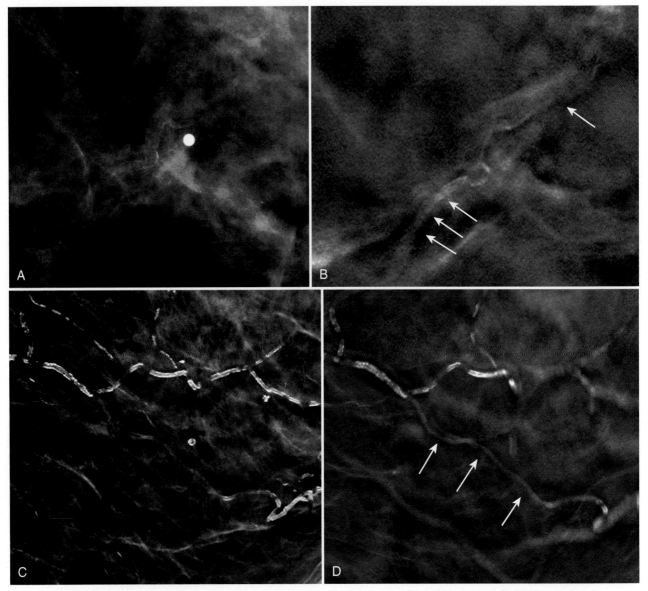

FIG. 3.18 Tomosynthesis slices visualize noncalcified vessels leading to vascular calcifications. (A and B) Conventional 2D mammogram (A) showing vascular calcifications and tomosynthesis 1-mm slice (B) of A. (C and D) Tomosynthesis-synthesized 2D (C) and tomosynthesis 1-mm slice (D) of C in another patient. In both cases, tomosynthesis slices (B and D) visualize noncalcified vessels (*arrows*) and their connection to calcified vessels more clearly than 2D or tomosynthesis-synthesized 2D mammograms (A and C). Tomosynthesis may be helpful when 2D mammograms leave a diagnosis of vascular calcifications in question simply by showing a noncalcified blood vessel leading directly to the calcified portion of the blood vessel. See a tomosynthesis movie of the second case (D) in Video 3.3.

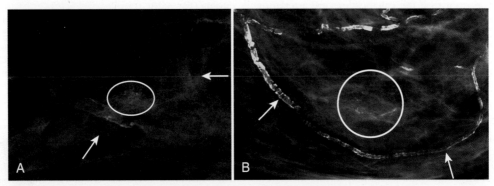

FIG. 3.19 Vascular calcifications with adjacent suspicious grouped calcifications. (A) Grouped amorphous calcifications (*circle*) are distinct from nearby vascular calcifications (*arrow*). Biopsy showed atypical ductal hyperplasia. (B) Grouped amorphous calcifications (*circle*) next to vascular calcification (*arrows*) are easily distinguished as suspicious. Biopsy shows ductal carcinoma in situ. Suspicious calcifications near vascular calcifications are sometimes confused as early faint vascular calcifications.

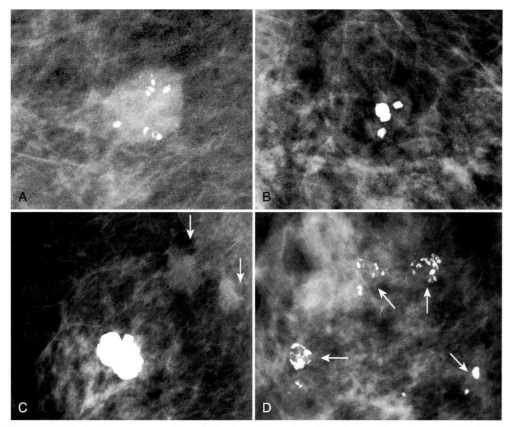

FIG. 3.20 Typically benign: popcorn-like calcifications. Examples of involuting fibroadenoma (FA). (A) Coarse calcifications are seen in the periphery of a circumscribed mass, which is a typical FA calcification location. (B) Typical dense, sharply marginated, round calcifications within a circumscribed FA mass. (C) Dense popcorn-like calcification occupies almost the entire FA mass. Notice the ill-defined cancer masses representing cancer in the axillary tail (*arrows*). (D) Multiple involuting FAs. Notice the coarse heterogeneous or popcorn-like calcifications (*arrows*) in different stages of FA calcification development.

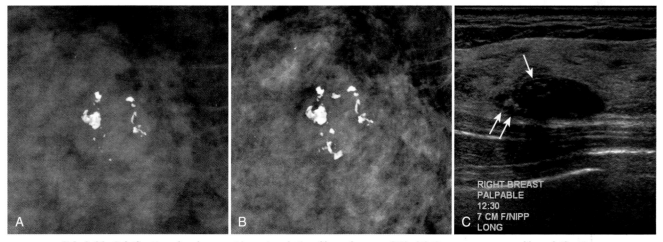

FIG. 3.21 Calcification development in an involuting fibroadenoma (FA). (A) Coarse or popcorn-like calcifications in the periphery of a benign-appearing mass suggest an FA. (B) Two years later from A, the calcifications increase in size. (C) On ultrasonography, bright echoes within the circumscribed oval FA mass indicate calcifications in the mass periphery (*arrows*).

Large Rodlike Calcifications (Secretory Disease, Plasma Cell Mastitis, and Duct Ectasia)

Benign secretory disease, duct ectasia, or plasma cell mastitis is a benign, common asymptomatic periductal or intraductal inflammation of breast ducts in older women that may be unilateral or bilateral. Intraductal inflammation results in calcifications filling the ducts and producing solid, large dense rodlike or thinner rodlike dense calcifications that have sharp margins oriented along breast ducts (Figs. 3.22 and 3.23A–C). Periductal secretory disease inflammation results in dense, sharply marginated sausage-like calcifications with radiolucent centers (Fig. 3.23D). These calcifications usually point at the nipple and line up in the ducts like cars in a train (Figs. 3.24 and 3.25).

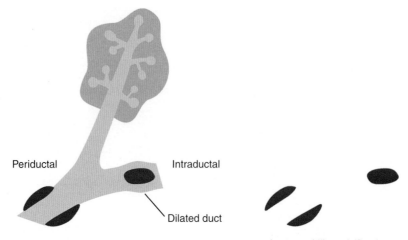

FIG. 3.22 Schematic of typically benign large rodlike calcifications from secretory disease or duct ectasia. This type of large rodlike calcification includes the intraductal type, forming in a dilated duct, and the periductal type, developing along the wall of a duct.

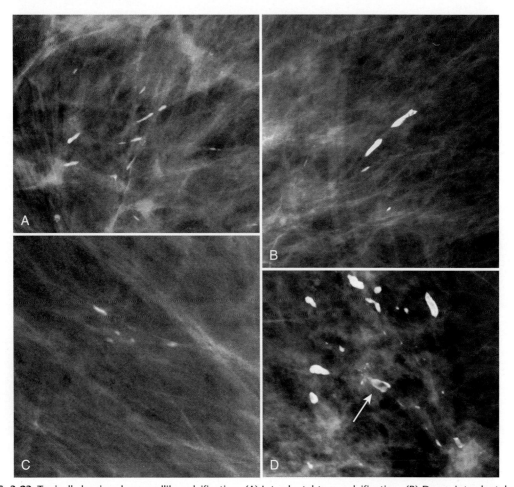

FIG. 3.23 Typically benign: large rodlike calcification. (A) Intraductal-type calcification. (B) Dense intraductal calcification. (C) Early stage of large rodlike calcification. Unlike ductal carcinoma in situ, secretory disease does not usually have many smaller calcific particles associated with the larger calcifications on magnification views. (D) Periductal type calcification (*arrow*). Calcification in the wall of the ducts makes the central lucent appearance.

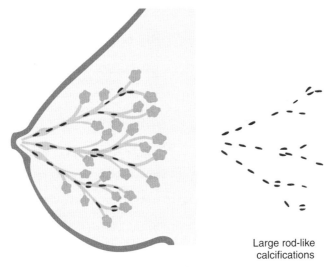

FIG. 3.24 Schematic of large rodlike calcification: distribution. Typically benign large rodlike calcifications of secretory disease are oriented along the breast ducts pointing at the nipple, can usually be seen without magnification, and branch widely over the breast.

Large rod-like calcifications

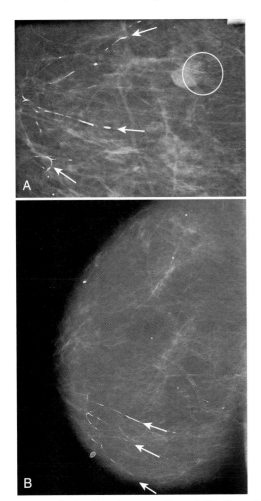

FIG. 3.25 Typically benign: large rodlike calcification, distribution. (A) Large rodlike calcifications (*arrows*) line up toward the nipple and are large, dense, and sharply marginated. Note that there are grouped fine pleomorphic calcifications adjacent that are proven to be infiltrating cancer with ductal carcinoma in situ (*circle*). (B) Large rodlike calcifications (*arrows*) line up in the lower quadrant of the breast in a segmental distribution. However, the calcifications can be dismissed as benign because of the typical appearance of the individual large rodlike calcification shapes.

TABLE 3.1 Secretory Disease versus Ductal Carcinoma In Situ Calcifications

Secretory Disease	DCIS
Lined up along ducts	Lined up along ducts
Point at nipple	Point at nipple
Linear, sometimes branching	Linear, sometimes branching, pleomorphic
Branches over a wide area	Branches many times over 1 cm (ducts are smaller)
No tiny additional calcifications	Magnification shows many more small calcifications
Big calcifications—can be seen without a magnifier	Big and small calcifications
Coarse, rodlike calcifications	Fine, linear calcifications
Sharply marginated	Indefinite margins

DCIS, ductal carcinoma in situ.

Benign large rodlike calcifications can be distinguished from DCIS even though both entities line up in breast ducts and have linear configurations. Benign rodlike secretory calcifications are large, coarse and are so big and dense that they can be seen on the mammogram without a magnifier. They branch widely over the breast, and their individual dense calcifications are separated by millimeters or centimeters (Table 3.1). On the other hand, DCIS calcifications are much smaller and less dense than benign rodlike calcifications, with tiny fine-linear or linear-branching shapes so small that they are best seen with magnifiers. Also, there are so many calcifications within a centimeter of each other that they branch quickly within their group.

Occasionally, duct ectasia, plasma cell mastitis, or secretory disease causes nipple discharge or an associated spiculated mass that simulates carcinoma, resulting in biopsy. Most often, however, the classic features of large rodlike calcifications on the mammogram are well recognized as a benign entity that should be left alone.

Round Calcifications (0.5 mm or Less Is Punctate)

Round calcifications form in round benign terminal breast acini or lobules and are benign (Fig. 3.26). Round calcifications take on the round shape of the acini in which they form, are regular in shape, densely calcified and sharply marginated, and are commonly <1 mm in size but can vary in size if grouped (Box 3.9; Fig. 3.27). Round calcifications are called punctate if they are 0.5 mm or less in size. Round or punctate calcifications can be located anywhere within the breast (Fig. e3.2). Their characteristic appearance suggests a benign diagnosis. They are often in diffuse (Fig. 3.28), scattered, or regional distributions and are associated with fibrocystic change. If they are in a single group and are non-palpable they may be categorized as BI-RADS category 3 Probably Benign and undergo short-term follow-up mammography. However, if they are increasing or new, or in a suspicious distribution (linear or segmental), or associated with a cancer they should be biopsied. On tomosynthesis, some round calcifications can be accompanied with shadow artifacts above and below the calcification, especially if they are quite dense (Fig. 3.29). These artifacts can vary depending on the vendor.

Rim Calcifications (with Radiolucent Centers)

Rim calcifications are eggshell-type calcifications with radiolucent centers and are virtually always benign. They are usually round or oval and calcify along their edges, with the radiolucent center darker than the white calcified rim (Fig. 3.30). They can be small (such as skin calcifications) or a few centimeters in size (such as fat necrosis). Isolated rim calcifications can form around debris in ducts within in the breast tissue, simulating skin calcifications at the breast periphery.

Oil cysts and fat necrosis caused by blunt trauma or surgery appear dark and fatty on mammograms before they calcify and later calcify along their edges from saponification, forming typical rim calcifications (Fig. 3.31). On the edge, the rim calcifications appear curvilinear. En face, the calcifications are sheetlike. Calcified oil cysts distributed diagonally across the breast may be caused by seat belt or steering wheel injuries.

In surgical beds, rim calcifications may be hard to distinguish from calcifications in malignancy. The radiologist should look at the old mammograms to establish where the surgery occurred and see if there was an oil cyst or fat in the area in which the calcifying fat necrosis has now formed to make sure it is indeed benign rim calcification.

Dystrophic Calcifications

Dystrophic calcifications occur in surgical beds of both benign and malignant disease and in areas of trauma. They are common in lumpectomy beds after radiation therapy. Dystrophic calcifications are coarse, sheetlike, and are occasionally accompanied by fat necrosis with lucent centers (Fig. 3.32 and Fig. e3.3). Unlike rim calcifications, dystrophic calcifications do not always have central lucent fat on mammograms. A history of previous surgical biopsy or trauma, when correlated with a surgical scar or area of trauma, should reveal that the calcifications are dystrophic.

On tomosynthesis, the lucent center may be more clearly visualized than on conventional mammograms (see Fig. 3.32), but the margin of the dense calcification may be accentuated by a

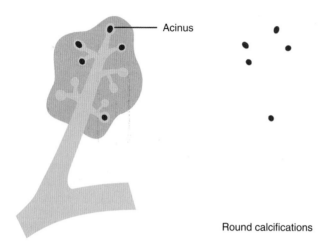

FIG. 3.26 Schematic of round calcifications. Calcifications in benign disease form in the acini or lobules of the duct, so they look round.

BOX 3.9 Typical Size of Round and Punctate Calcification

Round 0.5–1 mm
Punctate <0.5 mm

BOX 3.10 Methods to Identify Posttraumatic Dystrophic Calcifications

Metallic scar marker to show the biopsy site
Look for fat on old films in the region where calcifications now project
Look at old films for biopsied lesions; correlate the scar site with the current location of calcifications

---

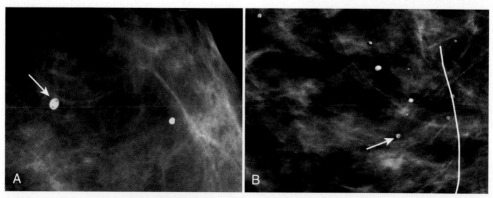

FIG. 3.27 Typically benign: round calcification, examples of primarily round calcifications (0.5–1 mm in size). Dense and sharply marginated round calcifications are scattered in the breast and vary in size (A and B). Some calcifications show a rim appearance (A and B; *arrows*) that may represent calcified dilated ductal structures or oil cysts that are clearly uncharacteristic of malignancy.

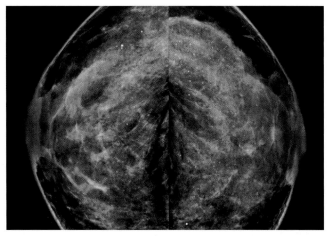

FIG. 3.28 Typically benign: round calcifications, distribution. Bilateral craniocaudal views show round and punctate calcifications in bilateral and diffuse distribution suggesting their benign entity.

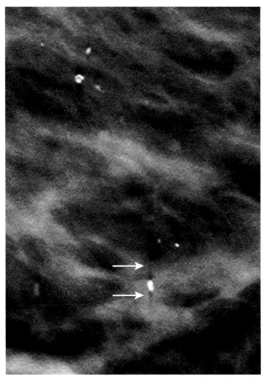

FIG. 3.29 Round calcifications on tomosynthesis. Tomosynthesis may be helpful in distinguishing intraparenchymal calcifications from skin calcifications and to determine whether they are grouped or scattered when scrolling through the tomosynthesis data asset. Note the typical shadow artifacts (*arrows*) above and below a fairly large round calcification.

tomosynthesis artifact, depending on the vendor (see Fig. e3.3). To determine whether suspect dystrophic calcifications are from scarring, some facilities place a radiopaque linear scar marker directly on the patient's skin scar to see if it correlates with apparent postbiopsy scarring on the mammogram (Box 3.10).

Calcifying sutures or benign fat necrosis usually develops 2 years or later after surgery and radiation therapy, with the exception of those forming in accelerated partial breast irradiation (APBI) or intraoperative radiation therapy (IORT), which can form as early as 6 months after radiation. Dystrophic calcifications in postradiation settings may be difficult to distinguish from cancer unless the classic sheetlike calcifications are seen or unless the calcifications calcify densely over time (Fig. 3.33).

Calcifications discovered in lumpectomy beds may also be calcifications in cancer missed at surgery or may be new. Comparing the current study with the prebiopsy, immediate postbiopsy, and specimen mammograms will determine whether all of the calcifications were removed at surgery, were missed, or are new.

The differential diagnosis for new calcifications in a cancer biopsy site is benign postbiopsy dystrophic calcification/fat necrosis calcifications versus recurrent cancer. Radiation therapy fails at a rate of about 1% per year, resulting in failure rates of about 5% at 5 years and 10% after 10 years. If the new calcifications are fine linear or fine-linear branching, fine pleomorphic, or increasing, biopsy should be performed

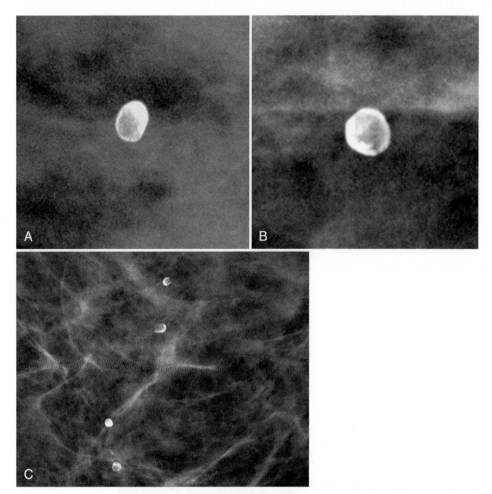

FIG. 3.30 Typically benign: rim calcifications, examples of rim (formerly eggshell) calcifications. (A–C) Magnification views show typically benign small eggshell-like rim calcifications with a radiolucent center that are surrounded by relatively a dense calcific edge.

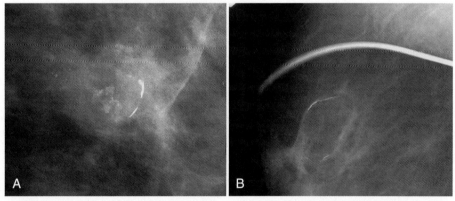

FIG. 3.31 Typically benign: rim calcifications, examples of oil cysts. (A) A photographically magnified view of an oil cyst shows partial rim calcification around a radiolucent center, with plaquelike calcifications seen en face in the calcified oil cyst wall. (B) Lateromedial spot magnification mammogram in another patient shows a thin rim of calcification around a mostly radiolucent oil cyst.

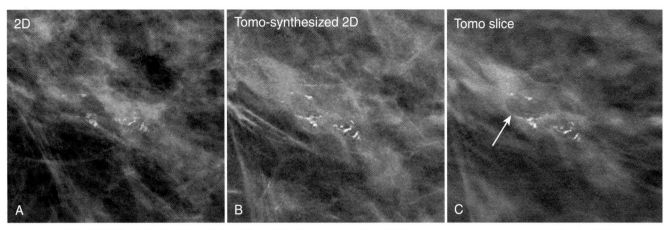

FIG. 3.32 Typically benign: dystrophic calcification, conventional 2D mammogram versus tomosynthesis. (A) Conventional 2D mammogram. (B) Tomosynthesis-synthesized 2D mammogram. (C) Tomosynthesis 1-mm slice. Amorphous calcification surrounding a radiolucent center represents dystrophic calcification in the biopsy site as well as around an oil cyst after breast reduction surgery. The fatty radiolucent center (C; *arrow*) is more clearly visualized on tomosynthesis slice (C) than 2D (A) and tomosynthesis-synthesized 2D (B).

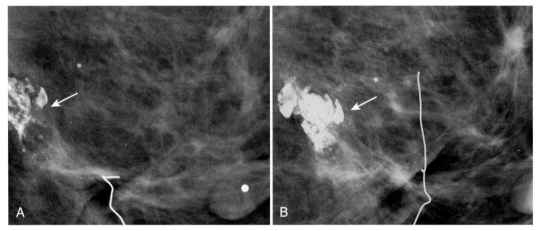

FIG. 3.33 Typically benign: dystrophic calcification, time course. (A) Seven years after intraoperative radiation therapy (IORT). (B) Eight years after IORT in the same patient. Dystrophic calcification (*arrows*) developed and became denser over 1 year.

to exclude recurrent tumor. Because of the problem of recurrent breast cancer in the cancer biopsy site, biopsy may be required for benign dystrophic calcifications that do not have a classic appearance.

A special type of calcification forms after IORT. These are typically tiny, round, and incredibly dense dystrophic calcifications in the biopsy bed. They are so dense they almost look like metal shavings (Fig. 3.34). Unlike whole-breast radiation, which fractionates the dose over 6 weeks over the entire breast, IORT uses more intense, concentrated radiation for several minutes on only the biopsy site and a small margin of tissue around it during the operation. Because breast cancer recurrences most often occur in or around the biopsy site, the rationale for IORT is that it sterilizes only the biopsy bed and surrounding tissues in which the cancer may recur. The advantage of IORT is that it treats the biopsy bed without the collateral radiation of surrounding tissues from whole-breast radiation therapy. Good results with few cancer recurrences have been shown with IORT when synchronous ipsilateral cancers are excluded during patient selection.

Milk of Calcium

Milk of calcium describes sedimented calcifications within tiny benign cysts that are linear on the lateral view (with the x-ray beam directed horizontally) and smudgy on the CC view (with

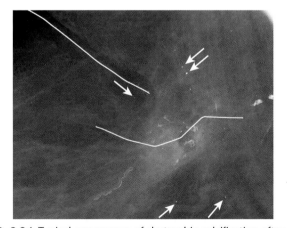

FIG. 3.34 Typical appearance of dystrophic calcification after intraoperative radiation therapy (IORT) in a postbiopsy scar for cancer surgery. There are multiple characteristic extremely dense tiny but scattered calcifications (*arrows*) spread around the dystrophic sheetlike and fat necrosis type calcifications in the surgical bed. These tiny dense punctate calcifications are typical for IORT calcifications and form within 1 year of IORT. Note two metallic linear scar markers over the biopsy site on the patient's skin and two calcified blood vessels inferior to the biopsy site.

Dilated acini or lobules

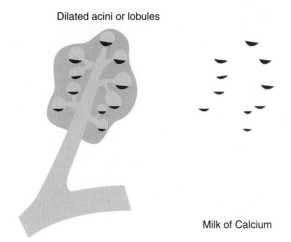

Milk of Calcium

FIG. 3.35 Schematic of milk of calcium. Milk of calcium is sedimented calcifications within tiny benign cysts, enlarged fluid-filled acini, or ductules. Note the crescentic or teacup shape of the calcifications falling to the bottom of the tiny cysts.

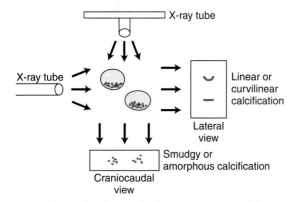

FIG. 3.36 Schematic of milk of calcium in craniocaudal (CC) and lateral views. The schematic shows the sedimented calcium particles appearing linear or curvilinear on the lateral view. En face the calcifications look smudgy on the CC view.

the x-ray bean directed vertically; Fig. 3.35). Milk of calcium is benign and should be left alone. The unique appearance of milk of calcium is caused by tiny fluid-filled cysts containing calcifications that float around the cyst like fake snow swirling in a snow globe. On the mediolateral mammogram in an upright patient, milk of calcium calcifications layer dependently, settling to the bottom of tiny imperceptible cysts (Figs. 3.36 and 3.37; Fig. e3.4). The settled calcifications appear dense, linear, or curvilinear and are always parallel to the floor on the mediolateral mammogram. On the CC projection, the en face calcifications have a cloudlike or smudgy appearance like tea leaves in the bottom of a teacup. In macrocystic milk of calcium, lateral views show both the cyst itself and a typical layering of semilunar, linear, or curvilinear calcifications in the bottom of the cyst. In other cases, cysts in milk of calcium are too small to be seen, and only the characteristic settled linear calcifications on the lateral view indicate their presence. Milk of calcium should be suspected when calcifications are plainly seen on the lateral or mediolateral oblique view but are hard to see or look like a vague smudge on the standard or even magnified CC views.

To diagnose suspected milk of calcium, technologists have the patient stand upright for a minute in light compression in the mediolateral projection, allowing the calcifications to layer dependently in the cysts. The fully compressed mediolateral mammogram will show linear and curvilinear calcification in the bottom of the cysts. Milk of calcium is seen best on magnification 2D digital mammography or the tomosynthesis-generated 2D synthesized view: sometimes the characteristic milk of calcium shapes may not be as apparent on tomosynthesis (Fig. e3.5).

Milk of calcium and DCIS are look-alikes on the mediolateral view but can be distinguished from each other on the CC view. On the lateral view both entities have linear shapes. On the CC view, milk of calcium is amorphous or smudgy, whereas DCIS calcifications retain their linear shapes, distinguishing them from milk of calcium (Table 3.2).

Even though milk of calcium is typically benign and should not undergo biopsy, unrecognized milk of calcium may be recommended for stereotactic core biopsy by accident. The biopsy can be stopped in time if one recognizes milk of calcium in the prone projection. Because patients undergoing stereotactic core biopsy lie prone on the stereotactic table for quite a long time, settled milk of calcium may layer dependently, changing its appearance from that seen on scout lateral views. On the upright lateral view, the linear calcifications are perpendicular to the chest wall and parallel to the floor. On the prone stereotactic mammogram, the

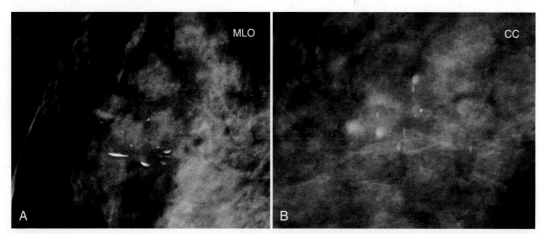

FIG. 3.37 Typically benign: milk of calcium. (A) On the mediolateral oblique view, sedimented calcifications take a linear or curvilinear appearance. Generally, the lateral views are best to see the typical linear or curvilinear appearance, but often oblique views, commonly used in screening mammography, provide enough information to make the diagnosis. (B) En face the calcifications look smudgy on the craniocaudal (CC) view.

linear calcifications are parallel to the chest wall and parallel to the floor. Thus milk of calcium should be suspected if the calcifications change from perpendicular to parallel to the chest wall on lateral versus prone stereotactic mammograms, allowing the radiologist to stop the biopsy.

Suture

Suture calcifications (Fig. 3.38) look like linear or tubular calcifications that sometimes show a knot and represent calcified suture material in the biopsy bed.

TABLE 3.2   Milk of Calcium versus Ductal Carcinoma In Situ Calcifications

	Milk of Calcium	DCIS
Lateromedial mammogram	Linear	Linear
Craniocaudal mammogram	Smudgy	Linear

DCIS, ductal carcinoma in situ.

White Artifacts Simulating Calcifications

Radiopaque materials on the skin can simulate calcifications. The most common artifact is deodorant or antiperspirant in the axilla producing dense particles in axillary skin creases (Fig. 3.39). If one suspects deodorant artifact, the patient washes her armpit to remove any deodorant or antiperspirant and has a repeat mammogram. The deodorant artifact should disappear on the repeat study. Iodine-containing or other radiopaque medicines also produce white artifacts on the skin (Fig. 3.40).

Dermal lesions or warts can retain radiopaque salves in their crevices, simulating calcifications in a mass. Some facilities put radiopaque skin markers on all moles or skin tags to distinguish dermal lesions from masses in the breast (Fig. 3.41).

If the radiologist suspects that a calcified mass is a skin lesion, a look at the patient's breast history sheet to see if there is a skin lesion drawn on the breast diagram where the mass exists on the mammogram may help identify the skin lesion. A direct physical examination also will clear up any questions about skin lesions. If there is still uncertainty if a mass is on the skin or in the breast, a technologist can place a marker on the skin lesion in question and repeat the mammogram. The mammogram should show the BB on the mass, if it is the skin

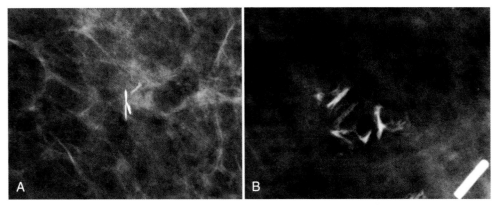

FIG. 3.38 Typically benign: suture calcification. (A) In this case, the suture calcification was observed at the place where a pacemaker was implanted and then removed. (B) In another case, suture calcifications was seen in an irradiated breast biopsy site after cancer.

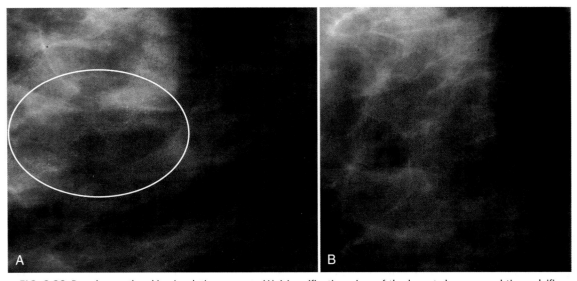

FIG. 3.39 Powder on the skin simulating cancer. (A) Magnification view of the breast shows round tiny calcific particles (*circle*) suggestive of ductal carcinoma in situ, but they were not seen on the orthogonal view. (B) Repeat mammogram after wiping the patient's skin shows no particles, confirming skin powder artifact.

lesion. If there are still questions, the technologist can take a mammogram with the beam tangential to the BB/skin lesion. This should show the mass/BB at the skin surface and no mass inside the breast. If the skin lesion/BB are at the skin surface and there is still a mass inside the breast, then the mass is within breast parenchyma and must be worked up.

Hair artifacts are white, thin, linear, and strandlike opacities near the chest wall (Fig. 3.42) caused when patients with long hair lean forward for their mammogram. Long hair overlaps into the field of view causing the artifact. A repeat mammogram with the patient's hair pulled away from the field of view will eliminate the strandlike artifacts on the mammogram.

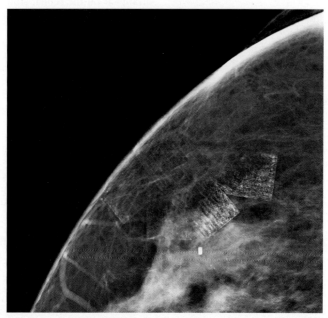

FIG. 3.40 Steri-Strip on skin. Iodine-containing medicine within two bandages placed after core biopsy make white artifacts on the skin. Note the postbiopsy metallic marker underneath the Steri-Strips in the core biopsy site, near calcifications showing ductal carcinoma in situ.

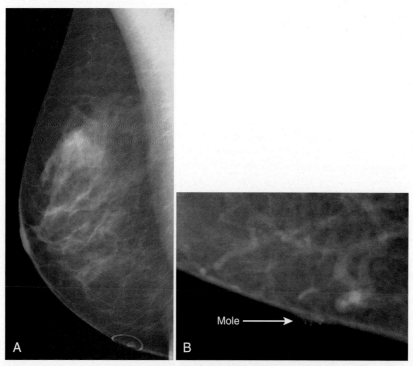

FIG. 3.41 Skin moles. (A) On the mediolateral oblique view, a breast "mass" can be diagnosed as a skin mole because it is marked by a radiopaque skin ring marker placed by the technologist. Visual inspection of the patient confirms a dermal mass and eliminates the possibility of an intraparenchymal lesion. (B) Magnification view of another mole (*arrow*) in tangent shows calcification as debris in the interstices of the mole. The calcifications appeared clustered and within the breast on the orthogonal view.

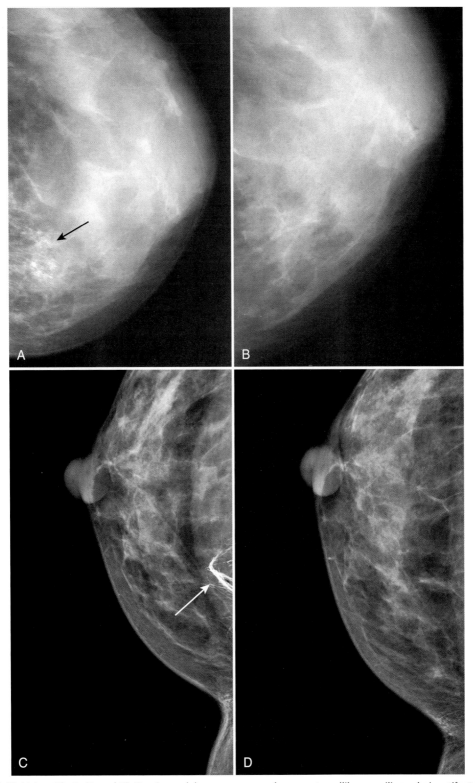

FIG. 3.42 Hair artifact. (A and B) Craniocaudal mammogram shows a strandlike, curvilinear hair artifact (A; *arrow*) near the chest wall over the pectoral muscle. After moving the patient's hair from the field of view, a repeat mammogram (B) shows no hair artifact. (C and D) In another patient, the CC view shows dense hair extensions (C; *arrow*) near the chest wall. The extension artifacts are gone after moving the patient's hair (D).

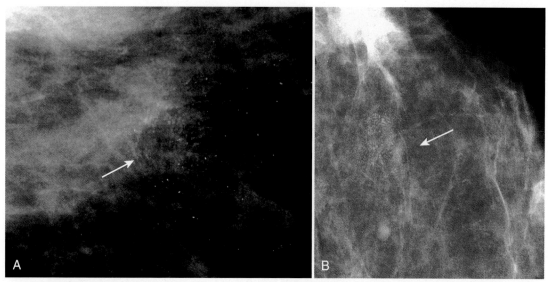

FIG. 3.43 Fingerprints on film-screen mammograms. Whorled curvilinear whitish artifacts on two mammograms (A and B) from two different patients represent characteristic fingerprints (*arrows*) caused by sticky fingers lifting the emulsion off sensitive mammography film.

Fingerprints are seen only on SFM and have a characteristic whorled appearance caused by sticky fingers handling sensitive mammographic films or film-intensifying screens (Fig. 3.43). A repeat film in the same projection after the screen has been cleaned will have no fingerprints in the same location, resolving the issue.

Calcifications from Foreign Bodies (Silicone Injections and Other)

Silicone injection foreign-body granulomas in the breast have a characteristic rim appearance associated with direct injections of silicone or paraffin-like substances into the breast for breast augmentation. Direct injections for augmentation occur in countries outside the United States, particularly in Southeast Asia (Fig. 3.44). Typical silicone injection calcifications appear as innumerable rim calcifications varying from a few millimeters in size up to a centimeter, are packed closely together, and may have a surrounding white fibrotic reaction. These injection granulomas often cause palpable breast masses. Silicone injection calcifications obscure the underlying breast on both mammography and ultrasound, making it difficult to evaluate the breast by physical examination or imaging.

Calcifications also form in fibrous capsules around breast implants. Fibrous capsule implant calcifications are characteristically dense, dystrophic calcifications that parallel the implant envelope (Fig. 3.45).

Objects inserted into the breast cause other foreign-body granulomas or can be seen because they are radiopaque. Foreign objects can be recognized by reading the patient history and by noting the foreign-body shape.

Suspicious Calcification Morphology

Calcifications that are not typically benign require analysis of their location, morphology, and distribution (Box 3.11). In terms of calcification morphologies, *amorphous, coarse heterogeneous, fine pleomorphic,* and *fine-linear or fine linear–branching* calcifications are worrisome for cancer and have positive predictive values for cancer of 21%, 13%, 29%, and 70%, respectively (Figs. 3.46 and 3.47; Table 3.3). Invasive ductal carcinoma (IDC) and

DCIS often contain suspicious calcifications, but calcifications are rare in invasive lobular cancer. Calcifications are also seen in papillary carcinoma, but this is a more rare form of cancer. The extremely rare osteogenic sarcoma of the breast contains calcifications that look like bone. The high-risk lesion, atypical ductal hyperplasia, often contains calcifications. Calcifications are not commonly seen in lobular carcinoma in situ (LCIS), which is a high-risk marker that usually has no mammographic findings and is often an incidental finding on a biopsy performed for another radiologic abnormality. However, there is a form of LCIS with pleomorphic features that does contain calcifications (Box 3.12).

The DCIS produces calcifications primarily within TDLUs that grow along ducts, resulting in a unique appearance of calcifications that can follow any one of the seven to nine ducts arborizing over a breast quadrant (see Figs. 3.6 and 3.7; Box 3.13). Calcifications associated with cancer also form in breast masses representing invasive cancers. The suspicious calcification types are described next.

Amorphous Calcifications

The BI-RADS term *amorphous* describes indistinct, hazy calcifications that are tiny, roundish, flake-shaped particles that are too small and vague to allow further characterization. If they are grouped, linear, or in a segmental distribution, they should be biopsied (positive predictive value [PPV] of approximately 21%, BI-RADS 2013) and fall into BI-RADS category 4B Suspicious (PPV >10% to <50%). However, amorphous calcifications may be thought to be benign if they are diffuse.

Both benign and malignant processes produce amorphous calcifications (see Box 3.7). Benign fibrocystic disease and sclerosing adenosis produce blunt duct extension and ductal dilatation that result in amorphous calcifications (Fig. 3.48). However, amorphous calcifications can also form in atypia (Fig. 3.49) or cancer including DCIS or IDC (Fig. 3.50). This overlap between benign- and malignant-appearing calcifications results in "false-positive" biopsies and contributes to the 75% of benign biopsy results that occur from procedures prompted by calcifications.

Amorphous calcifications are often very subtle and are the most difficult to detect by conventional 2D mammography views.

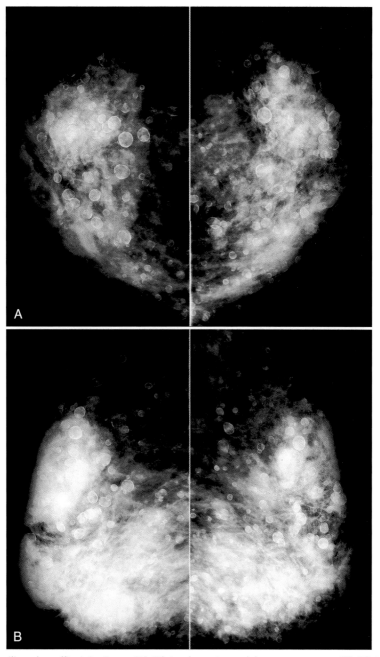

FIG. 3.44 Direct silicon/paraffin injections. (A) Bilateral craniocaudal mammograms. (B) Bilateral mediolateral oblique mammograms. Dense tissue and multiple rim (former eggshell-type) calcifications represent calcifications around silicone injection granulomas forming after silicone was injected into the breasts for augmentation. This procedure is performed outside of the United States.

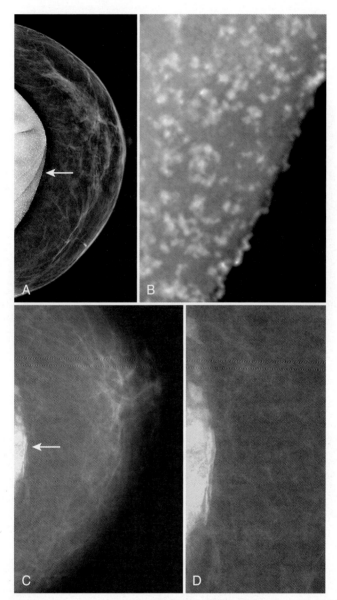

FIG. 3.45 Calcifications surrounding implants. (A and B) (B; photographically magnified view of A), Multiple tiny calcifications formed on the polyurethane-coated outer envelope of an intact saline implant (*arrow*). With the implant still in place, it is easily understood that these calcifications are associated with the implant envelope. (C and D) (D; photographically magnified view of C), This patient's implants were removed but the fibrous capsule that formed around the implant was left in the breast near the chest wall. The mammogram shows the typical sheetlike dystrophic calcification forming in the fibrous capsule that originally surrounded the implant at the edge of the image (*arrow*).

BOX 3.11   Terms for Suspicious Calcifications

INDIVIDUAL CALCIFICATION FORM

Amorphous
Coarse heterogeneous
Fine pleomorphic
Fine linear or fine-linear branching

CALCIFICATION CLUSTER SHAPE

Grouped
Linear (or linear-branching)
Segmental

From ACR BI-RADS Mammography, In *ACR BI-RADS atlas, breast imaging reporting and data system*, Reston, VA, 2013, American College of Radiology.

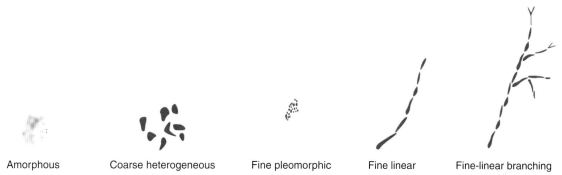

| Amorphous | Coarse heterogeneous | Fine pleomorphic | Fine linear | Fine-linear branching |

FIG. 3.46 BI-RADS suspicious morphology. Suspicious calcification morphology descriptors include *amorphous, coarse heterogeneous, fine pleomorphic,* and *fine linear or fine-linear branching.* (From ACR BI-RADS Mammography, In *ACR BI-RADS atlas, breast imaging reporting and data system,* Reston, VA, 2013, American College of Radiology.)

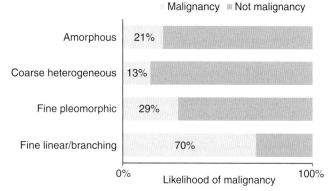

FIG. 3.47 Likelihood of malignancy according to calcification morphology. The values are presented as the percentage of cancer cases among all cases biopsied. (Based on the studies of Libernman et al., Berg et al., Burnside et al., and Bent et al. Modified From ACR BI-RADS Mammography, In *ACR BI-RADS atlas, breast imaging reporting and data system,* Reston, VA, 2013, American College of Radiology.)

TABLE 3.3   Suspicious Morphology of Calcifications Based on the Breast Imaging Reporting and Data System

BI-RADS Term	Morphology	Typical Size	Likelihood of Malignancy
Amorphous	Small and/or hazy appearance that is more specific, particle shape cannot be determined		21%
Coarse heterogeneous	Irregular, conspicuous calcification	0.5–1 mm	13%
Fine pleomorphic	Irregular, more conspicuous than amorphous, no linear shapes	<0.5 mm	29%
Fine linear or fine-linear branching	Thin, linear, irregular	<0.5 mm	70%

BI-RADS, Breast Imaging Reporting and Data System.
From ACR BI-RADS Mammography, In *ACR BI-RADS atlas, breast imaging reporting and data system,* Reston, VA, 2013, American College of Radiology.

BOX 3.12   Cancers Commonly Containing Calcifications[a]

Ductal carcinoma in situ
Papillary carcinoma
Invasive ductal cancer

[a]In invasive lobular cancer, calcifications are very rare.

BOX 3.13   Ductal Carcinoma in Situ

Beware of clusters containing:
A linear calcification (fine-linear or fine linear–branching morphology, linear distribution or both)
Many more calcifications on magnification than initially suspected on the screening mammogram

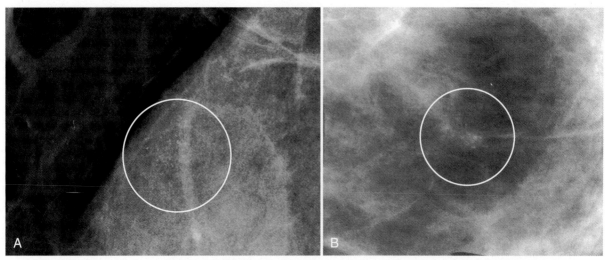

FIG. 3.48 Suspicious morphology: amorphous. Final diagnosis: benign, after biopsy. (A) Benign sclerotic breast tissue (*circle*). (B) Proliferative fibrocystic disease (*circle*).

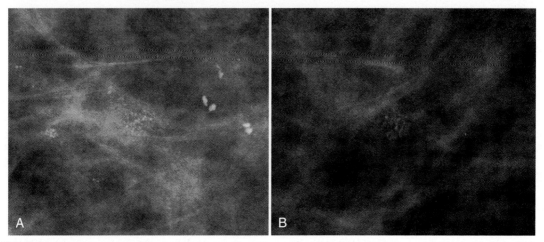

FIG. 3.49 Suspicious morphology: amorphous. Final diagnosis: high risk, after biopsy. (A) Flat epithelial atypia. (B) Atypical ductal hyperplasia.

Both amorphous calcifications and associated noncalcified duct dilatation or masses may be seen by tomosynthesis, but the best way to analyze amorphous calcifications is with 2D magnification mammograms (Fig. 3.51; Fig. e3.6).

Coarse Heterogeneous

Coarse heterogeneous describes irregularly shaped calcific particles that vary in size between 0.5 and 1 mm in size. Coarse heterogeneous calcifications are denser and more conspicuous than amorphous calcifications and tend to merge into each other (Fig. 3.52). They may form inside pockets of necrotic tumors, such as the micropapillary or cribriform forms of DCIS, but are also often seen in early calcifying fibroadenomas or dystrophic calcifications (Fig. 3.53). Although multiple bilateral grouped coarse heterogeneous calcifications may represent bilateral fibroadenomas or other benign entities, an isolated cluster containing coarse heterogeneous calcifications has a PPV of about 13% for cancer (BI-RADS 2013) and should be biopsied if it is not in a fibroadenoma.

Fine Pleomorphic

Fine pleomorphic calcifications are more visible and obvious than amorphous calcifications and are tiny (<0.5 mm or smaller),

but unlike amorphous calcifications they have discrete, individual irregular shapes and do not contain fine-linear shapes, which distinguishes them from the *fine-linear or fine linear–branching (casting) calcifications* (Fig. 3.54). Because fine pleomorphic calcifications have a PPV of 29% for malignancy (BI-RADS 2013), they fall into the BI-RADS category 4B Suspicious (PPV >10% to <50%) and should undergo biopsy. Fine pleomorphic calcifications develop in DCIS or invasive ductal cancer and may grow in breast ducts. Fine pleomorphic calcifications are rarely seen in lobular carcinoma (Fig. 3.54F) but are more commonly seen in atypical breast lesions (Fig. 3.55).

Fine Linear or Fine Linear–Branching

Fine-linear or fine linear–branching calcifications have the highest PPV for breast cancer (70%, BI-RADS 2013) and should be placed into BI-RADS category 4C Suspicious (PPV >50% to <95%). These faint, thin calcifications have linear forms because DCIS grows in branching ducts and the calcifications form within the DCIS, making tiny irregular casts of the duct. They look like little broken needles with pointy ends or may have a "dot-dash" appearance with both round and linear shapes (Fig. 3.56). Calcific casts of tumors growing in duct branches form X-, Y-, or Z-shaped calcifications. All fine-linear or fine linear–branching calcifications should undergo biopsy.

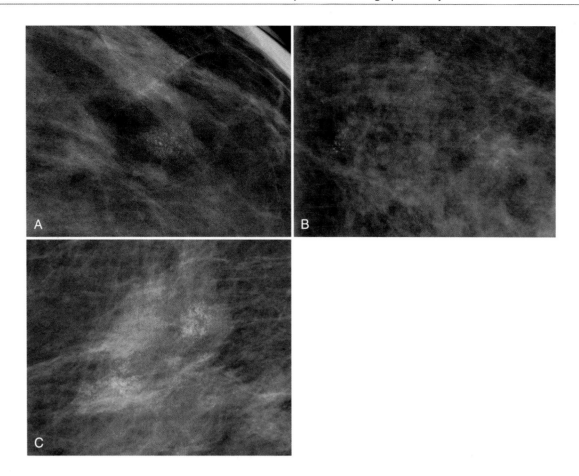

FIG. 3.50 Suspicious morphology: amorphous. Final diagnosis: malignancy, after biopsy. (A) Ductal carcinoma in situ (DCIS). (B) Invasive ductal carcinoma with atypical ductal hyperplasia. (C) DCIS.

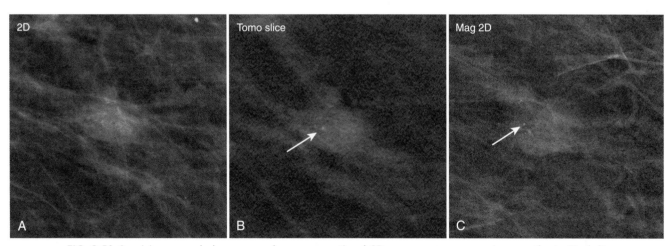

FIG. 3.51 Suspicious morphology: amorphous, conventional 2D mammogram versus tomosynthesis. Final diagnosis: invasive ductal carcinoma and ductal carcinoma in situ. (A) Conventional 2D mammogram, (B) Tomosynthesis key slice, (C) Magnification 2D mammogram. On conventional 2D mammogram (A), amorphous calcification is difficult to be identified. However, tomosynthesis (B) visualizes amorphous calcification more clearly. Magnification 2D view (C) confirms the amorphous calcifications and shows them more sharply.

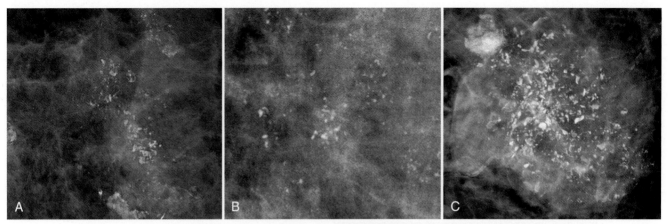

FIG. 3.52 Suspicious morphology: coarse heterogeneous. Final diagnosis: malignancy. (A) Ductal carcinoma in situ. (B) Invasive ductal carcinoma (IDC). (C) IDC.

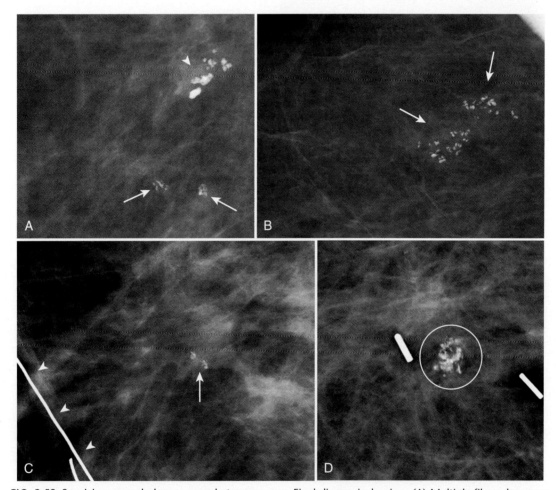

FIG. 3.53 Suspicious morphology: coarse heterogeneous. Final diagnosis: benign. (A) Multiple fibroadenomas. Cluster coarse heterogeneous calcifications (*arrows*) near the typical popcorn calcification (*arrowhead*) were proven to be fibroadenomas by biopsy. (B) Multiple fibroadenomas. Clusters of coarse heterogeneous calcifications (*arrows*) were proven to be fibroadenomas by biopsy. (C) Benign dystrophic calcification. Ten years after surgery and radiation therapy for right breast cancer, a new coarse calcification (*arrow*) was identified at the lumpectomy sited during the annual follow-up. Stereotactic biopsy showed benign calcification without carcinoma. Note that there is a skin marker (*arrowheads*) representing the surgical scar on the skin surface. (D) Benign dystrophic calcification in irradiated breast tissue (*circle*). Note the metal clips after surgery.

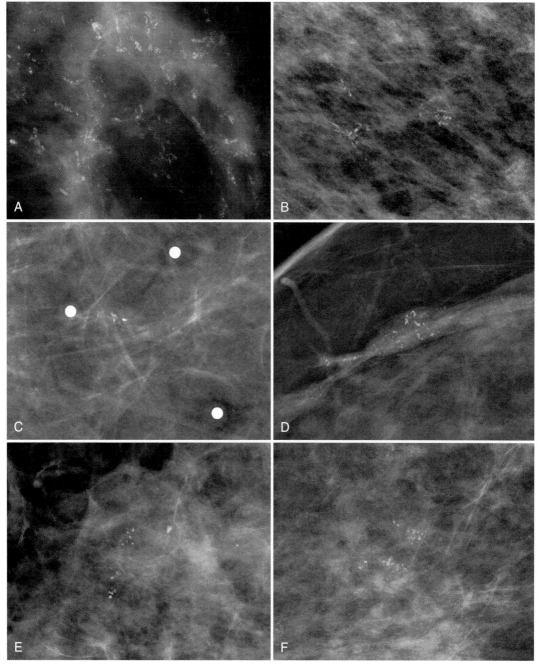

FIG. 3.54 Suspicious morphology: fine pleomorphic. Final diagnosis: malignancy. (A) Ductal carcinoma in situ (DCIS). The fine pleomorphic and amorphous calcifications line up in linear or branching patterns, suggesting intraductal spread of cancer. In addition to the fine pleomorphic calcifications, adjacent groups may be fine-linear and fine linear–branching calcifications. It is not unusual to have more than one calcification morphology in any particular group or distribution. (B) DCIS. The fine pleomorphic calcifications form in tight groups. Some calcifications seem like fine-linear and fine linear–branching calcifications. (C) DCIS. Note three BB markers on the skin. (D) Invasive ductal cancer (IDC) and DCIS. The grouped fine pleomorphic calcifications are accompanied with a small density. (E) IDC. (F) Invasive lobular carcinoma and lobular carcinoma in situ with pleomorphic features. Note that this is a rare case, because calcification is usually not seen in lobular carcinomas.

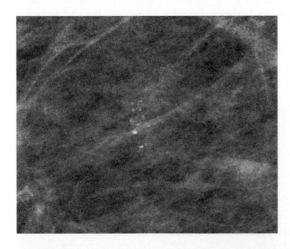

FIG. 3.55 Suspicious morphology, fine pleomorphic. Final diagnosis: high risk. Grouped fine pleomorphic, amorphous and punctate calcifications were atypical ductal hyperplasia by biopsy.

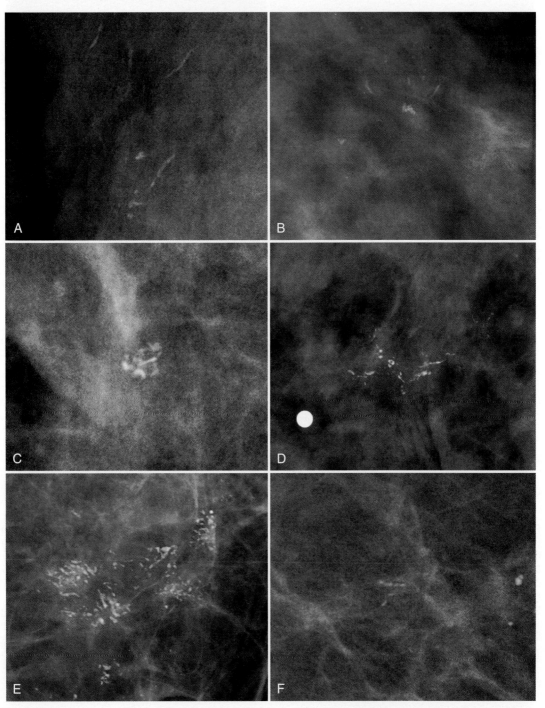

FIG. 3.56 Suspicious morphology: fine linear or fine-linear branching. Final diagnosis: malignancy. This morphology has the highest risk of cancer. (A) Ductal carcinoma in situ (DCIS). (B) DCIS. (C) DCIS and invasive ductal carcinoma (IDC). (D) IDC and DCIS. Note a BB skin marker. (E) DCIS with microscopic IDC and lobular carcinoma in situ. (F) IDC.

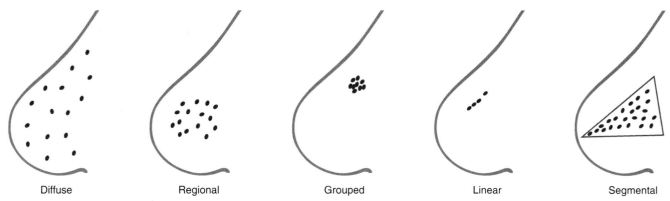

FIG. 3.57 BI-RADS Calcification Distributions. Distribution of calcifications is classified into the five types, including diffuse, regional, grouped, linear, and segmental. (From ACR BI-RADS Mammography, In *ACR BI-RADS atlas, breast imaging reporting and data system,* Reston, VA, 2013, American College of Radiology.)

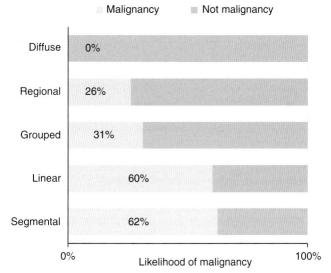

FIG. 3.58 Likelihood of malignancy according to the distribution pattern of calcifications. The values are presented as the percentage of cancer cases among all cases biopsied, based on the studies of Libernman et al., Burnside et al., and Bent et al. (Modified from ACR BI-RADS Mammography, In *ACR BI-RADS atlas, breast imaging reporting and data system,* Reston, VA, 2013, American College of Radiology.)

TABLE 3.4   Distribution of Calcifications Based on Breast Imaging Reporting and Data System

BI-RADS Term	Distribution	Typical Dimension	Likelihood of Malignancy
Diffuse	Throughout the breast		0%
Regional	In a large proportion of breast tissue	>2 cm in greatest dimension	26%
Grouped	In a small portion of breast tissue	<2 cm in greatest dimension (minimum 5 calcifications within 1 cm)	31%
Linear	In a line		60%
Segmental	In a segmental distribution area of concern		62%

BI-RADS, Breast Imaging Reporting and Data System.
From ACR BI-RADS Mammography, In *ACR BI-RADS atlas, breast imaging reporting and data system,* Reston, VA, 2013, American College of Radiology.

Calcification Distribution

The ACR BI-RADS lexicon terms for the arrangement of calcifications in the breast include *diffuse, regional, grouped, linear,* and *segmental* (Fig. 3.57). Among them, terms suspicious for cancer are *grouped, linear* (calcifications in a line that may show branching), and *segmental* (Fig. 3.58; Table 3.4). This is because the calcifications in these distributions may reflect cancer growing in diseased breast ducts within a specific breast lobe, the so-called "sick lobe," as described by Tot and Gere (2008). Generally, the decision to biopsy calcifications is based on the worst features of the individual calcification forms, their distribution within the breasts, if they are new or increase in number, the clinical scenario, and whether they are associated with a palpable mass.

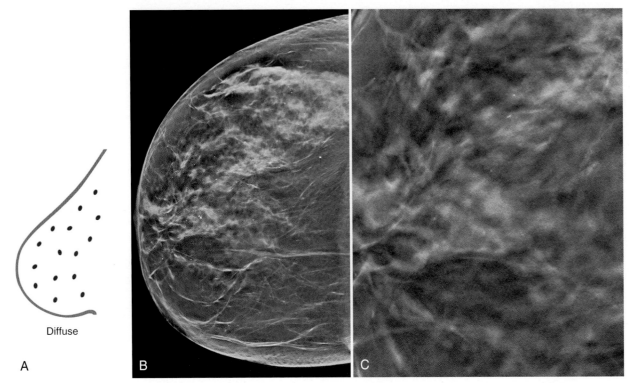

FIG. 3.59 Diffuse distribution of calcifications. (A) Schematic of diffuse distribution of calcifications. Diffusely distributed calcifications are not uncommon in the breasts bilaterally and are almost always benign. (B and C) A case with diffuse calcifications. Tomosynthesis-synthesized 2D view (B) shows diffuse, scattered calcifications. A tomosynthesis 1-mm slice (C) confirms that the calcifications lie within the breast parenchyma and not the skin, are diffuse and scattered throughout the breast, and are not grouped.

Grouped intraparenchymal calcifications are more suspicious for cancer than *diffuse* scattered calcifications. BI-RADS terms suggesting benign calcification distributions include *diffuse* and *regional.*

Diffuse

The *diffuse* pattern suggests innumerable scattered and occasionally clustered calcifications widely dispersed over the breasts and often reflects benign processes, which are also often spread widely throughout both breasts (Fig. 3.59). Calcifications widely distributed in both breasts are usually caused by fibrocystic change. Diffuse extensive benign-appearing calcifications in both breasts rarely represent breast cancer. Sigfusson et al. (1983) also showed that if there were immense numbers of calcifications, and particularly if they were diffusely scattered throughout the breast, they were most likely benign. This is true only if the individual calcification shapes are also benign in appearance.

Regional

Regional calcifications extend over more than one ductal distribution and are typically >2 cm in the greatest dimension and occupy a fairly large breast volume (Box 3.14; Fig. 3.60). On tomosynthesis, thick slabs or a synthesized 2D view may be helpful in identifying their distribution compared with thin slices (Fig. e3.7). However, the analysis of regional calcifications should include the individual calcification forms as well as their distribution to decide if they are benign.

Grouped

Grouped calcifications are clustered calcifications, typically covering <2 cm in their greatest dimension, with comparatively few calcific particles that cluster close to each other within 1 cm

of each other or form a group (Fig. 3.61). Isolated calcification groups suggest an isolated disease process in a small volume of tissue, representing DCIS, invasive cancer, fibrocystic change, papilloma, or sclerosing adenosis. The PPV for grouped calcifications is 31% (BI-RADS 2013).

To be considered a suspicious *group,* the calcifications should be grouped on two orthogonal views. Calcifications grouped on one view and dispersed on the orthogonal view are a fake group (Fig. 3.62). To prove that clustered calcifications are truly grouped together, the radiologist looks for similar-appearing clustered calcifications over the same volume of tissue at the same distance from the nipple on two 90-degree views. If the cluster is tightly packed on orthogonal views, it is a true cluster and should be assessed further. If the group is tightly packed on one view and scattered on the other view, it represents a superimposition of calcifications (a fake group) and can be dismissed. Grouped versus dispersed calcifications can also be confirmed on tomosynthesis, with grouped calcifications lying close together on orthogonal tomosynthesis views and dispersed calcifications being far apart on individual slices.

Calcifications forming in a localized malignancy are tightly clustered, vary in size and shape, and have bizarre irregular or linear forms. A suspicious cluster consists of at least five discrete particles smaller than 0.5 mm distributed over a 1-cm^3 region (see Box 3.14). Calcifications that meet these criteria and do not have a characteristic benign appearance should be viewed with suspicion and undergo biopsy (Fig. 3.63).

BOX 3.14 Typical Dimension of Regional and Grouped Calcification

Regional >2 cm
Grouped <2 cm (minimum five calcifications within 1 cm)

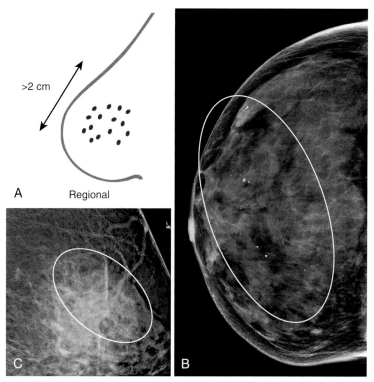

FIG. 3.60 Regional distribution of calcifications. (A) Schematic of regional distribution of calcifications. The greatest dimension is >2 cm. (B) Representative case with round and punctate calcifications in a regional distribution, suggesting the benign entity. (C) Another case of regional punctate calcification. Biopsy showed benign calcification.

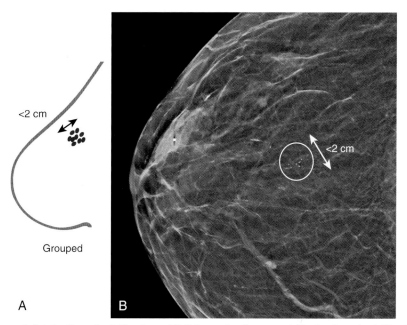

FIG. 3.61 Grouped distribution of calcifications. (A) Schematic of grouped distribution of calcifications. Grouped calcifications means relatively few calcifications that occupy a small portion of breast tissue within 2 cm of each other. The lower limit for use of this descriptor is five calcifications grouped within 1 cm of each other or when a definable pattern is identified. (B) Representative case with grouped calcifications. Note a BB marker on the skin surface near the nipple.

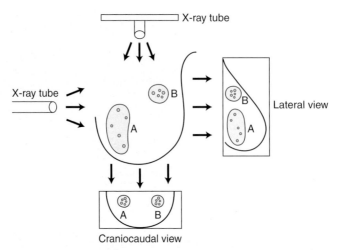

FIG. 3.62 Grouped calcifications must be seen on both orthogonal 2D views to prove they are a group. In this example, the craniocaudal (CC) mammogram shows the scattered calcifications (lesion *A*) and grouped calcifications (lesion *B*) as tightly clustered. This is because the scattered calcifications in *A* superimpose on each other, making a fake group on the CC view. On the lateral view, scattered calcifications in *A* are dispersed and no longer hang together, proving that they are a fake group. On the other hand, the true group *B* persists as a tight cluster on both the lateral and the CC view.

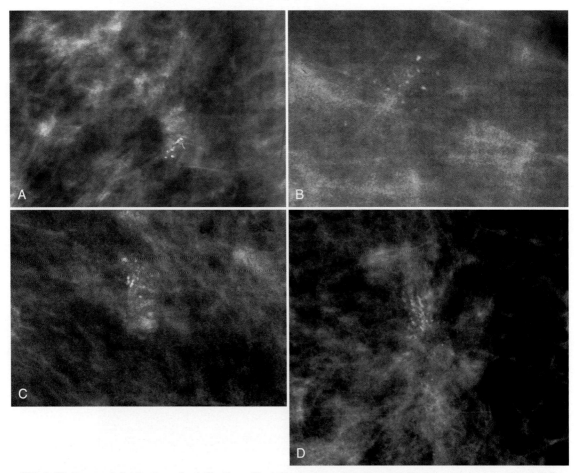

FIG. 3.63 Grouped distribution of calcifications. Final diagnosis: malignancy. (A) Ductal carcinoma in situ (DCIS). (B) DCIS. (C) Lobular carcinoma in situ. (D) Invasive ductal carcinoma. In all cases (A–D), these grouped calcifications include fine pleomorphic calcifications that should be biopsied. In addition, suspicious architectural distortion is observed in D. Grouped calcifications that are new or increasing in number, or whose individual calcification morphologies are not typically benign, should be viewed with suspicion and biopsied.

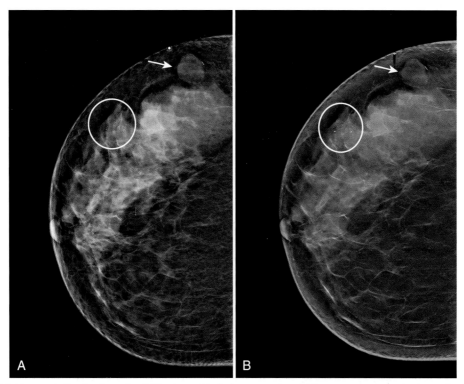

FIG. 3.64 Grouped distribution of calcifications *(circles):* conventional 2D versus tomosynthesis-synthesized 2D. (A) Right craniocaudal (CC) conventional mammogram. (B) Right CC tomosynthesis-synthesized 2D view. The contrast of grouped calcification against the background breast tissue is better on tomosynthesis-synthesized 2D mammogram (B) compared with conventional 2D mammogram (A). The brightness of calcifications can be selectively enhanced in tomosynthesis with its image-processing algorithm. A 7-mm area of grouped fine pleomorphic calcification was proven to be invasive ductal cancer by biopsy. A low-density mass in the outer breast was a cyst *(arrows).*

When analyzing a calcific group, one looks at both the individual calcification forms and the overall cluster shape. Lanyi (1988) suggested that the overall cluster shape is especially suspicious if it has a swallowtail, or V, shape, because it suggests cancer in tumor-packed branching ducts. On the other hand, calcifications forming in round clusters may be forming in acini and be benign, especially if the individual calcifications within the cluster are also benign appearing.

The number of calcifications in a group is as important as the individual calcification shapes. Sigfusson et al. (1983) reviewed thousands of calcification clusters on mammograms and showed that clusters containing fewer than five calcifications rarely represented cancer on biopsy. Based on this observation, biopsy of these calcification clusters is unlikely to yield cancer. Biopsy of a cluster containing fewer than five calcifications should be undertaken only if the individual calcification forms are extremely suspicious or if the calcifications present themselves within a suspicious clinical scenario.

Sigfusson et al. (1983) also showed that cancer was more likely with increased numbers of calcifications in the cluster. In clinical practice, calcifications are particularly worrisome if magnification shows many more tiny calcifications than originally suspected on the standard mammogram or if one or more of the calcifications has fine-linear or linear-branching forms.

It is not easy to find small groups of calcifications, especially when they have amorphous or fine pleomorphic shapes. Along with spot magnification views (see Fig. 3.11), tomosynthesis or tomosynthesis-synthesized 2D views might be helpful in detecting grouped calcifications, because tomosynthesis can enhance the brightness of calcifications against background breast tissue with the advanced image processing algorithms (Fig. 3.64).

Linear

The ACR BI-RADS distribution term *linear* is suspicious because it suggests a process within a duct and its branches and has a high PPV for cancer (60%, BI-RADS 2013). This term describes calcifications in a line and can contain any type of calcification morphology (Fig. 3.65). Linear calcifications can represent tumor in a duct (Fig. 3.66) or a focal benign process. Calcifications with suspicious individual morphologies in a linear distribution should be biopsied, and, on tomosynthesis, occasionally may display the noncalcified tumor-packed duct around the suspicious calcifications. Both large rodlike calcifications and vascular calcifications may be arrayed in a line, but their morphology should distinguish them as typically benign and allow them to be ignored. Early vascular calcification can simulate cancer if the artery calcifies on only one edge. To avoid doing an unnecessary biopsy on a vascular calcification, look for a sharply marginated noncalcified blood vessel approaching the suspect linear calcification to see if it lines up with an arterial wall.

Segmental

A *segmental* distribution is suspicious for cancer because it suggests a process within a branch and its ducts and has the highest PPV for cancer (62%, BI-RADS 2013; Fig. 3.67). Segmental calcifications cover slightly less than a quadrant and form in a triangle with its apex pointing at the nipple (Fig. e3.8). Although typically benign calcifications like large rodlike calcifications frequently distribute in a segmental distribution, their characteristic morphology allows them to be dismissed. However, fine pleomorphic or coarse heterogeneous calcifications, or even amorphous or punctate calcifications, should be viewed with suspicion for extensive multifocal cancer, especially if the calcifications are asymmetric and localized to one segment.

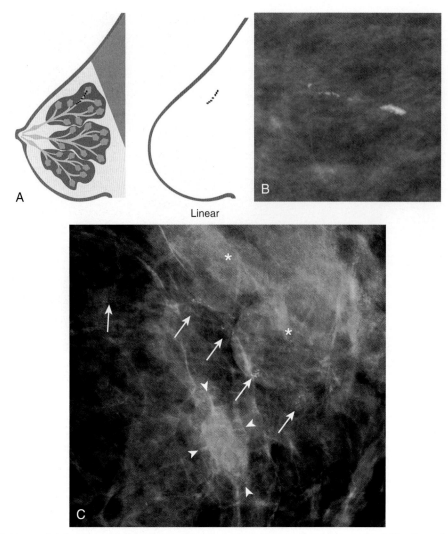

Linear

FIG. 3.65 Linear distribution of calcifications. (A) Schematic of linear distribution of calcifications. A linear distribution indicates extension of pathology along the mammary ducts. (B) Representative case with fine-linear or fine linear–branching and amorphous calcification in a linear distribution. Biopsy showed ductal carcinoma in situ (DCIS). (C) Another representative case with multiple grouped calcifications in a linear distribution (*arrows*). Each calcification particle shows fine pleomorphic and fine-linear or fine linear–branching morphology. Pathology showed DCIS associated with an invasive ductal cancer mass (*arrowheads*). Low-density masses with smooth margins were cysts on ultrasound (*asterisks*).

STABLE SUSPICIOUS CALCIFICATIONS

Although the stability of *benign-appearing* calcifications over time on several mammograms usually indicates that the calcifications are associated with a benign process, the stability of *suspicious calcifications* does not indicate they are benign. Although it is true that calcifications in cancer are usually new or increase over time, suspicious calcifications in cancer can be stable over time even if they have suspicious morphologies as described earlier.

A study by Lev-Toaff et al. (1994) looked at old mammograms of suspicious calcifications in DCIS or invasive cancer to see how long the suspicious calcifications were present and if they increased on serial mammograms. They showed that suspicious calcifications could be stable over a 6- to 50-month period, and yet they were still cancer when finally biopsied. The suspicious calcifications were more likely to be associated with invasive cancer than with DCIS if they increased in number. These findings indicate that suspicious calcifications should be biopsied, even if present on prior mammograms, and even if they are stable.

BREAST IMAGING REPORTING AND DATA SYSTEM CATEGORY 3 CALCIFICATIONS (GROUPED PUNCTATE) AND MANAGEMENT

Solitary grouped punctate calcifications may be classified into BI-RADS category 3 Probably Benign if they are nonpalpable, stable, or seen for the first time, and have been evaluated with magnification mammography. Brenner and Sickles (1989) showed that periodic mammographic follow-up for lesions thought to be benign is an acceptable management strategy if the findings fulfill all criteria for the probably benign lesion (Box 3.15). Specifically, the finding must be nonpalpable and one of three types: (1) a solitary group of round or punctate benign-appearing calcifications, (2) a noncalcified circumscribed solitary solid mass, or (3) an asymmetry (previously a focal asymmetry in BI-RADS 2004) without other associated mammographic abnormality. Periodic follow-up at 6 months and yearly follow-up for 2 to 3 years is the standard of care for BI-RADS category 3 calcifications if they have no malignant features and are stable at surveillance. At the

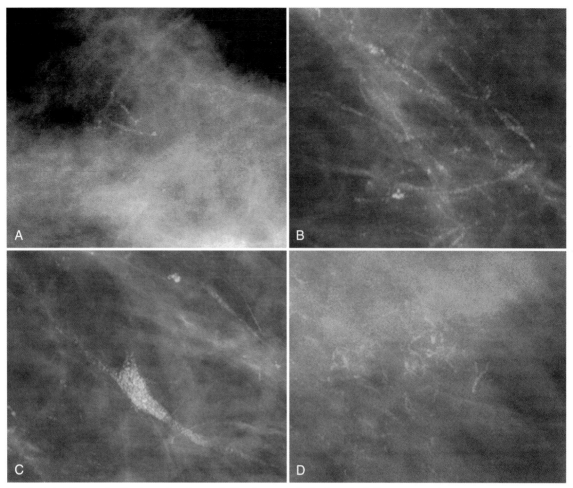

FIG. 3.66 Linear distribution of various calcification morphologies. Final diagnosis: malignancy. (A) Amorphous calcifications are growing in a V-shaped linear pattern. Note the oil cyst and other nonspecific calcifications near the ductal carcinoma in situ (DCIS). (B) DCIS. Amorphous calcifications in a linear distribution with a branch. (B and C) DCIS associated with invasive ductal cancer. Amorphous calcifications growing in a linear distribution with several branches (B) and in a Y-shaped linear pattern (C), suggesting calcifications packed in a duct. In this patient (B and C), the linear patterns extended into a larger segmental distribution. (D) DCIS. Fine-linear or fine linear–branching and fine pleomorphic calcifications in linear patterns suggesting branching ducts.

BOX 3.15   Probably Benign Lesions (All Nonpalpable, *Not* New, Terminology Modified to Accommodate 2013 American College of Radiology Breast Imaging Reporting and Data System Lexicon)

Solitary group of round or punctate calcifications
Solitary well-defined circumscribed noncalcified solid masses
Single areas of asymmetry without accompanying mammographic abnormality

From Sickles EA, Periodic mammographic follow-up of probably benign lesions: results in 3,184 consecutive cases, *Radiology* 179(2):463-468, 1991.

end of follow-up the calcifications should be changed to BI-RADS category 2 Benign.

New, palpable, increasing, or pleomorphic calcifications do not fulfill criteria for the "probably benign" BI-RADS category 3 and should be biopsied. Two studies, one by Lehman et al. (2008) and another by Rosen et al. (2002), looked at BI-RADS category 3 lesions that were later found to be cancer. They found that the "BI-RADS category 3" lesions actually did *not* fit "probably benign" criteria in retrospect. These cancers mistakenly categorized as BI-RADS category 3 had new or increasing calcifications, masses that were suspicious, had a new or growing mass, had palpable findings, or had asymmetries with spiculations or suspicious calcifications.

Short-term follow-up is an option for grouped punctate calcifications only if the likelihood is high that the calcifications will *not* change and the patient is likely to return for periodic imaging. If this alternative is chosen, careful documentation of each follow-up visit is especially important in practices that accept self-referred women for legal reasons. In self-referred cases, the radiologist becomes the "referring physician" and assumes primary care of the woman.

ULTRASOUND IN EVALUATION OF CALCIFICATIONS

Scientific studies show that high-resolution ultrasound can detect calcifications in the breast (Fig. 3.68) or detect masses that have caused the calcifications (Fig. 3.69). Often, however, the normal background speckle of breast parenchyma on ultrasound masks calcifications, especially if the calcifications are alone and there is no mass associated with them. Some investigators suggest that ultrasound scans in the region of calcifications are helpful if the

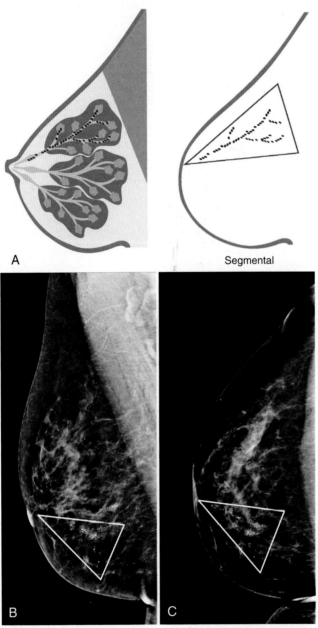

FIG. 3.67 Segmental distribution of calcifications. (A) When ductal carcinoma in situ (DCIS) grows and calcifies in an entire breast duct of a lobe (*left*), the resulting calcifications on mammography can show a segmental distribution that looks like a triangle pointing at the nipple (*right*). (B and C) Representative case with calcifications in segmental distribution. In both mediolateral oblique (B) and craniocaudal (C) views, calcifications are growing in a segmental pattern, suggesting a triangle with the apex pointing at the nipple. This case had DCIS with microscopic invasive ductal carcinoma and lobular carcinoma in situ.

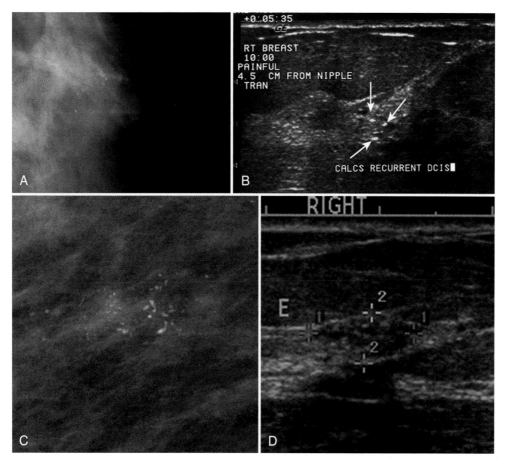

FIG. 3.68 Ultrasonographic appearance of calcifications in ductal carcinoma in situ (DCIS). (A and B) DCIS. Loosely grouped granular and amorphous calcifications on mammography (A) are observed as tiny white, high echoic spots (*arrows*) on ultrasound (B). Note that although calcifications can be seen, they might be difficult to detect without previous knowledge of their location, masked by the normal speckled appearance of the breast on ultrasound. (C and D) DCIS with foci of invasive ductal carcinoma. Grouped fine pleomorphic calcifications on mammography (C) are seen as multiple tiny echogenic spots in the hypoechoic DCIS lesion on ultrasound (D).

scan shows the suspicious mass representing the cancer causing the calcifications or if it pinpoints the calcifications for percutaneous biopsy or needle localization.

DUCTAL CARCINOMA IN SITU APPEARANCE ON MAMMOGRAPHY VERSUS MAGNETIC RESONANCE IMAGING

On mammography, suspicious calcifications are the most common indicator of DCIS, although noncalcified DCIS presents as an asymmetry, focal asymmetry, or asymmetric nodules on mammography. On contrast-enhanced magnetic resonance imaging (MRI), DCIS is typically displayed as clumped nonmass enhancement or clustered ring enhancement, and kinetics may show a persistent, plateau, or washout late phase. To achieve complete surgical removal, evaluation for DCIS extent is important but challenging on MRI. In some DCIS, the extent may be visualized as larger by mammographic calcifications than by MRI (Fig. 3.70). In some DCIS, the true extent may be larger on MRI (Fig. 3.71). Because MRI may miss DCIS shown by mammography calcifications in up to 25% of cases, suspicious calcifications should undergo biopsy, even if the MRI is negative.

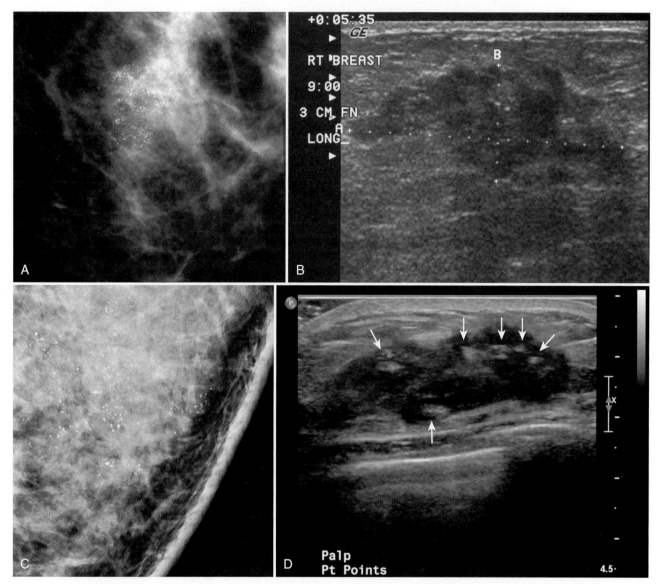

FIG. 3.69 Ultrasound for suspicious calcifications: detection of a mass. (A and B) Mammography (A) shows suspicious clustered pleomorphic calcifications in a patient with Paget disease of the nipple. Ultrasound (B) visualizes a hypoechoic, irregular mass containing calcifications. Pathologic examination showed invasive lobular and ductal cancer and ductal carcinoma in situ with calcifications. (C and D) In another case, on mammography (C) there are fine pleomorphic and coarse heterogeneous calcifications. Ultrasound shows a hypoechoic mass associated with multiple bright echogenic calcifications (D) that was hidden by adjacent dense tissue. Pathology showed invasive ductal carcinoma. Ultrasound may be helpful if the scan shows a mass in a location known to have calcifications.

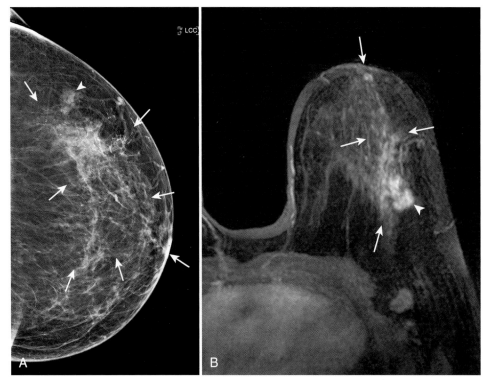

FIG. 3.70 Ductal carcinoma in situ (DCIS): mammography versus magnetic resonance imaging (MRI). (A) Left craniocaudal (CC) mammogram. (B) Contrast-enhanced axial MRI. In this case fine-linear and fine linear–branching calcifications on left CC mammogram (A; *arrows*) are more extensive and specific in estimating the transverse extent of DCIS, especially medially compared with linear/segmental nonmass enhancement on contrast-enhanced MRI (B; *arrows*). It is known that up to 25% of calcifications representing DCIS show no abnormal enhancement on MRI. This means that if there are suspicious calcifications on mammography, biopsy should be done even if the MRI is negative. Note that the mass in the outer deep breast on mammogram (A; *arrowhead*) and MRI (B; *arrowhead*) represents invasive ductal carcinoma.

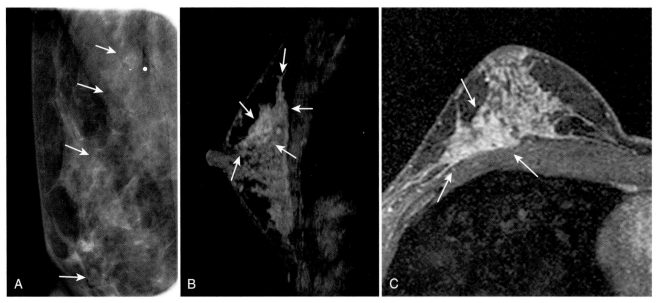

FIG. 3.71 Ductal carcinoma in situ (DCIS): mammography versus magnetic resonance imaging (MRI). (A) Right craniocaudal spot magnified mammogram. (B) Contrast-enhanced sagittal MRI. (C) Contrast-enhanced axial MRI. In this case there are scattered calcifications on mammography (A; *arrows*) to indicate DCIS, yet there is much more DCIS as shown by the extent of segmental nonmass enhancement (*arrows*) in the right breast on MRI (B and C; *arrows*). Unlike Fig. 3.70, the extent of the DCIS is seen better by MRI than by calcifications on mammography, and mammography underestimates the extent of the DCIS. In an individual case, DCIS may be seen better by either mammography or MRI, and management should be guided by the worst-looking images, the clinical scenario, and proof of malignancy by core biopsy.

Key Elements

Calcifications that are fine pleomorphic or fine linear or linear-branching in shape without a mass are significant because they may represent ductal carcinoma in situ or invasive ductal cancer.

Calcifications are not a feature of invasive lobular carcinoma and are rarely a feature of lobular carcinoma in situ.

Use a hand or optical magnifier to seek calcifications on standard mammograms.

Use air-gap magnification views with a 0.1-mm focal spot to work up calcifications.

Recognize "don't touch" calcifications and leave them alone. "Don't touch" calcifications include skin, vascular, coarse or popcorn-like (in fibroadenomas), large rodlike (in secretory disease), round, punctate, rim, dystrophic, milk of calcium, and suture calcifications.

Other benign calcifications include calcifying implant capsules, silicone injection calcifications, and artifacts that simulate calcifications.

Tangential views identify and diagnose skin calcifications.

Calcifications in malignancy occur in breast parenchyma.

Both the individual calcification forms and the distribution of the calcifications are clues for finding cancer.

Amorphous, coarse heterogeneous, fine pleomorphic, fine-linear or fine linear–branching individual calcification forms are worrisome for malignancy.

Grouped, linear, and segmental calcification distributions are suspicious for cancer, depending on the individual calcification forms within them.

Calcifications that have linear forms within the cluster need biopsy unless they are milk of calcium or secretory disease.

Know the Breast Imaging Reporting and Data System terms and positive predictive value for calcification shapes and distribution.

SUGGESTED READINGS

Adair FE: Plasma cell mastitis—lesion simulating mammary carcinoma: clinical and pathologic study with a report of 10 cases, *Arch Surg* 26:735–749, 1933.

Adair FE, Munzer JT: Fat necrosis of the female breast, *Am J Surg* 74:117–128, 1947.

Albayrak ZK, Onay HK, Karatag GY, et al.: Invasive lobular carcinoma of the breast: mammographic and sonographic evaluation, *Diagn Interv Radiol* 17(3):232–238, 2011.

Barreau B, de Mascarel I, Feuga C, et al.: Mammography of ductal carcinoma in situ of the breast: review of 909 cases with radiographic-pathologic correlations, *Eur J Radiol* 54(1):55–61, 2005.

Bassett LW, Gold RH, Mirra JM: Nonneoplastic breast calcifications: development after excision and primary irradiation, *AJR Am J Roentgenol* 138:335–338, 1982.

Bazzocchi M, Zuiani C, Panizza P, et al.: Contrast-enhanced breast MRI in patients with suspicious microcalcifications on mammography: results of a multicenter trial, *AJR Am J Roentgenol* 186(6):1723–1732, 2006.

Bent CK, Bassett LW, D'Orsi CJ, et al.: The positive predictive value of BI-RADS microcalcification descriptors and final assessment categories, *AJR Am J Roentgenol* 194(5):1378–1383, 2010.

Berkowitz JE, Gatewood OM, Donovan GB, Gayler BW: Dermal breast calcifications: localization with template-guided placement of skin marker, *Radiology* 163:282, 1987.

Black JW, Young B: A radiological and pathological study of the incidence of calcification in diseases of the breast and neoplasms of other tissues, *Br J Radiol* 38:596–598, 1965.

Brenner RJ, Sickles EA: Acceptability of periodic follow-up as an alternative to biopsy for mammographically detected lesions interpreted as probably benign, *Radiology* 171:645–646, 1989.

Chansakul T, Lai KC, Slanetz PJ: The postconservation breast: part 1, expected imaging findings, *AJR Am J Roentgenol* 198(2): 321–230 2012.

Chansakul T, Lai KC, Slanetz PJ: The postconservation breast: part 2, imaging findings of tumor recurrence and other long-term sequelae, *AJR Am J Roentgenol* 198(2):331–343, 2012.

Coren GS, Libshitz HI, Patchefsky AS: Fat necrosis of the breast: mammographic and thermographic findings, *Br J Radiol* 47:758–762, 1974.

Della Sala SW, Pellegrini M, Bernardi D, et al.: Mammographic and ultrasonographic comparison between intraoperative radiotherapy (IORT) and conventional external radiotherapy (RT) in limited-stage breast cancer, conservatively treated, *Eur J Radiol* 59(2):222–230, 2006.

Dershaw DD, Abramson A, Kinne DW: Ductal carcinoma in situ: mammographic findings and clinical implications, *Radiology* 170:411–415, 1989.

Dershaw DD, Chaglassian TA: Mammography after prosthesis placement for augmentation or reconstructive mammoplasty, *Radiology* 170(Pt 1):69–74, 1989.

Dershaw DD, Shank B, Reisinger S: Mammographic findings after breast cancer treatment with local excision and definitive irradiation, *Radiology* 164:455–461, 1987.

Destounis SV, Arieno AL, Morgan RC: Preliminary clinical experience with digital breast tomosynthesis in the visualization of breast microcalcifications, *J Clin Imaging Sci* 3:65, 2013.

DiPiro PJ, Meyer JE, Frenna TH, Denison CM: Seat belt injuries of the breast: findings on mammography and sonography, *AJR Am J Roentgenol* 164:317–320, 1995.

D'Orsi CJ, Feldhaus L, Sonnenfeld M: Unusual lesions of the breast, *Radiol Clin North Am* 21:67–80, 1983.

Egan RL, McSweeney MB, Sewell CW: Intramammary calcifications without an associated mass in benign and malignant diseases, *Radiology* 137(Pt 1):1–7, 1980.

Engel D, Schnitzer A, Brade J, et al.: Are mammographic changes in the tumor bed more pronounced after intraoperative radiotherapy for breast cancer? Subgroup analysis from a randomized trial (TARGIT-A), *Breast J* 19(1):92–95, 2013.

Fallenberg EM, Dimitrijevic L, Diekmann F, et al.: Impact of magnification views on the characterization of microcalcifications in digital mammography, *Rofo* 186(3):274–280, 2014.

Gershon-Cohen J, Ingleby H, Hermel MB: Calcification in secretory disease of the breast, *AJR Am J Roentgenol* 76:132–135, 1956.

Giess CS, Raza S, Birdwell RL: Distinguishing breast skin lesions from superficial breast parenchymal lesions: diagnostic criteria, imaging characteristics, and pitfalls, *Radiographics* 31(7):1959–1972, 2011.

Gilbert FJ, Tucker L, Gillan MG, et al.: Accuracy of digital breast tomosynthesis for Depicting Breast Cancer Subgroups in a UK Retrospective Reading Study (TOMMY Trial), *Radiology* 277:697–706, 2015.

Gilbert FJ, Tucker L, Gillan MG, et al.: The TOMMY trial: a comparison of TOMosynthesis with digital MammographY in the UK NHS Breast Screening Programme—a multicentre retrospective reading study comparing the diagnostic performance of digital breast tomosynthesis and digital mammography with digital mammography alone, *Health Technol Assess* 19:1–136, 2015. i–xxv.

Graf O, Berg WA, Sickles EA: Large rodlike calcifications at mammography: analysis of morphologic features, *AJR Am J Roentgenol* 200(2):299–303, 2013.

Gunhan-Bilgen I, Oktay A: Management of microcalcifications developing at the lumpectomy bed after conservative surgery and radiation therapy, *AJR Am J Roentgenol* 188(2):393–398, 2007.

Harnist KS, Ikeda DM, Helvie MA: Abnormal mammogram after steering wheel injury, *West J Med* 159:504–506, 1993.

Haygood TM, Arribas E, Brennan PC, Atkinson EN, Herndon M, Dieber J, et al.: Conspicuity of microcalcifications on digital screening mammograms using varying degrees of monitor zooming, *Acad Radiol* 16(12):1509–1517, 2009.

Helvie MA, Rebner M, Sickler EA, et al.: Calcifications in metastatic breast carcinoma in axillary lymph nodes, *AJR Am J Roentgenol* 151:921–922, 1988.

Hofvind S, Iversen BF, Eriksen L, Styr BM, Kjellevold K, Kurz KD: Mammographic morphology and distribution of calcifications in ductal carcinoma in situ diagnosed in organized screening, *Acta Radiol* 52(5):481–487, 2011.

Holland R, Hendriks JH: Microcalcifications associated with ductal carcinoma in situ: mammographic-pathologic correlation, *Semin Diagn Pathol* 11:181–192, 1994.

Holmberg L, Wong YN, Tabar L, et al.: Mammography casting-type calcification and risk of local recurrence in DCIS: analyses from a randomised study, *Br J Cancer* 108(4):812–819, 2013.

Hunter TB, Roberts CC, Hunt KR, et al.: Occurrence of fibroadenomas in postmenopausal women referred for breast biopsy, *J Am Geriatr Soc* 44:61–64, 1996.

Ikeda DM, Sickles EA: Mammographic demonstration of pectoral muscle microcalcifications, *AJR Am J Roentgenol* 151:475–476, 1988.

Kang SS, Ko EY, Han BK, et al.: Breast US in patients who had microcalcifications with low concern of malignancy on screening mammography, *Eur J Radiol* 67(2):285–291, 2008.

Kopans D, Gavenonis S, Halpern E, Moore R: Calcifications in the breast and digital breast tomosynthesis, *Breast J* 17(6):638–644, 2011.

Kopans DB, Meyer JE, Homer MJ, Grabbe J: Dermal deposits mistaken for breast calcifications, *Radiology* 149:592–594, 1983.

Kopans DB, Nguyen PL, Koerner FC, et al.: Mixed form, diffusely scattered calcifications in breast cancer with apocrine features, *Radiology* 177:807–811, 1990.

Krishnamurthy R, Whitman GJ, Stelling CB, et al.: Mammographic findings after breast conservation therapy, *Radiographics* 19:S53–S63, 1999.

Lai KC, Slanetz PJ, Eisenberg RL: Linear breast calcifications, *AJR Am J Roentgenol* 199(2):W151–W157, 2012.

Lanyi M: *Diagnosis and differential diagnosis of breast calcifications*, Berlin, 1988, Springer-Verlag.

Lehman CD, Rutter CM, Eby PR, et al.: Lesion and patient characteristics associated with malignancy after a probably benign finding on community practice mammography, *AJR Am J Roentgenol* 190(2):511–515, 2008.

Leung JW, Sickles EA: Developing asymmetry identified on mammography: correlation with imaging outcome and pathologic findings, *AJR Am J Roentgenol* 188(3):667–675, 2007.

Lev-Toaff AS, Feig SA, Saitas VL, et al.: Stability of malignant breast microcalcifications, *Radiology* 192(1):153–156, 1994.

Linden SS, Sickles EA: Sedimented calcium in benign breast cysts: the full spectrum of mammographic presentations, *AJR Am J Roentgenol* 152:967–971, 1989.

Mercado CL, Koenigsberg TC, Hamele-Bona D, Smith SJ: Calcifications associated with lactational changes of the breast: mammographic findings with histologic correlation, *AJR Am J Roentgenol* 179:685–689, 2002.

Millis RR, Davis R, Stacey AJ: The detection and significance of calcifications in the breast: a radiological and pathological study, *Br J Radiol* 49:12-26, 1976.

Murphy WA, DeSchryver-Kecskemeti K: Isolated clustered microcalcifications in the breast: radiologic-pathologic correlation, *Radiology* 127:335-341, 1978.

Orson LW, Cigtay OS: Fat necrosis of the breast: characteristic xeromammographic appearance, *Radiology* 146:35-38, 1983.

Pinsky RW, Rebner M, Pierce LJ, et al.: Recurrent cancer after breast-conserving surgery with radiation therapy for ductal carcinoma in situ: mammographic features, method of detection, and stage of recurrence, *AJR Am J Roentgenol* 189(1):140-144, 2007.

Rebner M, Pennes DR, Adler DD, et al.: Breast microcalcifications after lumpectomy and radiation therapy, *Radiology* 170(Pt 1):691-693, 1989.

Rosen EL, Baker JA, Soo MS: Malignant lesions initially subjected to short-term mammographic follow-up, *Radiology* 223(1):221-228, 2002.

Ross BA, Ikeda DM, Jackman RJ, Nowels KW: Milk of calcium in the breast: appearance on prone stereotactic imaging, *Breast J* 7:53-55, 2001.

Sapino A, Frigerio A, Peterse JL, et al.: Mammographically detected in situ lobular carcinomas of the breast, *Virchows Arch* 436(5):421-430, 2000.

Scaranelo AM, Eiada R, Bukhanov K, et al.: Evaluation of breast amorphous calcifications by a computer-aided detection system in full-field digital mammography, *Br J Radiol* 85(1013):517-522, 2012.

Scoggins M, Krishnamurthy S, Santiago L, Yang W: Lobular carcinoma in situ of the breast: clinical, radiological, and pathological correlation, *Acad Radiol* 20(4):463-470, 2013.

Sickles EA: Breast calcifications: mammographic evaluation, *Radiology* 160:289-293, 1986.

Sickles EA: Further experience with microfocal spot magnification mammography in the assessment of clustered breast microcalcifications, *Radiology* 137(Pt 1):9-14, 1980.

Sickles EA: Mammographic detectability of breast microcalcifications, *AJR Am J Roentgenol* 139:913-918, 1982.

Sickles EA: Mammography screening and the self-referred woman, *Radiology* 166 (Pt 1):271-273, 1988.

Sickles EA: Periodic mammographic follow-up of probably benign lesions: results in 3,184 consecutive cases, *Radiology* 179(2):463-468, 1991.

Sickles EA, Abele JS: Milk of calcium within tiny benign breast cysts, *Radiology* 141:655-658, 1981.

Sickles EA, D'Orsi CJ, Bassett LW, et al.: ACR BI-RADS® Mammography. In *ACR BI-RADS® atlas, breast imaging reporting and data system*, Reston, VA, 2013, American College of Radiology.

Sigfusson BF, Andersson I, Aspegren K, et al.: Clustered breast calcifications, *Acta Radiol Diagn (Stockholm)* 24:273-281, 1983.

Spangler ML, Zuley ML, Sumkin JH, et al.: Detection and classification of calcifications on digital breast tomosynthesis and 2D digital mammography: a comparison, *AJR Am J Roentgenol* 196(2):320-324, 2011.

Spring DB, Kimbrell-Wilmot K: Evaluating the success of mammography at the local level: how to conduct an audit of your practice, *Radiol Clin North Am* 25:983-992, 1987.

Stomper PC, Connolly JL: Ductal carcinoma in situ of the breast: correlation between mammographic calcification and tumor subtype, *AJR Am J Roentgenol* 159:483-485, 1992.

Tot T, Gere M: Radiological-pathological correlation in diagnosing breast carcinoma: the role of pathology in the multimodality era, *Pathol Oncol Res* 14(2):173-178, 2008.

Tse GM, Tan PH, Cheung HS, Chu WC, Lam WW: Intermediate to highly suspicious calcification in breast lesions: a radio-pathologic correlation, *Breast Cancer Res Treat* 110(1):1-7, 2008.

Tse GM, Tan PH, Pang AL, et al.: Calcification in breast lesions: pathologists' perspective, *J Clin Pathol* 61(2):145-151, 2008.

Wang LC, Sullivan M, Du H, et al.: US appearance of ductal carcinoma in situ, *Radiographics* 33(1):213-228, 2013.

Weigel S, Decker T, Korsching E, et al.: Calcifications in digital mammographic screening: improvement of early detection of invasive breast cancers? *Radiology* 255(3):738-745, 2010.

Witten D: *The breast. An atlas of tumor radiology*, Chicago, 1969, Year Book.

Yamada T, Mori N, Watanabe M, et al.: Radiologic-pathologic correlation of ductal carcinoma in situ, *Radiographics* 30(5):1183-1198, 2010.

Chapter 4

Mammographic and Ultrasound Analysis of Breast Masses

Kanae K. Miyake and Debra M. Ikeda

A breast mass is one of the most frequent presenting features of breast carcinoma. Benign masses usually have round or oval shapes with pushing or circumscribed borders and do not invade normal surrounding tissue. Malignant masses are often irregularly shaped with indistinct or spiculated margins produced by the tumor infiltrating adjacent normal tissue. Thus radiologists look carefully at mass shapes and margins to determine whether the mass is malignant.

Ultrasound (US) goes hand-in-hand with mammography in breast mass evaluation and shows whether the mass is cystic or solid. US provides real-time evaluation of mass shapes, borders, orientation, and internal characteristics to determine whether the mass is malignant or benign. Detailed principles and interpretation of ultrasonography are explained further in Chapter 5. This chapter reviews mammographic and US analysis of breast masses.

MAMMOGRAPHY FOR EVALUATING NONPALPABLE MASSES, ASYMMETRIES, AND PALPABLE MASSES

In asymptomatic women, screening mammography is a primary screening method for breast cancers in women 40 years of age or older and potentiates the detection of early, clinically occult cancers. When screening mammography detects suspicious findings, such as masses, focal asymmetries, and architectural distortion, diagnostic mammography is generally performed for further evaluation of nonpalpable mammographic findings, as detailed in the American College of Radiology (ACR) Appropriateness Criteria for Nonpalpable Mammographic Findings.

In women with clinically detected palpable masses, diagnostic mammography is the initial imaging modality of choice for evaluating the palpable breast masses in those 40 years of age

or older, as indicated in the ACR Appropriateness Criteria for Palpable Breast Masses (Harvey, 2013). For women 30 to 39 years old, either diagnostic mammography or US may be used for initial evaluation, but US is the initial imaging modality in a woman younger than 30 years old.

A true mass is a ball-shaped object that is approximately the same size, shape, and density in orthogonal mammographic projections. Radiologists detect masses because they are whiter than surrounding fibroglandular tissue, are an asymmetric finding compared with the contralateral breast, or display unique distinguishing characteristics from normal background tissue. For example, masses may have distinct edges, are higher density (whiter) than surrounding tissue, are new, or have spiculated margins that make them unique from normal breast tissue.

On two-dimensional (2D) mammography, the radiologist first detects masses because they are different from the surrounding tissue by a distinct mass edge, have higher density, have interval appearance, have architectural distortion, or because there is an asymmetry (Fig. 4.1). The radiologist determines whether the finding is a true mass or overlapping fibroglandular tissue (a fake mass) using mammographic techniques described in Chapter 2. If the finding is a true mass, the radiologist triangulates its position in the breast and then uses 2D fine-detail spot compression magnification mammography to characterize the mass' shape, margin, and associated findings such as calcifications (Newell, 2010). Two-dimensional mammography shows mass shapes and borders best when the mass is displayed against fat, thus, the optimal projection to perform spot magnification mammograms is where the mass lies in fat. If the mass is present or is still suspected, radiologists use US to confirm or exclude a mass lesion and to determine whether detected masses require a histologic diagnosis.

Radiologists reading 2D mammograms often struggle with findings seen on only one standard mammographic projection. Their dilemma is whether the one-view finding is a fake mass produced by overlapping normal tissue, called a *summation artifact*, or if it is a real mass hidden on the orthogonal view. One-view findings are often focal densities (a white finding that is whiter than the background tissue) called *asymmetries*, because the focal density is whiter than a mirror image area on the contralateral side. A study by Sickles (1998) shows that greater than 80% of mammographic asymmetries at screening are summation artifacts. His large prospective study of 61,273 screening mammograms showed that 3.3% (2023 cases) of mammographic screens had one view–only findings. Dr. Sickles' analysis showed that 54.7% (1086/2023 cases) of one-view findings were confidently dismissed as overlapping tissue by simply seeing the orthogonal view, whereas 29% (587/2023) were recalled and dismissed as normal after diagnostic imaging. None of these findings were cancer at follow-up. In the remaining 36 cases, cancer was found at diagnostic imaging, and 33% of these cancers were lobular cancer. The 2D

diagnostic mammographic methods to determine whether one-view findings are masses or normal tissue include repeating the same mammographic view to see if the finding persists, comparing studies with old mammograms, or a 2D diagnostic fine-detail workup including 2D rolled mammographic views, spot compression or spot compression magnification views, and step oblique mammography (Pearson et al., 2000; Sickles, 1988, Ikeda and Sickles, 1988; Sickles, 2007; Price, 2015). Targeted US (Leung, 2007a) and tomosynthesis (Andersson et al., 2008) can also be especially helpful to detect true masses. The Breast Imaging Reporting and Data System (BI-RADS) 2013 definitions of asymmetries and their workup will be discussed in the next section, and the remainder of this section will concentrate on true masses.

Breast tomosynthesis is a useful technique for evaluating masses and possible masses (see Fig. 4.1C; see Video 4.1). Studies show that breast tomosynthesis has an advantage over digital mammography in breast cancer diagnosis, with higher cancer detection rates and lower patient recall rates at screening (Ciatto et al., 2013; Skaane et al., 2014; Lang et al., 2015; Friedewald et al.,

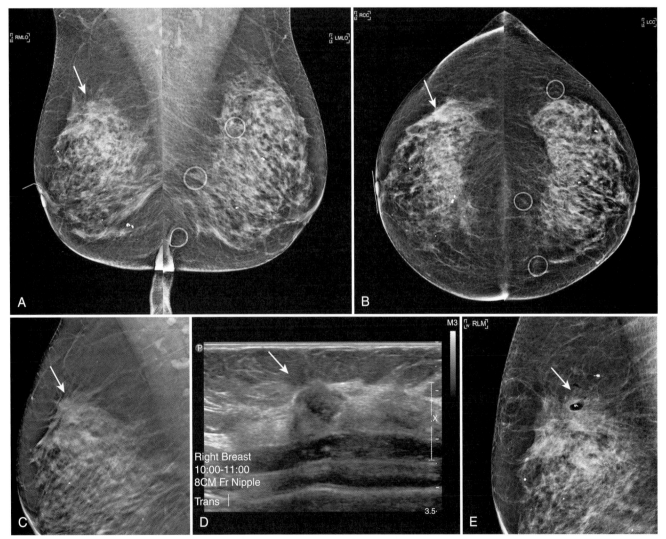

FIG. 4.1 Mammographic technique for evaluating masses. (A and B) Paired 2D mediolateral oblique (MLO) (A) and craniocaudal (B) mammogram show a possible spiculated mass (*arrow*) that overlies fibroglandular tissue. (C) Right MLO tomosynthesis slice (see also Video 4.1) shows the mass and spiculations. Note the mass and fibroglandular density contrast has a more narrow gray scale than the 2D mammogram, and the spiculations are enhanced by the reconstruction algorithm. (D) The corresponding ultrasound shows a hypoechoic mass with indistinct margins. (E) Two-dimensional lateromedial mammogram after biopsy with marker placement shows a metallic marker within an air bubble, showing the final location of the biopsied mass in the upper right breast. Biopsy showed invasive lobular carcinoma.

2014). In the diagnostic setting tomographic slices detect masses hidden on 2D mammograms by uncovering overlapping breast tissue. Tomosynthesis also displays morphologic mass features, helps localize masses, characterizes mass features, and shows the extent of disease in malignancies (Peppard et al., 2015; Yang et al., 2013). In both the screening and diagnostic settings, tomosynthesis also helps clarify if a suspected mass or asymmetry represents a true mass or a summation artifact (Baker and Lo, 2011), resulting in decreased screening recall rates of 15% to 17% in published studies (Ciatto et al., 2013; Skaane et al., 2014; Lang et al., 2015; Friedewald et al., 2014). Tomosynthesis at diagnostic workup is especially helpful to characterize masses that may not show on 2D spot compression (Roth, 2014) and to localize lesions for US targeting for biopsy (Cohen, 2014; Kopans, 2014; see Fig. 4.1 D–E).

In contrast, tomosynthesis does not show all masses, particularly masses that have a round shape, are circumscribed, or have an indistinct border in a dense breast. Masses are detected against mammographic backgrounds if they have unique imaging characteristics distinct from the surrounding tissue such as spiculated margins or pleomorphic calcifications. Tomosynthesis is exquisitely sensitive for mass spiculations (see Fig. 4.1C; see Video 4.1). Masses not seen by tomosynthesis usually are equal density to normal breast tissue and have nonspiculated borders that blend in with the surrounding tissue so there is no distinct mass margin detectable against the normal breast background (Andersson et al., 2008). Similar to the silhouette sign of pneumonia against the heart border, a nonspiculated breast mass edge is obscured or silhouetted by glandular tissue, making the mass undetectable. In Andersson's series, cancers missed by tomosynthesis were found because the patient felt something or the cancer was detected by US or magnetic resonance imaging (MRI). Clinically, this means that palpable findings should undergo US even if the tomosynthesis is negative, especially if the finding lies within dense tissue. The corollary is that a highly suspicious US or MRI finding should undergo histologic sampling even if 2D mammogram or tomosynthesis studies are negative.

Both diagnostic 2D mammography and tomosynthesis are commonly used to evaluate palpable masses under a radiologist's supervision, as detailed in the ACR Appropriateness Criteria for Palpable Breast Masses (Harvey et al., 2013). Usually, a technologist places a radiopaque skin marker over the palpable finding and obtains standard craniocaudal and mediolateral views including the marker to show the palpable finding. Special fine-detail mammograms (tangential views, spot compression, or magnification views) may show more detail of the palpable finding. US is used commonly to evaluate palpable breast masses and is the initial imaging modality of choice for women under the age of 30, whereas either diagnostic mammography or US is used as the initial examination for women 30 to 39 years of age. Further details of diagnostic workups of palpable masses are described in later.

DESCRIPTION OF MASSES, ASYMMETRY, AND ARCHITECTURAL DISTORTION BASED ON BREAST IMAGING REPORTING AND DATA SYSTEM 2013 MAMMOGRAPHY

Masses

The ACR BI-RADS lexicon defines a breast mass as a three-dimensional (3D) space-occupying lesion seen on at least two mammographic projections. Mass *shapes* are categorized as *oval, round,* or *irregular* (Figs. 4.2 and 4.3; Table 4.1). The probability of cancer increases as the mass shape becomes more irregular.

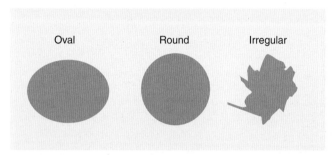

FIG. 4.2 Schematic of mass shapes: oval, round, and irregular. An oval mass is elliptical and can have two or three undulations. A round mass is spherical in shape. An irregular mass usually implies a suspicious lesion.

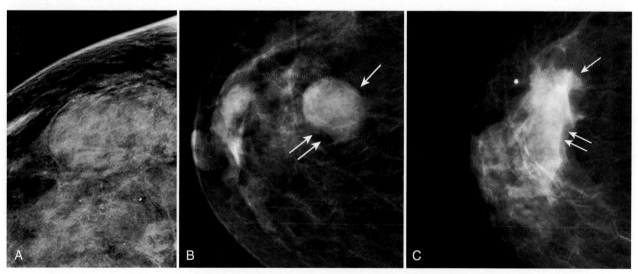

FIG. 4.3 Mass shapes: oval, round, and irregular. (A) Oval shape. Mammogram shows a low-density oval mass with circumscribed margins representing a simple cyst. Incidentally noted are scattered benign round/punctate calcifications in the breast tissue. (B) Round shape. Mammogram shows a high-density round mass with mostly circumscribed (*arrow*) and partly indistinct (*double arrow*) borders, representing invasive ductal cancer. (C) Irregular shape. Mammogram shows a palpable high-density irregular mass in the upper breast marked with a skin marker that has partly spiculated and indistinct margins (*arrow*) and obscured borders on its inferior aspect (*double arrows*), representing invasive ductal cancer.

The ACR BI-RADS lexicon defines mass margins as *circumscribed* (well defined or sharply defined), *microlobulated, obscured* by surrounding glandular tissue, *indistinct,* or *spiculated* (Fig. 4.4; see Table 4.1). As the mass margin becomes more spiculated, the probability of cancer increases. Masses with well-circumscribed borders are more likely to be benign (Fig. 4.5; Video 4.2). Sharply marginated borders indicate no invasion of the surrounding tissue; few cancers have smooth, well-circumscribed borders. An obscured mass has a border hidden by overlapping adjacent fibroglandular tissue, and that border cannot be assessed (Fig. 4.6). Microlobulated masses have small border undulations, like petals on a flower, and are more worrisome for cancer than are masses with circumscribed margins (Fig. 4.7). An indistinct mass has a margin that can be seen but is fuzzy. Indistinct margins are worrisome for carcinoma because the fuzzy border suggests tumor infiltration of surrounding tissue (Fig. 4.8). Finally, spiculated masses are characterized by thin lines radiating from the central portion of the mass and are especially worrisome for cancer (Fig. 4.9; Video 4.3). When caused by cancer, mass spiculations are caused by productive tumor fibrosis (desmoplastic reaction) or actual tumor infiltration. Tomosynthesis and the synthesized mammograms reconstructed from the tomosynthesis slices are especially sensitive for detecting spiculated masses (Fig. 4.10; Video 4.4).

Mass *density* describes the mass whiteness compared with an equal volume of fibroglandular tissue (Figs. 4.11 and 4.12; see Table 4.1).

High-density masses are whiter than fibroglandular tissue, and low-density masses are darker than fibroglandular tissue. High-density masses are especially worrisome for cancer, because they may contain cells with a higher atomic number than normal glandular tissue and fat. Low-density masses and masses with density equal to that of surrounding fibroglandular tissue are less worrisome for cancer. However, low-density cancers, such as mucinous cancers, do exist and mimic breast cysts. These cancers are low density because they contain mucin, which is fluid density.

Fat-containing masses on 2D mammography are almost always benign, except for the rare liposarcoma or tumors surrounding fat on tomosynthesis. Fat-containing masses include lymph nodes, oil cysts (see Fig. 4.12D), hamartomas, and fat necrosis, all of which are benign. However, tomosynthesis may show fat in both benign and malignant masses, and the fat seen on tomosynthesis may not be evident on 2D mammography (Freer et al., 2014). Cancers may appear to contain fat if the cancer shape is very irregular and has trapped fat in between arms of the tumor. This means that the old mammographic rule that masses containing fat are always benign does not apply to tomosynthesis. To avoid misdiagnosis of cancers that contain fat on tomosynthesis slices, radiologists analyze the mass for suspicious margins or shapes and proceed with biopsy based on the worst mass features, even if the mass contains fat (see section: Masses Containing Fat).

Asymmetry

The ACR BI-RADS mammography lexicon term *asymmetry* is used for mammography and not for US or MRI, although enhancing *findings* at MRI may be called symmetric or asymmetric. On mammography, asymmetries are white areas, more in one breast than in the other, and may represent asymmetric fibroglandular tissue or masses obscured by adjacent tissue. The finding must be included in the field of view on two orthogonal projections to

TABLE 4.1 American College of Radiology 2013 Breast Imaging Reporting and Data System Mammography Lexicon Descriptors for Masses

Shape	Oval	Elliptical or egg-shaped (may include 2–3 undulations)
	Round	Spherical, ball-shaped, circular, or globular
	Irregular	Neither round nor oval
Margin	Circumscribed	At least 75% of the margin is sharply demarcated, with an abrupt transition between the lesion and surrounding tissue
	Obscured	25% or more of the margin is hidden by superimposed or adjacent fibroglandular tissue
	Microlobulated	A margin characterized by short-cycle undulations
	Indistinct	No clear demarcation of the entire margin or any portion of it from the surrounding tissue
	Spiculated	Margin is characterized by lines radiating from the mass
Density	High density	X-ray attenuation of the mass is greater than the expected attenuation of an equal volume of fibroglandular breast tissue
	Equal density	X-ray attenuation of the mass is the same as the expected attenuation of an equal volume of fibroglandular breast tissue
	Low density	X-ray attenuation of the mass is less than the expected attenuation of an equal volume of fibroglandular breast tissue
	Fat containing	Includes all masses containing fat, such as oil cyst, lipoma, or galactocele, as well as mixed-density lesions such as hamartoma

From American College of Radiology: ACR BI-RADS®—Mammography. In *ACR BI-RADS atlas, breast imaging reporting and data system*, ed 5, Reston, VA, 2013, American College of Radiology.

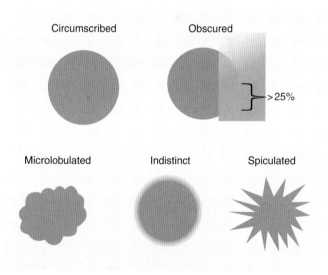

FIG. 4.4 Schematic of mass margins: circumscribed, obscured, microlobulated, indistinct, and spiculated. A circumscribed margin is sharply demarcated from the surrounding tissue. Obscured, is used when more than 25% of the entire margin of a mass is hidden by overlapping or adjacent tissue; this descriptor is used usually when the remaining unhidden mass margins are circumscribed. Margins with short-cycle undulations are described as microlobulated margins. When no clear demarcation of the entire margin is seen, the margin is categorized as indistinct (historically "ill-defined"). Spiculated margins are those with thin lines radiating center of the lesion, usually indicating cancer. The probability of cancer increases as mass margin progresses from circumscribed to spiculated.

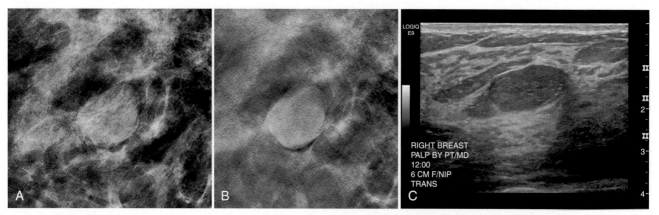

FIG. 4.5 Mass margin: circumscribed. (A) Photographically magnified mammogram shows a mass with a circumscribed margin. The most of the margin is sharply defined. Part of the margin is obscured by overlapping breast tissue, but is limited to less than 25%, making the use of the descriptor circumscribed appropriate. (B) With tomosynthesis, the entire circumscribed margin is more easily visible (see Video 4.2). (C) Ultrasonography shows that the corresponding mass is oval, hypoechoic, and has a circumscribed margin with posterior acoustic enhancement. Pathology was fibroadenoma.

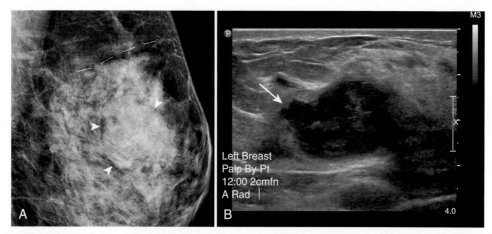

FIG. 4.6 Mass margin: obscured. (A) Photographically magnified mammogram shows a round high-density mass. The identifiable parts of the margin are circumscribed (*arrowheads*), but more than 25% of the margin is obscured by overlapping breast tissue. Thus the use of the descriptor obscured is appropriate for this mass. (B) The corresponding ultrasonography shows an irregular, hypoechoic mass with circumscribed superficial and deep margins, and an angular margin (*arrow*) that is suspicious for malignancy. Biopsy showed invasive ductal carcinoma.

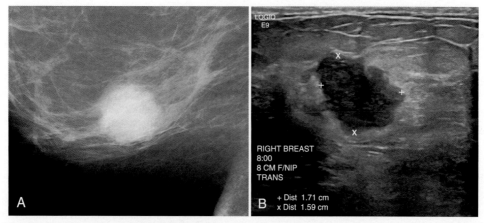

FIG. 4.7 Mass margin: microlobulated. (A) Photographically magnified mammogram shows a high-density, round irregular mass with microlobulated margins. (B) The corresponding ultrasound shows a hypoechoic irregular mass with microlobulated margins. Biopsy showed invasive ductal carcinoma.

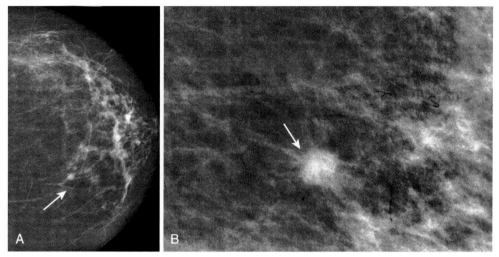

FIG. 4.8 Mass margin: indistinct. (A) Craniocaudal mammogram shows a round mass in the medial left breast (*arrow*). The differential is a focal area of glandular tissue, a cyst, or a solid mass. (B) Magnification mammogram shows the mass has indistinct margins rather than circumscribed borders (*arrow*). This shows the importance of fine-detail views and of being suspicious of medial breast masses. A biopsy showed invasive ductal cancer.

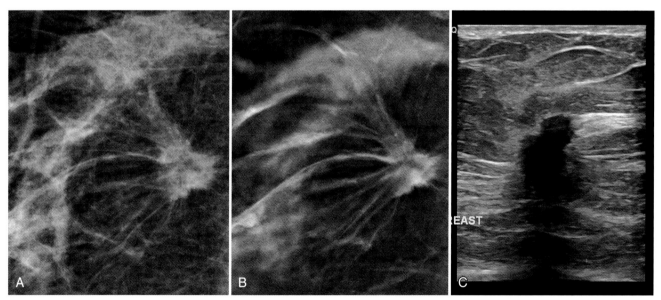

FIG. 4.9 Mass margin: spiculated. (A) Photographically magnified mammogram shows an irregular mass with a spiculated margin characterized by numerous fine lines radiating from the mass. There are a few associated pleomorphic calcifications along the superior margin. (B) Tomosynthesis (see Video 4.3) visualizes the radiating lines from the mass with less overlapping tissue. (C) Corresponding ultrasound shows a hypoechoic irregular mass with spiculated and indistinct margins. Biopsy showed invasive ductal carcinoma.

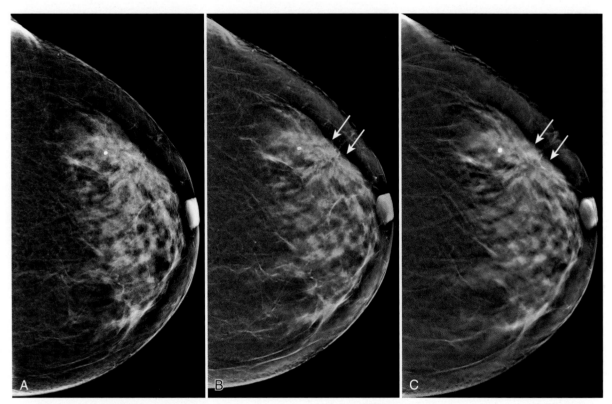

FIG. 4.10 Spiculation and distortion shown better on synthesized views and tomosynthesis. (A) Craniocaudal (CC) 2D mammogram of dense tissue shows possible spiculation and flattening of the normally scalloped glandular tissue edge of the outer left breast. (B) Synthesized 2D CC mammogram reconstructed from tomosynthesis slices shows distortion (*arrows*) in the outer breast better than the conventional 2D mammogram. (C) Tomosynthesis slice shows a spiculated mass (*arrows*) in the outer left breast, causing the distortion and flattening of the adjacent tissue, better than on conventional 2D (A) or synthesized 2D mammograms (B). Biopsy showed invasive lobular cancer (see also Video 4.4).

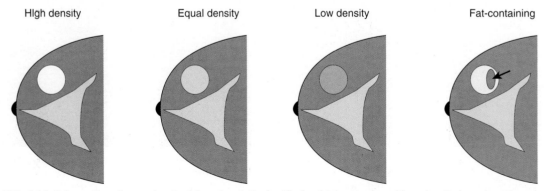

High density   Equal density   Low density   Fat-containing

FIG. 4.11 Schematics of mass density. Mass density is classified as high, equal, and low density based on the relative mass density compared with an equal volume of normal breast tissue. A fat-containing mass contains very low density identical to fat density (*arrow*). The fat density may comprise the entire mass, such as an oil cyst or lipoma, or part of the mass, as in a lymph node or hamartoma.

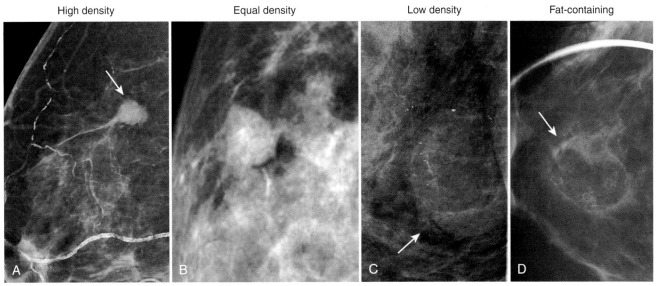

High density   Equal density   Low density   Fat-containing

FIG. 4.12 Mass density: high-density, equal-density, low-density, and fat-containing masses. (A) Mammogram shows a high-density mass (*arrow*) with spiculated margins, representing invasive ductal cancer. (B) Equal density. Mammogram shows an equal-density oval mass with mostly circumscribed margins, representing invasive ductal cancer. (C) Low density. Mammogram shows a low-density mass adjacent to the pectoralis (*arrow*), representing a simple cyst. Note scattered benign round/punctate calcifications in the breast tissue. (D) Fat containing. Spot compression magnification view shows a fat-containing, thin-walled mass with a radiolucent center and faint calcifications along its rim (*arrow*) in the area of a previous biopsy, representing an oil cyst.

qualify as an asymmetry. Asymmetries themselves do not qualify as masses on mammography. The ACR lexicon divides asymmetries into four categories: *asymmetry, global asymmetry, focal asymmetry*, and *developing asymmetry* (Table 4.2; Fig. 4.13). A focal asymmetry and developing asymmetry have a higher likelihood of representing true masses, including breast cancer.

The first category of asymmetries is *asymmetry*, which is a small area (less than one quadrant of the breast volume) of fibroglandular-density tissue seen only on one mammographic projection. The asymmetry is either invisible or looks like normal fibroglandular tissue on the orthogonal view. Most one-view asymmetries represent overlapping tissues producing a "fake mass" or summation artifact (Fig. 4.14; Video 4.5).

Because some asymmetries proved to be cancer, radiologists often recalled women with asymmetries from 2D screening mammography. Breast tomosynthesis decreases asymmetry recalls from screening because tomosynthesis either shows the mass as a true finding by removing glandular tissue in front of and behind the mass, or proves that the mass is fake, comprised of superimposed tissue on contiguous slices (see Fig. 4.14; see Video 4.5). However, not all asymmetries that persist as asymmetries/possible masses on tomosynthesis are true masses on workup. A possible mass may represent a summation artifact even on tomosynthesis, especially if there is suboptimal compression. These summation artifact asymmetries will spread out into their normal glandular components if there is sufficient compression, as with spot compression tomosynthesis (Fig. 4.15; Video 4.6). This means that tomosynthesis examinations require good compression to correctly demonstrate asymmetries as normal overlapping glandular tissue.

A large study from England (Gilbert et al., 2015) demonstrated a tendency for higher specificity for 2D plus tomosynthesis compared with 2D alone for distortion/asymmetry because tomosynthesis showed either overlapping tissue or an underlying mass. In another study (Nam KJ et al., 2015), lesions on tomosynthesis were seen as a more specific and localized pattern (eg, mass or focal asymmetry rather than asymmetry) than those on 2D

mammogram; cancers were more often constantly visible on tomosynthesis than on 2D mammography, and asymmetries were more often classified as focal asymmetry on tomosynthesis. Decreased recalls from screening in the author's own practice were often caused by tomosynthesis showing overlapping tissue that could be dismissed as benign, versus true distortion/mass that might be cancer.

Kopans et al. (1989) showed that asymmetries that represent normal, benign overlapping tissue are nonpalpable, contain no mass and no architectural distortion, and have no associated suspicious calcifications. Their study showed that asymmetries (formerly called asymmetric breast tissue) are present on mammograms in up to 3% of cases, and if benign, are stable on consecutive studies (see Fig. 4.14). In reviewing 8406 2D mammograms, Kopans et al. (1989) showed that 221/8406 (3%) screens had

TABLE 4.2 American College of Radiology Breast Imaging Reporting and Data System Mammography Lexicon Descriptors for Asymmetry

Asymmetry	An area of fibroglandular-density tissue that is seen in one standard mammographic view and likely represents summation
Global asymmetry	An area of fibroglandular-density tissue that occupies at least one quadrant and likely represents normal asymmetry between breasts
Focal asymmetry	An area of fibroglandular-density tissue that is seen in two mammographic views but does not fulfill criteria of mass
Developing asymmetry	A focal asymmetry that is new, larger, or more conspicuous than on a previous examination, 15% are cancer (Leung and Sickles, 2007a)

From American College of Radiology: ACR BI-RADS®—Mammography. In *ACR BI-RADS atlas, breast imaging reporting and data system*, ed 5, Reston, VA, 2013, American College of Radiology; Leung JWT, Sickles EA. Developing asymmetry identified on mammography: correlation with imaging outcomes and pathologic findings. *AJR Am J Roentgenol* 188:667-675.

Asymmetry visible on only one view

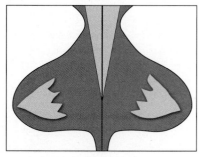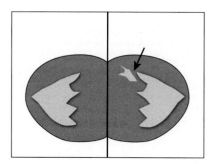

Global Asymmetry visible on 2 views, >1 quadrant in volume

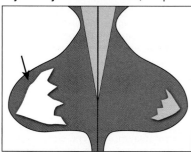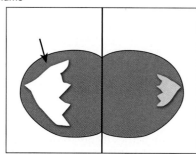

Focal Asymmetry visible on 2 views, <1 quadrant in volume

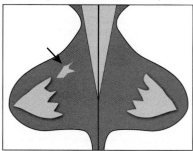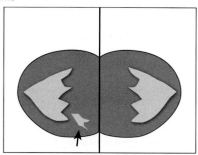

Developing Asymmetry new, visible on 2 views, <1 quadrant in volume

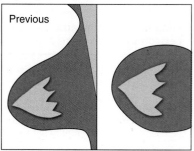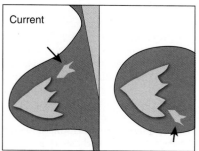

Previous

Current

FIG. 4.13 Schematics of asymmetry: asymmetry, global asymmetry, focal asymmetry, and developing asymmetry.

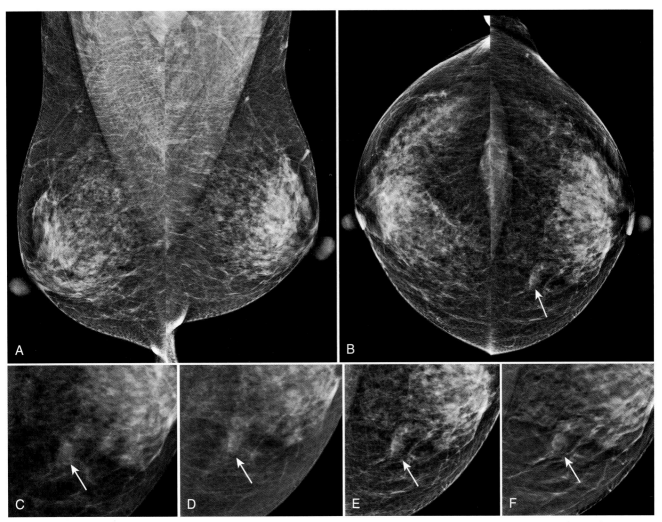

FIG. 4.14 Asymmetry: asymmetry—summation artifact, stable. (A and B) Paired mediolateral oblique (A) and craniocaudal (CC) (B) screening mammograms shows an asymmetry (*arrow*) in the left inner breast that is visible only on left CC view. (C–E) Photography magnified left CC views of annual screening mammograms (2-year [C] and 1-year [D] prior studies and the current study [E]) show this one-view asymmetry has been stable over years, which supports the diagnosis as a summation artifact of normal breast tissue. (F) On tomosynthesis (photography magnified left CC projection), this asymmetry has no central density, unlike a typical mass (see also Video 4.5).

asymmetric breast tissue and were not cancer if the asymmetry did not form a mass, was nonpalpable, and had no architectural distortion or calcifications. During the 36- to 42-month follow-up study period, 20 patients underwent excisional biopsy for clinical findings showing two breast cancer and one lymphoma cases, all of which were palpable. The remaining 17 biopsies were benign, and there were no breast cancers found in the remaining 201 patients with asymmetries. The study abstract concluded with the statement:

> *...an asymmetric volume of breast tissue, asymmetrically dense breast tissue, or asymmetrically prominent ducts that do not form a mass, do not contain microcalcifications, or do not produce architectural distortion should be view with concern only when associated with a palpable asymmetry, and are otherwise normal variations.*

BI-RADS 2013 states that a *global asymmetry* is large, containing one quadrant or more of fibroglandular-like breast tissue compared with the same location in the contralateral breast, and

is a real finding because it is displayed on two orthogonal projections. Global asymmetries are usually interspersed with fat and have no convex outward borders to suggest a mass. Similar to the smaller benign asymmetry, global asymmetries are benign if they are not new and have no associated architectural distortion, palpable findings, or suspicious calcifications. The nonpalpable global asymmetry is either an intrinsic normal variant (Fig. 4.16A) or is caused by surgical removal of glandular tissue in the contralateral breast (Fig. 4.16B). If nonpalpable, the global asymmetry can be assessed as a BI-RADS 2 Benign Finding and returned to screening. However, if the finding is new, palpable, or is actually a mass instead of a global asymmetry, it may represent cancer and needs workup.

A *focal asymmetry* is defined as a more fibroglandular-like density in one breast compared with the other, both in a corresponding location, is seen on two orthogonal views, and is less than one quadrant in size (smaller than the global asymmetry). The focal asymmetry also lacks outward convex borders seen in masses, and may be interspersed with fat. It may be challenging

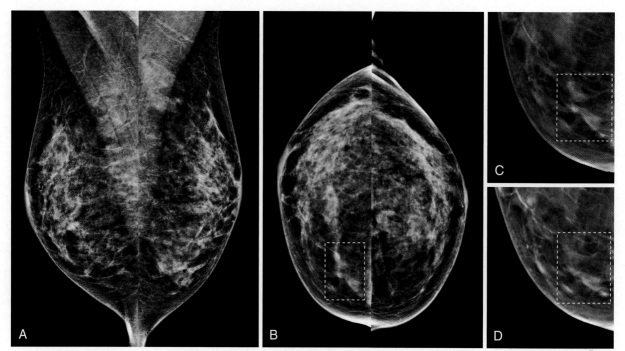

FIG. 4.15 Asymmetry: asymmetry—summation artifact. (A and B) Paired mediolateral oblique (A) and craniocaudal (CC; B) screening mammograms show an asymmetry (*box*) in the inner right breast that is visible only on the right CC view. (C) The one-view asymmetry (*box*) persists on the tomosynthesis slice (also see Video 4.6A–B) of the right CC projection caused by inadequate compression. (D) Spot compression right CC tomosynthesis study slice using greater compression on the asymmetry (also see Video 4.6C–D) shows normal overlapping normal tissue at the corresponding area (*box*), and US of the right breast was negative. The asymmetry was diagnosed as a summation artifact of overlapping normal breast tissue and shows the importance of good compression with tomosynthesis.

to identify focal asymmetries, because comparison to the contralateral breast is especially important to identify the asymmetry on two views, and the findings must be included in the field of view on both projections. Some focal asymmetries may be dismissed as benign at screening (Fig. 4.17), whereas others require workup. Scientific publications assess the focal asymmetry as a BI-RADS category 3 Probably Benign finding if called back from screening and is worked up, with a 0.5% to 1% probability of cancer if there are no masses at workup and it is stable over a 2-to 3-year mammographic follow-up period (Sickles, 1991; Varas et al., 1992, 2002; Vizcaino et al., 2001).

As stated in BI-RADS 2013, focal asymmetries that are less than 1 cm are of concern because they may represent nonpalpable cancers (Fig. 4.18; Video 4.7). It is of particular concern if the focal asymmetry recalled from screening has associated architectural distortion or calcifications. On occasion a focal asymmetry is found to be a true mass at diagnostic mammography or targeted US and might be cancer (Fig. 4.19).

A *developing asymmetry* is a focal asymmetry that, when compared with older mammograms, is new, larger, or more conspicuous than on prior studies (BI-RADS 2013; Fig. 4.20).

The 2007 study by Leung and Sickles (2007a) showed that developing asymmetries were present in 0.16% (292 cases) of 180,801 screening mammograms and 0.11% (32 cases) of diagnostic mammograms. At screening mammography, 12.8% of the developing asymmetries were cancer. The Leung and Sickles study and a follow-up study by Venkatesan et al. (2009) showed that the developing asymmetry in the diagnostic setting has a likelihood of 26.7% of malignancy if found in follow-up of BI-RADS category 3 lesions, if shown after a benign concordant biopsy or if developing in the first 5 years after breast

conservation. Because the percentage of cancer is above the 2% Probably Benign category 3 threshold, developing asymmetries should undergo biopsy if they are not normal overlapping tissue at workup.

Occasionally, nonpuerperal (nonlactating) mastitis may show a developing asymmetry with rare associated architectural distortion (Tan H, 2013), which can be difficult to distinguish from breast carcinoma. Puerperal or postpartum mastitis caused by lactation also produces the same radiologic features as developing asymmetry but clinically, women present with a clinical history of fever and pain, and their mammograms commonly show breast edema with the developing asymmetry.

Architectural Distortion

Architectural distortion is defined as linear alterations of breast parenchyma pulled into a central focus, without a definite visible mass, resulting in radiating spiculations or thin lines pointing toward the center, like a star (Fig. 4.21). Distortion also describes the pulling in or straightening of any edge of the glandular tissue boundary with fat (see Fig. 4.10). This was called the "tent sign" and attributed to Dr. Lazslo Tabar. When associated with asymmetry or calcifications, architectural distortion is even more suspicious for cancer. In contrast, architectural distortion associated with a history of surgical biopsy represents a postbiopsy scar and is benign. Because postbiopsy scars can be indicated by placement of a linear metallic marker on the skin over the postbiopsy scar, many facilities place radiopaque skin markers on skin scars to show that underlying distortion represents a benign scar. However, architectural distortion is suspicious for malignancy or radial scar if there is no history of trauma or surgery, and it

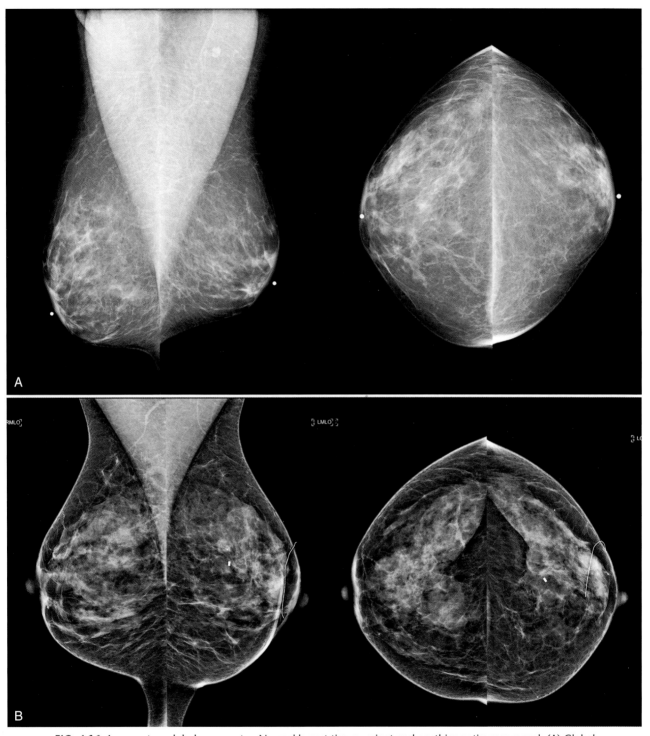

FIG. 4.16 Asymmetry: global asymmetry. Normal breast tissue variant and postbiopsy tissue removal. (A) Global asymmetry as a normal variant. Paired mediolateral oblique (MLO; *left*) and craniocaudal (CC; *right*) screening mammograms show more fibroglandular tissue in the right breast than the left, of greater than 25% of the breast volume (global asymmetry), and unchanged for 2 years. Note BB markers on the nipples. (B) Global asymmetry caused by surgery. Paired MLO (*left*) and CC (*right*) screening mammograms show more fibroglandular tissue in the right breast than the left, also of greater than 25% of the breast volume, and caused by surgical removal of breast tissue in the lower left breast (pathology showed papilloma, calcifications, and usual ductal hyperplasia). Given the clinical history, these are benign findings. Note the left linear skin scar marker and a postbiopsy metallic marker from benign biopsy in the left breast.

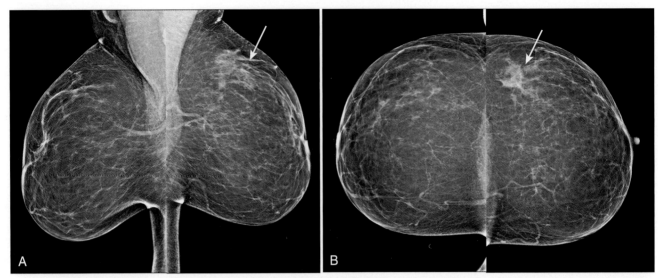

FIG. 4.17 Asymmetry: focal asymmetry. Summation artifact. (B) Paired mediolateral oblique (MLO; A) and craniocaudal (CC; B) screening mammograms show a focal asymmetry with upper outer left breast (*arrows*). It is more obvious on the CC view because it is a summation of overlapping tissue that is spread out on the MLO view and stable for 24 months. Unlike a true mass, which is more conspicuous on both views and has convex outward borders, this benign asymmetry has concave outward borders and is interspersed with fat.

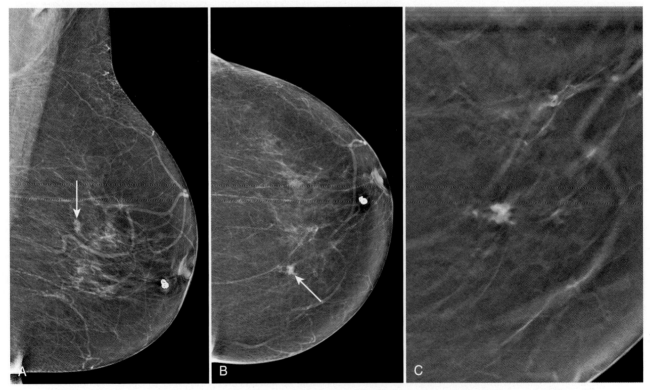

FIG. 4.18 Asymmetry: focal asymmetry/mass. Atypical ductal hyperplasia. (A and B) Mediolateral oblique (A) and craniocaudal (B) mammograms of left breast show a focal asymmetry (*arrows*). (C) This focal asymmetry persists as a mass of the same density and size on spot compression tomosynthesis (see also Video 4.7), unlike the summation artifact demonstrated in Fig. 4.15 and Video 4.6, which spread out into normal glandular elements. Wire-localized excisional biopsy showed atypical ductal hyperplasia.

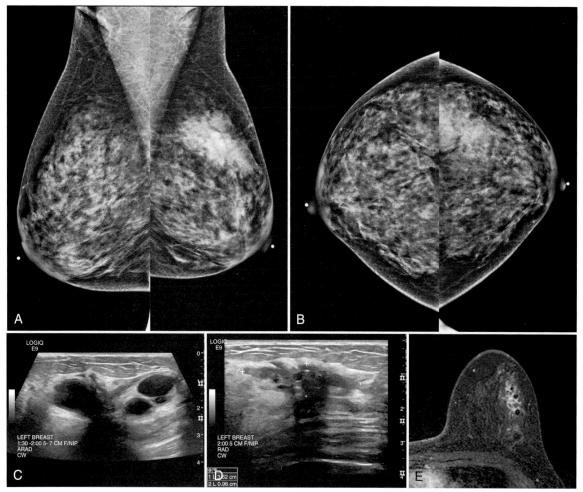

FIG. 4.19 Asymmetry: focal asymmetry. Breast cancer and cysts. (A and B) Paired mediolateral oblique (A) and craniocaudal (B) screening mammograms show a focal asymmetry with possible architectural distortion in the left upper outer breast. (C and D) Ultrasound shows multiple cysts (C) and a 3.6-cm irregular hypoechoic shadowing mass (D). (E) Contrast-enhanced magnetic resonance image shows a 3.1-cm segmental clumped nonmass enhancement with rapid initial and washout delayed kinetics and adjacent low signal cysts. Biopsy showed invasive carcinoma with desmoplastic stroma. In retrospect, the focal asymmetry consisted of breast cancer and multiple cysts.

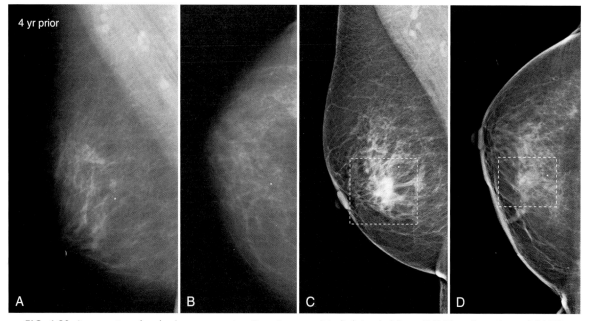

FIG. 4.20 Asymmetry: developing asymmetry. Breast cancer. Mediolateral oblique (MLO) and craniocaudal (CC) screening mammograms of the right breast 4 years before (A and B) and currently (C and D) show a new increased density (focal asymmetry; *box*) that looks like a mass behind the nipple on the MLO view but partly spreads out in the inner breast on the CC view, hidden by adjacent tissue. Workup showed a mass and biopsy showed tubular cancer.

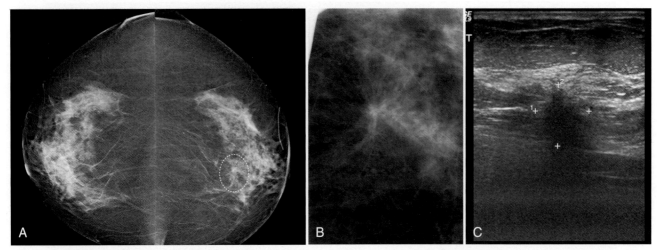

FIG. 4.21 Architectural distortion: breast cancer. (A) Paired craniocaudal (CC) mammograms show architectural distortion (*circle*) and possible focal asymmetry in the central left breast. (B) Spot compressed magnified CC view better depicts the distortion as a suspicious spiculated finding. (C) Ultrasound shows a hypoechoic irregular mass with indistinct margins with acoustic shadowing. Biopsy showed invasive ductal carcinoma.

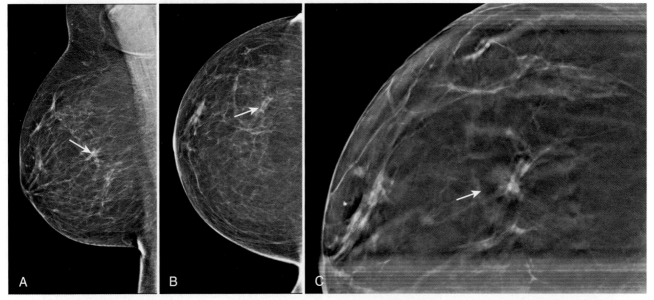

FIG. 4.22 Architectural distortion: radial scar. (A and B) Mediolateral oblique (A) and craniocaudal (CC) (B) screening mammograms show architectural distortion (*arrows*) in the outer right breast. (C) Spot compressed CC tomosynthesis slice (see also Video 4.8) shows distortion and a possible 7-mm mass not seen by US. Wire-localized biopsy showed radial scar.

requires biopsy. Architectural distortion is seen on 2D mammography and is even more exquisitely depicted on tomosynthesis. Architectural distortion seen on tomosynthesis may be invisible or subtle on 2D mammography, but still represents cancer or radial scar (Fig. 4.22; Video 4.8).

For findings seen only on tomosynthesis and undetected by US, biopsy may be done under tomosynthesis guidance (Freer et al., 2015). Architectural distortion may be a finding by itself or may be an associated finding (see section: Associated Features of Masses).

Associated Features of Masses

Associated findings of masses worrisome for cancer (Box 4.1) include skin or nipple retraction (Figs. 4.23 and 4.24; Video 4.9), skin thickening (Fig. 4.25), or trabecular thickening (Fig. 4.26);

BOX 4.1   American College of Radiology Breast Imaging Reporting and Data System Associated Findings

Skin retraction
Nipple retraction
Skin thickening
Trabecular thickening
Skin lesion
Axillary adenopathy
Architectural distortion
Calcifications

From American College of Radiology: ACR BI-RADS®—Mammography. In *ACR BI-RADS atlas, breast imaging reporting and data system*, ed 5, Reston, VA, 2013, American College of Radiology.

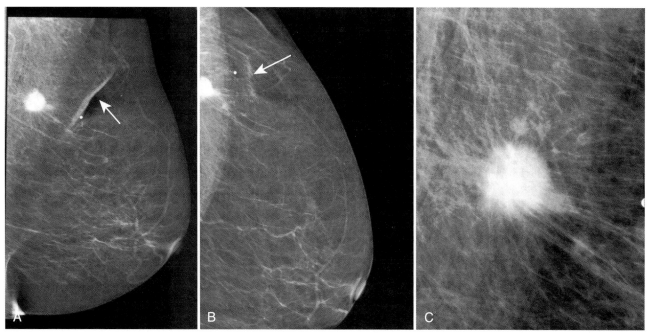

FIG. 4.23 Associated feature: skin retraction. Breast cancer. (A and B) Mediolateral oblique (MLO; A) and cranio-caudal (B) mammograms show a skin marker over a high-density palpable spiculated mass in the upper outer left breast causing skin retraction (*arrows*). (C) Magnification MLO view shows a high-density mass with spiculations extending to the skin, causing the skin tethering. Biopsy showed invasive ductal cancer.

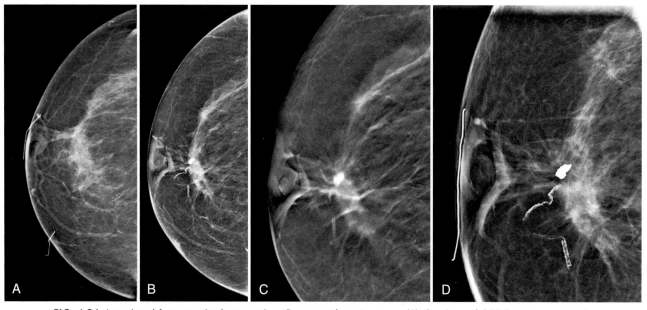

FIG. 4.24 Associated feature: nipple retraction. Recurrent breast cancer. (A) Craniocaudal (CC) mammogram in a patient with a previous history of right lumpectomy and radiation therapy for cancer shows linear scar markers and mild postbiopsy distortion in the retroareolar region. (B–D) Nine years after (A) diagnostic mammogram was performed because she developed lump and nipple inversion. Right CC mammogram (B) shows a retroareolar developing asymmetry with nipple retraction. Right CC tomosynthesis slice (C; see also Video 4.9) and spot compressed magnification CC mammogram with scar marker (D) depict an irregular mass with spiculations extending to the nipple. Note a normal dense calcification and vascular calcifications on B–D, new from the previous study (A). Biopsy showed invasive ductal carcinoma.

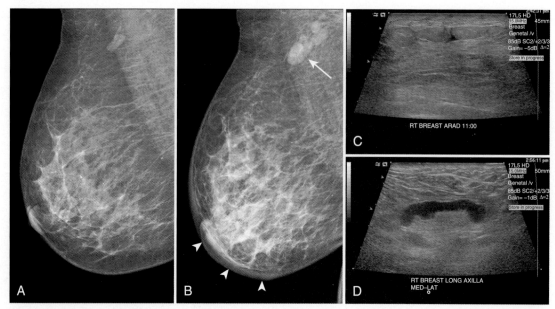

FIG. 4.25 Associated features: skin thickening. Inflammatory cancer. (A) Previous right mediolateral oblique (MLO) mammogram obtained 1 year prior shows no apparent abnormality. (B) The patient presented with skin redness and thickening of the central two-thirds of the right breast. Current right MLO mammogram shows widespread breast edema, trabecular thickening, and diffuse skin thickening most readily apparent in the lower breast (*arrowheads*). Axillary lymph nodes (*arrow*) are enlarged compared with the previous study. (C and D) Ultrasound shows diffuse abnormal increased echogenicity throughout the right breast (C), skin thickening, and an enlarged lymph node (D) with a lobulated border and impingement of the fatty hilum. Although a specific breast mass was not identified, biopsy of the skin showed angiolymphatic spaces containing carcinoma cells compatible with the clinical diagnosis of inflammatory cancer. Axillary lymph node biopsy showed metastatic carcinoma, consistent with ductal carcinoma of the breast.

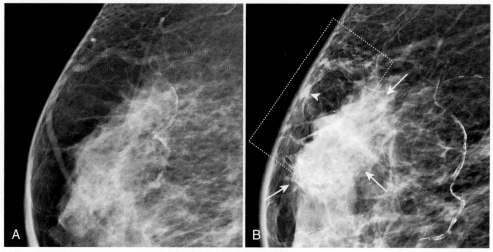

FIG. 4.26 Associated features: skin thickening and trabecular thickening. (A) Prior mediolateral oblique mammogram shows normal tissue and the normal dark fat below the skin with thin Cooper's ligaments. (B) Current lateromedial mammogram shows a new irregular high-density mass (*arrows*) with new trabecular thickening (*box*), shown by coarser white strands in the normally black subcutaneous fat and scalloping of the normally straight skin line (*arrowhead*). Biopsy of the mass showed invasive ductal carcinoma.

axillary adenopathy (Fig. 4.27); architectural distortion; and calcifications (Fig. 4.28).

Associated calcifications within or adjacent to a suspect mass are important for two reasons. First, suspicious, pleomorphic calcifications *inside* a *benign-appearing mass* may be the only clue that the mass is a cancer. Second, if the mass is cancer, calcifications around it may represent ductal carcinoma in situ (DCIS). Patient management includes sampling both the mass and surrounding suspicious calcifications (Box 4.2). If both

prove to be cancer, the surgeon will excise the extent of the suspicious calcifications to remove the cancer in its entirety (see Fig. 4.28B–C).

At histology, DCIS constituting more than 25% of an invasive ductal cancer is called an extensive intraductal component (EIC); such a cancer is called EIC-positive (EIC$^+$). Because EIC tumors have an increased risk of local recurrence, breast-conserving surgery is less successful. This is one of the reasons to always look for calcifications when a suspicious mass is present.

Other important associated mammographic findings suggestive of cancer are skin thickening, which may indicate breast edema or focal tumor invasion; skin retraction or nipple retraction as a result of focal tumor tethering; axillary adenopathy indicating axillary lymph node metastases; and architectural distortion.

FURTHER CHARACTERIZATION OF MASSES WITH ULTRASONOGRAPHY

US goes hand-in-hand with mammography in breast mass evaluation. A major advantage of US is the ability to directly correlate the clinical and imaging findings. It provides real-time evaluation of mass shapes, borders, orientation, and internal characteristics to determine whether the mass is cystic or solid or malignant or benign. Many masses that are not well characterized on mammography can be characterized as benign using US. US is often used for further assessment of possible masses after mammography and is the initial imaging modality in the evaluation of clinically detected palpable masses in a women younger than 30 years of age. Detailed principles and interpretation of ultrasonography are explained further in Chapter 5.

Ultrasound Technique and Analysis of Masses

The ACR BI-RADS US lexicon describes terms and features of breast masses that are key for the diagnosis of cancer (Table 4.3). As shown by Stavros et al. (1995), ultrasonographic features are basically different between malignant and benign solid masses (Box 4.3). Illustrations of these features are shown in Chapter 5, with the most important US features of cancer detailed under the categories of mass shape (irregular), margin (not circumscribed), and orientation (not parallel to the chest wall).

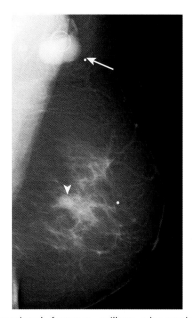

FIG. 4.27 Associated features: axillary adenopathy. Metastatic lymph node from breast cancer. Left breast mediolateral oblique view shows a 3.5-cm oval high-density left axillary mass (*arrow*) near a BB marker and circular mole marker, representing a metastatic lymph node. The primary invasive ductal cancer is an oval mass with indistinct margins (*arrowhead*) under another BB marker in the mid left breast that is much smaller than the metastasis. Note that lymphadenopathy may be a dominant or an only indicator of breast cancer, because even small cancers can metastasize.

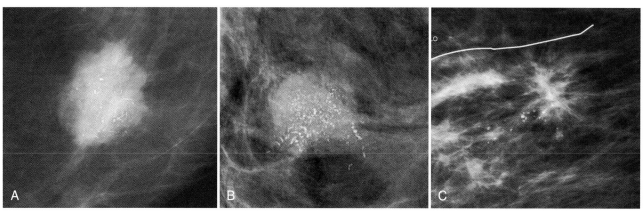

FIG. 4.28 Associated features: calcifications. Three different cases with breast cancer. (A) Cropped magnified mammogram shows a suspicious irregular mass containing pleomorphic calcifications, representing grade II invasive ductal cancer (IDC) and ductal carcinoma in situ (DCIS). (B) Another patient has a suspicious dense mass and fine pleomorphic calcifications within and adjacent to the mass. Excisional biopsy showed high-grade DCIS. (C) Spiculated mass, representing IDC, has fine-linear and pleomorphic calcifications within it and extending into the surrounding tissue, representing DCIS. Note the linear scar marker overlying this breast cancer recurrence near the prior postbiopsy scar. Radiologists report both the mass and calcification extent to ensure the surgeon removes all suspicious findings.

US evaluation of breast masses begins with determining whether the mass is cystic or solid. Simple cysts are anechoic (all black inside), round or oval shaped with circumscribed margins, have an abrupt interface with surrounding tissue, have a thin posterior wall, and are enhanced through sound transmission (have a white tail on the side of the mass opposite of the transducer, like a comet tail). Simple cysts are dismissed as benign.

In contrast, solid breast masses have internal echoes and could be either malignant or benign. To determine whether a mass is cancer on US, the radiologist evaluates the mass shape, margins, and orientation. The most suspicious mass shape is irregular. The most suspicious mass margin is *not circumscribed,* including margins that are indistinct (including echogenic halo), angular, microlobulated, and spiculated. The most suspicious orientation is not-parallel orientation in which the long axis of the mass is perpendicular to the chest wall. Not parallel is also known as "taller than wide" by Stavros criteria (1995) and is of concern that the mass is growing through normal tissue planes. Other suspicious descriptors are a *heterogeneous* or *complex cystic and solid* internal echo pattern, *posterior acoustic shadowing,* or *architectural distortion* of the surrounding breast tissue. The presence and location of associated calcifications are helpful in describing masses on US.

After scanning, the technologist takes representative pictures of the mass and labels the images to clarify the mass' location in the breast. The ACR Practice Parameter for the Performance of a Breast Ultrasound Examination, Labeling, includes facility name and location, examination date, patient's first and last name, which breast was scanned (left or right), position of the mass in terms of breast clock face or diagram annotation, the finding's location in centimeters from the nipple, and the technologist's initials. Other information helpful in finding the mass on subsequent studies includes the scan angle (radial or antiradial and transverse or longitudinal). The technologist captures the image without and with measuring calipers on the mass (Box 4.4). It is also helpful to indicate whether the mass is palpable or nonpalpable. The ACR Practice Parameter encourages real-time scanning

by the interpreter. Many facilities capture cine or moving images in addition to static images.

Benign US findings include no malignant features, oval or round shape, an abrupt circumscribed margin, intense homogeneous internal hyperechogenicity, fewer than four gentle lobulations, parallel (wider than tall) configuration (parallel to the chest wall), no posterior acoustic shadowing, and a thin echogenic capsule (Stavros et al., 1995). Because benign and malignant features in solid masses overlap, common sense plays a major role in patient management for solid masses, especially if the mass looks benign but the clinical scenario is suspicious (for example, new benign-appearing mass in a patient with a strong family history of breast cancer).

Correlating Palpable and Nonpalpable Masses on Mammography and Ultrasound

A common clinical problem is the palpable breast mass. The ACR Appropriateness Criteria for Palpable Breast Masses (Harvey et al., 2013) specifies guidelines to tailor imaging examinations for palpable masses. For example, the ACR Criteria recommends initial mammography for women aged ≥40 years old, usually with US as the second test. For pregnant or lactating women, or women aged ≤30 years old, US is the first study. Either US or mammography can be done first in women between these ages.

When US is the only study for a *palpable* mass, one correlates US findings with the palpable mass at real-time imaging. One method to correlate US findings to the mass is to place an examining finger or a cotton-tipped swab directly on the palpable mass and scan over the finger or cotton-tipped swab on the mass to generate a ring-down shadow. Subsequent removal of the finger or cotton-tipped swab from under the probe produces a scan of the palpable finding. Then the radiologist, technologist, and patient have no doubt that the palpable finding has been scanned, because this technique ensures that the transducer is placed directly on the palpable finding.

To correlate *palpable* US and mammographic findings when US is the first study, the radiologist or technologist scans the palpable mass and if there is a US-detected mass, the sonographer places a finger or cotton-tipped swab on the skin over the mass. The sonographer then marks the skin with indelible ink and places a metallic skin marker, such as a BB, over the palpable finding. Subsequently, the mammography technologist performs the mammogram. If the marker is at or near the mammographic finding, the palpable, mammographic, and US findings all correlate with each other.

BOX 4.2 Masses and Microcalcifications

Beware of pleomorphic calcifications adjacent to a suspicious breast mass that is biopsy-proven invasive cancer. The adjacent calcifications should undergo biopsy because the calcifications may represent ductal carcinoma in situ.

TABLE 4.3 **American College of Radiology Breast Imaging Reporting and Data System Ultrasound Lexicon Descriptors for Masses**

Shape	Orientation	Margin	Echo Pattern	Posterior Acoustic Features	Associated Features	Calcifications
Oval	Parallel	Circumscribed	Anechoic	None	Architectural distortion	Calcifications in a mass
Round	Not parallel	Not circumscribed	Hyperechoic	Enhancement	Duct changes	Calcifications outside
Irregular		Indistinct	Complex	Shadowing	Skin changes	of a mass
		Angular	Hypoechoic	Combined	Skin thickening	Intraductal
		Microlobulated	Isoechoic		Skin retraction	calcifications
		Spiculated	Heterogeneous		Edema	
					Vascularity	
					Absent	
					Internal vascularity	
					Vessels in rim	
					Elasticity assessment	
					Soft	
					Intermediate	
					Hard	

BOX 4.3 Ultrasound Features of Solid Breast Masses: Malignant versus Benign

MALIGNANT

Irregular shape
Not-parallel orientation (taller than wide)
Not-circumscribed margin (indistinct, angulated, microlobulated, and spiculated)
Very hypoechoic
Acoustic shadowing
Microcalcifications
Duct extension
Branch pattern
Hard elasticity assessment

BENIGN

Oval shape
Parallel orientation (wider than tall)
Circumscribed margin
Intense homogeneous hyperechogenicity
Four or fewer gentle lobulations
Thin echogenic pseudocapsule/ellipsoid shape
No malignant characteristics

Modified from Stavros AT, Thickman D, Rapp CL, et al: Solid breast nodules: use of sonography to distinguish between benign and malignant lesions, *Radiology* 196:123–134, 1995.

BOX 4.4 American College of Radiology Recommendations for Breast Ultrasound Labeling[a]

Right or left breast
Mass position in terms of clock face or quadrant
Number of centimeters from the nipple
Scan plane (radial/antiradial and transverse/long)
Initials of person performing the scan
Orthogonal images of mass without and with measuring calipers

[a]2014 ACR Practice Parameter for the Performance of the Breast Ultrasound Examination

To correlate nonpalpable US findings with mammographic findings when mammography is the first study, the sonographer looks at the mammogram to determine where to scan and what to expect on US. If there is a US finding that might correlate with the mammographic finding, the sonographer places a finger, cotton-tipped swab, or large unwound paper clip under the transducer so that a ring-down shadow is superimposed over the finding. The sonographer removes the transducer, marks the skin over the mass with an indelible ink marker, and places a metallic skin marker on the ink spot. The mammography technologist takes orthogonal mammographic views. The skin marker over the US finding should be in the same location as the mammographic finding on the films. It should be expected that even if the mammogram and US findings are the same, the mammographic finding might be 1 cm or more away from the skin marker on the films because the skin marker will be compressed away from the mass on the mammogram by the compression paddle.

Sometimes it is still uncertain whether a US and mammographic finding are one and the same even after US/mammography skin marking. If the patient agrees to a biopsy of the US finding, the radiologist places a metallic marker into the mass using a US-guided, percutaneously placed needle after the biopsy (Fig. 4.29). Postbiopsy mammograms will show the marker in the mass if the US and mammography findings are the same. If the mass was only seen by tomosynthesis, marker placement in the mass should be confirmed by postbiopsy tomosynthesis.

Alternatively, a retractable hookwire may be placed in the mass under US. A mammogram with the wire in place will show that the US finding and the mammographic finding represent the same mass. The radiologist can subsequently remove the retractable hookwire.

The mammography and US report for a breast mass should describe if the mass is palpable; the size, shape, margin, and density of the mass; its location and associated findings; and any change from previous examinations, if known. The report should also include US finding descriptors and whether it correlates with the mammographic finding. Finally, each report that includes a mammogram should be assigned an ACR BI-RADS final assessment code indicating the level of suspicion for cancer and follow-up management recommendations (Box 4.5).

MAMMOGRAPHIC AND ULTRASOUND ATLAS OF MASSES

Masses with Spiculated Borders and Sclerosing Features

Masses with spiculated borders and sclerosing features suggest malignancy (Box 4.6). The benign (but high-risk) radial scar also appears as a spiculated mass on both 2D mammography and tomosynthesis and is a common cause of false-positive breast biopsies. On occasion, inflammatory or fibrotic lesions also may appear as spiculated masses

Cancer

Invasive Ductal Carcinoma. Invasive ductal carcinoma is the most common breast cancer and accounts for approximately 90% of all cancers. Also known as invasive ductal carcinoma not otherwise specified (NOS), invasive ductal carcinoma usually grows as a hard irregular mass in the breast (Fig. 4.30; Video 4.10). The classic appearance of invasive ductal carcinoma is a high-density irregular or spiculated mass, occasionally containing or associated with adjacent pleomorphic calcifications representing DCIS. On the mammogram, the mass should be about the same size and density on two orthogonal mammographic views. Spot compression magnification views may show unsuspected calcifications in or around the mass or unsuspected irregular borders.

Mammographic spiculated masses are often round, irregular, or spiculated on US and commonly produce acoustic shadowing as a result of either productive fibrosis or tumor extension. When present, acoustic spiculation looks like thin radiating lines extending from the tumor into surrounding breast structures, occasionally causing tissue distortion. In a dense white breast, the US spicules are dark against the white glandular tissue. In a fatty breast, the spicules are white against the dark fatty background.

On MRI, the usual appearance of invasive ductal cancer is a brightly enhancing irregular mass with or without spiculation; enhancement is initially rapid, with a late-phase plateau or washout curve. Rim enhancement and heterogeneous enhancement are other worrisome signs for invasive ductal cancer on MRI.

Invasive Lobular Carcinoma. Invasive lobular carcinoma (ILC) is most commonly seen as an equal-density or high-density noncalcified mass, occasionally showing spiculations or ill-defined borders (Fig. 4.31; see also Fig. 4.1). Johnson et al. (2015) and Hilleren et al. (1991) showed that 50% of ILC may have a density equal or lower than surrounding glandular tissue and Mendelson et al. (1989) showed that some ILC may contain lucent areas. ILC has a higher rate of bilaterality and multifocality than does invasive ductal cancer. It accounts for less than 10% of all invasive cancers, but historically it is the most difficult

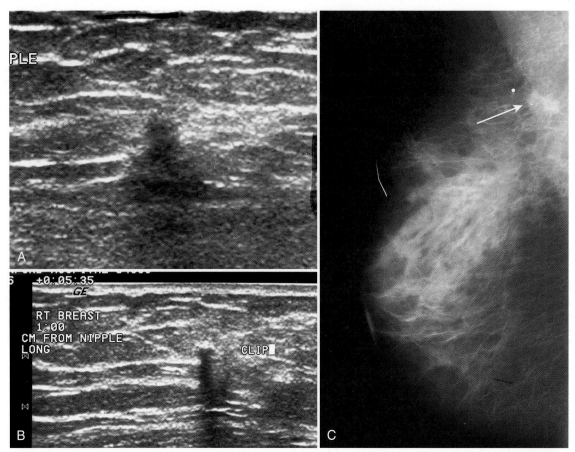

FIG. 4.29 Ultrasound (US)-guided marker placement to correlate nonpalpable US and mammography findings. (A) A patient with a nonpalpable mass seen only on the mediolateral oblique (MLO) view underwent US, showing an indistinct, not-parallel mass with an echogenic rim and acoustic shadowing. (B) After US-guided core biopsy with marker placement in the mass, a BB skin marker was placed over the skin where US showed the mass. (C) The MLO view shows the mass and marker (*arrow*) and the skin BB over the mass, proving the US-detected finding represents mammographic mass. Biopsy showed invasive ductal carcinoma. Note the metallic linear scar marker on the skin over a previous biopsy.

BOX 4.5   American College of Radiology Breast Imaging Reporting and Data System Mass Reporting

Size and location
Mass type and modifiers (shape, margin, and density)
Associated calcifications
Associated findings
How changed if previously present
Summary and BI-RADS code (0–6)

BI-RADS, Breast Imaging Reporting and Data System.
From American College of Radiology: ACR BI-RADS®—Mammography. In *ACR BI-RADS atlas, breast imaging reporting and data system,* ed 5, Reston, VA, 2013, American College of Radiology.

BOX 4.6   Differential Diagnosis of Spiculated Masses

Invasive ductal carcinoma
Invasive lobular carcinoma
Tubular cancer
Postbiopsy scar
Radial scar
Fat necrosis (atypical)
Sclerosing adenosis
Proliferative fibrocystic change (rare)

---

breast cancer to see on mammograms (Box 4.7). ILC gives radiologists a bad name because it can be missed by mammography, at a rate reported by Brem et al. (2009) to be as high as 21%. This failure can be partly explained by the growth pattern of the carcinoma. Classically, ILC grows in single lines of tumor cells infiltrating the surrounding glandular tissue and may not produce a mass, making it difficult to see by mammography and difficult to feel by physical examination. It usually does not contain microcalcifications. It often infiltrates the breast, is often seen on only one view, and may cause only subtle distortion of the surrounding glandular tissue. When actually seen on the mammogram, ILC masses are often of equal or higher density than fibroglandular tissue and are seen because of the mass itself or its effect on surrounding tissue, such as architectural distortion and straightening of Cooper's ligaments. As with any mass, distortion, flattening, and tenting of glandular tissue caused by ILC are most easily seen in locations in which Cooper's ligaments extend out into surrounding fat, such as in the retroglandular fat or along the edge of the normal, scalloped fibroglandular tissue (see Figs. 4.10 and 4.25).

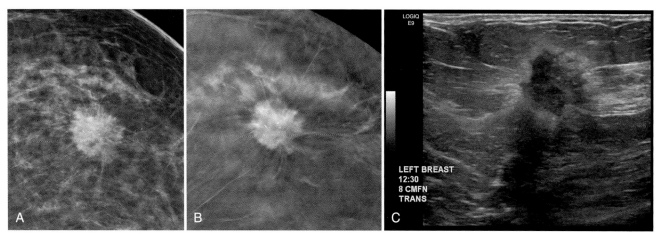

FIG. 4.30 Spiculated mass: invasive ductal carcinoma. (A) Magnification craniocaudal (CC) mammogram shows a spiculated mass. (B) Tomosynthesis of left CC projection slice (see also Video 4.10) shows spiculations and microcalcifications within the mass more clearly. (C) The corresponding ultrasound shows a hypoechoic mass with indistinct, spiculated margins. Biopsy showed invasive ductal carcinoma.

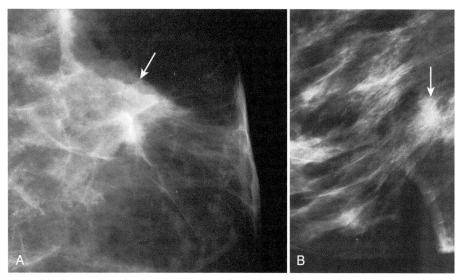

FIG. 4.31 Spiculated mass: invasive lobular cancer in two different cases. (A) Spot compression craniocaudal mammogram shows a spiculated mass causing distortion (*arrow*) and flattening of the nipple. Thin straight lines extend from the tumor into subcutaneous fat, indicating its presence. (B) In another patient, there is a spiculated mass (*arrow*) at the edge of the film at the chest wall on a right mediolateral oblique view. The cancer looks very similar to the rest of the breast tissue and is seen only because of the spiculations extending into the fat, and also because it is a density in "no man's land" in which there is usually only fat near the chest wall.

BOX 4.7 Features of Invasive Lobular Carcinoma

10% of all breast cancers
Grows in single-cell files
Hardest tumor to see on mammography
Often seen on one view
Causes mass or architectural distortion
Calcifications not a feature

On US, ILC is a hypoechoic, irregular, spiculated, or ill-defined mass that may or may not have acoustic shadowing. When ILC becomes very large, only the acoustic shadowing may be apparent; the mass itself can be difficult to see because of its large size. On MRI, ILC looks like a spiculated mass but may have variable enhancing patterns; it can look like a mass, like a distortion of tissue, or like nodular regions connected by strands of tissue. Its enhancement kinetics can be similar to those of normal breast tissue and can thus be a cause of false-negative MRI examinations. However, ILC is detected more readily by MRI compared with mammography and US, rendering ILC a common indication for breast MRI when assessing extent of disease. In a 2015 study, Debald et al. (2015) showed that women with ILC were significantly associated with having other foci of cancer in the involved breast when evaluated with MRI ($p = 0.02$).

Tubular Carcinoma. Tubular carcinoma is a generally slow-growing tumor with a bilateral incidence of 12% to 40%. On mammography, tubular cancer is a dense or equal-density spiculated mass with occasional microcalcifications (Fig. 4.32). On occasion it may be apparent on the previous mammogram because of its slow growth. Although controversial, some pathologists believe that radial scars may be a precursor to tubular carcinoma. Generally, tubular carcinoma has a good prognosis and a lower

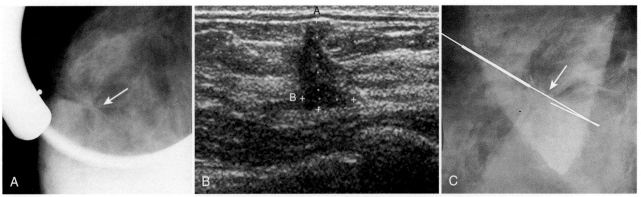

FIG. 4.32 Spiculated mass: tubular cancer with mammographic and ultrasound correlation. (A) Spot compression mammogram shows a palpable spiculated mass (*arrow*) under a BB skin marker in extremely dense tissue. (B) Ultrasound shows a not-parallel spiculated irregular mass. (C) Specimen radiograph better shows the typical spiculations radiating from the mass (*arrow*) around a localizing hookwire.

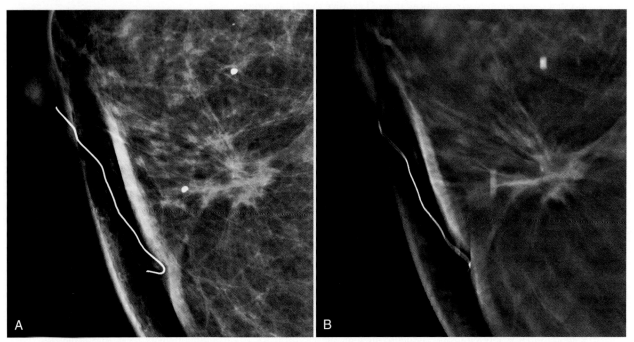

FIG. 4.33 Spiculated mass: postbiopsy scar. (A) Photographic magnification 2D mammogram shows a spiculated mass directly under a linear scar marker over a postbiopsy site, representing a postbiopsy scar. (B) Tomosynthesis slice (see also Video 4.11) shows the postbiopsy scar to greater advantage.

incidence of metastases than does invasive ductal cancer. On US, tubular cancers are hypoechoic, irregular masses that occasionally produce acoustic shadowing.

Postbiopsy Scar

On mammograms, a new postbiopsy scar is round, ill-defined, and contains air and fluid; after healing, an old postbiopsy scar looks like a spiculated mass that is impossible to distinguish from cancer. In the immediate postoperative period, postbiopsy scars show air and fluid in a round or oval mass at the biopsy site, with adjacent skin thickening where the surgeon has closed the skin. Because the surgeon does not close the excised cavity with sutures, the cavity is left to fill with fluid (seroma) that may contain blood. The fluid is resorbed to varying degrees over time, with fluid occasionally persisting for several years as a round or oval mass in the biopsy site. In other cases the

fluid resorbs completely, and the surrounding glandular tissue is drawn into a central dense nidus of scar tissue. As a result, the mammogram shows a centrally dense spiculated mass (the scar) with straightening of the surrounding Cooper's ligaments and indrawing of normal glandular tissue, simulating a spiculated breast cancer (Fig. 4.33; Video 4.11). In some patients, no dense central nidus occurs, and the scar appears as a focal architectural distortion with radiating thin white lines from a central point. On US, a postbiopsy scar is a hypoechoic mass with acoustic spiculation and shadowing, similar to cancer. There should be thickening of the patient's skin where the skin scar lies and distortion of subcutaneous tissue extending from the patient's skin scar, down the plane of the incision, and finally leading to the postbiopsy scar.

The postbiopsy scar is not of concern for cancer if it occupies a surgical site (Box 4.8). To distinguish postbiopsy scars from cancer, the radiologist reviews surgical biopsy locations on the

To determine whether a spiculated mass is a postbiopsy scar, correlate the "scar" to a linear scar marker on the skin showing the location of the previous biopsy, and correlate the scar location with the targeted finding on old prebiopsy mammograms. If the postbiopsy scar is nowhere near the linear scar marker, or if the scar has developed in a location other than the targeted, excised finding, it is not a scar and should undergo biopsy.

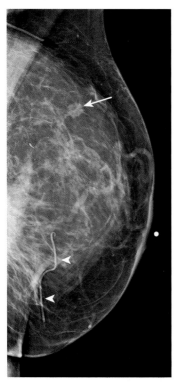

FIG. 4.34 Spiculated mass: postbiopsy scar and new cancer away from scar marker. Mediolateral oblique mammogram shows a postbiopsy scar (*arrowheads*) from resection of a papillary cancer with a new spiculated mass (*arrow)* in the upper breast. The new mass in the upper breast cannot represent a postbiopsy scar because it is far away from the linear scar marker. Biopsy showed invasive ductal cancer.

breast history form and reviews older films to see if the scar is at the same location as the resected finding. Some facilities place a radiopaque linear metallic scar marker on the patient's skin scar to show the skin scar location on the mammogram (see Fig. 4.33; see Video 4.11). The metallic linear scar marker should be on top of the architectural distortion thought to represent postbiopsy scar. If the mammographic scar does not correspond to a postbiopsy site, it is a mass, should be considered suspicious, and should undergo workup and biopsy (Fig. 4.34). However, increased density, growth, or changing of the normally convex postbiopsy scar to a concave margin suggests breast cancer recurrence and needs workup (see Chapter 8).

Radial Scar

A radial scar has nothing to do with a postbiopsy scar but is a common name for a benign proliferative breast lesion that looks like a spiculated cancerous mass or postbiopsy scar on mammograms. Both radial scars and their larger variants, called complex sclerosing lesions, may include adenosis and hyperplasia. In

autopsy series, small radial scars are common but often may not be apparent on 2D mammography. The central part of a radial scar undergoes atrophy, resulting in a scarlike formation, with pulling in of the surrounding glandular tissue that produces a spiculated mass. On occasion, because of entrapment of breast ductules, the radial scar may be difficult for pathologists to distinguish from infiltrating ductal carcinoma. However, both epithelial and myoepithelial cells in benign radial scars distinguish them from breast cancer. Radial scars may contain or be associated with atypical ductal hyperplasia, atypical lobular hyperplasia, lobular carcinoma in situ, or cancer. This is one of the rationales for surgical excision. Some pathologists believe that a radial scar may be a precursor to tubular carcinoma and should be excised, although this position is controversial.

On mammography, a radial scar appears as a spiculated mass with either a dark or white central area that may or may not have associated microcalcifications (Figs. 4.35 and 4.36; Video 4.12). It is a myth that radial scars have dark centers in the mass on mammography and can be distinguished from breast cancers, which have white-centered masses. Scientific studies have shown that radial scars and breast cancer can both have either white or dark centers on mammograms. This means that all spiculated masses not representing a postbiopsy scar should be sampled histologically (Box 4.9).

Because tomosynthesis is extremely sensitive in detecting spiculation or distortion, many radial scars are now found by tomosynthesis that were invisible on 2D mammography. Unfortunately, a radial scar cannot be distinguished from cancer even on tomosynthesis, thus it requires a biopsy and is a cause for false-positive studies.

On US, a radial scar is a hypoechoic mass, with or without acoustic shadowing (see Figs. 4.35 and 4.36; Linda et al., 2010, 2012).

Fat Necrosis, Sclerosing Adenosis, and Other Benign Breast Disease

Fat necrosis is caused by saponification of fat from previous trauma, usually from surgery or blunt trauma from an injury, such as from a steering wheel or seat belt in an automobile accident. On mammography, fat necrosis typically contains a fatty lipid center and is round, but occasionally it has a spiculated appearance. Other appearances include asymmetric opacity, round opacity, and dystrophic or pleomorphic calcifications. The diagnosis may be established by eliciting a history of blunt trauma or previous surgery. On occasion, fat necrosis contains a dense or equal-density central nidus with radiating folds extending from its center, similar to cancer, prompting biopsy. On US, fat necrosis can appear cystic with or without posterior acoustic enhancement or has internal echoes in about 30% of the cases, showing increased echogenicity in 27% and solid in approximately 14%, as reported by Bilgen et al. (2001). With true fat necrosis, follow-up should show a decrease in size of masses; the occasional increasing fat necrosis lesion should undergo biopsy, leading to the diagnosis.

Sclerosing adenosis is a proliferative benign lesion resulting from mammary lobular hyperplasia. It is characterized by the formation of fibrous tissue that distorts and envelops the glandular tissue. The resulting process may produce a masslike tissue with or without infiltrating margins to the surrounding tissue caused by sclerosis. The small duct lumens can contain microcalcifications. Thus on mammography and ultrasonography, sclerosing adenosis manifests as various appearances, including spiculated masses, circumscribed masses, microlobulated masses, masses with indistinct margins, asymmetries, and microcalcifications (pleomorphic, amorphous and punctate shapes, etc.) and can mimic cancers (Fig. 4.37; Gill et al., 2003; Günhan-Bilgen et al., 2002).

Like sclerosing adenosis, proliferative fibrocystic change occasionally has a slightly spiculated appearance on mammography

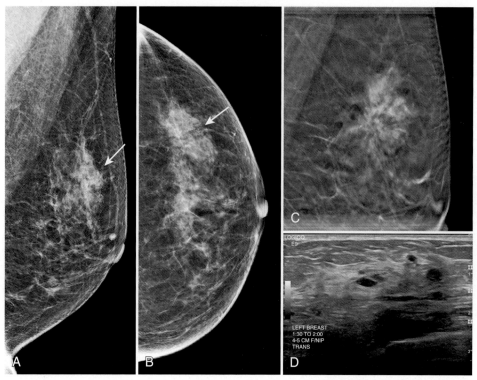

FIG. 4.35 Spiculated mass: radial scar with spot compression tomosynthesis studies. (A and B) Left mediolateral oblique (MLO; A) and craniocaudal (B) views show a focal asymmetry with possible architectural distortion (*arrows*) in the upper outer left breast. (C) Spot compressed MLO tomosynthesis slice shows architectural distortion more clearly (also see Video 4.12). (D) Corresponding ultrasound shows heterogeneous hypoechoic area surrounded by several cysts. Excisional biopsy showed radial scar. Obstruction of mammary ducts by radial scar likely caused the surrounding cysts.

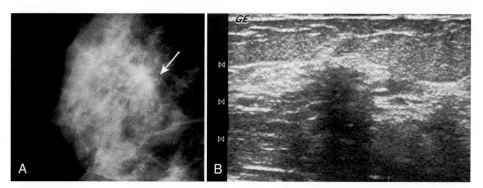

FIG. 4.36 Spiculated mass: radial scar with mammographic and ultrasound correlation. (A) Photographically magnified mammogram shows a vague spiculated mass (*arrow*) with a dense white center in the upper part of the breast. (B) Ultrasound shows an irregular hypoechoic mass, simulating cancer. Biopsy showed radial scar, which is indistinguishable from cancer on imaging.

BOX 4.9   Radial Scar versus Cancer

Radial scars cannot be distinguished from cancer on mammography. Spiculated masses not representing postbiopsy scar tissue require a histologic diagnosis.

---

and occasionally contains calcifications, simulating cancer and requiring biopsy.

If these benign entities have suspicious appearances, such as spiculations and microcalcifications, fat necrosis, sclerosing adenosis, and proliferative fibrocystic disease, they may undergo biopsy, resulting in false-positive practice audits.

Masses with Round/Oval Shapes or Expansile Borders

Masses with round/oval shapes or expansile borders include both malignant and benign disease entities (Box 4.10). Generally, masses with this feature represent benign disease entities, such as cysts and fibroadenomas. However, on occasion, malignant tumors (the most commonly, invasive ductal carcinomas) may appear as round/oval masses and mimic benign masses.

Cyst and Cystic Mass

Cystic masses, such as simple cysts, complex cysts, intracystic papillomas, and intracystic carcinomas, often present as masses

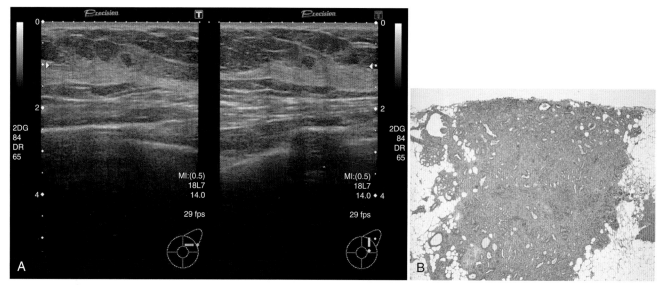

FIG. 4.37 Sclerosing adenosis. (A) Transverse and longitudinal views of ultrasonography show a small irregular, hypoechoic mass with microlobulated and indistinct margins. (B) Photography of biopsied specimen (hematoxylin and eosin stain) demonstrates a masslike area consisting of proliferated glands and fibrosis, which has an irregular border against the surrounding fat tissue. Sclerosing adenosis is the diagnosis. (Courtesy Shotaro Kanao, M.D., Ph.D., Kyoto University, Kyoto, Japan).

BOX 4.10   Differential Diagnosis of Round Masses

Cyst (includes complicated cysts, intracystic papilloma, or carcinoma)
Fibroadenoma
Papilloma
Invasive Ductal Cancer (uncommon form of most common cancer)
Medullary cancer
Mucinous (colloid) carcinoma
Papillary carcinoma
Adenoid cystic carcinoma
Phyllodes tumor
Breast metastasis
Lactating adenoma

---

with rounded or expansile borders on mammography. Simple cysts are the most common disease entity within the mammographic round/oval mass category. Radiologists use US to identify cyst fluid and to distinguish cystic from solid masses. The further details of cysts and cystic masses are discussed later (see section: Fluid Containing Masses).

Fibroadenoma

Fibroadenoma is the most common solid benign tumor in young women. It is thought to arise from the terminal ductal lobular unit via localized hypertrophy. Fibroadenomas can be single or multiple. A fibroadenoma contains structures suggesting breast ductules and also has stromal tissue, which can be quite cellular in young women. Fibroadenomas may also undergo adenosis or hyperplasia and proliferation and may contain fibrous bands or septations. DuPont et al. (1994) described fibroadenomas containing such proliferation or cysts with the nomenclature complex fibroadenomas. *Giant fibroadenomas* are 8 cm or larger in size. *Juvenile fibroadenomas* occur in

adolescents and can grow rapidly, stretch the skin, and become huge. Because juvenile fibroadenomas may grow to such a large size, they are often also giant fibroadenomas, but not all giant fibroadenomas are juvenile fibroadenomas. The usual treatment for the giant juvenile fibroadenoma is excision with preservation of the nipple/areolar complex and developing breast tissue (Sosin et al., 2015).

On mammograms, the classic fibroadenoma is an oval, equal-density mass with circumscribed margins, and up to three to four gentle lobulations (Fig. 4.38). In young patients, fibroadenomas are very cellular but are usually oval and circumscribed. As the fibroadenoma ages, it may become sclerotic and less cellular. Popcorn-like calcifications may develop at the periphery of the mass and occasionally replace the entire mass so it looks like a "breast rock."

On US, fibroadenomas are oval, well-circumscribed homogeneous masses, usually growing parallel to the chest wall and between Cooper's ligaments (wider than tall). They are hypoechoic, homogeneous masses but may occasionally contain cystic spaces or dark internal septations. Posterior acoustic enhancement is increased, equal, or shadowing. Fibroadenomas occasionally display irregular borders, heterogeneous internal characteristics, or not-parallel orientation (taller than wide), so biopsy is necessary to distinguish these atypical-appearing fibroadenomas from cancer (Fig. 4.39).

Because fibroadenomas contain ductal elements, ductal or lobular carcinoma in situ occurs in fibroadenomas rarely. For this reason, suspicious change in a fibroadenoma should prompt biopsy

On MRI, fibroadenomas have the classic appearance of an enhancing oval or lobulated mass with well-circumscribed borders. In 20% they contain dark internal septations. Kinetic data show a gradual initial enhancement rate and a late persistent enhancement curve (Fig. 4.40). The initial enhancement rate in fibroadenomas can be slow or rapid but unlike cancer, which shows late plateau or washout curves, the late enhancement curve of a fibroadenoma is persistent (Uematsu, 2009; Kuhl et al., 1999).

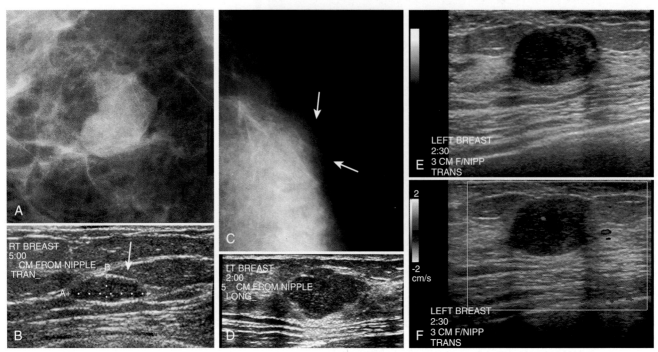

FIG. 4.38 Typical fibroadenoma in three different cases. (A and B) Mammogram (A) shows an oval well-circumscribed mass. Corresponding ultrasound (US; B) shows an oval well-circumscribed parallel homogenous almost isoechoic mass, which is typical for fibroadenoma. (C and D) Mammogram (C) in a young woman shows an equal-density, circumscribed oval but mostly obscured mass (*arrows*). Corresponding US (D) shows an oval, lobulated, well-circumscribed homogenous mass not as typical for fibroadenoma. (E and F) Ultrasound (E) of a palpable mass in a young woman shows a well-circumscribed parallel homogeneous mass typical of fibroadenoma. Doppler US (F) shows vascularity within the fibroadenoma.

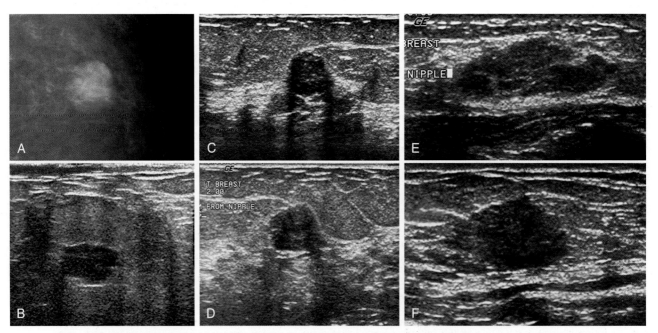

FIG. 4.39 Atypical appearances of fibroadenoma mimicking cancer in three different cases. (A and B) Mammogram (A) shows a round equal-density mass, but on ultrasound (US; B) this mass has margins that are not circumscribed and is very hypoechoic, similar to cancer. (C and D) Transverse (A) and longitudinal (B) view show a taller than wide microlobulated mass with internal echogenic foci, possibly calcifications. Biopsy showed fibroadenoma. (E and F) Other atypical appearances of biopsy-proven fibroadenoma on US.

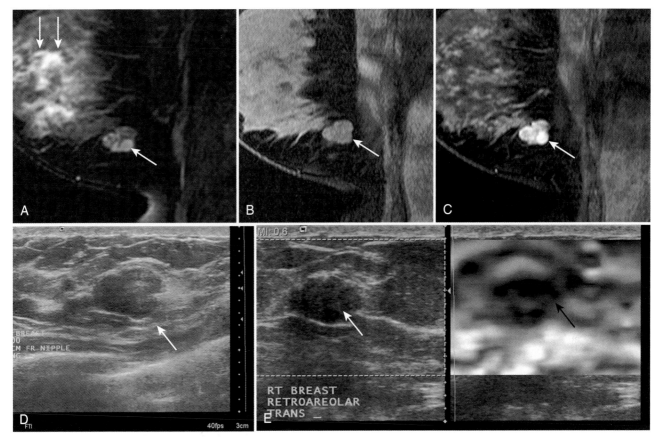

FIG. 4.40 Fibroadenoma on magnetic resonance imaging (MRI) and elastography. (A) T2-weighted sagittal noncontrast MRI image shows a slightly high signal intensity (*arrow*) lobulated mass in the lower breast and fluid in benign breast ducts (*double arrows*). Precontrast (B) and postcontrast (C) sagittal 3D spectral-spatial excitation magnetization transfer MRIs show an oval enhancing mass with dark septations and circumscribed margins (*arrow*). Enhancement kinetics showed a slow uptake and late persistent curve, suggesting fibroadenoma. (D) MRI-directed ultrasound (US) shows an oval circumscribed homogeneous mass (*arrow*) in the area of the MRI-detected mass. (E) B-mode (*left image*) and elastography (*right image*) US images show that the mass (*arrows*) is about the same size on the strain view, suggesting a benign finding. Biopsy showed fibroadenoma.

Papilloma

Papillomas are either solitary or multiple. In young patients, papillomas are called juvenile papillomas. Solitary papillomas are either central or peripheral, originate in the ductal epithelium, and are often seen in the subareolar region or in subareolar ducts. Tumors starting in the terminal ducts further from the nipple are called peripheral papillomas and are considered a risk factor for breast cancer. Multiple papillomas are usually in a more peripheral location in younger women. Juvenile papillomatosis occurs in young women, but multiple papillomas can also be seen in much older women. Papillomas grow on fibrovascular stalks, which can twist and lead to ischemia, necrosis, and blood extending into the duct. The bleeding papilloma results in the classic symptom of bloody nipple discharge, similar to a symptom of DCIS, causing patients to seek advice. Clinically, papillomas can also cause new, spontaneous clear or serous nipple discharge. Papillomas are usually excised to exclude DCIS or papillary cancer.

On mammography, papillomas are round, well-circumscribed, and equal-density masses that occasionally contain calcifications, They are usually located in the subareolar region, but they can be located in the breast periphery (Fig. 4.41). In papillomatosis, papillomas can be multiple and peripherally located. Occasionally, papillomas are not seen on mammography or US despite the symptom of bloody or clear nipple discharge. On US, papillomas are solid round, oval, or microlobulated hypoechoic masses. Small internal cystic spaces are seen occasionally in juvenile papillomatosis. In patients with nipple discharge, US may show papilloma as a solid mass in a fluid-filled subareolar duct. On galactography, the papilloma produces an intraductal filling defect (see Fig. 10.23).

On MRI, papillomas are round enhancing masses, with a rapid initial rise and a late plateau as washout on kinetic curves, indistinguishable from invasive ductal cancers (Fig. 4.42). Bright T2-weighted signal in ducts on precontrast studies, when seen, represents fluid-filled ducts. If a papilloma is present, the high signal in the duct may obscure an enhancing papilloma within it.

The finding of a round solid mass suspected to be papilloma requires a histologic diagnosis. Follow-up for papillomas diagnosed by core biopsy is controversial. However, surgical excisional biopsy is universally advised for papillomas with papillary carcinoma, atypia, or nonconcordant imaging findings. Surgical excisional biopsy for papillomas without atypia or malignancy diagnosed by core biopsy is variable, but many investigators recommend excision, particularly if the patient is at high risk for breast cancer, or if any atypia or other high-risk lesions found at surgery will prompt chemoprevention therapy and change patient management.

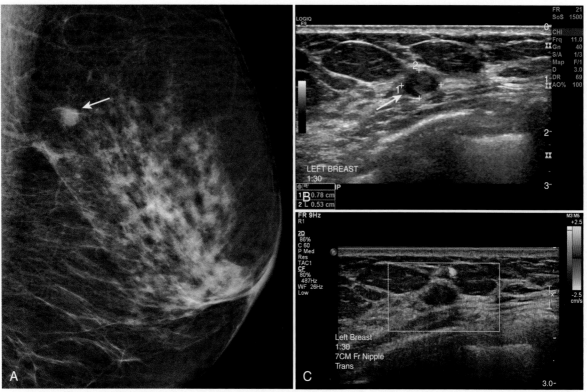

FIG. 4.41 Papilloma. (A) Left mediolateral oblique mammogram shows a small round mass (*arrow*) with indistinct margins in the posterior upper breast. (B and C) Corresponding ultrasound shows an oval hypoechoic mass containing a cystic space at its periphery (B; *arrow*), with no apparent increased vascularity (C). Biopsy showed a peripheral papilloma with focal atypia.

Cancer

Invasive Ductal Cancer. Invasive ductal cancer is the most common round breast cancer (Fig. 4.43). The "round" invasive ductal carcinoma is an uncommon form of the most common cancer, invasive ductal carcinoma. Invasive ductal carcinoma represents approximately 90% of all invasive breast cancers. Even though invasive ductal carcinomas are not often round, there are so many invasive ductal carcinomas that the most common round cancer is ductal carcinoma (uncommon round form of the most common breast cancer; Box 4.11).

The classic invasive ductal carcinoma is a dense spiculated or irregular mass on mammography. The much less common round invasive ductal carcinoma may grow so rapidly that it does not produce spiculated margins; instead, it has smooth or pushing borders (Fig. 4.44). This is especially true of triple negative (ER, PR, HER2 receptor negative) breast cancers, which are often round (M.Y. Kim, 2013). On screening mammography, round invasive ductal carcinoma may appear to have a circumscribed border. However, the mass borders may be obscured by surrounding breast tissue, or the standard mammogram may not have the resolution to reveal abnormal margins. Magnification views may show irregular, microlobulated, or indistinct borders, suggesting invasion of surrounding tissue and the true diagnosis. This is why new round masses on screening mammography are tricky and should be recalled from screening. A new round invasive ductal carcinoma mimics benign cysts or fibroadenomas, and the radiologist can mistakenly think the round mass is benign until the mass undergoes magnification.

On US, the round invasive cancer may be circumscribed, or may show suspicious indistinct or angular margins, and not-parallel orientation (taller than wide) or may have a thick echogenic rim. The not parallel or taller than wide orientation is an important ultrasonographic sign in the diagnosis

of breast cancer. Taller than wide is a US term described by Stavros et al. (1995) for masses invading through the normal horizontal tissue. It means that the cancer grows up toward the skin and violates normal tissue planes rather than growing horizontally between Cooper's ligaments (like benign tumors). The corresponding BI-RADS term is *not parallel*. Benign masses growing between Cooper's ligaments are called *parallel* in orientation in BI-RADS (parallel to Cooper's ligaments, or wider than tall).

Medullary Carcinoma. Medullary carcinoma is an invasive breast cancer that commonly has a round or pushing border. It occasionally has a surrounding lymphoid infiltrate and has a better prognosis than infiltrating ductal cancer (NOS). They are common in BRCA1-associated carcinomas. Atypical medullary carcinomas have the same prognosis as infiltrating ductal cancer. On screening mammography, medullary carcinoma is a high-density or equal-density round mass whose margins may appear well circumscribed, suggestive of a cyst or fibroadenoma (Fig. 4.45). On US, medullary carcinomas are round, solid, and homogeneous. Because they are homogeneous, medullary carcinomas occasionally cause posterior acoustic enhancement and it is important pay attention to scanning parameters to not mistake the solid medullary carcinoma for a cyst. Color or power Doppler US may show internal vascularity, unlike an anechoic simple cyst. The pushing expansile growth of medullary carcinoma may produce circumscribed mass borders, similar to fibroadenoma, and is a cause for misdiagnosis. This means that a new round solid mass should be biopsied, even if it is circumscribed.

Mucinous (Colloid) Carcinoma. This rare, round or oval cancer contains malignant tumor cells that float in mucin within a solid tumor rim. The mucinous portion can have fibrovascular bands segregating the mucinous compartments that comprise the tumor and give it its name. The amount of mucin versus solid

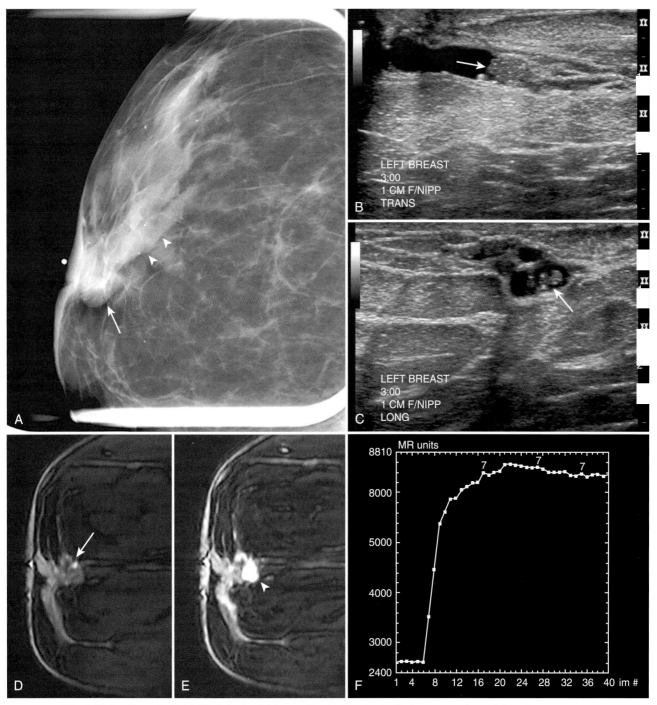

FIG. 4.42 Papilloma in fluid-filled ducts. (A) In a patient with nipple discharge, craniocaudal spot mammogram with nipple marker shows dilated ducts (*arrowheads*) and a possible retroareolar mass (*arrow*). (B and C) Ultrasound shows an intraductal mass in a fluid-filled duct in transverse (B) and longitudinal (C) images (*arrows*) suggesting papilloma, papillary cancer, or ductal carcinoma in situ. (D–F) Dynamic contrast magnetic resonance imaging (MRI) was performed. On precontrast T1-weighted fat-suppressed sagittal MRI (D), there is a precontrast high signal intensity retroareolar dot (*arrow*), which may represent debris in a fluid-filled duct. Postcontrast 3D spectral-spatial excitation magnetization transfer sagittal MRI (E) shows an enhancing mass in the retroareolar region (*arrowhead*). The kinetic curve of the mass (F) shows rapid initial enhancement and delayed washout, suggesting invasive ductal cancer or a papilloma. Biopsy showed papilloma.

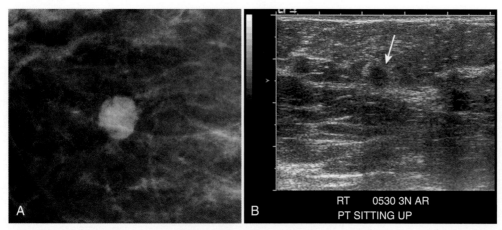

FIG. 4.43 Round invasive ductal carcinoma. (A) Photographically magnified mammogram shows a circumscribed, round high-density mass, simulating a fibroadenoma. (B) On ultrasound the mass borders are indistinct (*arrow*). Biopsy showed invasive ductal carcinoma.

BOX 4.11   Round Breast Cancers

The most common round breast cancer is invasive ductal cancer (IDC), which is more often seen as a spiculated mass or as pleomorphic calcifications. Because IDC is the most common breast cancer (90% of all cancers), its uncommon round form is seen more often than other cancers. For example, although medullary and mucinous cancers are quite often round in form, they are very uncommon.

---

tumor components vary from tumor to tumor, and account for the variable appearance of mucinous carcinoma on mammography and US. On mammography, mucinous carcinomas containing mostly mucin show a well-circumscribed low-density round mass that can suggest a cyst or fibroadenoma and can occasionally have lobulated margins (Fig. 4.46). Mixed-type mucinous carcinomas may be of higher density and have ill-defined or spiculated margins. On US, the tumor mass is round and may be isoechoic to fat, occasionally contains fluid-filled hypoechoic spaces, and may have posterior acoustic enhancement (see Fig. 4.46). The mass can simulate a cyst on US, but unlike the cyst it will not be entirely anechoic. Thus new round masses on a mammogram that have solid components or do not meet all the specific criteria for a simple cyst on US should be considered for biopsy.

Papillary Carcinoma. This rare tumor accounts for only 1% to 2% of all cancers and is the malignant form of benign intraductal papilloma. Papillary cancers may be single or multiple, and DCIS is sometimes seen in surrounding breast tissue. Classically, these masses are round, oval, or lobulated on mammography, sometimes containing calcifications, and are solid on US. If associated with nipple discharge and detected by US, papillary cancers are solid intraductal masses outlined by a fluid-filled structure and are difficult to distinguish from a benign intraductal papilloma (Fig. 4.47).

Adenoid Cystic Carcinoma. A very rare tumor that clinically manifests as a palpable firm mass, the adenoid cystic carcinoma, has a mixture of glandular and stromal elements that infiltrate the normal fibroglandular tissue in approximately 50% of cases. The tumor has a good prognosis if completely resected; however, recurrence is possible if the mass is not entirely excised. Imaging characteristics vary because of the rarity of reported cases and range from a well-circumscribed lobulated mass to ill-defined masses or focal asymmetries.

Phyllodes Tumor

Phyllodes tumors used to be called cystosarcoma phyllodes, which is a misnomer because most of these uncommon tumors are benign. Classically, the phyllodes tumor occurs in women in their fifth decade, with a median age of 45 years, and can be quite large, up to 5 cm in size when first detected. In the clinic, most often women with a phyllodes tumor seek advice for a rapidly growing palpable mass. Because the phyllodes tumor can have a biphasic growth pattern, some women report growth of a mass that has been stable for many years. A phyllodes tumor has both stromal and epithelial elements, in contrast to fibroadenoma. The phyllodes tumor also has fluidlike spaces containing solid growth of cellular stroma and epithelium in a leaf-like configuration, from which the tumor gets its name (Fig. 4.48). The preferred treatment is wide surgical excision. Incomplete excision of either benign or malignant phyllodes tumors may result in local recurrence in 15% of cases, and they may be excised again and again, only to grow back. About 25% of phyllodes tumors are malignant, and 20% of the malignant subtype may metastasize. No distinguishing imaging features can be used to differentiate malignant phyllodes tumors from the more common benign form.

On mammography, a phyllodes tumor is a dense round, oval, or lobulated noncalcified mass with smooth borders (Fig. 4.49). On US, a phyllodes tumor is a smoothly marginated inhomogeneous mass that occasionally contains cystic spaces producing acoustic posterior enhancement, and it can be mistaken for a fibroadenoma or circumscribed cancer. The goal of imaging is to identify the tumor for wide excision and to search for recurrence in the biopsy bed after surgery when the patient returns.

Breast Metastasis

Axillary or intramammary lymph node metastasis from breast cancer, lymphoma, or other malignancy makes the normal benign lymph node change its appearance from a circumscribed oval or kidney bean–shaped mass with a central radiolucency (fatty hilum) to a rounder, bigger, and denser mass with loss of the fatty hilum as the abnormal cells expand the lymph node cortex, eventually obliterating the central fatty hilum. This results in a round, dense mass in the axilla. Metastases in breast lymph nodes, including in intramammography lymph nodes, can occur from breast cancer, lymphoma, leukemia, melanoma, and other adenocarcinomas, even mesothelioma.

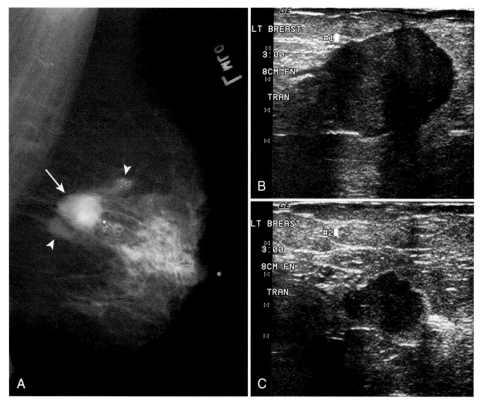

FIG. 4.44 Round invasive ductal carcinomas with calcifications. (A) Mediolateral oblique mammogram shows a round dense mass (*arrow*) with associated pleomorphic calcifications and suggestion of adjacent smaller irregular masses (*arrowheads*). (B and C) Ultrasound shows an oval partly circumscribed mass (B), corresponding to the round mass on mammography (A; *arrow*), and a second multilobulated mass (C). Both represented invasive ductal cancer.

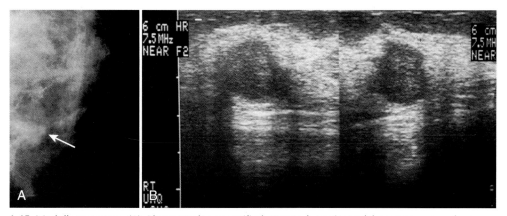

FIG. 4.45 Medullary cancer. (A) Photography magnified cropped craniocaudal mammogram shows a round mass (*arrow*) with circumscribed and partly obscured margins in the inner left breast. (B) Corresponding ultrasound shows a round mass with microlobulated and occasional angular margins with acoustic enhancement.

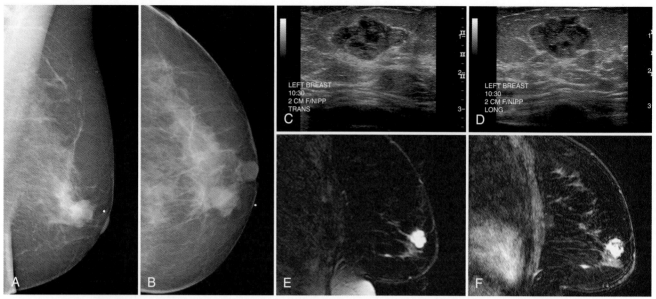

FIG. 4.46 Mucinous carcinoma. (A and B) Left mediolateral oblique (A) and craniocaudal (B) mammograms show an equal-density lobulated mass (*arrows*) near the nipple with a BB skin marker. (C and D) On ultrasound, a microlobulated heterogeneous mass containing cystic structures is seen on transverse (C) and longitudinal (D) views, worrisome for cancer or a heterogeneous fibroadenoma. (E and F) On magnetic resonance imaging (MRI), unenhanced T2-weighted sagittal MRI (E) shows a high signal intensity mass with dark septations within the mass, suggesting either fibroadenoma or mucinous cancer. Postcontrast fat-suppressed T1-weighted sagittal image (F) shows an irregular round mass with either dark septations or central necrosis. The irregular mass margin and thick irregular internal dark septations suggest cancer instead of fibroadenoma (in fibroadenoma the septations are thinner and regular, and the mass border is usually circumscribed). Core biopsy showed mucinous cancer.

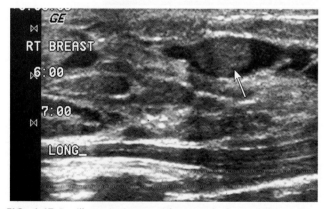

FIG. 4.47 Papillary carcinoma. Ultrasound of a papillary cancer shows a fluid-filled dilated duct with a solid oval intraductal mass (*arrow*) that cannot be distinguished from a benign intraductal papilloma on the scan.

Hematologically spread metastases are single or multiple, round, usually circumscribed, and appear as very dense round masses in one or both breasts (Fig. 4.50). If multiple, the masses vary in size as a result of the various lengths of time that the metastases have had to grow in breast tissue after hematogenous spread. Typically, the appearance of multiple new solid masses all over the breast in a nonductal pattern is worrisome for hematogenous spread of cancer from a nonbreast site, similar to pulmonary metastases. Melanoma and renal cell carcinoma were reported to metastasize to the breast in this manner. The differential diagnosis of multiple solid breast masses includes multiple fibroadenomas or papillomas, or metastases in appropriate clinical settings (Box 4.12).

Lactating Adenoma

Occurring in young pregnant patients in the second or third trimester, lactating adenomas are solid well-circumscribed masses that can enlarge rapidly during pregnancy and may be solitary or multiple and bilateral. Patients seek clinical evaluation because of a growing palpable mass that may or may not have been felt previously. The lactating adenoma has been reported as an oval mass with circumscribed margins and may be equal or higher in density than normal tissue on mammography (Parnes et al., 2013). On US, a lactating adenoma is oval or lobular, smoothly marginated, and can contain cystic or necrotic spaces sometimes with posterior acoustic enhancement, but infarcted lactating adenomas may have atypical irregular margins, and posterior acoustic shadowing (Vashi et al., 2013). Biopsy by either fine-needle aspiration or core needle biopsy is used for evaluation as clinically warranted (Fig. 4.51). The mass may regress in size in the postpartum period.

Masses with Indistinct Margins

Masses with indistinct margins are suggestive of malignancy, because cancer cell infiltration to the surrounding tissue blurs the tumor edge and produces indistinct mammographic borders (Box 4.13). Rarely, benign lesions, such as pseudoangiomatous stromal hyperplasia (PASH), or inflammation may produce this appearance.

Cancer

Invasive Ductal Carcinoma. On mammography, the indistinct margins of invasive ductal carcinoma are caused by infiltration of the surrounding glandular tissue by tumor. The mass margin can appear unsharp or smudged, similar to a line partially erased by a pencil eraser. The indistinct margin is best seen on spot magnification views against a fatty background. On US, the

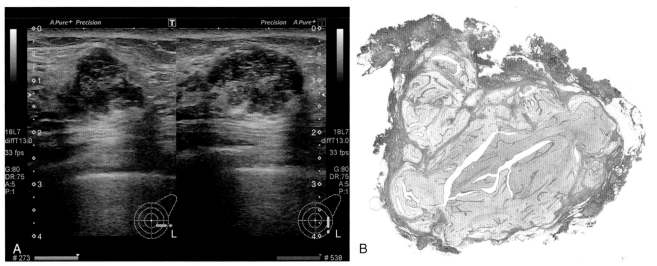

FIG. 4.48 Phyllodes tumor. (A) Ultrasound of phyllodes tumors in a young woman shows an oval partly circumscribed heterogeneous mass. (B) Pathologic photomicrograph show the leaflike projections of the phyllodes tumor that gives this fibroepithelial tumor its name. (Courtesy Shotaro Kanao, M.D., Ph.D., Kyoto University, Kyoto, Japan).

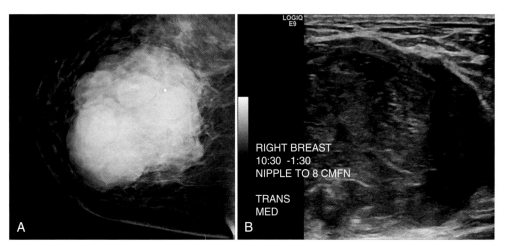

FIG. 4.49 Phyllodes tumor. (A) Mammogram shows a high-density lobulated circumscribed mass under a skin BB marker on the palpable finding. (B) Ultrasound reveals a lobulated circumscribed heterogeneous hypoechoic mass containing fluid spaces. Excisional biopsy showed a phyllodes tumor.

indistinct tumor mass occasionally has an echogenic rim or halo that suggests the diagnosis (Fig. 4.52).

Invasive Lobular Carcinoma. Often seen on only one view, lobular carcinoma may appear as an indistinct mass without microcalcifications. A more typical appearance of ILC is a spiculated mass or architectural distortion without calcifications.

Squamous Cell Carcinoma. Squamous cell tumor is the most common type of metaplastic breast carcinoma and belongs to a group of rare breast cancers. Squamous cell tumors produce large, round, noncalcified, and ill-defined masses. Other reports describe well-defined masses. On US, the masses are hypoechoic, with some reports describing central cystic spaces. They are located in breast tissue and are not found near the skin. The diagnosis of a primary squamous cell carcinoma should be established after the exclusion of the possibility of metastasis from another site, such as either a primary skin cancer or cancer at a distant site such as cervical carcinoma.

Sarcoma

Breast sarcomas are rare. Typically, they contain malignant stromal elements but, on occasion, may contain fibrous elements, as seen in the rare fibrosarcoma. Even more rarely, a breast sarcoma contains osseous elements and bone. As in invasive ductal cancer, these tumors are usually solid masses with ill-defined margins on both mammography and US.

Lymphoma

When it appears in the breast, lymphoma most commonly involves axillary breast lymph nodes, causing lymphadenopathy. On mammography, bilateral lymphadenopathy is the most common appearance of lymphoma involving the breast, appearing as dense lymph nodes in the axilla that have lost their fatty hila and become bigger and rounder (Fig. 4.53).

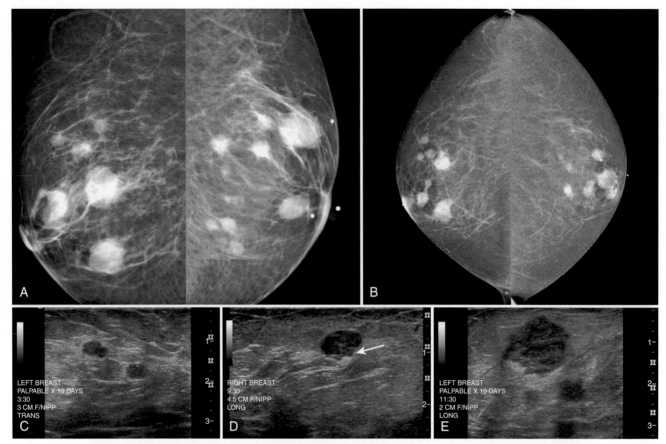

FIG. 4.50 Breast metastases. (A and B) Bilateral mediolateral oblique (A) and craniocaudal (B) mammograms in a patient with neuroendocrine cervical cancer show multiple dense masses of varying sizes in the retroareolar regions. The differential diagnosis includes multiple cysts, fibroadenomas, cancers, papillomas, and metastases. (C–E) On breast ultrasound, the masses are solid, some are round or oval (C), but others have at least one microlobulated border (*arrow*; D) or irregular borders (E), excluding the diagnosis of cysts or fibroadenomas. Core biopsy showed bilateral breast metastases.

BOX 4.12   Differential Diagnosis of Multiple Round Masses

Cysts
Fibroadenomas
Multiple round invasive breast cancers
Metastases: vary in size and nonductal growth pattern
Papillomas: may grow in a ductal pattern
False multiple masses: skin lesions such as moles or skin tags

---

Primary or secondary breast lymphoma is rare, occurs within breast parenchyma, and is usually caused by non-Hodgkin lymphomatous infiltration in breast tissue and not in a lymph node. It is a rare cause of a solitary oval or round mass with circumscribed or microlobulated margins without calcifications (Surov et al., 2012) that occasionally looks like invasive ductal cancer on mammography (Fig. 4.54). The borders of the lymphomatous mass occasionally may be irregular or indistinct because of lymphomatous infiltration into the surrounding glandular tissue, show architectural distortion, or may not be seen at all (Surov, 2013). On US, primary or secondary breast lymphomas in the breast tissue appear as solitary round or oval masses with circumscribed or ill-defined margins that have homogeneous or mixed hypo to hyper internal echoes with a posterior acoustic enhancement.

Without a diagnosis of lymphoma elsewhere in the body, the diagnosis of primary breast lymphoma is often unsuspected until percutaneous biopsy is performed on the breast mass. Primary breast lymphoma is treated by chemotherapy and radiation therapy, and not by surgical excisional biopsy, which distinguishes lymphoma treatment from breast cancer treatment. If a patient has a primary diagnosis of lymphoma elsewhere in the body and presents with a new ill-defined breast mass, the first and foremost diagnosis for the breast mass should be primary breast cancer, with a secondary but important differential diagnosis of breast lymphoma. Because breast cancer and lymphoma of the breast are treated differently, fine-needle or core biopsy should be done to establish a diagnosis and determine patient management.

Pseudoangiomatous Stromal Hyperplasia

PASH is a rare benign cause of a growing ill-defined noncalcified round or oval mass (Fig. 4.55). It occurs in premenopausal women or in postmenopausal women receiving exogenous hormone therapy. Occasionally, the mass may be well circumscribed. This entity is of unknown etiology and is composed of stromal and epithelial proliferation; it occasionally shows rapid growth on mammography and requires biopsy. On US, PASH is a mixed or hypoechoic mass with ill-defined borders in 62%, as reported by Wieman et al. in 2008. It is thought that there is a hormonal influence on its development, and PASH is more often seen in premenopausal women or postmenopausal women receiving

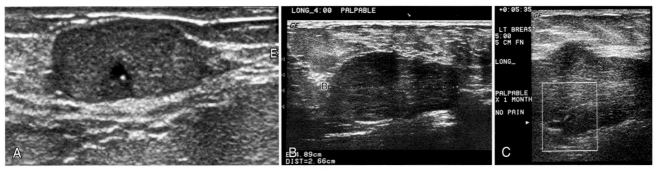

FIG. 4.51 Lactating adenoma in two different cases. (A) Periareolar, well-circumscribed oval mass containing one calcification in a 7-month pregnant woman grew in the previous few weeks and was confirmed to be a lactating adenoma on biopsy. (B and C) A 4.8-cm heterogeneous circumscribed oval mass (B) is shown in another pregnant patient with a lactating adenoma that contains blood vessels on Doppler ultrasonography (C).

BOX 4.13 Solid Masses with Indistinct Margins

Invasive ductal cancer
Invasive lobular carcinoma
Squamous cell carcinoma
Breast sarcoma
Primary or secondary non-Hodgkin lymphoma
Pseudoangiomatous stromal hyperplasia

---

hormone therapy. Fine-needle aspiration and core needle biopsy can be inconclusive. Because low-grade angiosarcoma can mimic PASH on core biopsy, excisional biopsy is recommended if the mass grows. The relationship of PASH to breast cancer risk is small (Degnim et al., 2010).

Masses Containing Fat

Masses containing fat are basically benign (Box 4.14). However, on tomosynthesis, radiologists should pay attention to mass shapes and margins even if the mass contains fat, because malignant tumors occasionally engulf the fat in the breast.

Lymph Nodes

The lymph nodes draining the breast are typically seen in the axilla, near the upper outer quadrant, and adjacent to a blood vessel. They are round or oval, circumscribed, and contain a radiolucent fatty center (Fig. 4.56). Benign lymph nodes may be of any size, have a smooth solid cortex, and contain a fatty hilum. An intramammary lymph node has the same appearance as lymph nodes in the axilla; it is often located in the upper outer quadrant of the breast along blood vessels but can be located anywhere in the breast and should not be mistaken for a malignancy. Both tomosynthesis and spot magnification views demonstrate a well-circumscribed oval kidney bean–shaped mass and, importantly, its fatty hilum in possible lymph nodes seen on standard 2D mammograms. On breast US, the lymph node has a hypoechoic bean-shaped cortex surrounding an echogenic center. On color Doppler US, the lymph node hilum or fatty center will contain a pulsating blood vessel. On MRI, the lymph node kinetics shows rapid initial enhancement with late washout, similar to cancer, caused by its central blood vessel. However, its typical appearance on MRI, which shows a solid mass with the fatty hilum and high signal on T2-weighted images, should distinguish it from cancer, which has no fatty hilum and commonly has a low signal on T2-weighted images.

Hamartoma

The benign hamartoma, known as a fibroadenolipoma, is a benign mass containing fat and normal parenchymal fibroglandular tissue. On physical examination, a hamartoma may not be felt distinctly if it contains mostly fat and glandular tissue. The classic mammographic appearance of a hamartoma is that of an oval mass containing fat and fibroglandular tissue within a thin capsule or rim, or a "breast within a breast" appearance (Fig. 4.57). Breast hamartomas have a variable appearance, depending on the amount of fat and stromal elements they contain. On occasion, a hamartoma may have mostly stromal and glandular elements and appear as a dense mass rather than one containing mostly fat and glandular elements. Because cancer develops in breast epithelial elements and ducts, it can develop in hamartomas. Biopsy should be performed on hamartomas only if they contain suspicious microcalcifications or masses developing within them. Otherwise, a classic breast-within-a-breast hamartoma is benign and should be left alone.

Oil Cyst

An oil cyst is a sequela of fat necrosis after blunt trauma or surgery. A benign oil cyst is a radiolucent circumscribed oval or round mass containing fatty fluid with a thin radiodense rim (Fig. 4.58). Oil cysts may calcify and result in rim or eggshell-type calcifications surrounding the fatty oil center. On US, oil cysts are round or oval and contain liquefied fat that is usually hypoechoic or isoechoic. The oil cyst is benign and is one of the "don't touch" lesions that should be left alone.

Lipoma

Breast lipomas are similar to lipomas elsewhere in the body. They produce a soft mass or a mass that may not be felt at all. On mammography, a lipoma is a circumscribed round or oval fatty mass containing a radiolucent center that may have a distinguishable thin discrete rim separating it from the surrounding glandular tissue, or may have no rim at all (Fig. 4.59). Unlike a posttraumatic oil cyst, a lipoma never calcifies. Typically, a lipoma is discovered because the patient feels a soft mass. If a technologist places a skin marker (BB) over the palpable lipoma, a spot compression view of the mass shows only fat below the skin marker. US of a lipoma shows only fatty tissue in a well-circumscribed oval or round mass. Lipomas are benign and should be left alone.

Steatocystoma Multiplex

This is a rare, autosomal dominantly inherited condition that is characterized by multiple and extensive intradermal oil cysts

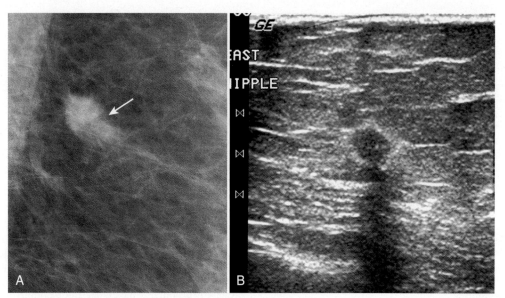

FIG. 4.52 Invasive ductal cancer with indistinct margins. (A) Mammography shows a round mass (*arrow*) with an indistinct margin and an upper partly spiculated border displayed against a fatty background. (B) Corresponding ultrasound shows a round mass with indistinct margins and a thin echogenic halo.

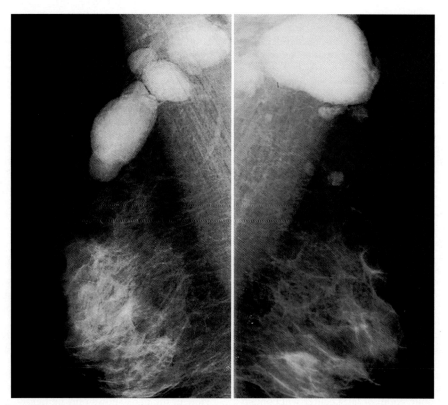

FIG. 4.53 Breast lymphoma involving the axillary lymph nodes. Bilateral mediolateral oblique mammograms show large oval high-density axillary lymph nodes that have lost their fatty hila, representing lymphadenopathy from lymphoma. Bilateral lymphadenopathy suggests systemic disease, such as lymphoma, leukemia, metastatic disease, systemic infection, or collagen vascular disease.

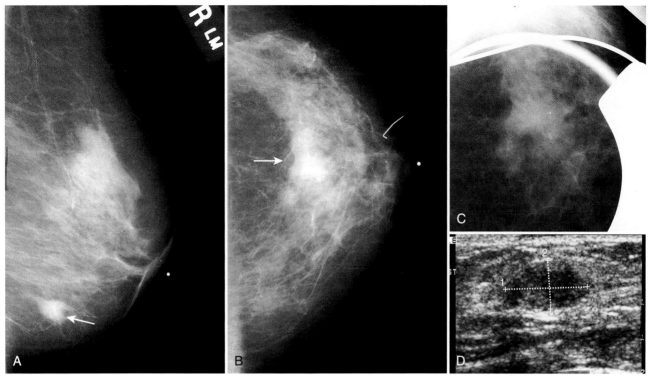

FIG. 4.54 Primary breast lymphoma with indistinct margins. (A and B) Lateromedial (A) and craniocaudal (CC; B) mammograms show an equal-density, ill-defined mass (*arrows*) in the lower central part of the breast that is indistinguishable from breast cancer. Note the linear scar marker showing a previous biopsy site. (C) The CC spot compression shows that the mass persists. (D) Ultrasound reveals a hypoechoic mass, and biopsy showed primary breast lymphoma. Imaging is indistinguishable from invasive breast cancer.

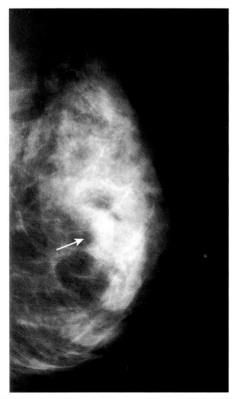

FIG. 4.55 Pseudoangiomatous stromal hyperplasia (PASH). Mediolateral oblique mammogram shows a high-density, partly obscured mass in the midportion of the breast (*arrow*). Biopsy showed PASH.

BOX 4.14 Differential Diagnosis of Masses Containing Fat

Lymph node
Hamartoma
Oil cyst
Lipoma
Steatocystoma multiplex
Invasive breast cancer containing fat on tomosynthesis (hint: margins or shape are suspicious)
Liposarcoma
Galactocele (rarely seen fat/fluid level on upright mammogram)

---

bilaterally. The oil cysts may be palpable or nonpalpable. Mammography shows extensive bilateral well-circumscribed radiolucent masses with a typical appearance of oil cysts, but unlike posttraumatic intraparenchymal oil cysts, the oil cysts in steatocystoma multiplex are intradermal in location, innumerable, and bilateral without a history of trauma. In 40% of affected patients, a typical family history of steatocystoma multiplex confirms the diagnosis.

Fat-Containing Cancer on Tomosynthesis

Freer et al. (2014) showed that growing breast cancers may engulf existing breast fat, producing a "fat-containing" cancer that has encapsulated normal fatty tissue, or shows fat interspersed along spicules. Pathologies that infiltrate in this way included both invasive ductal cancer and lobular cancer. In particular, their article warns against "nonencapsulated fat-containing masses (including nonencapsulated lobulated masses and especially spiculated

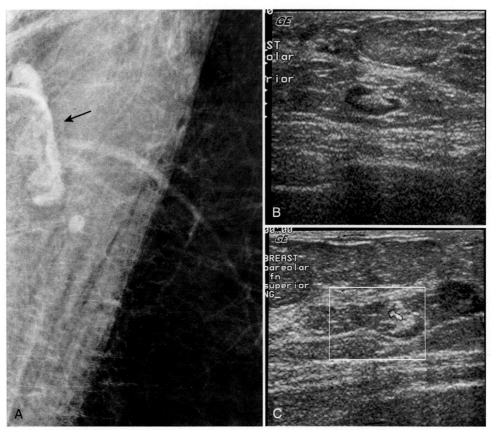

FIG. 4.56 Normal lymph node in two different cases. (A) Mediolateral oblique mammogram shows fat-containing lymph nodes (*arrow*) in the left axilla. (B and C) In another patient, ultrasound (US) of a normal lymph node shows the characteristic oval hypoechoic mass with an echogenic center (B). Doppler US (C) shows the typical pulsating blood vessel in the middle of the fatty hilum.

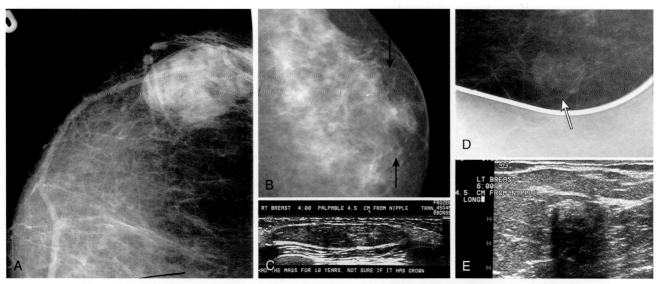

FIG. 4.57 Typical hamartomas in three different cases. (A) Craniocaudal mammogram shows an oval mass containing fibroglandular and fatty tissue, typical of a hamartoma. (B and C) Mammogram (B) shows an oval mass containing mostly fat and little fibroglandular tissue within a thin capsule (*arrows*). Ultrasound (C) shows an oval circumscribed mass containing mostly fat. (D and E) Spot magnification mammogram (D) shows an oval partly circumscribed, partly indistinct mass that may contain fat (*arrow*). Ultrasound (E) shows a partly echogenic, partly hypoechoic shadowing mass that was a hamartoma on biopsy. Hamartomas have a variable appearance, depending on their composition of fat and glandular tissue.

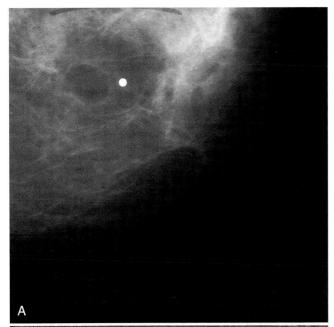

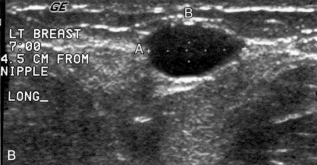

FIG. 4.58 Oil cyst. (A) Mammogram shows a palpable fat-containing thin-walled mass marked with a skin BB marker. (B) Corresponding ultrasound shows a hypoechoic, oval, and well-circumscribed mass typical for oil cyst.

fat-containing masses) which should be considered suspicious until proved otherwise." Specifically, the illustrations in the article show spiculated or irregular masses that contain a small amount of fat, or larger tumors that infiltrate surrounding fat and have fat between the infiltrating cancer spicules or associated desmoplastic reaction. An analysis of the mass shape and margin would lead to a diagnosis of breast cancer, and the article states that the mere presence of fat within a suspicious mass should not deter biopsy.

Liposarcoma

Liposarcoma is the only fat-containing malignancy and is extremely rare. A fat-containing, but rapidly growing, mass should raise suspicion of the rare liposarcoma.

Fluid-Containing Masses

Fluid-containing masses in breast include benign cysts, necrotic or cystic malignant tumors, and abscesses (Box 4.15). Radiologists should evaluate masses containing fluid for the presence of thickened wall or solid portions on US to exclude cancer.

Cyst

A simple cyst occurs in 10% of all women and is frequently seen in women receiving exogenous hormone replacement therapy.

Caused by obstruction and dilatation of the terminal ducts with fluid trapped within them, a cyst can enlarge with the patient's menstrual cycle and decrease after the onset of menses. Cysts may be asymptomatic or may become painful and produce a palpable lump. They may be single or multiple, and they can regress or grow spontaneously and rapidly.

Because cysts often produce a palpable mass, they are a frequent cause of symptoms for which patients seek advice. On mammography, cysts are round or oval, well-circumscribed, and are low density or equal in density to fibroglandular tissue. Tomosynthesis or spot compression magnification will show an equal-density or low-density round or oval mass with a circumscribed, sharply marginated border in which they are not obscured by adjacent dense glandular tissue.

Breast US shows an anechoic mass with imperceptible walls, a sharp back wall, and enhanced posterior transmission of sound (Fig. 4.60). Cysts may have internal echoes as a result of debris. They may be left alone (Box 4.16) or can be aspirated by palpation or under US guidance if symptomatic, but they have no malignant potential. If a cyst is causing a palpable mass, the palpable finding should resolve after cyst aspiration. On MRI, cysts have a high T2-weighted signal and show no enhancement. Occasionally, inflamed cysts show rim enhancement and can be a cause of a false-positive MRI. However, the bright T2-weighted signal, no enhancement of the cyst centrally after contrast injection, and a thin rim should differentiate the inflamed cyst from cancer on MRI.

Hematoma/Seroma

Breast hematomas and seromas occur after biopsy or trauma, and their diagnosis is established by correlating the hematoma/seroma to the clinical history. On mammography, a hematoma is usually round or oval in shape, but may have a circumscribed, obscured, irregular, or ill-defined border depending on surrounding healing and may be high density or equal density (Fig. 4.61 A–B). In the acute phase, surrounding hemorrhage may obscure hematomas. A hematoma will become smaller with time as the blood resorbs. Initially on US, a hematoma is a fluid-filled mass (Fig. 4.61C). Later, as the hematoma evolves, the US may show that the previously hypoechoic blood-filled mass changes to serous fluid, sometimes containing debris, solid components, fluid/fluid levels, or thin strands of fibrin that float in the seroma cavity. Occasionally, the biopsy site fills only with a seroma without blood products.

Abscess

A breast abscess occurs after mastitis. Staphylococcus aureus or Streptococcus is the usual pathogen in abscess. In a nursing mother, the infection develops as a result of bacterial entry through a cracked nipple. In teenagers, infection may occur during sexual contact. In older women, those who are diabetic or immunocompromised are especially at risk for mastitis and abscess. Typically, an abscess is a painful hard mass that is tender to touch, with overlying red, edematous skin and surrounding cellulitis, and the patient may have a fever.

On mammography, an abscess is usually subareolar; appears as a dense or equal-density noncalcified mass, distortion, or asymmetry with focal or diffuse skin thickening (Joshi et al., 2013); and may be obscured by surrounding breast edema.

On US, an abscess is a hypoechoic complex cystic fluid-filled mass or masses with indistinct margins and posterior acoustic enhancement occasionally containing debris or septations (Fig. 4.62). The surrounding edema blurs the normal adjacent breast structures, makes the adjacent fat gray, and causes skin thickening. A breast abscess usually does not contain air. Bright echoes or specular reflectors may represent air in the abscess after attempted drainage.

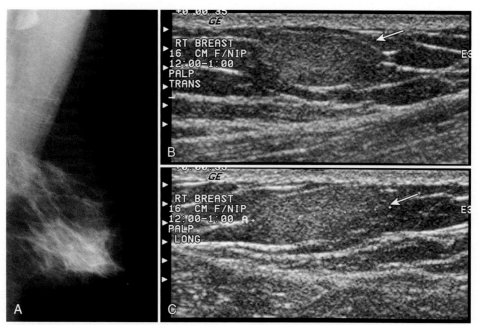

FIG. 4.59 Lipomas. (A) The rim of the palpable lipoma is not identifiable high in the breast on the mediolateral oblique mammogram where only fat is present. (B and C) However, ultrasound shows a hypoechoic fatty mass corresponding to the palpable finding on transverse (B) and longitudinal (C) views (*arrows*). This mass was proved to be a lipoma on excisional biopsy. Note that the lipoma blends into the surrounding fat and is hard to see.

<table>
<tr><td colspan="2">

BOX 4.15   Differential Diagnosis of Fluid-Containing Masses

Cyst
Hematoma/Seroma
Abscess
Intracystic papilloma
Galactocele
Necrotic cancer
Intracystic carcinoma
Sebaceous cyst (are not cysts but on or near the skin)

</td></tr>
</table>

BOX 4.16   Benign Masses That Should be Left Alone

Simple cyst
Benign postbiopsy scar
Lymph node
Hamartoma
Oil cyst
Lipoma
Hematoma
Seroma
Sebaceous cysts
Galactocele

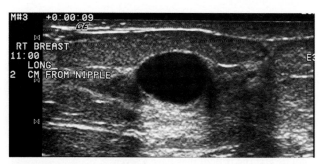

FIG. 4.60 Typical cyst. A well-circumscribed anechoic mass with an imperceptible back wall and enhanced transmission of sound is a simple cyst and needs no further follow-up.

Treatment involves antibiotic therapy and drainage of the abscess by either percutaneous or surgical methods. Surgery usually involves incision and debridement, leaving the abscess cavity open to heal by granulomatous formation by second intention. Percutaneous needle aspiration without catheter placement is usually unsuccessful as the only method of drainage if the abscess is large (>2.4–3 cm) or septated, or if incompletely

drained pockets are left in the surrounding breast tissue. In these cases, percutaneous needle drainage without an indwelling catheter may be palliative. Women with a chronic subareolar abscess caused by chronic duct obstruction are in a special category and require duct excision as well as abscess treatment. The chronic subareolar abscess may have an adjacent skin fistula. Successful treatment of this type of abscess requires excision of the fistula as well as incision and debridement of the abscess.

Intracystic Papilloma

This tumor is also rare and appears as a round mass on mammogram. On US, an intracystic papilloma is a solid mural nodule or mass in a round fluid-filled mass, with a similar appearance to that of the rare intracystic carcinoma.

Galactocele

Typically seen in lactating women, a galactocele represents a focal collection of breast milk that occasionally causes a palpable mass and is caused by an obstructed duct with distention of lobular structures proximal to the obstruction. On mammography, a galactocele is a low-density or equal-density, oval or round,

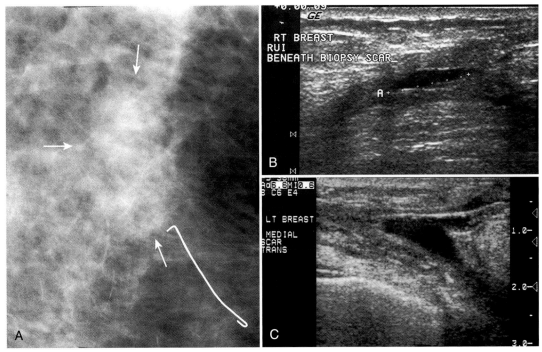

FIG. 4.61 Hematoma/seroma in two different cases. (A and B) Magnification mammogram (A) shows a density (arrows) near a linear metallic scar marker 5 months after biopsy of a benign tumor. Corresponding ultrasound (US; B) shows a fluid-filled biopsy cavity with healing hypoechoic breast tissue surrounding it. (C) In another patient, biopsy site US shows a V-shaped fluid-filled cavity, with the upper portion of the V representing fluid tracking along the incision toward the skin.

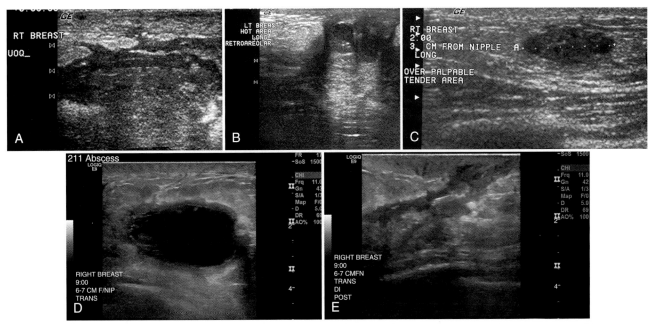

FIG. 4.62 Abscesses in four different cases. (A) Ultrasound (US) shows an irregular heterogeneous mass with extensions of fluid into tissue, with thickened skin and indistinct breast tissue structures from cellulitis. (B) In another patient, two hot retroareolar, painful, round, well-organized fluid-filled abscesses were surrounded by a less well-organized infection. (C) In a third patient, the abscess is a well-formed, encapsulated oval mass with septated fluid and debris. (D and E) In the fourth patient, US (D) shows a well-encapsulated hypoechoic mass with fluid/scant debris, representing abscess, with adjacent breast edema. Ultrasound after partial breast abscess drainage (E) shows collapse of the abscess cavity. Complete drainage was done with a percutaneous catheter in the interventional radiology department because the pus was too thick to be drained through a needle.

well-circumscribed mass, but it can be of higher density, depending on resorption of its fluid contents and the residual solid milky component. On an upright mammogram, a classic but rarely seen finding of a fat/fluid level in the mass represents fat rising to the top of the galactocele while the other milk components layer dependently below. On US, a galactocele may look like a well-defined hypoechoic cystlike mass. Galactoceles containing more solid elements simulate a solid mass that occasionally displays posterior acoustic shadowing (Fig. 4.63). On aspiration, milky fluid will be obtained. Atypical galactoceles with a round or irregular shape and nonparallel orientation mimicking suspicious solid masses on US requiring biopsy have also been reported (Kim, 2006).

Necrotic Cancer

Cancers with central necrosis or hemorrhage may contain fluid. Generally, on US necrotic tumors usually have a thick, irregular solid rim or solid components, distinguishing them from a thin-walled simple or complicated cyst (Fig. 4.64).

Intracystic Carcinoma

This extremely rare tumor produces a solid mass in a cyst wall, and the mass looks like a cyst on mammography. Because the tumor is mostly mucin, the mammographic mass is low density unless it has a denser solid component or has bled into the cystic portion to produce a dense mass. On US, an intracystic carcinoma is a solid mural mass surrounded by cystic fluid that yields fresh or old blood on aspiration (Fig. 4.65). On pneumocystography, the air inside the cyst wall will outline a solid mass along the border of the wall. Intracystic carcinomas must be excised, just as all other cancers are excised. The differential diagnosis for a solid intracystic mass includes intracystic carcinoma, intracystic papilloma, and a cyst with debris adherent to the cyst wall.

Masses on the Skin

Sebaceous and Epidermal Inclusion Cysts

Sebaceous cysts are not cysts at all, but result from keratin accumulation in plugged ducts. They have an epithelial cell lining from the sebaceous gland, whereas epidermal cysts have a true epidermal cell lining and no sebaceous glands. Because they have almost no malignant potential, biopsy is not required unless the patient desires removal.

Clinically, sebaceous cysts can produce a palpable mass or a blackhead that when squeezed will yield cheesy yellow or white material. On mammography, sebaceous and epidermal inclusion cysts are identical, with subcutaneous oval or round well-defined

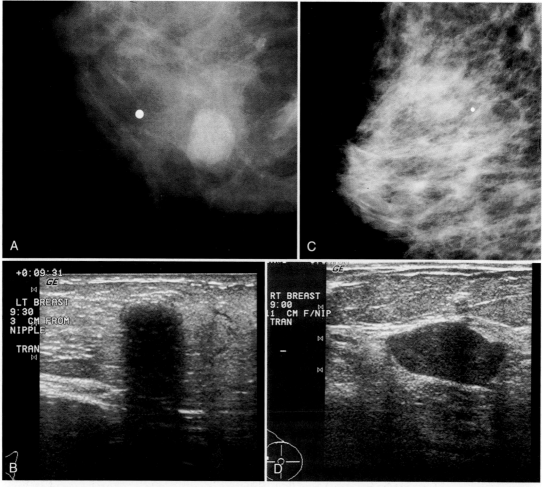

FIG. 4.63 Galactoceles in two different cases. (A and B) Mammogram (A) shows a dense round mass with corresponding ultrasound (B) showing an oval, shadowing mass. Excisional biopsy revealed a galactocele. Most likely the fluid components of the galactocele resorbed, resulting in the apparent solid mass. (C and D) Mammogram (C) shows a palpable equal-density mass under a skin marker that is difficult to see against the dense fibroglandular tissue. Ultrasound (D) shows an oval hypoechoic galactocele that yielded milk on aspiration.

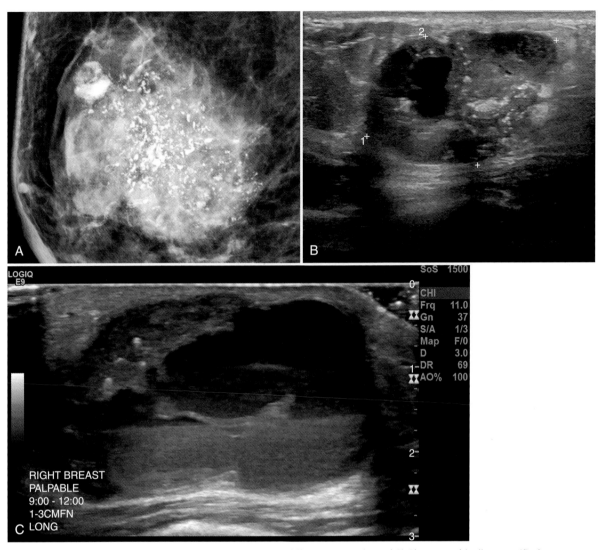

FIG. 4.64 Necrotic invasive ductal carcinoma in two different cases. (A and B) Photographically magnified mammogram (A) shows a high-density 4-cm irregular mass with mixed fine pleomorphic and coarse heterogeneous calcifications. Corresponding ultrasound (B) shows a complex cystic and solid mass with calcifications. Biopsy showed invasive ductal carcinoma. (C) Ultrasound of another patient with invasive ductal carcinoma shows a complex cystic and solid mass containing fluid. Note a fluid/fluid level is seen within the necrotic cavity.

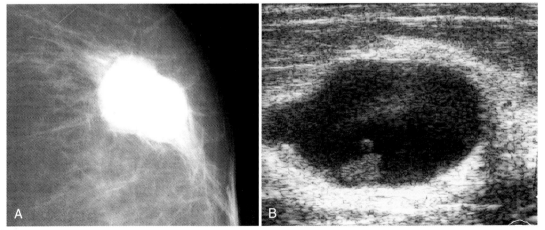

FIG. 4.65 Intracystic carcinoma. (A) Mammogram shows a dense oval mass. (B) Corresponding ultrasound shows a fluid-filled cyst with an irregular mural mass. Although this mass was an intracystic carcinoma, the differential diagnosis includes papilloma or debris in a benign cyst.

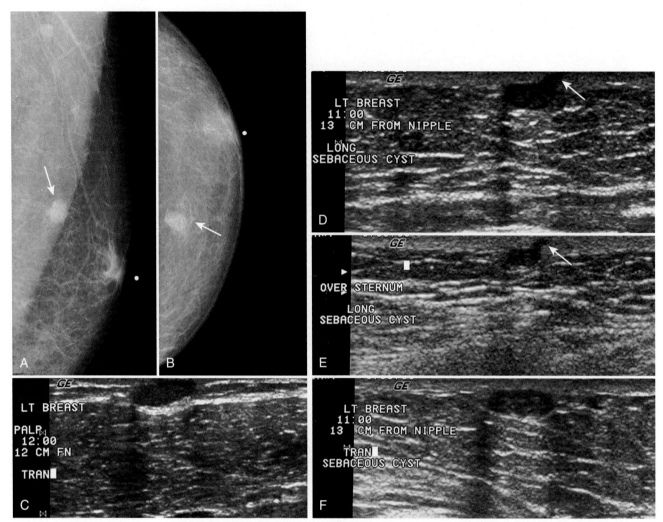

FIG. 4.66 Sebaceous cyst in two different cases. (A and B) Left mediolateral oblique (A) and craniocaudal (B) mammograms in a man with gynecomastia (under skin BB marker) show an upper inner quadrant mass (*arrows*) that was in the skin. Ultrasound (US; C) showed an oval, hypoechoic, well-circumscribed mass between the two bright lines of the skin. This is a sebaceous cyst. (D–F) In another patient, longitudinal US (D and E) shows an oval hypoechoic sebaceous cyst at the junction of the skin surface and subcutaneous fat, with the typical thin tail (*arrows*) extending into the skin. Note that on the transverse scan (F) this sebaceous cyst is an oval mass that appears to be below without the tail. The tail connecting the mass to the skin surface is seen only with careful scanning and clinches the diagnosis.

masses that are often overexposed because of their location near the skin surface (Fig. 4.66). They occasionally contain calcifications and US shows an oval, well-circumscribed, hypoechoic or anechoic mass in a subcutaneous location with a little tail extending into the skin, representing the dilated hair follicle (see Fig. 4.66 D-E).

Displacement of epidermal fragments from the skin surface to locations deep within the breast parenchyma cause epidermal inclusion cysts after percutaneous biopsy or surgery. The epidermal inclusion cyst produces a round or oval mass located within breast tissue far away from the skin surface. Because epidermal inclusion cysts have an epithelial lining, they can produce a growing mass on the mammogram as a result of accumulating inspissated material within them. Because they cause a growing solid mass, the epidermal inclusion cyst often requires biopsy to exclude cancer.

Key Elements

A mass is a three-dimensional object seen on at least two mammographic projections.

On mammography, the mass repeat includes a description of the shape, margins, density, location, associated findings, and how it has changed if previously present.

Mass shapes are round, oval, lobular, and irregular, with the probability of cancer increasing with increasing irregularity of the shape.

Mass margins are circumscribed, microlobulated, obscured, indistinct, or spiculated, with the probability of cancer increasing with increasing spiculation of the margin.

Fat-containing masses are almost never malignant.

Mass density is lower, equal to, or higher than an equal amount of fibroglandular tissue. High-density masses are suspicious for cancer.

The differential diagnosis for spiculated masses includes invasive ductal cancer, invasive lobular cancer, tubular cancer, postbiopsy scar, radial scar, fat necrosis, and sclerosing adenosis.

To determine whether a spiculated mass represents a postbiopsy scar, correlate the postbiopsy mammogram with the prebiopsy study showing where the finding was removed.

Spiculated masses that do not represent postbiopsy scars should undergo biopsy to exclude cancer.

Radial scars cannot be distinguished from spiculated breast cancer on mammography.

Invasive lobular cancer accounts for approximately 10% of all cancers but is one of the hardest to see on mammography because of its single-file cellular growth pattern.

The differential diagnosis for solid masses with round or expansile borders includes fibroadenoma, cancer, phyllodes tumor, papilloma, lactating adenoma, tubular adenoma, metastases, sebaceous cyst, and epidermal inclusion cyst.

The most common round cancer is invasive ductal cancer, an uncommon form of the most common breast cancer.

Medullary and mucinous breast cancers are commonly round in shape, but they are much rarer than invasive ductal cancer.

Fat-containing masses include lymph nodes, hamartoma, oil cyst, lipoma, and the rare liposarcoma.

Normal lymph nodes are oval, have an echogenic fatty hilum, and may contain a central pulsating blood vessel on color or power Doppler US in the fatty hilum.

Abnormal lymph nodes lose their fatty hilum and become larger and rounder than previously.

Fluid-containing masses include cysts, hematoma/seroma, necrotic cancer, intracystic carcinoma, intracystic papilloma, abscess, and galactocele.

Hamartomas look like a breast within a breast and should be left alone.

Galactoceles may rarely show a fat/fluid level on upright mammographic views.

Know the typical appearance of "don't touch" benign lymph nodes, hamartomas, oil cysts, lipomas, galactoceles, cysts, and postbiopsy scars.

SUGGESTED READINGS

Abdelhadi MS: Giant juvenile fibroadenoma: experience from a university hospital, *J Family Community Med* 12:91–95, 2005.

Accurso A, Pettinato G, Ciancia G, et al.: Pure primary squamous cell carcinoma of the breast presenting as an intracystic tumor, *Breast J* 18:608–609, 2012.

Adler DD, Helvie MA, Oberman HA, et al.: Radial sclerosing lesion of the breast: mammographic features, *Radiology* 176:737–740, 1990.

Adler DD, Hyde DL, Ikeda DM: Quantitative sonographic parameters as a means of distinguishing breast cancers from benign solid breast masses, *J Ultrasound Med* 10:505–508, 1991.

Aiello Bowles EJ, Miglioretti DL, Sickles EA, et al.: Accuracy of short-interval follow-up mammograms by patient and radiologist characteristics, *AJR Am J Roentgenol* 190:1200–1208, 2008.

Akladios CY, Roedlich MN, Bretz-Grenier MF, et al.: Intracystic papillary carcinoma of the breast: a diagnostic challenge with major clinical impact, *Anticancer Res* 34:5017–5020, 2014.

Alakhras MM, Brennan PC, Rickard M, et al.: Effect of radiologists' experience on breast cancer detection and localization using digital breast tomosynthesis, *Eur Radiol* 25:402–409, 2015.

Albayrak ZK, Onay HK, Karatag GY, et al.: Invasive lobular carcinoma of the breast: mammographic and sonographic evaluation, *Diagn Interv Radiol* 17:232–238, 2011.

American College of Radiology (ACR): The ACR practice parameter for the performance of a breast ultrasound examination. www.acr.org/~/media/52d58307e93e45898b09d4c4d407dd76.pdf Accessed October 13, 2015.

Andacoglu O, Kanbour-Shakir A, Teh YC, et al.: Rationale of excisional biopsy after the diagnosis of benign radial scar on core biopsy: a single institutional outcome analysis, *Am J Clin Oncol* 36:7–11, 2013.

Andersson I, Ikeda DM, Zackrisson S, et al.: Breast tomosynthesis and digital mammography: a comparison of breast cancer visibility and BIRADS classification in a population of cancers with subtle mammographic findings, *Eur Radiol* 18:2817–2825, 2008.

Ayyappan AP, Crystal P, Torabi A, et al.: Imaging of fat-containing lesions of the breast: a pictorial essay, *J Clin Ultrasound* 41:424–433, 2013.

Bae MS, Park SY, Song SE, et al.: Heterogeneity of triple-negative breast cancer: mammographic, US, and MR imaging features according to androgen receptor expression, *Eur Radiol* 25:419–427, 2015.

Baker JA, Lo JY: Breast tomosynthesis: state-of-the-art and review of the literature, *Acad Radiol* 18:1298–1310, 2011.

Baker JA, Soo MS, Breast US: assessment of technical quality and image interpretation, *Radiology* 223:229–238, 2002.

Baker TP, Lenert JT, Parker J, et al.: Lactating adenoma: a diagnosis of exclusion, *Breast J* 7:354–357, 2001.

Baum JK, Hanna LG, Acharyya S, et al.: Use of BI-RADS 3-probably benign category in the American College of Radiology Imaging Network Digital Mammographic Imaging Screening Trial, *Radiology* 260:61–67, 2011.

Berg WA, Sechtin AG, Marques H, et al.: Cystic breast masses and the ACRIN 6666 experience, *Radiol Clin North Am* 48:931–987, 2010.

Bernardi D, Caumo F, Macaskill P, et al.: Effect of integrating 3D-mammography (digital breast tomosynthesis) with 2D-mammography on radiologists' true-positive and false-positive detection in a population breast screening trial, *Eur J Cancer* 50:1232–1238, 2014.

Bilgen IG, Ustun EE, Memis A: Fat necrosis of the breast: clinical, mammographic and sonographic features, *Eur J Radiol* 39:92–99, 2001.

Bowles EJ, Sickles EA, Miglioretti DL, et al.: Recommendation for short-interval follow-up examinations after a probably benign assessment: is clinical practice consistent with BI-RADS guidance? *AJR Am J Roentgenol* 194:1152–1159, 2010.

Brem RF, Ioffe M, Rapelyea JA, et al.: Invasive lobular carcinoma: detection with mammography, sonography, MRI, and breast-specific gamma imaging, *AJR Am J Roentgenol* 192:379–383, 2009.

Brenner RJ: Follow-up as an alternative to biopsy for probably benign mammographically detected abnormalities, *Curr Opin Radiol* 3:588–592, 1991.

Brookes MJ, Bourke AG: Radiological appearances of papillary breast lesions, *Clin Radiol* 63:1265–1273, 2008.

Buch KA, Qureshi MM, Carpentier B, et al.: Surveillance of probably benign (BI-RADS 3) lesions in mammography: what is the right follow-up protocol? *Breast J* 21:168–174, 2015.

Cardenosa G, Doudna C, Eklund GW: Mucinous (colloid) breast cancer: clinical and mammographic findings in 10 patients, *AJR Am J Roentgenol* 162:1077–1079, 1994.

Carney PA, Abraham L, Cook A, et al.: Impact of an educational intervention designed to reduce unnecessary recall during screening mammography, *Acad Radiol* 19:1114–1120, 2012.

Cawson JN, Law EM, Kavanagh AM: Invasive lobular carcinoma: sonographic features of cancers detected in a BreastScreen Program, *Australas Radiol* 45:25–30, 2001.

Cawson JN, Nickson C, Evans J, et al.: Variation in mammographic appearance between projections of small breast cancers compared with radial scars, *J Med Imaging Radiat Oncol* 54:415–420, 2010.

Celliers L, Wong DD, Bourke A: Pseudoangiomatous stromal hyperplasia: a study of the mammographic and sonographic features, *Clin Radiol* 65:145–149, 2010.

Chang CB, Lvoff NM, Leung JW, et al.: Solitary dilated duct identified at mammography: outcomes analysis, *AJR Am J Roentgenol* 194:378–382, 2010.

Chapellier C, Balu-Maestro C, Bleuse A, et al.: Ultrasonography of invasive lobular carcinoma of the breast: sonographic patterns and diagnostic value: report of 102 cases, *Clin Imaging* 24:333–336, 2000.

Chetlen A, Nicholson B, Patrie JT, et al.: Is screening detected bilateral axillary adenopathy on mammography clinically significant? *Breast J* 18:582–587, 2012.

Chopra S, Evans AJ, Pinder SE, et al.: Pure mucinous breast cancer—mammographic and ultrasound findings, *Clin Radiol* 51:421–424, 1996.

Chung CS, Giess CS, Gombos EC, et al.: Patient compliance and diagnostic yield of 18-month unilateral follow-up in surveillance of probably benign mammographic lesions, *AJR Am J Roentgenol* 202:922–927, 2014.

Ciatto S, Houssami N, Bernardi D, et al.: Integration of 3D digital mammography with tomosynthesis for population breast-cancer screening (STORM): a prospective comparison study, *Lancet Oncol* 14:583–589, 2013.

Cohen MA, Morris EA, Rosen PP, et al.: Pseudoangiomatous stromal hyperplasia: mammographic, sonographic, and clinical patterns, *Radiology* 198:117–120, 1996.

Cohen SL, Margolies LR, Szabo JR, et al.: Introductory pictorial atlas of 3D tomosynthesis, *Clin Imaging* 38:18–26, 2014.

Cohen Y: Tomosynthesis assisting in localization of breast lesions for ultrasound targeting seen on one mammographic view only, *AJR Am J Roentgenol* 203:W555, 2014.

Cole-Beuglet C, Soriano RZ, Kurtz AB, et al.: Fibroadenoma of the breast: sonomammography correlated with pathology in 122 patients, *AJR Am J Roentgenol* 140:369–375, 1983.

Cucci E, Santoro A, Di Gesu C, et al.: Sclerosing adenosis of the breast: report of two cases and review of the literature, *Pol J Radiol* 80:122–127, 2015.

Da Costa D, Taddese A, Cure ML, et al.: Common and unusual diseases of the nipple-areolar complex, *Radiographics* 27(Suppl 1):S65–S77, 2007.

Daly CP, Bailey JE, Klein KA, et al.: Complicated breast cysts on sonography: is aspiration necessary to exclude malignancy? *Acad Radiol* 15:610–617, 2008.

Dang PA, Freer PE, Humphrey KL, et al.: Addition of tomosynthesis to conventional digital mammography: effect on image interpretation time of screening examinations, *Radiology* 270:49–56, 2014.

Darling ML, Smith DN, Rhei E, et al.: Lactating adenoma: sonographic features, *Breast J* 6:252–256, 2000.

Debald M, Abramian A, Nemes L, et al.: Who may benefit from preoperative breast MRI? A single-center analysis of 1102 consecutive patients with primary breast cancer, *Breast Cancer Res Treat* 153:531–537, 2015.

Degnim AC, Frost MH, Radisky DC, et al.: Pseudoangiomatous stromal hyperplasia and breast cancer risk, *Ann Surg Oncol* 17:3269–3277, 2010.

Denison CM, Ward VL, Lester SC, et al.: Epidermal inclusion cysts of the breast: three lesions with calcifications, *Radiology* 204:493–496, 1997.

Destounis S, Arieno A, Morgan R: Initial experience with combination digital breast tomosynthesis plus full field digital mammography or full field digital mammography alone in the screening environment, *J Clin Imaging Sci* 4:9, 2014.

Destounis SV, Morgan R, Arieno A: Screening for dense breasts: digital breast tomosynthesis, *AJR Am J Roentgenol* 204:261–264, 2015.

Domchek SM, Hecht JL, Fleming MD, et al.: Lymphomas of the breast: primary and secondary involvement, *Cancer* 94:6–13, 2002.

Doyle EM, Banville N, Quinn CM, et al.: Radial scars/complex sclerosing lesions and malignancy in a screening programme: incidence and histological features revisited, *Histopathology* 50:607–614, 2007.

Dupont WD, Page DL, Pari FF, et al.: Long-term risk of breast cancer in women with fibroadenoma, *N Engl J Med* 351:10–15, 1994.

Durand MA, Haas BM, Yao X, et al.: Early clinical experience with digital breast tomosynthesis for screening mammography, *Radiology* 274:85–92, 2015.

Eiada R, Chong J, Kulkarni S, et al.: Papillary lesions of the breast: MRI, ultrasound, and mammographic appearances, *AJR Am J Roentgenol* 198:264–271, 2012.

Elson BC, Helvie MA, Frank TS, et al.: Tubular carcinoma of the breast: mode of presentation, mammographic appearance, and frequency of nodal metastases, *AJR Am J Roentgenol* 161:1173–1176, 1993.

Elson BC, Ikeda DM, Andersson I, et al.: Fibrosarcoma of the breast: mammographic findings in five cases, *AJR Am J Roentgenol* 158:993–995, 1992.

Farshid G, Rush G: Assessment of 142 stellate lesions with imaging features suggestive of radial scar discovered during population-based screening for breast cancer, *Am J Surg Pathol* 28:1626–1631, 2004.

Feder JM, de Paredes ES, Hogge JP, et al.: Unusual breast lesions: radiologic-pathologic correlation, *Radiographics* 19:S11–S26, 1999. Spec No: S11–26; quiz S260.

Fisher B, Anderson S, Bryant J, et al.: Twenty-year follow-up of a randomized trial comparing total mastectomy, lumpectomy, and lumpectomy plus irradiation for the treatment of invasive breast cancer, *N Engl J Med* 347:1233–1241, 2002.

Fornage BD, Lorigan JG, Andry E: Fibroadenoma of the breast: sonographic appearance, *Radiology* 172:671–675, 1989.

Freer PE, Niell B, Rafferty EA: Preoperative tomosynthesis-guided needle localization of mammographically and sonographically occult breast lesions, *Radiology* 275:377–383, 2015.

Freer PE, Wang JL, Rafferty EA: Digital breast tomosynthesis in the analysis of fat-containing lesions, *Radiographics* 34:343–358, 2014.

Friedewald SM, Rafferty EA, Rose SL, et al.: Breast cancer screening using tomosynthesis in combination with digital mammography, *JAMA* 311:2499–2507, 2014.

Geller BM, Bogart A, Carney PA, et al.: Educational interventions to improve screening mammography interpretation: a randomized controlled trial, *AJR Am J Roentgenol* 202:W586–W596, 2014.

Gennaro G, Hendrick RE, Toledano A, et al.: Combination of one-view digital breast tomosynthesis with one-view digital mammography versus standard two-view digital mammography: per lesion analysis, *Eur Radiol* 23:2087–2094, 2013.

Gilbert FJ, Tucker L, Gillan MG, et al.: Accuracy of digital breast tomosynthesis for depicting breast cancer subgroups in a UK Retrospective Reading Study (TOMMY Trial), *Radiology* 277:697–706, 2015.

Gilbert FJ, Tucker L, Gillan MG, et al.: The TOMMY trial: a comparison of TOMosynthesis with digital MammographY in the UK NHS Breast Screening Programme—a multicentre retrospective reading study comparing the diagnostic performance of digital breast tomosynthesis and digital mammography with digital mammography alone, *Health Technol Asses* 19:i–xxv, 2015.

Gill HK, Ioffe OB, Berg WA: When is a diagnosis of sclerosing adenosis acceptable at core biopsy? *Radiology* 228:50–57, 2003.

Gkali CA, Chalazonitis AN, Feida E, et al.: Primary non-Hodgkin lymphoma of the breast: ultrasonography, elastography, digital mammography, contrast-enhanced digital mammography, and pathology findings, *Ultrasound Q* 31:79–282, 2015.

Graf O, Helbich TH, Fuchsjaeger MH, et al.: Follow-up of palpable circumscribed noncalcified solid breast masses at mammography and US: can biopsy be averted? *Radiology* 233:850–856, 2004.

Graf O, Helbich TH, Hopf G, Graf C, Sickles EA: Probably benign breast masses at US: is follow-up an acceptable alternative to biopsy? *Radiology* 244:87–93, 2007.

Greenberg JS, Javitt MC, Katzen J, et al.: Clinical performance metrics of 3D digital breast tomosynthesis compared with 2D digital mammography for breast cancer screening in community practice, *AJR Am J Roentgenol* 203:687–693, 2014.

Gresik CM, Godellas C, Aranha GV, et al.: Pseudoangiomatous stromal hyperplasia of the breast: a contemporary approach to its clinical and radiologic features and ideal management, *Surgery* 148:752–757, 2010.

Gruber R, Jaromi S, Rudas M, et al.: Histologic work-up of non-palpable breast lesions classified as probably benign at initial mammography and/or ultrasound (BI-RADS category 3), *Eur J Radiol* 82:398–403, 2013.

Günhan-Bilgen I, Memis A, Ustun EE: Metastatic intramammary lymph nodes: mammographic and ultrasonographic features, *Eur J Radiol* 40:24–29, 2001.

Günhan-Bilgen I, Memis A, Ustün EE: Sclerosing adenosis: mammographic and ultrasonographic findings with clinical and histopathological correlation, *Eur J Radiol* 44:232–238, 2002.

Günhan-Bilgen I, Zekioglu O, Ustun EE, et al.: Invasive micropapillary carcinoma of the breast: clinical, mammographic, and sonographic findings with histopathologic correlation, *AJR Am J Roentgenol* 179:927–931, 2002.

Gur AS, Unal B, Edington H, et al.: Pseudoangiomatous stromal hyperplasia (PASH) of the breast: intraductal appearance, *J Obstet Gynaecol Res* 35:816–818, 2009.

Haas BM, Kalra V, Geisel J, et al.: Comparison of tomosynthesis plus digital mammography and digital mammography alone for breast cancer screening, *Radiology* 269:694–700, 2013.

Hakim CM, Catullo VJ, Chough DM, et al.: Effect of the availability of prior full-field digital mammography and digital breast tomosynthesis images on the interpretation of mammograms, *Radiology* 276:65–72, 2015.

Hardesty LA, Kreidler SM, Glueck DH: Digital breast tomosynthesis utilization in the United States: a survey of physician members of the Society of Breast Imaging, *J Am Coll Radiol* 11:594–599, 2014.

Hargaden GC, Yeh ED, Georgian-Smith D, et al.: Analysis of the mammographic and sonographic features of pseudoangiomatous stromal hyperplasia, *AJR Am J Roentgenol* 191:359–363, 2008.

Harnist KS, Ikeda DM, Helvie MA: Abnormal mammogram after steering wheel injury, *West J Med* 159:504–506, 1993.

Harvey JA, Mahoney MC, Newell MS, et al.: ACR appropriateness criteria palpable breast masses, *J Am Coll Radiol* 10:742–749, 2013.

Harvey JA, Moran RE, Maurer EJ, et al.: Sonographic features of mammary oil cysts, *J Ultrasound Med* 16:719–724, 1997.

Harvey JA, Nicholson BT, Lorusso AP, et al.: Short-term follow-up of palpable breast lesions with benign imaging features: evaluation of 375 lesions in 320 women, *AJR Am J Roentgenol* 193:1723–1730, 2009.

Hilleren DJ, Andersson I, Lindholm K, et al: Invasive lobular carcinoma: mammographic findings in a 10-year experience, *Radiology* 178:149–154, 1991.

Hilton SV, Leopold GR, Olson LK, et al.: Real-time breast sonography: application in 300 consecutive patients, *AJR Am J Roentgenol* 147:479–486, 1986.

Ho JM, Jafferjee N, Covarrubias GM, et al.: Dense breasts: a review of reporting legislation and available supplemental screening options, *AJR Am J Roentgenol* 203:44–456, 2014.

Homer MJ: Proper placement of a metallic marker on an area of concern in the breast, *AJR Am J Roentgenol* 167:390–391, 1996.

Houssami N: Digital breast tomosynthesis (3D-mammography) screening: data and implications for population screening, *Expert Rev Med Devices* 12:377–379, 2015.

Houssami N, Macaskill P, Bernardi D, et al.: Breast screening using 2D-mammography or integrating digital breast tomosynthesis (3D-mammography) for single-reading or double-reading—evidence to guide future screening strategies, *Eur J Cancer* 50:1799–1807, 2014.

Ikeda DM, Sickles EA: Second-screening mammography: one versus two views per breast, *Radiology* 168:651–656, 1988.

Ilkay TM, Gozde K, Ozgur S, et al.: Diagnosis of adenoid cystic carcinoma of the breast using fine-needle aspiration cytology: a case report and review of the literature, *Diagn Cytopathol* 43:722–726, 2015.

Johnson K, Sarma D, Hwang ES: Lobular breast cancer series: imaging, *Breast Cancer Res* 17:94, 2015.

Joshi S, Dialani V, Marotti J, et al.: Breast disease in the pregnant and lactating patient: radiological–pathological correlation, *Insights Imaging* 4:527–538, 2013.

Kim MJ, Kim EK, Park SY, et al.: Galactoceles mimicking suspicious solid masses on sonography, *J Ultrasound Med* 25:145–151, 2006.

Kim MY, Choi N: Mammographic and ultrasonographic features of triple-negative breast cancer: a comparison with other breast cancer subtypes, *Acta Radiol* 54:889–894, 2013.

Kim SH, Cha ES, Park CS, et al.: Imaging features of invasive lobular carcinoma: comparison with invasive ductal carcinoma, *Jpn J Radiol* 29:475–482, 2011.

Kim SM, Kim HH, Kang DK, et al.: Mucocele-like tumors of the breast as cystic lesions: sonographic-pathologic correlation, *AJR Am J Roentgenol* 196:1424–1430, 2011.

Kopans DB: Digital breast tomosynthesis from concept to clinical care, *AJR Am J Roentgenol* 202:299–308, 2014.

Kopans DB, Swann CA, White G, et al.: Asymmetric breast tissue, *Radiology* 171:639–643, 1989.

Kuhl CK, Mielcareck P, Klaschik S, et al.: Dynamic breast MR imaging: are signal intensity time course data useful for differential diagnosis of enhancing lesions? *Radiology* 211:101–110, 1999.

Lang K, Andersson I, Rosso A, et al.: Performance of one-view breast tomosynthesis as a stand-alone breast cancer screening modality: results from the Malmo Breast Tomosynthesis Screening Trial, a population-based study, *Eur Radiol* 26:184–190, 2015.

Lang K, Andersson I, Zackrisson S: Breast cancer detection in digital breast tomosynthesis and digital mammography-a side-by-side review of discrepant cases, *Br J Radiol* 87:20140080, 2014.

Lee CH, Dershaw DD, Kopans D, et al.: Breast cancer screening with imaging: recommendations from the Society of Breast Imaging and the ACR on the use of mammography, breast MRI, breast ultrasound, and other technologies for the detection of clinically occult breast cancer, *J Am Coll Radiol* 7:18–27, 2010.

Lee CH, Giurescu ME, Philpotts LE, et al.: Clinical importance of unilaterally enlarging lymph nodes on otherwise normal mammograms, *Radiology* 203:329–334, 1997.

Lee CI, Cevik M, Alagoz O, et al.: Comparative effectiveness of combined digital mammography and tomosynthesis screening for women with dense breasts, *Radiology* 274:772–780, 2015.

Lee CI, Lehman CD: Digital breast tomosynthesis and the challenges of implementing an emerging breast cancer screening technology into clinical practice, *J Am Coll Radiol* 10:913–917, 2013.

Lee E, Wylie E, Metcalf C: Ultrasound imaging features of radial scars of the breast, *Australas Radiol* 51:240–245, 2007.

Lee KA, Zuley ML, Chivukula M, et al.: Risk of malignancy when microscopic radial scars and microscopic papillomas are found at percutaneous biopsy, *AJR Am J Roentgenol* 198:W141–W145, 2012.

Lei J, Yang P, Zhang L, et al.: Diagnostic accuracy of digital breast tomosynthesis versus digital mammography for benign and malignant lesions in breasts: a meta-analysis, *Eur Radiol* 24:595–602, 2014.

Leung JW, Sickles EA: Developing asymmetry identified on mammography: correlation with imaging outcome and pathologic findings, *AJR Am J Roentgenol* 188:667–675, 2007a.

Leung JW, Sickles EA: Multiple bilateral masses detected on screening mammography: assessment of need for recall imaging, *AJR Am J Roentgenol* 175:23–29, 2000.

Leung JW, Sickles EA: The probably benign assessment, *Radiol Clin North Am* 45:773–789, 2007b.

Linda A, Zuiani C, Furlan A, et al.: Nonsurgical management of high-risk lesions diagnosed at core needle biopsy: can malignancy be ruled out safely with breast MRI? *AJR Am J Roentgenol* 198:272–280, 2012.

Linda A, Zuiani C, Furlan A, et al.: Radial scars without atypia diagnosed at imaging-guided needle biopsy: how often is associated malignancy found at subsequent surgical excision, and do mammography and sonography predict which lesions are malignant? *AJR Am J Roentgenol* 194:1146–1151, 2010.

Lindfors KK, Kopans DB, Googe PB, et al.: Breast cancer metastasis to intramammary lymph nodes, *AJR Am J Roentgenol* 146:133–136, 1986.

Lopez JK, Bassett LW: Invasive lobular carcinoma of the breast: spectrum of mammographic, US, and MR imaging findings, *Radiographics* 29:165–176, 2009.

Lourenco AP, Barry-Brooks M, Baird GL, et al.: Changes in recall type and patient treatment following implementation of screening digital breast tomosynthesis, *Radiology* 274:337–342, 2015.

McCarthy AM, Kontos D, Synnestvedt M, et al.: Screening outcomes following implementation of digital breast tomosynthesis in a general-population screening program, *J Natl Cancer Inst* 106, 2014. pii:dju316.

Mendelson EB, Jarris KM, Doshi N, et al.: Infiltrating lobular carcinoma: mammographic patterns with pathologic correlation, *AJR Am J Roentgenol* 153:265–271, 1989.

Meyer JE, Amin E, Lindfors KK, et al.: Medullary carcinoma of the breast: mammographic and US appearance, *Radiology* 170:79–82, 1989.

Michael M, Garzoli E, Reiner CS: Mammography, sonography and MRI for detection and characterization of invasive lobular carcinoma of the breast, *Breast Dis* 30:21–30, 2008.

Mishra SP, Tiwary SK, Mishra M, et al.: Phyllodes tumor of breast: a review article, *ISRN Surg* 361469:2013, 2013.

Morel JC, Iqbal A, Wasan RK, et al.: The accuracy of digital breast tomosynthesis compared with coned compression magnification mammography in the assessment of abnormalities seen on mammography, *Clin Radiol* 69:1112–1116, 2014.

Nam KJ, Han BK, Ko ES, et al.: Comparison of full-field digital mammography and digital breast tomosynthesis in ultrasonography-detected breast cancers, *Breast* 24:649–655, 2015.

Nam SY, Ko ES, Han BK, et al.: Ultrasonographic hyperechoic lesions of the breast: are they always benign? *Acta Radiol* 56:18–24, 2015.

Neuhouser ML, Aragaki AK, Prentice RL, et al.: Overweight, obesity, and postmenopausal invasive breast cancer risk: a secondary analysis of the Women's Health Initiative Randomized Clinical Trials, *JAMA Oncol* 1:611–621, 2015.

Newell MS, Birdwell RL, D'Orsi CJ, et al.: ACR Appropriateness Criteria® on nonpalpable mammographic findings (excluding calcifications), *J Am Coll Radiol* 7:920–930, 2010.

Nicholson BT, Harvey JA, Cohen MA: Nipple-areolar complex: normal anatomy and benign and malignant processes, *Radiographics* 29:509–523, 2009.

Noroozian M, Hadjiiski L, Rahnama-Moghadam S, et al.: Digital breast tomosynthesis is comparable to mammographic spot views for mass characterization, *Radiology* 262:61–68, 2012.

Paramagul CP, Helvie MA, Adler DD: Invasive lobular carcinoma: sonographic appearance and role of sonography in improving diagnostic sensitivity, *Radiology* 195:231–234, 1995.

Park KY, Oh KK, Noh TW: Steatocystoma multiplex: mammographic and sonographic manifestations, *AJR Am J Roentgenol* 180:271–274, 2003.

Parnes AN, Akalin A, Quinlan RM, et al.: AIRP best cases in radiologic-pathologic correlation: lactating adenoma, *Radiographics* 33:455–459, 2013.

Partyka L, Lourenco AP, Mainiero MB: Detection of mammographically occult architectural distortion on digital breast tomosynthesis screening: initial clinical experience, *AJR Am J Roentgenol* 203:216–222, 2014.

Patel BK, Falcon S, Drukteinis J: Management of nipple discharge and the associated imaging findings, *Am J Med* 128:353–360, 2015.

Patterson SK, Neal CH, Jeffries DO, et al.: Outcomes of solid palpable masses assessed as BI-RADS 3 or 4A: a retrospective review, *Breast Cancer Res Treat* 147:311–316, 2014.

Pearson KL, Sickles EA, Frankel SD, et al.: Efficacy of step-oblique mammography for confirmation and localization of densities seen on only one standard mammographic view, *AJR Am J Roentgenol* 172:745–752, 2000.

Peppard HR, Nicholson BE, Rochman CM, et al.: Digital breast tomosynthesis in the diagnostic setting: indications and clinical applications, *Radiographics* 35:975–990, 2015.

Perou CM, Sorlie T, Eisen MB, et al.: Molecular portraits of human breast tumours, *Nature* 406:747–752, 2000.

Plaza MJ, Swintelski C, Yaziji H, et al.: Phyllodes tumor: review of key imaging characteristics, *Breast Dis* 35:79–86, 2015.

Porter AJ, Evans EB, Foxcroft LM, et al.: Mammographic and ultrasound features of invasive lobular carcinoma of the breast, *J Med Imaging Radiat Oncol* 58:1–10, 2014.

Price ER, Joe BN, Sickles EA: The developing asymmetry: revisiting a perceptual and diagnostic challenge, *Radiology* 274:642–651, 2015.

Rafferty EA, Park JM, Philpotts LE, et al.: Assessing radiologist performance using combined digital mammography and breast tomosynthesis compared with digital mammography alone: results of a multicenter, multireader trial, *Radiology* 266:104–113, 2013.

Rafferty EA, Park JM, Philpotts LE, et al.: Diagnostic accuracy and recall rates for digital mammography and digital mammography combined with one-view and two-view tomosynthesis: results of an enriched reader study, *AJR Am J Roentgenol* 202:273–281, 2014.

Ray KM, Turner E, Sickles EA: Suspicious findings at digital breast tomosynthesis occult to conventional digital mammography: imaging features and pathology findings, *Breast J* 21:538–542, 2015.

Ribeiro-Silva A, Mendes CF, Costa IS, et al.: Metastases to the breast from extramammary malignancies: a clinicopathologic study of 12 cases, *Pol J Pathol* 57:161–165, 2006.

Rose SL, Tidwell AL, Bujnoch LJ, et al.: Implementation of breast tomosynthesis in a routine screening practice: an observational study, *AJR Am J Roentgenol* 200:1401–1408, 2013.

Rose SL, Tidwell AL, Ice MF, et al.: A reader study comparing prospective tomosynthesis interpretations with retrospective readings of the corresponding FFDM examinations, *Acad Radiol* 21:1204–1210, 2014.

Rosen EL, Baker JA, Soo MS: Malignant lesions initially subjected to short-term mammographic follow-up, *Radiology* 223:221–228, 2002.

Roth RG, Maidment ADA, Weinstein SP, et al.: Digital breast tomosynthesis: lessons learned from early clinical implementation, *Radiographics* 34:E89–E102, 2014.

Salvador R, Salvador M, Jimenez JA, et al.: Galactocele of the breast: radiologic and ultrasonographic findings, *Br J Radiol* 63:140–142, 1990.

Samardar P, de Paredes ES, Grimes MM, et al.: Focal asymmetric densities seen at mammography: US and pathologic correlation, *Radiographics* 22:19–33, 2002.

Sanders LM, Sara R: The growing fibroadenoma, *Acta Radiol Open* 4, 2015. 2047981615572273.

Schrading S, Distelmaier M, Dirrichs T, et al.: Digital breast tomosynthesis-guided vacuum-assisted breast biopsy: initial experiences and comparison with prone stereotactic vacuum-assisted biopsy, *Radiology* 274:654–662, 2015.

Schwab FD, Burger H, Isenschmid M, et al.: Suspicious axillary lymph nodes in patients with unremarkable imaging of the breast, *Eur J Obstet Gynecol Reprod Biol* 150:88–91, 2010.

Seidenwurm D, Rosenberg R: Breast cancer screening with tomosynthesis and digital mammography, *JAMA* 312:1695, 2014.

Sharma SD, Barry M, O'Reilly EA, et al.: Surgical management of lobular carcinoma from a national screening program: a retrospective analysis, *Eur J Surg Oncol* 41:79–85, 2015.

Sheppard DG, Whitman GJ, Huynh PT, et al.: Tubular carcinoma of the breast: mammographic and sonographic features, *AJR Am J Roentgenol* 174:253–257, 2000.

Shin JH, Han BK, Ko EY, et al.: Probably benign breast masses diagnosed by sonography: is there a difference in the cancer rate according to palpability? *AJR Am J Roentgenol* 192:W187–W191, 2009.

Sickles EA: Findings at mammographic screening on only one stand projection: outcomes analysis, *Radiology* 208:471–475, 1998.

Sickles EA: Mammographic features of 300 consecutive nonpalpable breast cancers, *AJR Am J Roentgenol* 146:661–663, 1986.

Sickles EA: Periodic mammographic follow-up of probably benign lesions: results in 3,184 consecutive cases, *Radiology* 179:463–468, 1991.

Sickles EA: Practical solutions to common mammographic problems: tailoring the examination, *AJR Am J Roentgenol* 151:31–39, 1988.

Sickles EA: Probably benign breast lesions: when should follow-up be recommended and what is the optimal follow-up protocol? *Radiology* 213:11–14, 1999.

Sickles EA: Successful methods to reduce false-positive mammography interpretations, *Radiol Clin North Am* 38:693–700, 2000.

Sickles EA:The spectrum of breast asymmetries: imaging features, work-up, management, *Radiol Clin North Am* 45:765-771, 2007.

Sickles EA, D'Orsi CJ, Bassett LW, et al.: ACR BI-RADS® Mammography. In *ACR BI-RADS atlas, breast imaging reporting and data system*, Reston, VA, 2013, American College of Radiology.

Sickles EA, Herzog KA: Intramammary scar tissue: a mimic of the mammographic appearance of carcinoma, *AJR Am J Roentgenol* 135:349-352, 1980.

Skaane P, Bandos AI, Eben EB, et al.:Two-view digital breast tomosynthesis screening with synthetically reconstructed projection images: comparison with digital breast tomosynthesis with full-field digital mammographic images, *Radiology* 271:655-663, 2014.

Skaane P, Bandos AI, Gullien R, et al.: Comparison of digital mammography alone and digital mammography plus tomosynthesis in a population-based screening program, *Radiology* 267:47-56, 2013.

Skaane P, Bandos AI, Gullien R, et al.: Prospective trial comparing full-field digital mammography (FFDM) versus combined FFDM and tomosynthesis in a population-based screening programme using independent double reading with arbitration, *Eur Radiol* 23:2061-2071, 2013.

Sonnenblick EB, Margolies LR, Szabo JR, et al.: Digital breast tomosynthesis of gynecomastia and associated findings-a pictorial review, *Clin Imaging* 38:565-570, 2014.

Soo MS, Dash N, Bentley R, et al.:Tubular adenomas of the breast: imaging findings with histologic correlation, *AJR Am J Roentgenol* 174:757-761, 2000.

Sosin M, Pulcrano M, Feldman ED, et al.: Giant juvenile fibroadenoma: a systematic review with diagnostic and treatment recommendations, *Gland Surg* 4:312-321, 2015.

Sperber F, Blank A, Metser U:Adenoid cystic carcinoma of the breast: mammographic, sonographic, and pathological correlation, *Breast J* 8:53-54, 2002.

Stavros AT, Thickman D, Rapp CL, Dennis MA, Parker SH, Sisney GA: Solid breast nodules: use of sonography to distinguish between benign and malignant lesions, *Radiology* 196:123-134, 1995.

Sumkin JH, Perrone AM, Harris KM, Nath ME, Amortegui AJ, Weinstein BJ: Lactating adenoma: US features and literature review, *Radiology* 206:271-274, 1998.

Surov A: Imaging findings of hematologic diseases affecting the breast, *Semin Ultrasound CT MR* 34:550-557, 2013.

Surov A, Holzhausen HJ, Wienke A, et al.: Primary and secondary breast lymphoma: prevalence, clinical signs and radiological features, *Br J Radiol* 85:e195-e205, 2012.

Svahn T, Andersson I, Chakraborty D, et al.:The diagnostic accuracy of dual-view digital mammography, single-view breast tomosynthesis and a dual-view combination of breast tomosynthesis and digital mammography in a free-response observer performance study, *Radiat Prot Dosimetry* 139:113-117, 2010.

Svahn TM, Chakraborty DP, Ikeda D, et al.: Breast tomosynthesis and digital mammography: a comparison of diagnostic accuracy, *Br J Radiol* 85:e1074-1082, 2012.

Taira N, Aogi K, Ohsumi S, et al.: Epidermal inclusion cyst of the breast, *Breast Cancer* 14:434-437, 2007.

Takemura A, Mizukami Y, Takayama T, et al.: Primary malignant lymphoma of the breast, *Jpn J Radiol* 27:221-224, 2009.

Tan H, Li R, Peng W, et al.: Radiological and clinical features of adult non-puerperal mastitis, *Br J Radiol* 86, 2013. 20120657.

Tan M, Zheng B, Ramalingam P, et al.: Prediction of near-term breast cancer risk based on bilateral mammographic feature asymmetry, *Acad Radiol* 20:1542-1550, 2013.

Thibault F, Dromain C, Breucq C, et al.: Digital breast tomosynthesis versus mammography and breast ultrasound: a multireader performance study, *Eur Radiol* 23:2441-2449, 2013.

Thomassin-Naggara I, Perrot N, Dechoux S, et al.: Added value of one-view breast tomosynthesis combined with digital mammography according to reader experience, *Eur J Radiol* 84:235-241, 2015.

Uematsu T, Kasami M: MR imaging findings of benign and malignant circumscribed breast masses: part 1. Solid circumscribed masses, *Jpn J Radiol* 27:395-404, 2009.

Varas X, Leborgne F, Leborgne JH: Nonpalpable, probably benign lesions: role of follow-up mammography, *Radiology* 184:409-414, 1992.

Varas X, Leborgne JH, Leborgne F, et al.: Revisiting the mammographic follow-up of BI-RADS category 3 lesions, *AJR Am J Roentgenol* 179:691-695, 2002.

Vashi R, Hooley R, Butler R, et al.: Breast imaging of the pregnant and lactating patient: physiologic changes and common benign entities, *AJR Am J Roentgenol* 200:329-336, 2013.

Venkatesan A, Chu P, Kerlikowske K: Positive predictive value of specific mammographic findings according to reader and patient variables, *Radiology* 250:648-657, 2009.

Venta LA, Wiley EL, Gabriel H: Imaging features of focal breast fibrosis: mammographic-pathologic correlation of noncalcified breast lesions, *AJR Am J Roentgenol* 173:309-316, 1999.

Vijan SS, Hamilton S, Chen B, et al.: Intramammary lymph nodes: patterns of discovery and clinical significance, *Surgery* 145:495-499, 2009.

Vizcaino I, Gadea L, Andreo L, et al.: Short-term follow-up results in 795 nonpalpable probably benign lesions detected at screening mammography, *Radiology* 219:475-483, 2001.

Wahner-Roedler DL, Sebo TJ, Gisvold JJ: Hamartomas of the breast: clinical, radiologic, and pathologic features, *South Med J* 89:511-515, 1996.

Waldherr C, Cerny P, Altermatt HJ, et al.:Value of one-view breast tomosynthesis versus two-view mammography in diagnostic workup of women with clinical signs and symptoms and in women recalled from screening, *AJR Am J Roentgenol* 200:226-231, 2013.

Walsh R, Kornguth PJ, Soo MS, et al.:Axillary lymph nodes: mammographic, pathologic, and clinical correlation, *AJR Am J Roentgenol* 168:33-38, 1997.

Wan JM, Wong JS, Tee SI: Mammographic and sonographic findings of steatocystoma multiplex presenting as breast lumps, *Singapore Med J* 53:e261-e263, 2012.

Weigel RJ, Ikeda DM, Nowels KW: Primary squamous cell carcinoma of the breast, *South Med J* 89:511-515, 1996.

Wieman SM, Landercasper J, Johnson JM, et al.:Tumoral pseudoangiomatous stromal hyperplasia of the breast, *Am Surg* 74:1211-1214, 2008.

Woods ER, Helvie MA, Ikeda DM, et al.: Solitary breast papilloma: comparison of mammographic, galactographic, and pathologic findings, *AJR Am J Roentgenol* 159:487-491, 1992.

Yang TL, Liang HL, Chou CP, et al.:The adjunctive digital breast tomosynthesis in diagnosis of breast cancer, *Biomed Res Int* 597253:2013, 2013.

Youk JH, Kim EK, Ko KH, et al.:Asymmetric mammographic findings based on the fourth edition of BI-RADS: types, evaluation, and management, *Radiographics* 29:e33, 2009.

Zhang L, Jia N, Han L, et al.: Comparative analysis of imaging and pathology features of mucinous carcinoma of the breast, *Clin Breast Cancer* 15:e147-154, 2015.

Zuley ML, Bandos AI, Ganott MA, et al.: Digital breast tomosynthesis versus supplemental diagnostic mammographic views for evaluation of noncalcified breast lesions, *Radiology* 266:89-95, 2013.

Chapter 5
Breast Ultrasound Principles

Dipti Gupta and Ellen B. Mendelson

CHAPTER OUTLINE

Ultrasound (US) is a useful adjunct to mammography for diagnosis and management of benign and malignant breast disease. Technical advances have resulted in consistent, reproducible, high-resolution clinical US images. Although whole-breast automated scanners are now available and increasing in use, most practices rely on high-resolution handheld transducers. In women with dense breasts and additional risk factors, a screening breast US has been shown to detect additional cancers that may be occult on mammography. This chapter explores the major role of US in breast imaging.

TECHNICAL CONSIDERATIONS

B-Mode Gray Scale Image Optimization

Real-time handheld scanners can be used to differentiate between cysts and solid breast masses and to assess sonographic features used to characterize masses as benign, probably benign, or suspicious. Handheld units used for breast imaging should include a linear array, high-frequency transducer operating at a center frequency of 10 MHz or greater (Fig. 5.1), which provides good tissue penetration to 4 cm or 5 cm. The American College of Radiology (ACR) Practice Parameter for the Performance of a Breast Ultrasound Examination (2014) recommends use of a linear array transducer with a center frequency of at least 10 MHz. All scanners should also include a marking system to document and annotate US images.

Good sonographic image quality relies on the application of technical principles. Superficial lesions in the near field of the transducer can be imaged well by using a thin standoff pad or a thick layer of gel to bring the lesion into the focal zone of the transducer. Accurate diagnosis of deep lesions depends on appropriate power, gain, and focal zone settings. Improper adjustments of technical parameters can result in misdiagnosis, such as mistaking a cancer for a cyst by producing suboptimal images (Fig. 5.2).

The patient should be positioned to minimize the breast thickness to allow adequate tissue penetration. To flatten the breast tissue in the upper outer quadrant, the patient is scanned in a supine oblique position with the patient's hand behind the head and the back and shoulder supported by a wedge. For the inner breast, a supine position serves to flatten the medial breast tissue.

To ensure that the field of view includes all the breast tissue from the skin surface to the chest wall, the operator includes the pectoralis muscle and chest wall at the base of the image. Blank areas are caused by excessive depth; the field of view selected should be appropriate to the thickness of tissue in the area being scanned (Fig. 5.3).

Fine adjustments can be made to the time gain compensation (TGC) curve so that fat is uniformly gray from the subcutaneous tissues to the chest wall. A gentle downward slope enables accurate evaluation of masses as cystic or solid at any depth in the breast. Incorrect gain and contrast settings that make the fat look black (anechoic) may also erroneously make a solid mass look like an anechoic cyst.

Once the sonographer identifies an area of interest or a mass, he or she may zoom in on the area to fill the screen appropriately, because it is difficult to evaluate the features of a very small lesion. The sonographer then resets the focal zone to the center of the finding or depth range to include the lesion as well as the TGC curve for optimal characterization. When the indication for a breast US is evaluation of a palpable finding, the patient is asked to locate the mass or symptomatic area to ensure inclusion of the area of concern. If the patient is unaware of a physician-detected abnormality, the quadrant or area requested by the referring physician is scanned.

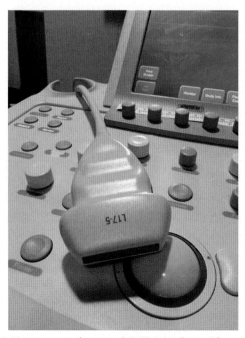

FIG. 5.1 Linear array ultrasound (US) transducer. There are several types of US transducers, including the linear array transducer, curved array transducer, phased array transducer, and sector scan transducer. Beam profile, image area, and beam frequency are different among transducers. For breast examination, use of a linear array transducer with a center frequency of at least 10 MHz is recommended by the ACR Practice Parameter for the Performance of a Breast Ultrasound Examination 2014.

In the ACR Practice Parameter for the Performance of the Breast Ultrasound Examination (2014), the ACR has made specific recommendations for US labeling. Labeling annotations should include laterality (right or left), clock face position, number of centimeters from the nipple (eg, "9 o'clock 5 cm fn"), scan plane such as radial or antiradial and longitudinal or transverse, and the initials of the person performing the scan (Box 5.1). In accordance with the Practice Parameter and ACR Breast US Accreditation instructions, orthogonal images of the mass with and without measuring calipers should be documented. Measuring calipers overlying the margin of a mass, particularly if it is small, may prevent definitive evaluation. Any other pertinent clinical information, such as whether or not the lesion is palpable, may also be helpful to note. It is important that any annotation not be placed on the image of the breast itself.

Doppler Sonography

The reflected echoes that form the US image have both frequency and amplitude. The frequency of US changes by the motion of red blood cells. This Doppler shift frequency, which is the difference between the *frequency* of the transmitted US and the reflected US, is used to form the B-mode color Doppler image. The power Doppler image, on the other hand, is formed by the *amplitude* of the frequency-shifted echoes. Unlike color Doppler imaging, power Doppler is independent of flow direction and relative flow velocity (Fig. 5.4). Power Doppler imaging is slightly more sensitive than color Doppler imaging and less affected by the Doppler angle. Technical aspects to remember include modest compression of the probe in the area of insonation, so as not to occlude flow, and selection of a sensitive frequency setting to enable low flow vascularity to be depicted.

Doppler sonography is used to assess the vascularity of a mass visualized on gray scale US and may be helpful in determining whether a nearly anechoic mass is solid. It is important to note that there is significant overlap between benign and malignant blood flow patterns. Color Doppler imaging does not always

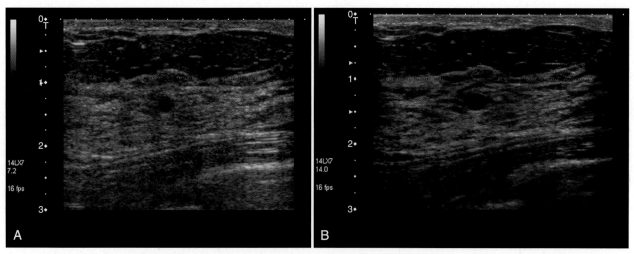

FIG. 5.2 Image quality: effects of higher frequency and compression. (A) Oval mass in sagittal view has indistinct margins at 7.2 MHz (linear transducer, frequency range 14–7 MHz). Diagnosis of a simple cyst cannot be made, and the patient would most likely have undergone aspiration. (B) Same mass imaged with same transducer but operating at 14 MHz is identifiable as a simple cyst. Additional compression of the tissue with the probe helps reduce refraction shadowing that is prominent in image. Improved image quality in the image (B) allowed BI-RADS assessment as benign. (From Mendelson EB, Böhm-Vélez M, Berg WA, et al: ACR BI-RADS® Ultrasound. In *ACR BI-RADS® atlas, breast imaging reporting and data system.* Reston, VA, 2013, American College of Radiology. Copyright by Helmut Madjar, MD.)

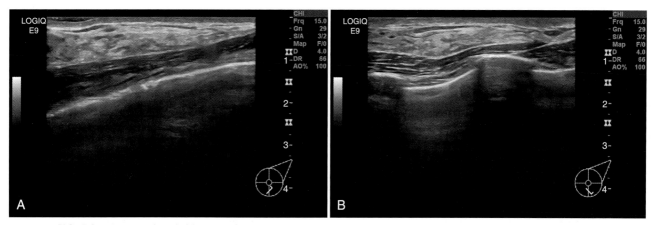

FIG. 5.3 Image quality: field of view (FOV). Two views (A and B) of the left breast at 6 o'clock with breast tissue occupying only 50% of the FOV. In these images, from the depth of 2 to 4 cm, there is no information. The focal range is set too deeply as well. (From Mendelson EB, Böhm-Vélez M, Berg WA, et al: ACR BI-RADS® Ultrasound. In *ACR BI-RADS® atlas, breast imaging reporting and data system.* Reston, VA, 2013, American College of Radiology. Copyright by Ellen B. Mendelson, MD, FACR.)

BOX 5.1 **Ultrasound Labeling**

Breast side (left or right)
Quadrant or clock position
Scan plane (radial or antiradial and transverse or longitudinal)
Number of centimeters from the nipple
Image of pertinent findings, with and without measuring calipers
Technologist's initials

---

detect increased flow in breast cancer, and absence of color flow should not dissuade biopsy of a mass with suspicious shape or margin. In the appropriate clinical setting, vascularity in the rim of a mass with suspicious marginal characteristics can suggest abscess (Fig. 5.5) rather than cancer. In such cases, US-guided aspiration should be the initial approach followed by core biopsy if aspiration is unsuccessful.

Elastography

Elastography is a measurement of the stiffness of a lesion compared with that of subcutaneous fat or fibroglandular tissue outside of the lesion at the same depth, independent of the lesion morphology. Usually cancers tend to be stiff (Fig. 5.6), whereas benign masses are softer (Fig. 5.7). The elastogram often shows a cancer to be larger compared with B-mode gray scale US imaging (see Fig. 5.6), whereas there is no significant difference in size of a benign mass on gray scale or elastographic depiction. At the current time, using elastography to increase specificity above that of gray scale morphology is operable only for Breast Imaging Reporting and Data System (BI-RADS) categories 3 and 4A; downgrading soft masses assessed as categories 4B, 4C, and 5 to avoid biopsy is not permitted. Other technologies such as optoacoustics are under study for improving the specificity of US but have not been validated for use.

Other Techniques

The use of contrast agents has been proposed as a means of improving the sensitivity of US vascular imaging. Three-dimensional gray scale US (Fig. 5.8), currently without either vascularity or elastographic assessment, is undergoing rapid development for whole-breast automated US in which the coronal view of the entire breast can enable rapid perception of architectural distortion and masses (see Fig. 5.8). Other new algorithms for use with high-resolution linear transducers have been in development, such as one that aids in the detection of microcalcifications.

BREAST ANATOMY

The breast is located on the chest wall between the second and the sixth ribs between the layers of the superficial pectoral fascia, the anterior layer lying beneath the skin, and the posterior layer just anterior to the pectoral muscle. Composed of fat and fibroglandular tissue, the breast is loosely organized into 8 to 20 ductal segments. Connective tissue support to the breast is provided by the curved arcs of Cooper's ligaments (Figs. 5.9 and 5.10).

Arterial supply to the breast is from the branches of the axillary artery, including the thoracoacromial, lateral thoracic, and subcapsular branches. The internal mammary artery arising from the subclavian artery also contributes to the vascular supply. The venous drainage is via the subareolar venous plexus, which drains into the intercostal, axillary, and internal thoracic veins.

Lymphatic drainage of the breast is predominantly into the ipsilateral axillary lymph nodes. Drainage to the contralateral axillary nodes may occur if there is extensive metastatic involvement of the ipsilateral axilla or if there are extensive postsurgical changes that occlude drainage of the ipsilateral axillary lymphatics. Axillary lymph nodes are classified by their relation to the pectoralis muscle, with level I lymph nodes lateral to the pectoralis minor, level II lymph nodes posterior to the pectoralis minor, and level III lymph nodes medial to the pectoralis minor muscle (Fig. 5.11).

The breast bud that develops into the adult breast lies beneath the nipple. In neonates, influenced by circulating maternal hormones, the breast bud may develop asymmetrically. The ensuing palpable mass can be mistakenly interpreted as abnormal (Fig. 5.12). This normal structure should not be removed surgically because breast development will be arrested on that side.

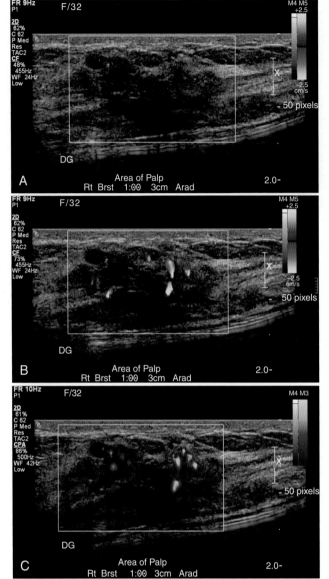

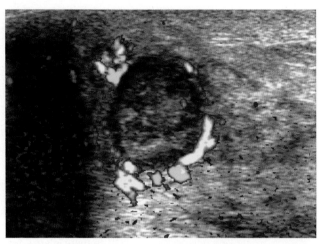

FIG. 5.5 Color flow Doppler: vessels in rim. Circumscribed 6-mm mass with rim and peripheral vascularity diagnosed as abscess. (From Mendelson EB, Böhm-Vélez M, Berg WA, et al: ACR BI-RADS® Ultrasound. In *ACR BI-RADS® atlas, breast imaging reporting and data system.* Reston, VA, 2013, American College of Radiology. Copyright by Giorgio Rizzatto, MD.)

FIG. 5.4 Color Doppler versus power Doppler. (A) The color flow sensitivity setting is inadequate and the compression with the probe is too great, occluding the small vessels in the mass. (B) The appropriate corrections have been made to sensitivity settings and compression. The vessels within the mass are now seen. (C) Amplitude-based power Doppler image shows vessels in pattern similar to that in (B) with a greater number depicted. Flow direction cannot be determined on power Doppler, but its sensitivity is higher than that of color flow. Mass containing small cysts and some calcifications is a biopsy-proven radial. (Copyright by Ellen B. Mendelson, MD, FACR.)

Tissue Composition

As in mammography and magnetic resonance imaging (MRI), US can depict the many variations in breast tissue composition. According to BI-RADS fifth edition for mammography, loosely correlating with the four densities are three US categories: *homogeneous background echotexture—fat; homogeneous background echotexture—fibroglandular;* and *heterogeneous background echotexture.*

The proportion of fat-to-fibroglandular parenchyma varies widely in the normal population variably dependent on the patient's age, hormonal influences, and individual characteristics. In young women the breast tissue is composed predominantly of fibroglandular tissue; in older women, breast tissue has a greater proportion of fat. However, there are substantial individual variations.

In breasts with homogeneous background echotexture—fat, most of breast tissue is occupied by oval fat lobules surrounded by a thin rim of connective tissue or Cooper's ligaments, which provide connective tissue support for the breast from the posterior layer of superficial pectoral fascia to the superficial layer lying just beneath the skin (Fig. 5.13). Breasts with homogeneous background texture—fibroglandular have a thick zone of homogeneously echogenic fibroglandular parenchyma beneath a layer of subcutaneous fat of variable thickness (Fig. 5.14). Many lesions, both benign and malignant, arise within the fibroglandular zone or at its junction with the layer of fat.

Heterogeneous background echotexture is characterized by multiple hyperechoic and hypoechoic areas, which can be focal or diffuse (Fig. 5.15). Heterogeneous parenchyma may confound interpretation of small hypoechoic areas of fat with small hypoechoic masses.

Masses

The BI-RADS lexicon suggests standardized reporting for masses using feature analysis. A mass has three dimensions and occupies space. It should be seen in two planes on two-dimensional imaging and in three planes with volumetric acquisitions. Using multiple sonographic descriptors when describing a mass increases specificity and diagnostic confidence. The three most important feature categories, taken together for assessment of likelihood of malignancy, are *shape, orientation,* and *margin.* Additional

ULTRASOUND LEXICON IN BREAST IMAGING REPORTING AND DATA SYSTEM FOR ULTRASOUND (2013)

The ACR BI-RADS US subcommittee developed a US lexicon to describe US findings in a manner that is standardized, clear, and concise (Table 5.1). Use of the terminology in the ACR BI-RADS lexicon helps standardize assessments, reduce confusion in interpretation and reporting, trigger appropriate management recommendations, and guide principles of an audit.

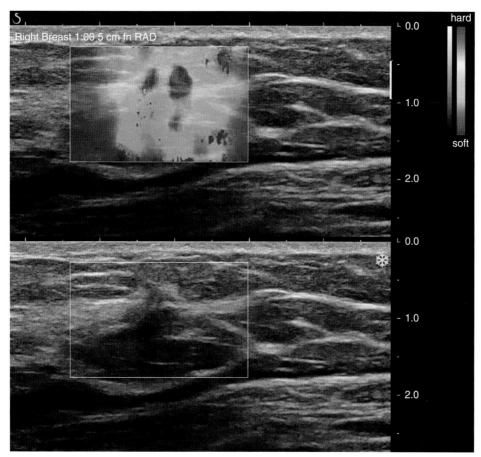

FIG. 5.6 Shear wave elastogram of a biopsy-proven invasive ductal carcinoma seen in the upper half of the image shows predominantly red, orange, and yellow colors at the stiff end of the color scale. B-mode image is seen in the lower half, and it shows a tiny irregular mass that might easily have been overlooked. (Copyright by Ellen Mendelson, MD, FACR.)

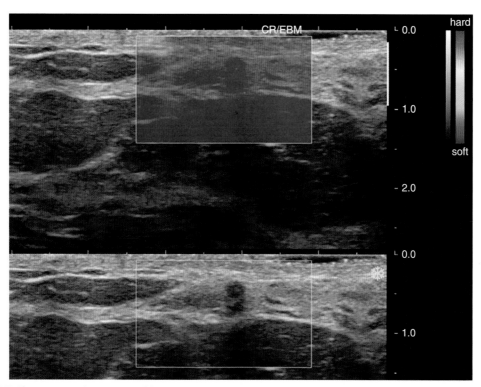

FIG. 5.7 Shear wave elastogram of benign mass boxed in the upper half of the image is all blue, soft, and distinctly recognizable through the blue overlay. B-mode image is seen in the lower half, and histopathology is apocrine metaplasia and microcysts. BI-RADS assessment in this case was category 3, probably benign, and the patient requested biopsy rather than follow-up. (From Mendelson EB, Böhm-Vélez M, Berg WA, et al: ACR BI-RADS® Ultrasound. In ACR BI-RADS® atlas, breast imaging reporting and data system. Reston, VA, 2013, American College of Radiology. Copyright by Ellen B. Mendelson, MD, FACR.)

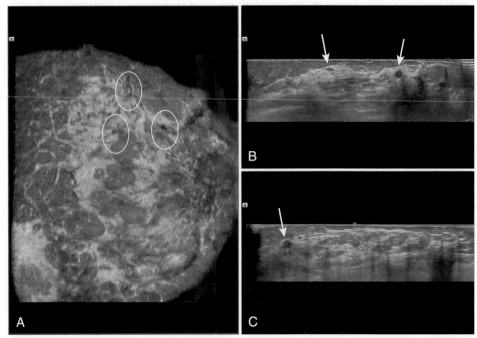

FIG. 5.8 Three-dimensional gray scale ultrasound (US) demonstrates architectural distortion. Coronal view (A) from automated whole-breast US demonstrates three masses (*circles*). The superior mass is irregular (C; *arrow*) and the two adjacent masses are oval (B; *arrows*) on the axial views. (Copyright by Ellen Mendelson, MD, FACR.)

Anatomy of the Breast

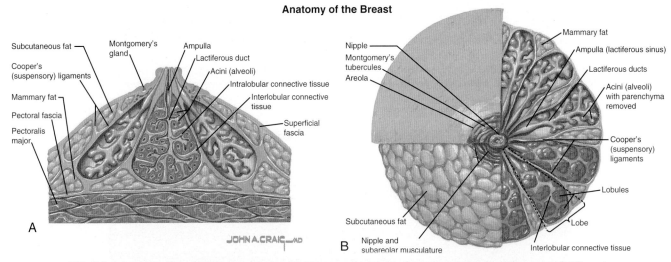

FIG. 5.9 Schematic of normal breast anatomy. (A) Diagram of a breast of a woman in supine (ultrasound [US]) position. (B) Anatomy of the breast in coronal plane, which is important view in automated US systems. (Netter medical illustration used with permission of Elsevier. All rights reserved.)

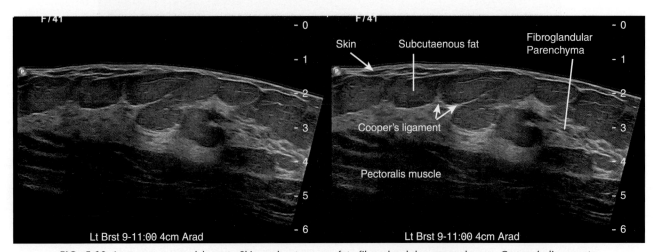

FIG. 5.10 Anatomy: normal breast. Skin, subcutaneous fat, fibroglandular parenchyma, Cooper's ligaments, and pectoralis muscle on extended field of view of a normal breast. (Copyright by Ellen Mendelson, MD, FACR.)

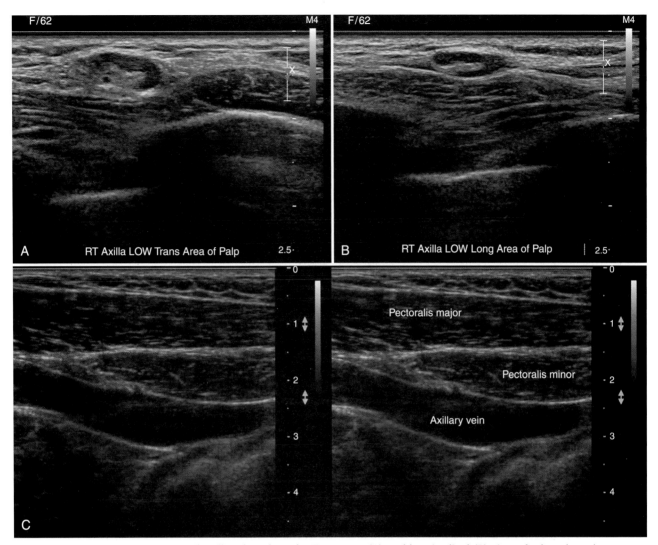

FIG. 5.11 Anatomy: normal axillary lymph node. Transverse (A) and longitudinal (B) view of a lymph node of normal size, cortical thickness, and echogenic hilum resembles a miniature kidney. (C) Normal axilla. Pectoralis major is shown anterior to pectoralis minor with axillary vein deep to both. Nodal levels are defined relative to the pectoralis minor, level I lateral to it, level II between the muscles, and level III, deep to it.*RT,* right. (From Mendelson EB, Böhm-Vélez M, Berg WA, et al: ACR BI-RADS® Ultrasound. In *ACR BI-RADS® atlas, breast imaging reporting and data system.* Reston, VA, 2013, American College of Radiology. Copyright by Ellen B. Mendelson, MD, FACR.)

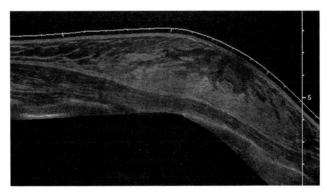

FIG. 5.12 Anatomy: normal breast bud in female adolescent. The breast at puberty resembles gynecomastia with hypoechoic tissue immediately posterior to the nipple. Because these young patients ordinarily do not undergo mammography, it is important not to misinterpret the hypoechoic retroareolar breast bud as an abnormality requiring biopsy. This area should be recognized as normal for this age group and if removed surgically, the breast will not develop. (From Mendelson EB, Böhm-Vélez M, Berg WA, et al: ACR BI-RADS® Ultrasound. In *ACR BI-RADS® atlas, breast imaging reporting and data system.* Reston, VA, 2013, American College of Radiology. Copyright by Helmut Madjar, MD.)

TABLE 5.1 American College of Radiology Breast Imaging Reporting and Data System Ultrasound Lexicon Descriptors

BREAST COMPOSITION	**CALCIFICATIONS**
Homogeneous background echotexture, fat	Calcifications in a mass
Homogeneous background echotexture, fibroglandular	Calcifications outside of a mass
Heterogeneous background echotexture	Intraductal calcifications
MASSES	**ASSOCIATED FEATURES**
Shape[a]	*Architectural distortion*
Oval	*Duct changes*
Round	*Skin changes*
Irregular	Skin thickening
Orientation[a]	Skin retraction
Parallel	Edema
Not parallel	*Vascularity*
Margin[a]	Absent
Circumscribed	Internal vascularity
Not circumscribed	Vessels in rim
Indistinct	*Elasticity assessment*
Angular	Soft
Microlobulated	Intermediate
Spiculated	Hard
Echo pattern	**SPECIAL CASES**
Anechoic	*Simple cyst*
Hyperechoic	*Clustered microcysts*
Complex cystic and solid	*Complicated cyst*
Hypoechoic	*Mass in or on skin*
Isoechoic	*Foreign body including implants*
Heterogeneous	*Lymph nodes, intramammary*
Posterior features	*Lymph nodes, axillary*
No posterior features	*Vascular abnormalities*
Enhancement	AVMs
Shadowing	Mondor disease
Combined pattern	*Postsurgical fluid collection*
	Fat necrosis

[a]Shape, margin, and orientation are the most important feature categories taken together for assessment of likelihood of malignancy.

From ACR BI-RADS® Ultrasound. In *ACR BI-RADS atlas, breast imaging reporting and data system*, Reston, VA, 2013, American College of Radiology.

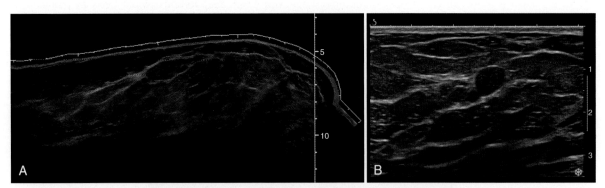

FIG. 5.13 Tissue composition: homogeneous background echotexture—fat. Two cases. (A) Homogeneously fatty tissue in a 59-year-old patient is easily characterized and compared with mammography using field of view or other ultrasound techniques that widen the field. For these images, the patient's head would be at the left and feet at the right. (B) In another patient, a fibroadenoma is seen within tissue with fatty composition. The fibroadenoma is distinguished by its oblique orientation in the midst of the horizontal oriented fat lobules. (From Mendelson EB, Böhm-Vélez M, Berg WA, et al: ACR BI-RADS® Ultrasound. In *ACR BI-RADS® atlas, breast imaging reporting and data system*. Reston, VA, 2013, American College of Radiology. A, Copyright by Helmut Madjar, MD. B, Copyright by Ellen B. Mendelson, MD, FACR.)

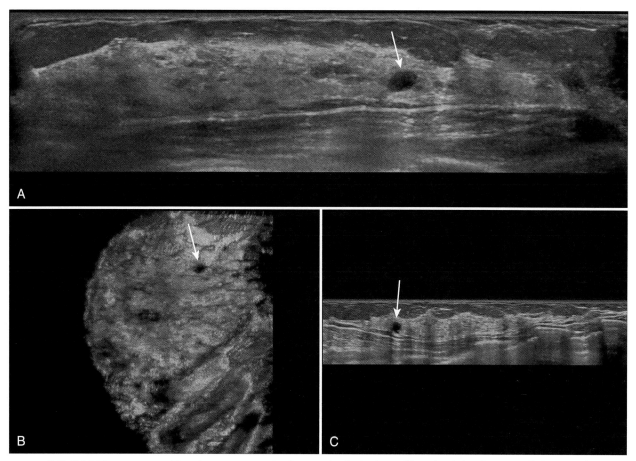

FIG. 5.14 Tissue composition: homogeneous background echotexture—fibroglandular. Automated ultrasound image (lateral view) of the left breast showing a small cyst within the homogeneous echogenic fibroglandular (FG) zone on each view (*arrows*), the 14 to 5 MHz linear acquisition, 14.5 cm wide (*top*), with the coronal (*bottom, left*) and vertical (*bottom, right*) reconstructions below. A thin layer of subcutaneous fat overlies the FG zone. (From Mendelson EB, Böhm-Vélez M, Berg WA, et al: ACR BI-RADS® Ultrasound. In *ACR BI-RADS® atlas, breast imaging reporting and data system.* Reston, VA, 2013, American College of Radiology. Copyright by Ellen B. Mendelson, MD, FACR.)

feature categories such as *echo pattern, posterior features,* and *architectural distortion* (included in *associated features*) may aid in assessing a mass.

Shape

Mass shapes are classified as *oval, round,* or *irregular* (Figs. 5.16 and 5.17). The descriptor *oval* is used for a mass that is elliptical and includes gentle lobulation with up to three undulations. A round mass is one that is spherical, ball shaped, circular, or globular. Round is the least common shape. With US, to call a mass round, it must be circular in perpendicular projections. By definition, a mass that is neither round nor oval is irregular.

Orientation

This feature is unique to US imaging. The orientation of a mass is categorized as *parallel* or *not parallel* (Fig. 5.18). Orientation is defined with reference to the skin surface. A parallel, or *wider-than-tall,* orientation is a property of most benign masses, but it may be seen with some cancers as well. Not parallel, or *taller-than-wide,* orientation indicates that a mass may be growing through the normal tissue planes and is the most

common orientation of malignant masses. Orientation alone should not be used in assessing a mass.

Margin

Margin is the edge or border of the lesion and is an important predictor of the likelihood of malignancy of a mass. Margins are *circumscribed* or *not circumscribed.* A circumscribed margin is one that is well defined or sharp, with an abrupt transition between the lesion and the surrounding tissue (Fig. 5.19). Because US is tomographic (thin slices), the margin of a mass cannot be obscured. For example, a mammographic depiction of a circumscribed mass only needs to display 75% or more of the margin; however, the entire margin must be circumscribed on US.

If any portion of the margin is not circumscribed, the margin of the mass should be reported as not circumscribed (Fig. 5.20). Not circumscribed includes *indistinct, angular, microlobulated,* and *spiculated.* Indistinct margin means there is no clear demarcation between any portion of the mass and surrounding tissue (Fig. 5.21). The boundary is poorly defined and includes masses such as some cancers and abscesses with an *echogenic rim,* which is historically called an "echogenic halo" (Fig. 5.22).

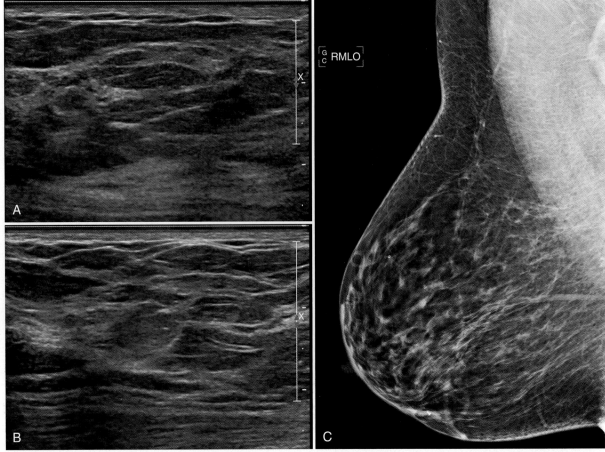

FIG. 5.15 Tissue composition: heterogeneous tissue composition. Two ultrasound images of the breast, one at 10 o'clock in the right breast (A) and a second at 12 o'clock (B), show an admixture of fat and fibroglandular (FG) tissue, not in separate homogeneous tissue layers as on Figs. 5.13 and 5.14. (C) The mammographic correlate is seen on a mediolateral oblique (*MLO*) image of this 57-year-old woman's breast described as BI-RADS® density category B, scattered areas of FG density. (From Mendelson EB, Böhm-Vélez M, Berg WA, et al: ACR BI-RADS® Ultrasound. In *ACR BI-RADS® atlas, breast imaging reporting and data system.* Reston, VA, 2013, American College of Radiology. Copyright by Ellen B. Mendelson, MD, FACR.)

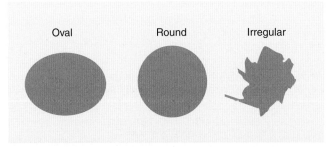

FIG. 5.16 Schematic of mass shapes: oval, round, and irregular.

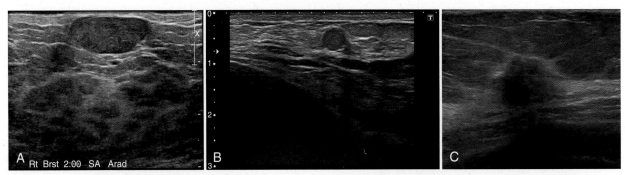

FIG. 5.17 Mass shape: oval, round, and irregular. (A) Oval. An oval, circumscribed solid mass likely represents a fibroadenoma. (B) Round. A small round hypoechoic mass is an intraductal papilloma (C) Irregular. An irregular hypoechoic mass with posterior shadowing is an invasive ductal cancer. (From Mendelson EB, Böhm-Vélez M, Berg WA, et al: ACR BI-RADS® Ultrasound. In *ACR BI-RADS® atlas, breast imaging reporting and data system.* Reston, VA, 2013, American College of Radiology. A, Copyright by Judith A. Wolfman, MD. B, Copyright by Ellen B. Mendelson, MD, FACR. C, Copyright by Marcela Böhm-Vélez, MD.)

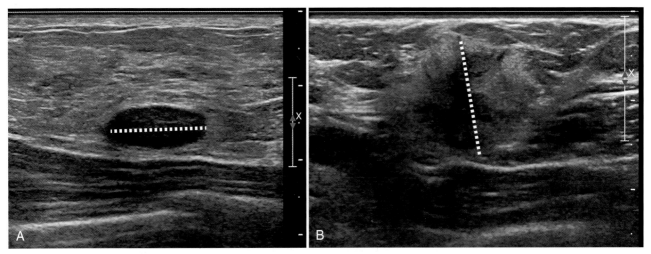

FIG. 5.18 Mass orientation: parallel and not parallel. (A) Parallel orientation. A circumscribed oval solid mass is wider than tall, with the longest axis (*dotted line*) parallel to the skin. This is a fibroadenoma. (B) Not-parallel orientation. An irregular-shaped hypoechoic mass is taller than wide, with the longest axis (*dotted line*) not parallel to the skin. This is an invasive ductal cancer. (From Mendelson EB, Böhm-Vélez M, Berg WA, et al: ACR BI-RADS® Ultrasound. In *ACR BI-RADS® atlas, breast imaging reporting and data system.* Reston, VA, 2013, American College of Radiology. Copyright by Ellen B. Mendelson, MD, FACR.)

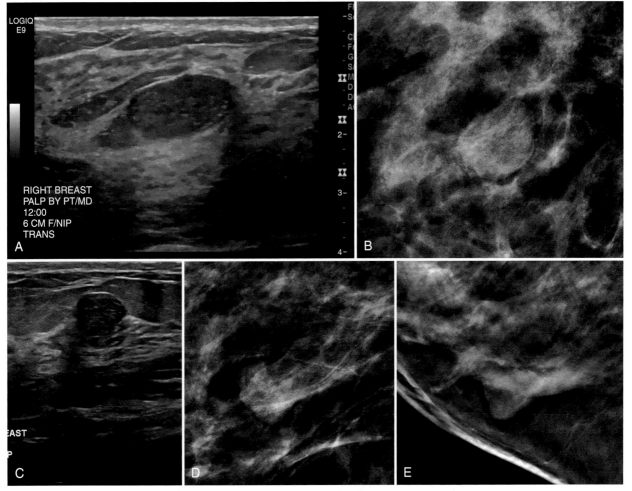

FIG. 5.19 Mass margin: circumscribed. Two cases. Ultrasound (A) of fibroadenoma shows a circumscribed, oval solid mass with posterior acoustic enhancement. The corresponding mammogram (B) also demonstrates circumscribed margins. (C) Ultrasound shows a circumscribed hypoechoic mass. Two-dimensional mammogram (D) and spot tomosynthesis slice (E) show partly obscured and circumscribed margins. On tomosynthesis, depending on how the mass is situated within breast, the margin may not be fully revealed. Core biopsy histopathology was fibroadenoma and atypical lobular hyperplasia, which was not upgraded at excision.

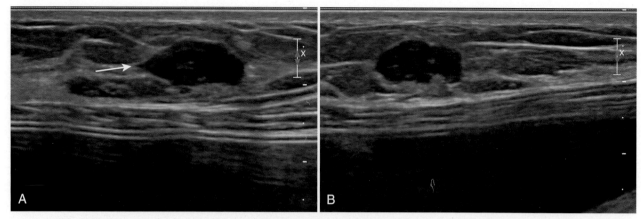

FIG. 5.20 Circumscribed or not circumscribed? On ultrasound (A), margins of a hypoechoic mass may appear circumscribed at first; however, close observation enables the identification of an angulation (*arrow*) of the margin (A) microlobulation of the margin (B). This mass should be categorized as a mass with a not-circumscribed margin. Histopathology: Invasive ductal carcinoma, grade 3. (Copyright by Ellen Mendelson, MD, FACR.)

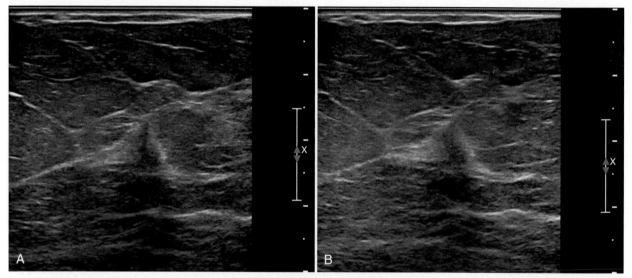

FIG. 5.21 Margin: not circumscribed, indistinct. Orthogonal ultrasound views (A and B) of a tiny invasive and intraductal carcinoma, grade 2, in a 65-year-old patient show an indistinct margin. (From Mendelson EB, Böhm-Vélez M, Berg WA, et al: ACR BI-RADS® Ultrasound. In *ACR BI-RADS® atlas, breast imaging reporting and data system*. Reston, VA, 2013, American College of Radiology. Copyright by Ellen B. Mendelson, MD, FACR.)

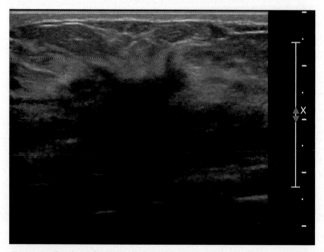

FIG. 5.22 Margin: not circumscribed, indistinct. Echogenic halo. This is a 37-year-old woman with thickening of her left breast. The biopsy-proven invasive lobular carcinoma demonstrates an irregular mass with an echogenic halo. (From Mendelson EB, Böhm-Vélez M, Berg WA, et al: ACR BI-RADS® Ultrasound. In *ACR BI-RADS® atlas, breast imaging reporting and data system*. Reston, VA, 2013, American College of Radiology. Copyright by Ellen B. Mendelson, MD, FACR.)

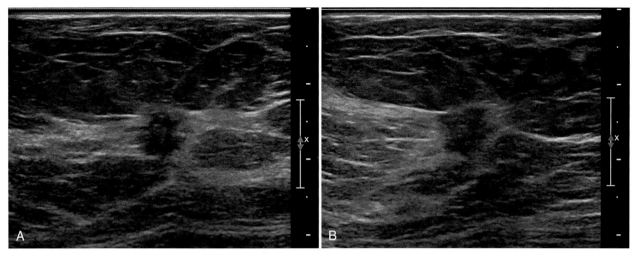

FIG. 5.23 Margin: not circumscribed, angular. (A and B) Orthogonal ultrasound views of an invasive ductal cancer show an irregularly shaped hypoechoic mass with angular margins. (From Mendelson EB, Böhm-Vélez M, Berg WA, et al: ACR BI-RADS® Ultrasound. In *ACR BI-RADS® atlas, breast imaging reporting and data system.* Reston, VA, 2013, American College of Radiology. Copyright by Ellen B. Mendelson, MD, FACR.)

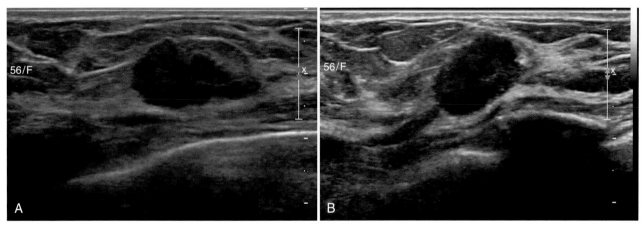

FIG. 5.24 Margin: not circumscribed, microlobulated. Invasive ductal carcinoma, grade 3, is parallel to the skin (A), and on both views the margin is not circumscribed. Several marginal descriptors apply here, including microlobulation, which is particularly well depicted on B; short spicules; and angulation. (From Mendelson EB, Böhm-Vélez M, Berg WA, et al: ACR BI-RADS® Ultrasound. In *ACR BI-RADS® atlas, breast imaging reporting and data system.* Reston, VA, 2013, American College of Radiology. Copyright by Ellen B. Mendelson, MD, FACR.)

An angular margin has sharp corners and often forms acute angles (Fig. 5.23). Microlobulated margins are characterized by short-cycle undulations (Fig. 5.24). A spiculated margin has sharp lines radiating from the mass and often indicates malignancy but also can be seen with radial scar or surgical scars (Fig. 5.25). Any or all of the four descriptors of margin can be used, but the significant marginal feature to be reported is *not circumscribed.*

Echo Pattern

The internal echo pattern is described as *anechoic, hyperechoic, complex cystic,* and *solid, hypoechoic, isoechoic* (equal), or *heterogeneous* (Fig. 5.26). Echogenicity of a mass is defined relative to the subcutaneous fat. An anechoic mass has no internal echoes and appears black inside. Hyperechoic, isoechoic, and hypoechoic masses are characterized as increased, equal, and decreased echogenicity, respectively, compared with subcutaneous fat. A complex cystic and solid mass is one consisting of both an anechoic cystic area and echogenic solid components such as an intracystic papilloma. Heterogeneous echotexture describes a mixture of echogenic patterns within a solid mass.

Echogenicity of most benign and malignant masses is hypoechoic relative to the subcutaneous fat. Most echogenic masses tend to be benign, although final assessment should be guided by margin descriptors as well. Lipomas are circumscribed with no architectural distortion of the surrounding tissues; they are more echogenic than subcutaneous fat lobules (Fig. 5.27). Some cancers are predominantly echogenic with small areas of hypoechogenicity within them; these masses are not circumscribed and should be carefully evaluated with US to avoid assessing them as benign (Fig. 5.28).

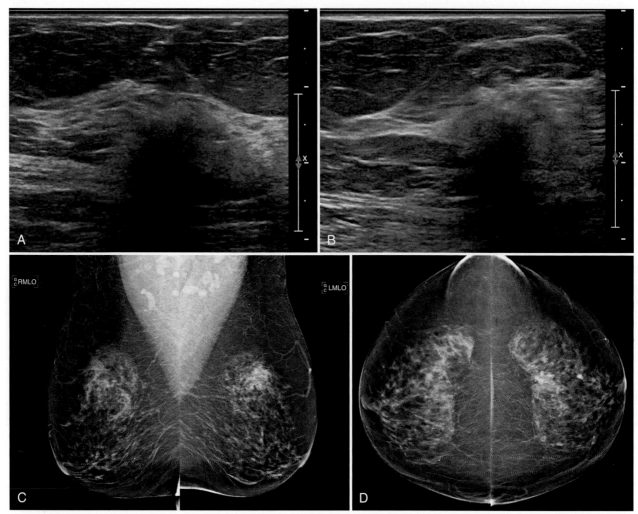

FIG. 5.25 Margin: not circumscribed, spiculated. (A and B) Hypoechoic mass with posterior shadowing has short spicules extending from it anteriorly. The sonogram was performed to characterize the mass observed at 12 o'clock in the left breast with similar features on screening mammograms (C and D; mediolateral oblique and craniocaudal views, respectively) and to provide biopsy guidance. Histopathology: invasive lobular carcinoma, grade 2. (Copyright by Ellen B. Mendelson, MD, FACR. A and B, From Mendelson EB, Böhm-Vélez M, Berg WA, et al: ACR BI-RADS® Ultrasound. In *ACR BI-RADS® atlas, breast imaging reporting and data system.* Reston, VA, 2013, American College of Radiology.)

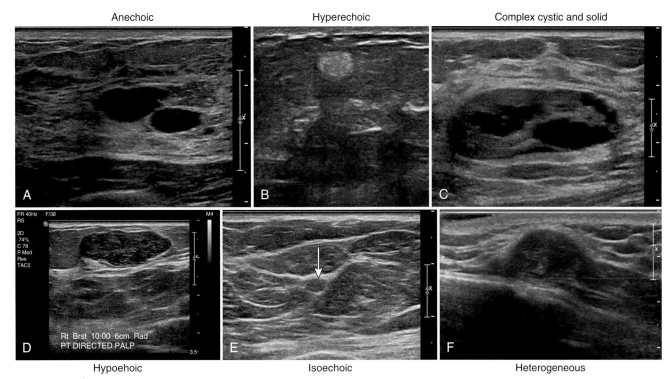

FIG. 5.26 Echo pattern: anechoic, hyperechoic, complex cystic and solid, hypoechoic, isoechoic, and heterogeneous. (A) Anechoic. Two adjacent anechoic masses meet all the criteria of simple, benign cysts. (B) Hyperechoic. Oval, circumscribed hyperechoic mass is a biopsy-proven hemangioma. (C) Complex cystic and solid mass in a 39-year-old patient contains yielded pseudoangiomatous hyperplasia (PASH). (D) Hypoechoic. This is a 38-year-old patient with a palpable oval, circumscribed, hypoechoic mass that likely represents a fibroadenoma. (E) Isoechoic. A small isoechoic mass (*arrow*) hides within fatty breast tissue. BI-RADS Assessment category 3, probably benign, was assigned. The patient requested biopsy. Histopathology: invasive ductal carcinoma with mucinous features, grade 1. (F) Heterogeneous. Palpable mass at the sternum on the left in a 43-year-old man. Histopathology from ultrasound-guided core biopsy specimens: granular cell tumor. (From Mendelson EB, Böhm-Vélez M, Berg WA, et al: ACR BI-RADS® Ultrasound. In *ACR BI-RADS® atlas, breast imaging reporting and data system.* Reston, VA, 2013, American College of Radiology. A, Copyright by Judith A. Wolfman, MD. B, Copyright by Wendie A. Berg, MD, PhD. C, Copyright by Ellen B. Mendelson, MD, FACR. E, Copyright by Marina I. Feldman, MD, MBA. F, Copyright by Ellen B. Mendelson, MD, FACR.)

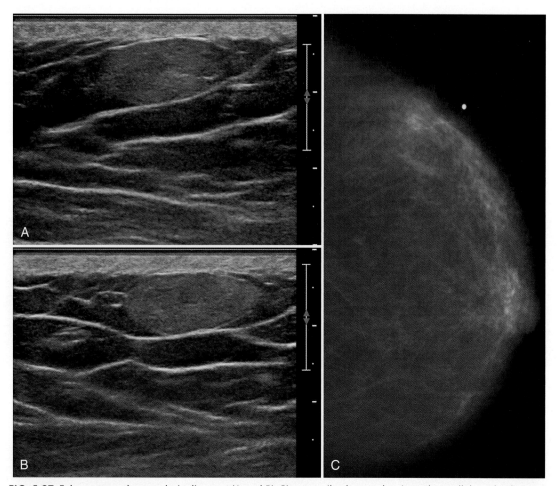

FIG. 5.27 Echo pattern: hyperechoic, lipoma. (A and B) Circumscribed mass that is oval, parallel, and echogenic is a lipoma within a fat lobule. Lipomas are hyperechoic compared with fat lobules. A fibroadenoma superficially located might have a similar appearance, but mammography could help to differentiate the lipoma, which is of fat density, as in this case, and the fibroadenoma of water density. (C) Mammogram taken tangential to a BB placed on the lipoma. (From Mendelson EB, Böhm-Vélez M, Berg WA, et al: ACR BI-RADS® Ultrasound. In *ACR BI-RADS® atlas, breast imaging reporting and data system.* Reston, VA, 2013, American College of Radiology. Copyright by Ellen B. Mendelson, MD, FACR.)

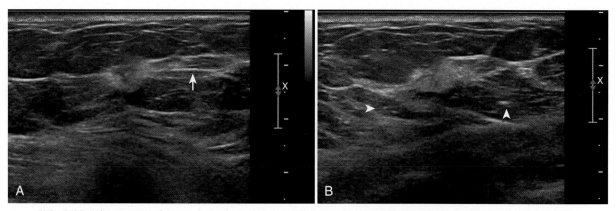

FIG. 5.28 Echo pattern: hyperechoic, breast cancer. Ill-defined echogenic area surrounded by fat, containing small curvilinear hypoechoic areas. This was detected on a screening mammography in a 75 year-old woman. The mass, small as it is, causes architectural distortion with tugging of the Cooper's ligaments (A; *arrow*) at the right lateral aspect of the mass. Calcifications (B; *arrowheads*) are seen around the mass. BI-RADS assessment should be 4C or 5. Histopathology: invasive and intraductal carcinoma, grade 2. (From Mendelson EB, Böhm-Vélez M, Berg WA, et al: ACR BI-RADS® Ultrasound. In *ACR BI-RADS® atlas, breast imaging reporting and data system.* Reston, VA, 2013, American College of Radiology. Copyright by Ellen B. Mendelson, MD, FACR.)

Posterior Features

Posterior features represent the attenuation characteristics of a mass with respect to its acoustic transmission. Posterior acoustic features are described as *no posterior acoustic features, enhancement, shadowing,* or a *combined pattern* (Fig. 5.29). In a mass with no posterior acoustic features, there is no enhancement or shadowing deep to the mass, which means that the echogenicity of the area just behind the mass is not different from that of adjacent tissues at the same depth.

Acoustic enhancement appears as a column deep to the mass that is more echogenic (whiter) than the adjacent tissue. Posterior enhancement occurs when the sound beam is not attenuated by the mass. Posterior acoustic enhancement is one criterion for the diagnosis of a simple cyst, but enhancement is not dependably a benign characteristic. Although many benign masses such as fibroadenomas will enhance or show no change in posterior features, some high-grade carcinomas may enhance as well (Fig. 5.30).

In contrast, posterior shadowing occurs when there is attenuation of sound beams and appears as an area posterior to the mass, which is hypoechoic (darker) compared with the adjacent tissue. Acoustic shadowing can be caused by fibrosis, which may occur with cancer as desmoplasia but is also seen with certain benign etiologies such as postsurgical scars (Fig. 5.31) or diabetic mastopathy.

A combined pattern is when there is more than one pattern of posterior attenuation. This is not commonly seen but may be present with lesions that are evolving like a postlumpectomy seroma. Although the seroma enhances posteriorly in its early stages, as the fluid resorbs and scarring develops, posterior shadowing is seen with developing fibrosis.

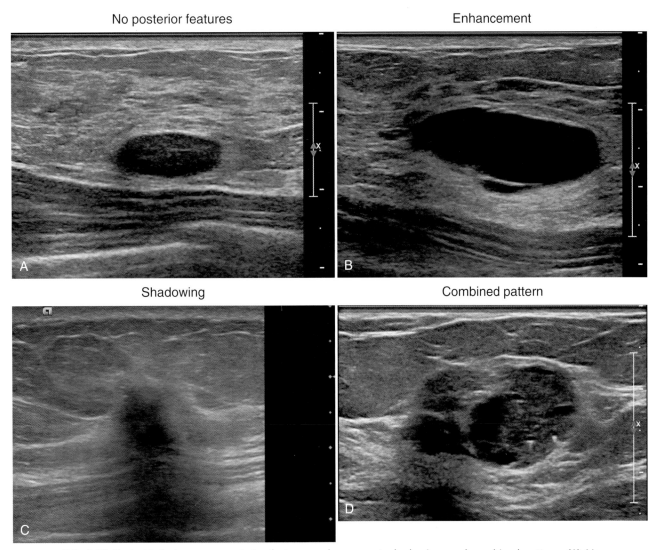

FIG. 5.29 Posterior features: no posterior features, enhancement, shadowing, and combined pattern. (A) No posterior features. Ultrasound of a fibroadenoma in a 35-year-old patient shows no posterior features. (B) Enhancement. A typical simple cyst shows a circumscribed, anechoic mass with marked posterior acoustic enhancement. (C) Shadowing. Ultrasound shows a taller than wide, spiculated mass with acoustic shadowing, representing invasive ductal cancer. (D) Combined pattern. Fibroepithelial lesion presenting as a mixed solid and cystic mass with calcifications showing both areas of shadowing and enhancement. (From Mendelson EB, Böhm-Vélez M, Berg WA, et al: ACR BI-RADS® Ultrasound. In *ACR BI-RADS® atlas, breast imaging reporting and data system.* Reston, VA, 2013, American College of Radiology. A, B, and D, Copyright by Ellen B. Mendelson, MD, FACR. C, Copyright by Marcela Böhm-Vélez, MD.)

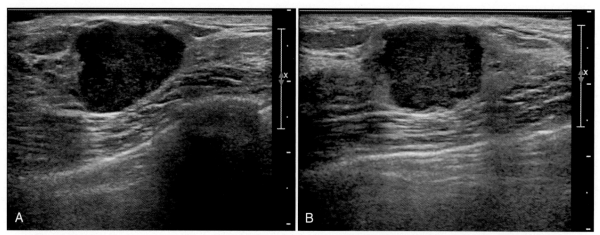

FIG. 5.30 Posterior acoustic features: enhancement, breast cancer. Palpable mass, in a 28-year-old woman has an irregular shape (A) and margins not circumscribed on orthogonal ultrasound views (A and B). The mass has a strong posterior acoustic enhancement. BI-RADS assessment, 4C. Histopathology: infiltrating ductal carcinoma, grade 3. (From Mendelson EB, Böhm-Vélez M, Berg WA, et al: ACR BI-RADS® Ultrasound. In *ACR BI-RADS® atlas, breast imaging reporting and data system.* Reston, VA, 2013, American College of Radiology. Copyright by Ellen B. Mendelson, MD, FACR.)

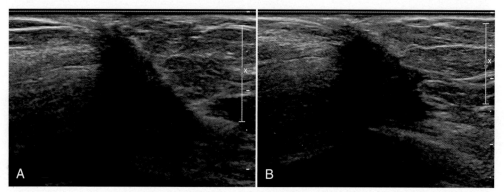

FIG. 5.31 Posterior acoustic features: shadowing, postsurgical scar. Scar in a 64-year-old patient following lumpectomy and radiation therapy for invasive mammary carcinoma 11 years earlier with prominent scar that shadows intensely, obscuring the posterior aspect of the scar on the radial view (A), with partial visibility of the chest wall on the oblique view (B). (From Mendelson EB, Böhm-Vélez M, Berg WA, et al: ACR BI-RADS® Ultrasound. In *ACR BI-RADS® atlas, breast imaging reporting and data system.* Reston, VA, 2013, American College of Radiology. Copyright by Ellen B. Mendelson, MD, FACR.)

Calcifications

Although mammography is better at characterizing calcifications, they are also identifiable on US. Microcalcifications are seen as echogenic foci on US and are not accompanied with acoustic shadowing because of their small size. Macrocalcifications can be accompanied with acoustic shadowing. According to BI-RADS 2013, calcifications are described as *calcifications in a mass* (Fig. 5.32), *calcifications outside of a mass,* or *intraductal calcifications* (Fig. 5.33).

When indeterminate calcifications are seen well enough to target, US-guided core biopsy may be performed, preferably using a vacuum-assisted biopsy device. In these cases, specimen radiography should always be obtained to confirm adequate sampling of the targeted calcifications.

Associated Features

Associated features include *architectural distortion, duct changes, skin changes, edema, vascularity,* and *elasticity assessment.*

Architectural distortion (Fig. 5.34) is the most important of the associated features, and in interpreting breast US images, one should always look first at the area surrounding a mass to see if the lesion has affected the tissue around it. Architectural distortion presents as disruption or blurring of normal anatomic planes. A mass causing the distortion may or may not be present. When the architectural distortion is not postsurgical, it is suspicious for malignancy or radial scar and needs to be biopsied.

Abnormal duct changes include duct ectasia (Fig. 5.35); cystic ductal dilatation; abnormal arborization patterns such as *beading*; extension of ducts to or from a suspicious mass; or the presence of an intraductal mass such as papilloma, thrombus, or detritus.

Skin changes include *skin thickening* and *skin retraction.* Skin thickening may refer to focally or diffusely thickened skin (>2 mm; Fig. 5.36) as may be seen in inflammatory processes, abscesses, and inflammatory carcinoma. Skin retraction is characterized by concave or ill-defined skin surface. The causes of skin retraction include breast cancer (Fig. 5.37), granular cell tumors, and scars.

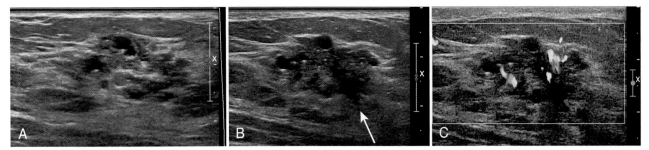

FIG. 5.32 Calcifications: calcifications in a mass. (A and B) Two orthogonal prebiopsy views of a microlobulated complex cystic and solid mass that contain microcalcifications predominantly within the small cystic components. The right posterior margin of the mass, on antiradial image (B), is spiculated (*arrow*). The color Doppler image (C) shows the distribution of vessels within the mass. BI-RADS assessment was 4B (11%–50% likelihood of malignancy). Core biopsy histopathology was sclerosing adenosis and radial scar, which was not upgraded at excision. (From Mendelson EB, Böhm-Vélez M, Berg WA, et al: ACR BI-RADS® Ultrasound. In *ACR BI-RADS® atlas, breast imaging reporting and data system.* Reston, VA, 2013, American College of Radiology. Copyright by Ellen B. Mendelson, MD, FACR.)

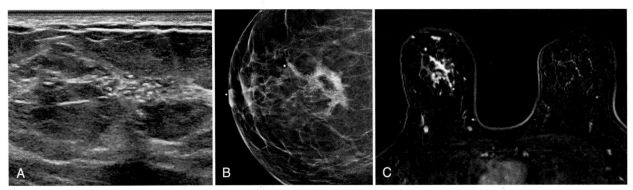

FIG. 5.33 Types of calcifications: intraductal calcifications. (A) Echogenic flecks within tiny round dark areas are microcalcifications within ducts. (B) Mammography confirms suspicious calcifications in a segmental distribution. (C) Magnetic resonance imaging performed for extent of disease shows asymmetric, clumped nonmass enhancement. (From Mendelson EB, Böhm-Vélez M, Berg WA, et al: ACR BI-RADS® Ultrasound. In *ACR BI-RADS® atlas, breast imaging reporting and data system.* Reston, VA, 2013, American College of Radiology. Copyright by Ellen B. Mendelson, MD, FACR.)

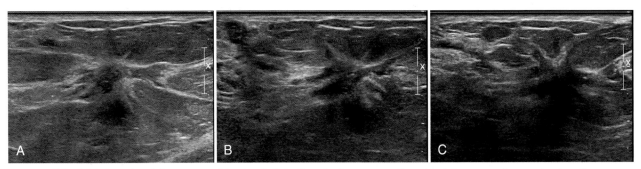

FIG. 5.34 Associated features: architectural distortion. In the narrow fibroglandular zone of a predominantly fatty breast, an invasive carcinoma with mixed ductal and lobular features, grade 2, extends itself in all directions. Three different views of the mass are shown (A–C), and the image quality is excellent. (Copyright by Ellen Mendelson, MD, FACR.)

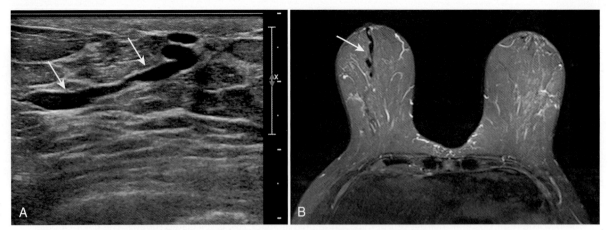

FIG. 5.35 Associated features: duct changes. This 64-year-old patient is noted to have a solitary dilated duct on screening mammography. Ultrasound (A) and magnetic resonance imaging (B) were performed showing fluid (*arrows*), was anechoic on ultrasound, and had low signal intensity on axial contrast-enhanced short TI inversion recovery (STIR) fat-suppressed T1-weighted image within the duct (B, *arrow*). Outside mammograms dating back a decade did not show change, and biopsy was canceled. (Copyright by Brandie Fagin, MD. A, From Mendelson EB, Böhm-Vélez M, Berg WA, et al: ACR BI-RADS® Ultrasound. In *ACR BI-RADS® atlas, breast imaging reporting and data system.* Reston, VA, 2013, American College of Radiology.)

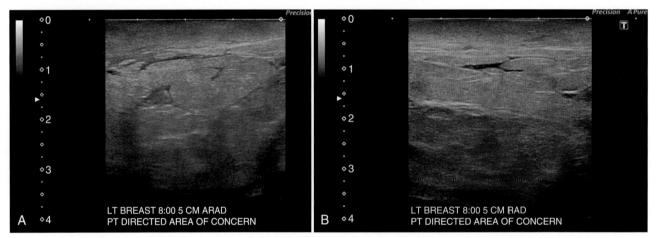

FIG. 5.36 Associated features: skin thickening. Thirty-five year old who had been breast feeding for 2 weeks presented with redness, pain, and fever. Radial (A) and anti-radial (B) images show skin thickening and breast edema, consistent with mastitis. No abscess was identified. (Copyright by Ellen Mendelson, MD, FACR.)

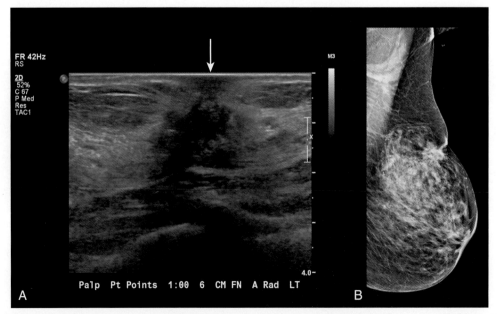

FIG. 5.37 Associated features: skin retraction and skin thickening. Ultrasound (A) shows skin retraction and focal skin thickening (*arrow*) from an irregular, hypoechoic mass. Mediolateral oblique view from the mammogram (B) also depicts that skin retraction is caused by a spiculated mass. This is a biopsy-proven invasive ductal carcinoma. (Copyright by Ellen Mendelson, MD, FACR.)

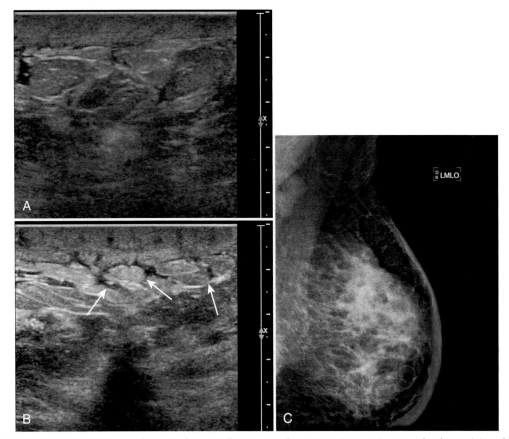

FIG. 5.38 Associated features: breast edema, inflammatory breast carcinoma. Increased echogenicity of surrounding tissue and reticulation. An angular network of hypoechoic lines (*arrows*) signifies edema associated with inflammatory breast cancer (A and B). Malignant masses are seen deep in the breast tissue (A and B), and the skin is thick on the mediolateral mammographic view (C), which also shows axillary lymphadenopathy. (Copyright by Ellen B. Mendelson, MD, FACR. A and B, From Mendelson EB, Böhm-Vélez M, Berg WA, et al: ACR BI-RADS® Ultrasound. In *ACR BI-RADS® atlas, breast imaging reporting and data system.* Reston, VA, 2013, American College of Radiology.)

Breast edema often accompanies skin thickening in inflammatory breast cancer (Figs. 5.38 and 5.39), mastitis, and systemic disorders such as congestive heart failure. It is indicated by increased echogenicity of the surrounding tissue and reticulation (angular network of hypoechoic lines representing dilated lymphatics or interstitial fluid).

Vascularity is classified as *absent, internal vascularity* (Fig. 5.40A–B), and *vessels in rim* (Fig. 5.40C; see section: Doppler Sonography for a more detailed discussion).

Elasticity assessment is categorized as soft, intermediate, and hard (see Figs. 5.6 and 5.7). Some additional elastographic features recently described include a larger area of involvement of elastography pattern compared with the gray scale lesion size (see Fig. 5.6).

Special Cases

Special cases include simple cyst; clustered microcysts; complicated cyst; mass in or on skin; foreign body, including implants; lymph nodes, intramammary and axillary; vascular abnormalities (arteriovenous malformation and Mondor disease); postsurgical

fluid collection; and fat necrosis. In reporting special cases, there is no need if the diagnosis is certain to describe the lesion using the feature descriptors that characterize it. An example would be to say "a simple cyst" rather than "an anechoic, oval, parallel, circumscribed mass consistent with a benign simple cyst." For fat necrosis, it is necessary, however, to characterize the suspected abnormality further and correlate it with mammography and clinical setting.

Reporting Ultrasound Findings Based on Breast Imaging Reporting and Data System 2013

The US report should be assigned an ACR BI-RADS final assessment code indicating the level of suspicion for cancer and follow-up management recommendations (Table 5.2). The use of category 3 Probably Benign is usually limited to a single solid mass with an oval shape, circumscribed margin, and parallel orientation (most commonly fibroadenoma); an isolated complicated cyst; and clustered microcysts. These assessments are being revisited, and multiple benign-appearing masses, cystic or solid, may now be assigned BI-RADS category 2.

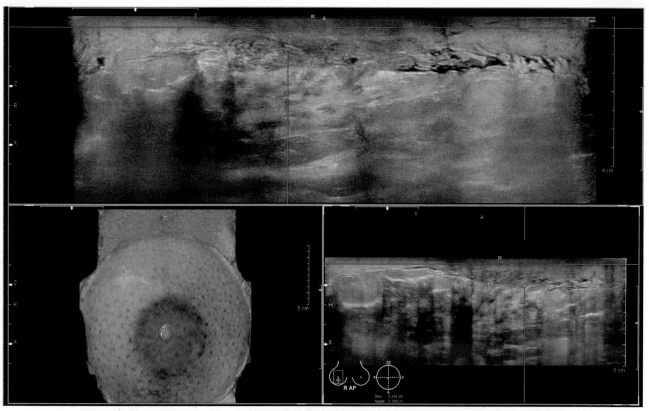

FIG. 5.39 Associated features: breast edema, inflammatory breast carcinoma. Automated ultrasound showing edema, skin thickening, and architectural distortion in inflammatory breast carcinoma on the linear wide field-of-view acquisition (*top*) with coronal (*bottom, left*) and sagittal (*bottom, right*) reconstructions. The hypoechoic areas deep to the markedly thickened skin are malignant masses, with refraction shadowing where the curved Cooper's ligaments interface with breast tissue. Skin pores are prominent on the coronal view for this patient whose breast clinically showed *peau d'orange.* These images in three planes are all orthogonal. (Copyright by Ellen Mendelson, MD, FACR.)

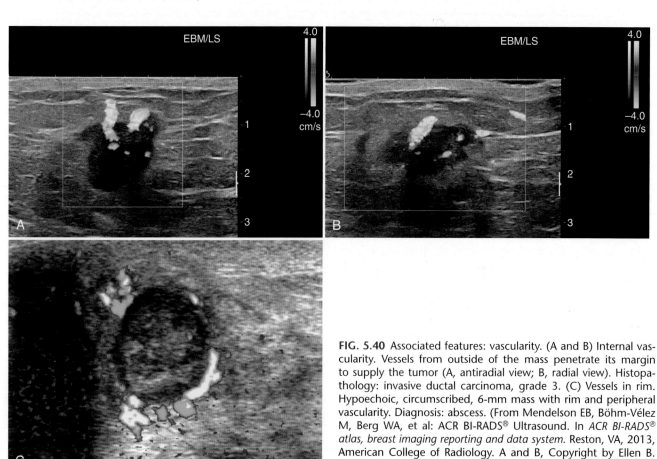

FIG. 5.40 Associated features: vascularity. (A and B) Internal vascularity. Vessels from outside of the mass penetrate its margin to supply the tumor (A, antiradial view; B, radial view). Histopathology: invasive ductal carcinoma, grade 3. (C) Vessels in rim. Hypoechoic, circumscribed, 6-mm mass with rim and peripheral vascularity. Diagnosis: abscess. (From Mendelson EB, Böhm-Vélez M, Berg WA, et al: ACR BI-RADS® Ultrasound. In *ACR BI-RADS® atlas, breast imaging reporting and data system.* Reston, VA, 2013, American College of Radiology. A and B, Copyright by Ellen B. Mendelson, MD, FACR. C, Copyright by Giorgio Rizzatto, MD.)

TABLE 5.2   American College of Radiology Breast Imaging Reporting and Data System Code Assessment Categories

BI-RADS Category	Definition	Likelihood of Malignancy	Management Recommendation
0	Incomplete	N/A	Recall for additional imaging
1	Negative	Essentially 0%	Routine screening
2	Benign	Essentially 0%	Routine screening
3	Probably benign[a]	>0% but ≤2%	Short-interval (6-month) follow-up or continued surveillance
4A	Low suspicion for malignancy	>2% to ≤10%	Tissue diagnosis
4B	Moderate suspicion for malignancy	>10% to ≤50%	Tissue diagnosis
4C	High suspicion for malignancy	>50% to <95%	Tissue diagnosis
5	Highly suggestive of malignancy	≥95%	Tissue diagnosis
6	Known biopsy-proven malignancy	N/A	Surgical excision when clinically appropriate

[a]A solid mass with an oval shape, circumscribed margin, and parallel orientation, an isolated complicated cyst, and clustered microcysts are placed in category 3.
From ACR BI-RADS®—Breast Ultrasound, in *ACR BI-RADS atlas, breast imaging reporting and data system*, Reston, VA, 2013, American College of Radiology.

> **BOX 5.2   Simple Cyst Criteria**
>
> Oval or round shape with circumscribed margins
> Anechoic
> Imperceptible wall
> Enhanced transmission of sound

MASSES: FEATURE ANALYTIC APPROACH

A cyst is the most common cause of a palpable breast abnormality. With appropriate technique, most cysts can be diagnosed on US.

Breast Cysts: Simple and Complicated Cysts

The criteria for a simple cyst include a round or oval shape (round less likely), circumscribed margin, anechogenicity, and posterior acoustic enhancement (Box 5.2; Fig. 5.41). Simple cysts usually have imperceptible walls. Simple cysts may be solitary, multiple, or septated (as long as the wall is thin; Fig. 5.42) and may occur in one or both breasts. Cysts smaller than 2 mm are called microcysts, and these dilated lobular acini may be grouped as *clustered microcysts* (Fig. 5.43). Cysts may be painful and may wax and wane with the patient's menstrual cycle. Simple cysts are completely benign, assessed as BI-RADS category 2, and do not require any intervention or follow-up to confirm the diagnosis. Symptomatic cysts are also characterized as BI-RADS category 2 but may be aspirated to relieve symptoms.

Complicated cysts, on the other hand, contain low-level internal echoes (Fig. 5.44) and may have a fluid-fluid level. The internal echoes may be caused by proteinaceous content. Despite their internal echoes, complicated cysts usually have posterior acoustic enhancement because they have increased transmission of sound waves (see Fig. 5.44). Low-level internal echoes within complicated cysts, depicted with high-resolution linear transducers, are real and should be recognized as such. It is important that the sonographic findings are not be manipulated with harmonic imaging to make the mass appear anechoic (Fig. 5.45). A solitary complicated cyst can be characterized as BI-RADS category 3, but several or multiple complicated cysts or complicated cysts in combination with simple cysts should receive a BI-RADS category 2 assessment (Fig. 5.46).

Fluid levels develop in cysts that contain fluids with different specific gravities and are most often seen when oil and water

fluid phases exist in the same cyst. The immiscible oily phase, which is generally more echogenic, floats on top of the watery phase. The fluid-fluid level is also seen with galactoceles, in which the fat-containing cream layer floats atop the watery component of the milk product. When the patient is moved from a supine to decubitus position, the fluid level moves slowly and shifts with gravity. Power Doppler US can also cause movement of particulate matter within complicated breast cysts.

Sometimes a solitary complicated cyst may resemble a fibroadenoma, and a definitive diagnosis of a complicated cyst cannot be made. If doubt exists, either cyst aspiration (Fig. 5.47) or short-interval follow-up may be performed. When a cyst is aspirated, it is standard practice to discard the fluid unless it is bloody or purulent (Fig. 5.48). If the aspirate is bloody, and the procedure has not been traumatic, the fluid should be sent for cytology with microbiology added as well for a purulent collection.

Complex Cystic and Solid Masses

The presence of a discrete solid component, including a solid mural nodule, differentiates a complicated cyst from complex cystic and solid mass (Fig. 5.49). Cystic and solid complex masses are often thick walled. In contrast to a complicated cyst, which does not need sampling, a complex cystic and solid mass is suspicious and must be biopsied.

A cyst should be examined in two perpendicular planes with attention to the cyst wall for any intracystic vegetation or focal wall thickening. Color Doppler flow within an intracystic nodule confirms a solid mass, which should be targeted at the time of biopsy.

The differential considerations for a complex cystic and solid mass include intracystic papilloma (Fig. 5.50), intracystic carcinoma, phyllodes tumor with a marked cystic component, and solid cancers with central necrosis. Benign masses such as a hematoma, fat necrosis, abscess (Fig. 5.51), galactocele, and seroma, can also present as complex cystic and solid masses; however, clinical history, and where appropriate, mammography would be needed to dissuade a biopsy.

Intracystic carcinomas are a rare subgroup of tumors that arise from the walls of a cyst and represent 0.5% to 1.3% of all breast cancers. These tumors have a better prognosis than other malignant breast neoplasms. On US, intracystic carcinomas often appear as solid mural excrescences projecting into the cyst fluid and may appear solid and circumscribed with the tumor completely replacing the fluid.

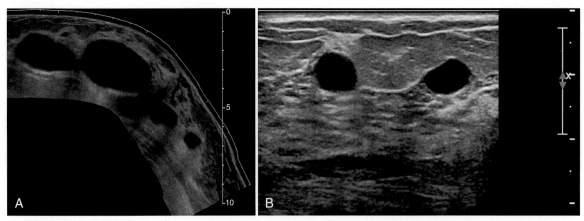

FIG. 5.41 Typical appearance of a simple cyst in two different patients. (A) Extended field-of-view scan shows numerous simple cysts within the fibroglandular tissue of this 46-year-old woman. (B) Two small simple cysts circumscribed and anechoic with posterior enhancement. BI-RADS assessment is benign, category 2. (From Mendelson EB, Böhm-Vélez M, Berg WA, et al: ACR BI-RADS® Ultrasound. In *ACR BI-RADS® atlas, breast imaging reporting and data system.* Reston, VA, 2013, American College of Radiology. A, Copyright by Helmut Madjar, MD. B, Copyright by Judith A. Wolfman, MD.)

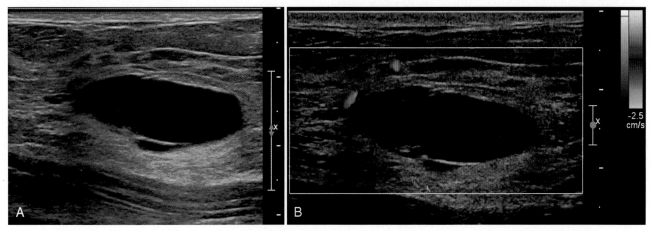

FIG. 5.42 Simple cyst with a septum. B-mode (A) shows a simple cyst with a septum. Color Doppler applied to the cyst (B) shows the cyst to be avascular with a small amount of flow in the tissue surrounding the cyst. Application of Doppler imaging is helpful in establishing identity of a mass as fluid filled, but for reliability, Doppler parameters must be optimized. (From Mendelson EB, Böhm-Vélez M, Berg WA, et al: ACR BI-RADS® Ultrasound. In *ACR BI-RADS® atlas, breast imaging reporting and data system.* Reston, VA, 2013, American College of Radiology. Copyright by Ellen B. Mendelson, MD, FACR.)

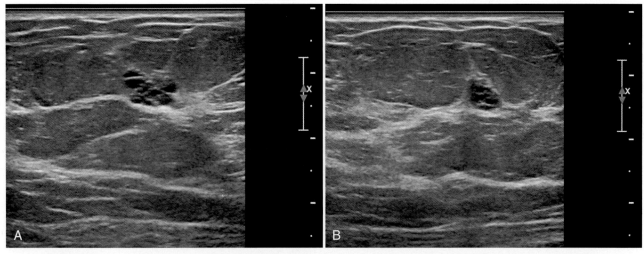

FIG. 5.43 Clustered microcysts. The groupings of cysts shown on perpendicular views (A and B) are minute. No solid component is present, and an assessment category of 3, probably benign, or category 2, benign, would be appropriate. (From Mendelson EB, Böhm-Vélez M, Berg WA, et al: ACR BI-RADS® Ultrasound. In *ACR BI-RADS® atlas, breast imaging reporting and data system.* Reston, VA, 2013, American College of Radiology. Copyright by Ellen B. Mendelson, MD, FACR.)

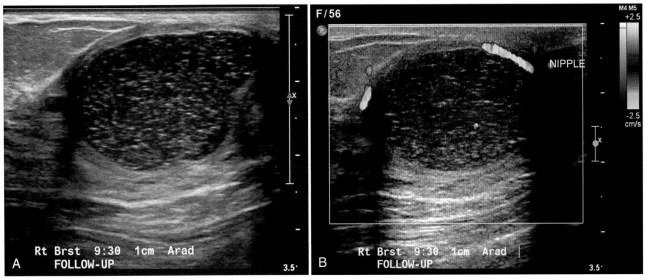

FIG. 5.44 Complicated cyst. This is a 56-year-old woman with palpable mass just lateral to her right nipple that contains low-level echoes throughout (A); rim vascularity, but none within (B); and is a complicated cyst. Note posterior acoustic enhancement behind the complicated cyst. (From Mendelson EB, Böhm-Vélez M, Berg WA, et al: ACR BI-RADS® Ultrasound. In *ACR BI-RADS® atlas, breast imaging reporting and data system.* Reston, VA, 2013, American College of Radiology. Copyright by Ellen B. Mendelson, MD, FACR.)

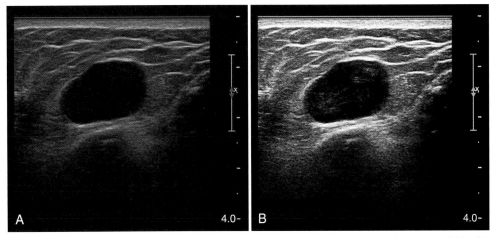

FIG. 5.45 A pitfall in the diagnosis of complicated cysts. With gain settings too low (A), echoes within this complicated cyst disappear and a diagnosis of simple cyst could be rendered mistakenly. The echoes in B are real and should be recognized as such. (Copyright by Ellen Mendelson, MD, FACR.)

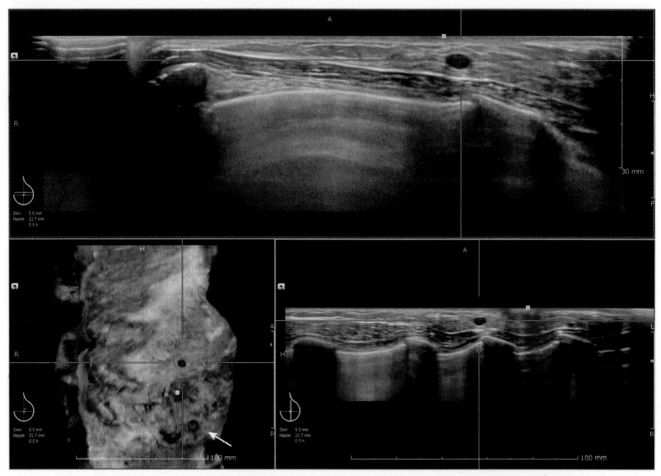

FIG. 5.46 Supine automated ultrasound, right anteroposterior view shows a straight fluid level in a small complicated cyst within the crosshairs on the transverse acquisition image (*top*). The cyst is seen in the coronal (*bottom, left*) and sagittal (*bottom, right*) reconstruction planes. Additional tiny cysts or ducts resembling small black holes are present on this image, and a larger cyst with its more echogenic rounded lower curvature is seen in the lower breast (*arrow*), coronal view. Its appearance is akin to that of milk of calcium seen on a mammographic craniocaudal view. Multiplicity of these findings with benign features supports a BI-RADS category 2 assessment with routine follow-up. (*Yellow square* on all three views denotes nipple). (Copyright by Ellen Mendelson, MD, FACR.)

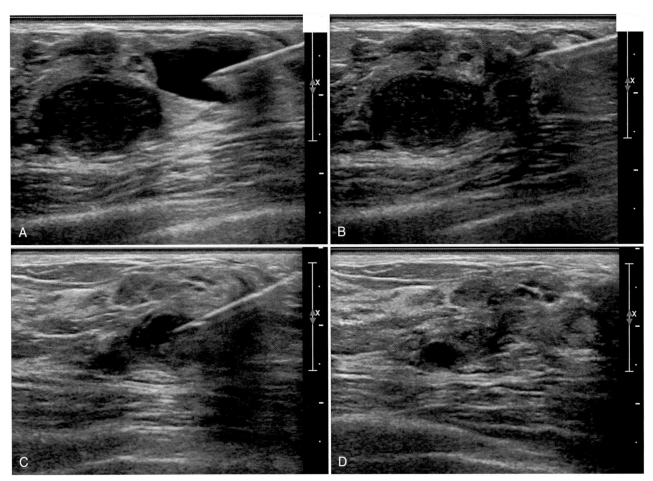

FIG. 5.47 Diagnosis of complicated cyst with ultrasound-guided aspiration. This 42-year-old patient experienced left breast tenderness localized to the outer central breast where simple (anechoic) and complicated (low-level internal echoes or fluid-fluid level) cysts were grouped (A). A needle is seen in the aspiration cavity after aspiration of the simple cyst shown in A (B). Within 2 minutes, most of the complicated cyst was aspirated, bringing relief to the patient (B and C). Postaspiration changes in the tissue are seen in D. (Copyright by Ellen Mendelson, MD, FACR.)

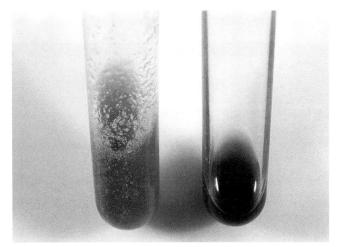

FIG. 5.48 Diagnosis of complicated cyst with ultrasound (US)-guided aspiration: fluid contents. The complicated cyst fluid in the left test tube, which contains debris consisting of particulate matter, causes speckles within the cyst on ultrasound. The simple cyst fluid in the right test tube is clear and contains no debris.

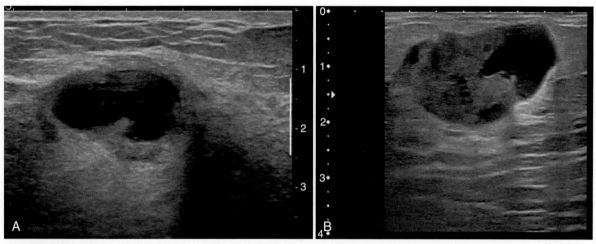

FIG. 5.49 Complex cystic and solid masses in two different patients. Cystic masses with solid components are in BI-RADS category 4, suspicious, unless the etiology is prior intervention, such as aspiration of a simple cyst with clot formation after the procedure. After aspiration of a small amount of the fluid, core biopsy was directed to the solid posterior echogenic component and thick wall of these complex masses (A and B). Histopathology of A: chronic inflammation and fat necrosis, consistent with ruptured duct. Histopathology of B: intracystic papillary carcinoma. (Copyright by Ellen B. Mendelson, MD, FACR. B, From Mendelson EB, Böhm-Vélez M, Berg WA, et al: ACR BI-RADS® Ultrasound. In *ACR BI-RADS® atlas, breast imaging reporting and data system.* Reston, VA, 2013, American College of Radiology.)

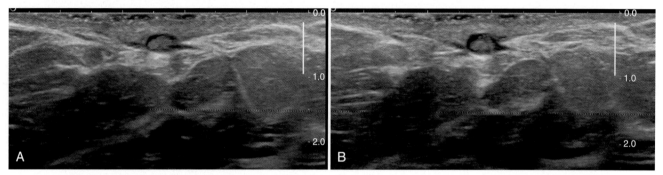

FIG. 5.50 Complex cystic and solid mass: intraductal papilloma. Complex cystic and solid mass in a 32-year-old woman with right nipple discharge has a small central oval echogenic component and anechoic rim, resembling a lymph node on both views (A and B). The linear extensions at the lateral borders are ducts, and the mass at biopsy was an intraductal papilloma. (Copyright by Ellen B. Mendelson, MD, FACR. A, From Mendelson EB, Böhm-Vélez M, Berg WA, et al: ACR BI-RADS® Ultrasound. In *ACR BI-RADS® atlas, breast imaging reporting and data system.* Reston, VA, 2013, American College of Radiology.)

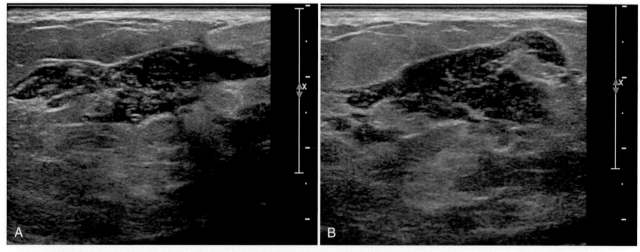

FIG. 5.51 Complex cystic and solid mass: abscess. Irregular mass parallel to the skin with cystic areas and septa in a 19-year-old patient was aspirated. Radial (A) and anti-radial (B) images are shown. Core biopsy histopathology was chronic granulomatous abscess. (From Mendelson EB, Böhm-Vélez M, Berg WA, et al: ACR BI-RADS® Ultrasound. In *ACR BI-RADS® atlas, breast imaging reporting and data system.* Reston, VA, 2013, American College of Radiology. Copyright by Ellen B. Mendelson, MD, FACR.)

Benign Solid Masses

In their 1995 study, Stavros et al. prospectively classified 750 solid breast masses as benign, indeterminate, or malignant based on sonographic features, and compared the sonographic classification with biopsy results. In this study, a mass was characterized as benign if it had an oval shape, less than three gentle lobulations, intense hyperechogenicity, and a thin echogenic capsule. More importantly, for a mass to be characterized as benign, it could have no suspicious findings including spiculation, angular margin, marked hypoechogenicity, shadowing, calcification, duct extension, branch pattern, or microlobulation. When these criteria were used, the study showed a negative predictive value of 99.5% and a sensitivity of 98.4%.

The goal of feature analysis is to determine a lesion's likelihood of malignancy to assign the appropriate BI-RADS category, which will trigger management. An oval, circumscribed, and parallel mass with no suspicious sonographic features seen for the first time can safely be assessed as probably benign, BI-RADS category 3, and when unchanged on a series of US examinations, BI-RADS category 2 Benign. If the area of the mass has been imaged previously and the mass is new, it should be biopsied, because up to 2% of cancers, including papillary, mucinous, medullary, and invasive ductal cancers, may be circumscribed, and a new circumscribed mass still warrants a biopsy (Box 5.3).

Fibroadenoma

Fibroadenomas are the most common benign breast tumor and predominantly affect women between 20 and 40 years of age. As they respond to circulating estrogen, many fibroadenomas form at the time of puberty or early adolescence, may enlarge during pregnancy and lactation, and rarely develop after menopause. They present clinically as firm, mobile masses.

Fibroadenomas and cysts arise from breast lobules. Once diagnosed, fibroadenomas may remain stable in 80% of cases, regress in about 15%, and grow in 5% to 10%. Fibroadenomas may be single or multiple and are called *giant fibroadenomas* if larger than 5 cm (Fig. 5.52).

On mammography, fibroadenomas are indistinguishable from cysts because both present as oval, circumscribed masses. On US, fibroadenomas are typically oval (including macrolobulated), circumscribed, and uniformly hypoechoic and have a parallel orientation (Fig. 5.53). They may have gentle lobulations and may sometimes be isoechoic. On Doppler images, fibroadenomas may show variety of vascularity, including no vascularity, hypovascularity, and hypervascularity (Fig. 5.54). When a mass identified on either mammography or physical examination meets these sonographic criteria, it should be assessed as probably benign and biopsy is not needed.

Fibroadenoma appearances, however, can be highly variable. Fibroadenomas may infrequently display irregular margins, inhomogeneous echotexture, not-parallel orientation, or posterior acoustic shadowing. Because masses that look like atypical fibroadenomas are often breast cancers (Figs. 5.55 and 5.56), masses with this appearance merit a biopsy. It is also important to scan masses in orthogonal planes and at multiple angles in real time to assess all the margins (see Fig. 5.56). A mass that appears round in one plane might actually be the cross section of an oval mass. When characterizing orientation, it should be from the view that depicts the longest axis of the lesion.

Other Benign or Benign-Appearing Masses

Although fibrocystic change is usually diffuse, it may form focal nodules that resemble fibroadenomas on imaging. As discussed earlier, a complicated or inspissated cyst may also be indistinguishable from a fibroadenoma on US. Lipoma and hamartoma are fat-containing masses and should be characterized as benign on mammography. Ultrasound may be performed for confirmation and demonstrates increased echogenicity of the fatty components. Hamartoma or fibroadenolipoma displays a thin capsule, heterogeneous septa, and a "breast within a breast" pattern that refers to a mixture of fat, glandular, and connective tissue within the mass (Fig. 5.57). Hemangiomas, neurofibromas, and granular cell tumors are other types of benign breast masses.

Another mass with similar sonographic appearance to a fibroadenoma is the phyllodes tumor, which can grow very rapidly. The average age of diagnosis is 45 years, although the range is wide. As phyllodes can recur locally, it should be surgically excised with wide margins. The sonographic appearance of these masses is similar to fibroadenomas, but they can often have cystic elements (Fig. 5.58). A phyllodes tumor should be considered if a benign-appearing mass shows unmistakable growth in a short period of time. The patient will usually present with this newly palpable or rapidly growing mass.

Malignant Solid Masses

Breast cancer is the most common malignancy in women and the second most common cause of cancer-related deaths in women. One in eight women in the United States will develop invasive breast cancer in their lifetime. The two biggest risk factors for developing breast cancer are the female gender and age. Nearly

---

BOX 5.3 Differential Diagnosis of Round or Oval Solid Breast Masses

Fibroadenoma
Phyllodes tumor
Invasive ductal cancer, not otherwise specified
Medullary cancer
Mucinous (colloid) carcinoma
Papillary carcinoma
Metastasis (not breast primary)
Papilloma

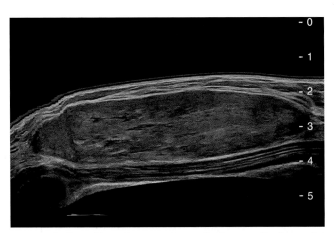

FIG. 5.52 Giant fibroadenoma. An oval, circumscribed, parallel mass in a 28-year-old woman is a giant fibroadenoma. Giant fibroadenomas are those greater than 5 cm in longest dimension. Extended field-of-view scan that depicts the entire extent of the mass, which is more than 9 cm on this medial-to-lateral image. (From Mendelson EB, Böhm-Vélez M, Berg WA, et al: ACR BI-RADS® Ultrasound. In *ACR BI-RADS® atlas, breast imaging reporting and data system.* Reston, VA, 2013, American College of Radiology. Copyright by Ellen B. Mendelson, MD, FACR.)

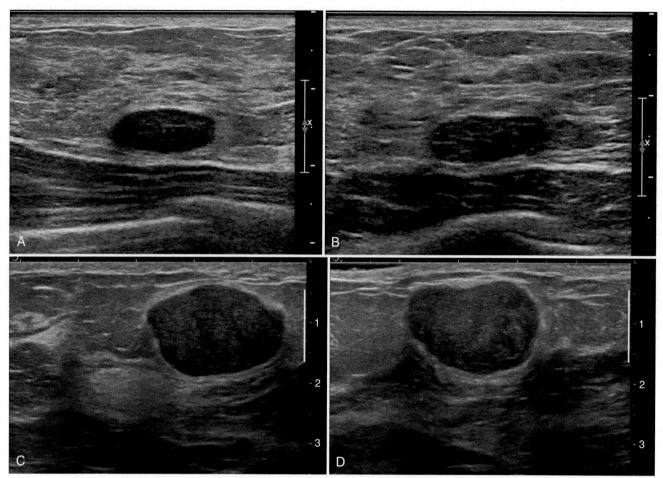

FIG. 5.53 Typical fibroadenoma in two different patients. (A and B) Fibroadenoma located within fibroglandular tissue is adjacent to the pectoral muscle in this 35-year-old patient. Antiradial (A) or radial (B) images of this benign mass. (C and D) Radial (C) and antiradial (D) images of an oval, circumscribed mass consistent with a biopsy-proven fibroadenoma. (From Mendelson EB, Böhm-Vélez M, Berg WA, et al: ACR BI-RADS® Ultrasound. In *ACR BI-RADS® atlas, breast imaging reporting and data system.* Reston, VA, 2013, American College of Radiology. Copyright by Ellen B. Mendelson, MD, FACR.)

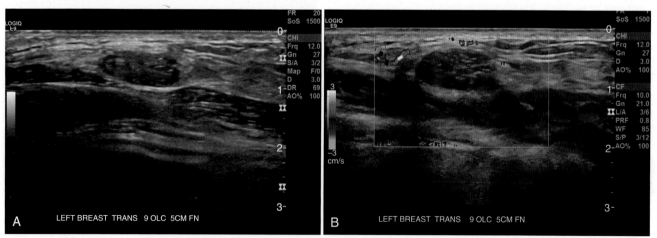

FIG. 5.54 Color Doppler imaging of fibroadenomas. Gray scale ultrasound (A) of a typical fibroadenoma shows a mass that is wider than tall, smooth, and homogeneous. Color Doppler image (B) shows a mild internal vascularity within the mass.

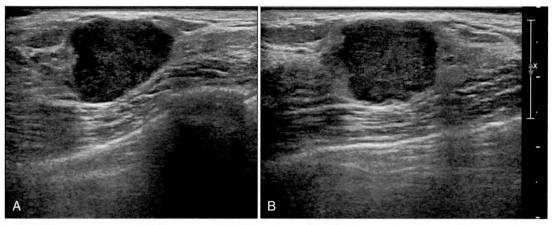

FIG. 5.55 Breast cancer mimicking an atypical fibroadenoma. Palpable mass in a 28-year-old woman has an irregular shape (A) and margins not circumscribed. The mass has strong posterior acoustic enhancement (B). BI-RADS Assessment, 4C. Histopathology: infiltrating ductal carcinoma, grade 3. (From Mendelson EB, Böhm-Vélez M, Berg WA, et al: ACR BI-RADS® Ultrasound. In *ACR BI-RADS® atlas, breast imaging reporting and data system.* Reston, VA, 2013, American College of Radiology. Copyright by Ellen B. Mendelson, MD, FACR.)

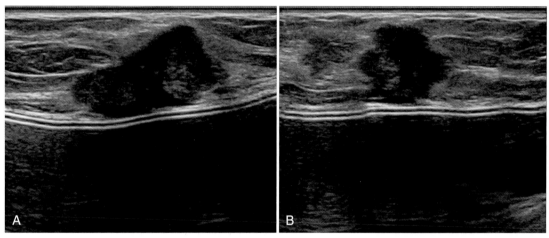

FIG. 5.56 Breast cancer mimicking an atypical fibroadenoma. A mass in a 46-year-old woman sits on the fibrous capsule, with a saline implant beneath. The mass has parallel orientation (A) like most fibroadenomas, but has an irregular shape and margins that are not circumscribed, and are best appreciated on the short axis view (B). Echogenic flecks clumped within the mass are microcalcifications. Histopathology: invasive ductal carcinoma, grade 2. It is important to evaluate a mass in orthogonal planes. Also note that the mass orientation is defined as parallel, although nonparallel orientation is shown in the short axis view (B). (From Mendelson EB, Böhm-Vélez M, Berg WA, et al: ACR BI-RADS® Ultrasound. In *ACR BI-RADS® atlas, breast imaging reporting and data system.* Reston, VA, 2013, American College of Radiology. Copyright by Ellen B. Mendelson, MD, FACR.)

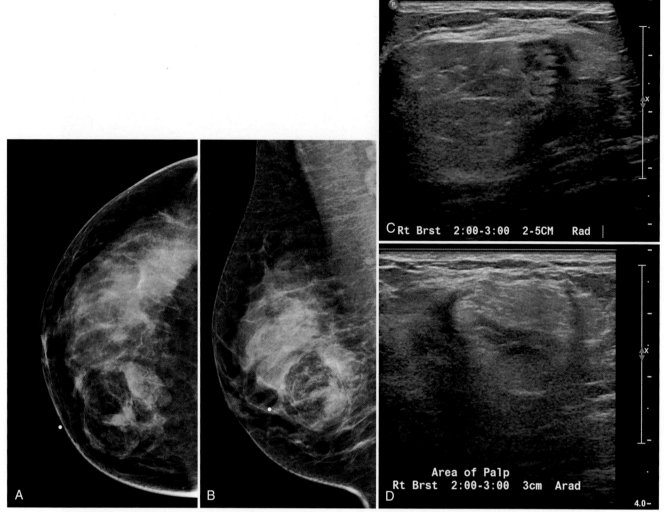

FIG. 5.57 Hamartoma. The round radiopaque marker in the right inner central breast marking the palpable abnormality correlates with a mixed density mass on mammogram (A and B) with a classic "breast within a breast pattern." Ultrasound (C and D) confirms a mixed echogenicity mass, which is mostly echogenic, consistent with a hamartoma. (Copyright by Ellen Mendelson, MD, FACR.)

half of diagnosed breast cancers (48%) occur in the upper outer quadrant, which is the site of greatest amount of fibroglandular parenchyma. However, all areas of the breast should be carefully examined.

Carcinomas have a wide variety of sonographic features. Typically, a malignant mass has an irregular shape (Fig. 5.59) and margins that are not circumscribed, which include *indistinct, angular, microlobulated,* and *spiculated margins* (Fig. 5.60). Although the echogenicity can vary, most cancers are hypoechoic. Approximately 60% of cancers have posterior acoustic shadowing caused by desmoplastic reaction, which is a fibrous response to the tumor (Fig. 5.61). When posterior acoustic shadowing is present, it supports a diagnosis of malignancy; however, absence of shadowing is not a reliable criterion for benignity. It is not uncommon in high-grade tumors that posterior enhancement is seen on ultrasonography. A not-parallel orientation, that is, if the mass is taller than wide or predominantly vertical, is also suspicious. It should be noted that although a not-parallel orientation signifies a high likelihood of malignancy, a parallel orientation is not necessarily benign and many malignancies may be oriented parallel to the

skin. As carcinomas infiltrate surrounding tissues, it is important to observe indirect signs, found in the Associated Features section of BI-RADS for US, such as architectural distortion (Fig. 5.62), disruption of Cooper's ligaments, and skin or nipple retraction. Inflammatory carcinoma may have all of these signs, but its sonographic hallmarks are marked attenuation of the sound beam caused by breast edema and skin thickening.

Malignant tumors can present with a variety of imaging findings and create atypical presentations of breast cancer. Although most cancers are irregular (see Figs. 5.59–5.62), some may present as round or oval circumscribed solid masses (Fig. 5.63). The most common round breast cancer is invasive ductal cancer (Box 5.4). Although the round, circumscribed sonographic feature pattern is uncommon, invasive ductal cancers are so common that a round cancer is statistically likely to be invasive ductal cancer. Other round, circumscribed malignancies include medullary, solid papillary, and colloid (mucinous) carcinomas. These cancers can simulate benign masses on US by appearing round or oval in shape with enhanced transmission of sound (see Fig. 5.63). Although the margin may appear circumscribed in one scan plane, it is important to scan real

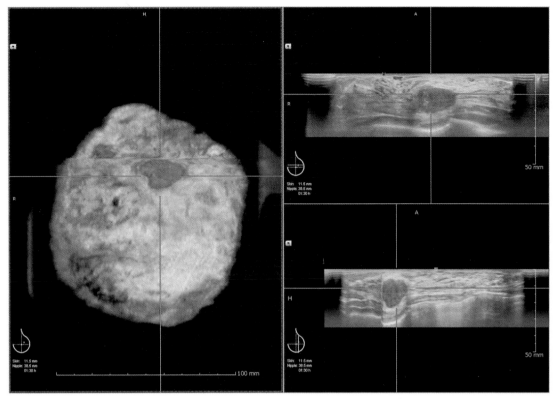

FIG. 5.58 Phyllodes tumor. Automated whole breast ultrasound (US) in coronal plane (*left*), axial plane (*upper right*), and saggital plane (*lower right*) demonstrates an oval, circumscribed mass similar in appearance to a fibroadenoma at the intersection of the lines. The mass was biopsied because it was new from the prior screening ultrasound examination and yielded a benign phyllodes tumor. (Copyright by Ellen Mendelson, MD, FACR.)

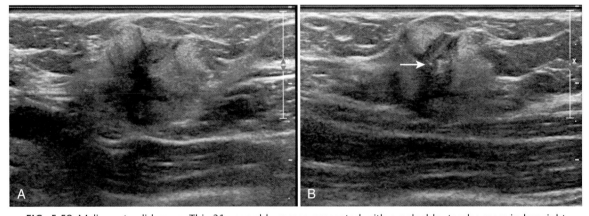

FIG. 5.59 Malignant solid mass. This 31-year-old woman presented with a palpable, tender mass in her right axilla. The mass has a very irregular shape, nonparallel orientation, and spiculated margin (A and B). Microcalcifications are seen within it (B; *arrow*), and surrounding the central hypoechoic components is a thick echogenic rim. Histopathology: infiltrating ductal carcinoma, grade 3. (From Mendelson EB, Böhm-Vélez M, Berg WA, et al: ACR BI-RADS® Ultrasound. In *ACR BI-RADS® atlas, breast imaging reporting and data system.* Reston, VA, 2013, American College of Radiology. Copyright by Ellen B. Mendelson, MD, FACR.)

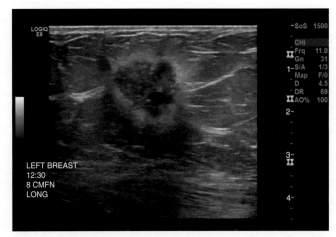

FIG. 5.60 Malignant solid mass. An ultrasound shows an irregular hypoechoic mass with heterogeneous internal echoes, speculated margins, echogenic halo, and posterior acoustic shadowing. The orientation is not parallel. This was an invasive ductal carcinoma.

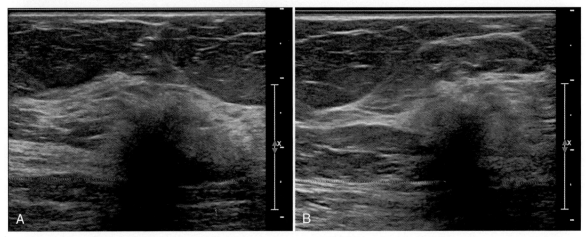

FIG. 5.61 Malignant solid mass with posterior shadowing. Radial (A) and antiradial (B) views of a hypoechoic mass with posterior shadowing are consistent with biopsy-proven invasive lobular carcinoma, grade 2. (From Mendelson EB, Böhm-Vélez M, Berg WA, et al: ACR BI-RADS® Ultrasound. In *ACR BI-RADS® atlas, breast imaging reporting and data system.* Reston, VA, 2013, American College of Radiology. Copyright by Ellen B. Mendelson, MD, FACR.)

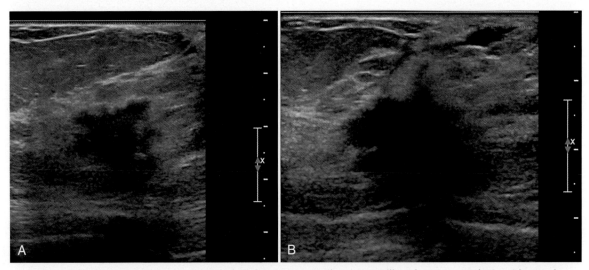

FIG. 5.62 Malignant solid mass. Invasive ductal carcinoma with micropapillary features, grade 3, with angular margins (A and B). Spiculated edges are also seen along with duct extension anteriorly in B with architectural distortion surrounding the mass. (From Mendelson EB, Böhm-Vélez M, Berg WA, et al: ACR BI-RADS® Ultrasound. In *ACR BI-RADS® atlas, breast imaging reporting and data system.* Reston, VA, 2013, American College of Radiology. Copyright by Ellen B. Mendelson, MD, FACR.)

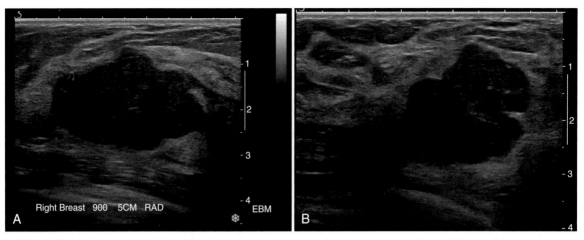

FIG. 5.63 Malignant solid mass with oval shape. Invasive ductal carcinoma, grade 3, in a 42-year-old woman has an oval shape; however, all of the margins are not circumscribed (A). Not uncommon in high-grade tumors is enhancement of the tissue posterior to the mass, which is well seen (B). (Copyright by Ellen Mendelson, MD, FACR.)

BOX 5.4   Round Breast Cancer

The most common round breast malignancy is invasive ductal cancer. It is an uncommon form of a very common tumor.

---

time in multiple planes to evaluate the entire mass. Also, any circumscribed solid mass that is new or enlarging significantly (more than 20% of its volume in a 6-month period) merits a biopsy to rule out a malignancy.

Although more than 90% of cancers are hypoechoic, certain cancers may appear echogenic. More diffuse lesions, such as invasive lobular carcinomas that infiltrate tissues, rarely appear hyperechoic. Necrosis or mucin within cancers may produce anechoic regions, resulting in posterior acoustic enhancement of sound, which may be mistaken for the enhanced transmission of sound seen in cysts.

Evaluation of lymph nodes for tumor involvement is helpful for surgical planning. Size is an unreliable predictor of an abnormal lymph node. Normal axillary lymph nodes resemble small kidneys with an echogenic hilum and a near anechoic cortex. An enlarged lymph node with a uniformly widened cortex measuring less than 3 mm is usually reactive. When a lymph node is eccentrically thickened and contains an area of altered echogenicity, metastatic disease may be the cause, especially when there is an ipsilateral breast cancer that is suspected or confirmed (Fig. 5.64). The normal hilum may be progressively compressed to a sliver or complete obliteration (Fig. 5.65). Although reactive and metastatic lymph nodes can at times be recognized on US, there is considerable overlap among normal, reactive, and metastatic nodes. If indeterminate lymph nodes are identified or it is clinically indicated, sampling may be performed with US-guided core biopsy or fine-needle aspiration. Sentinel axillary lymph node sampling performed at the time of surgery remains the standard of care when a lumpectomy is performed for invasive breast cancer.

As with mammography, approaches to sonographic interpretation of lymph nodes take into account unilaterality or bilaterality; mild versus extreme enlargement; single or multiple nodal enlargement; and an impression of whether the nodes represent a malignant process, cancer or lymphoma, or a systemic benign process such as sarcoid or rheumatoid arthritis. When mammography has been performed, US and mammographic findings should be correlated.

APPROPRIATENESS CRITERIA, AMERICAN COLLEGE OF RADIOLOGY PRACTICE PARAMETERS, AND OTHER GUIDELINES

The ACR publishes an evidence-based set of algorithms for various clinical scenarios such as palpable breast mass in young women. Some of these scenarios are listed later. They are referenced by some payers who use them to determine whether or not the imaging study being considered is indicated and thus reimbursable. The Practice Parameters are guides—not standards—to help the breast imaging practitioner. The Practice Parameters as well as the Appropriateness Criteria are updated periodically to incorporate new data. These documents, which are thoroughly vetted, go through a consensus process before publication.

Ultrasound's use is important for characterizing palpable breast masses as well as masses seen on mammography and breast MRI. The false-negative rate of mammography in detection of breast cancer has been reported to be approximately 10%. These mammographically occult malignancies are often found on physical examination with some on self-examination.

A palpable breast mass may be detected on breast self-examination or clinical breast examination. Palpable breast thickening, defined as greater firmness of an area of the breast compared with other areas in the same breast or the contralateral breast, may be associated with breast cancer in 5% of women and also warrants US investigation. Invasive lobular carcinoma's clinical presentation is as an area of thickening. Some benign and malignant palpable masses are difficult to differentiate on clinical examination, and imaging evaluation is necessary in all cases. Although the negative predictive value of mammography with US is over 97%, negative imaging findings should never dissuade biopsy of a clinically suspicious palpable mass.

Palpable Mass in Women 40 Years of Age or Older

The initial evaluation of a palpable abnormality in women 40 years of age or older starts with a diagnostic mammogram. If the patient has had a bilateral mammogram within the last 6 months, only the breast with the palpable mass needs to be imaged. If the patient can locate the palpable finding, it can be marked by a small radiopaque pellet placed on the skin. A spot tangential mammographic view can aid in confirming a mass by visualizing its anterior portion framed in subcutaneous fat and its posterior portion obscured by fibroglandular tissue.

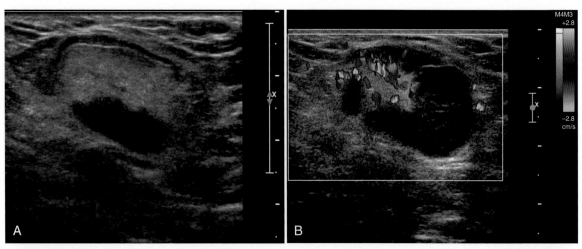

FIG. 5.64 Metastatic axillary lymphadenopathy. Metastatic involvement of this lymph node (A, B-mode; B, color Doppler) shows eccentric cortical thickening with a large area of hilar fat with scalloped contour impinged on by the cortical metastasis. The focal metastasis shows increased echogenicity and decreased vascularity on B. (From Mendelson EB, Böhm-Vélez M, Berg WA, et al: ACR BI-RADS® Ultrasound. In *ACR BI-RADS® atlas, breast imaging reporting and data system.* Reston, VA, 2013, American College of Radiology. Copyright by Ellen B. Mendelson, MD, FACR.)

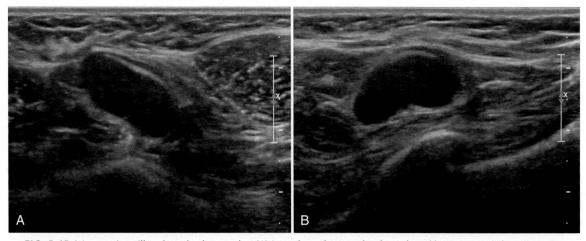

FIG. 5.65 Metastatic axillary lymphadenopathy. (A) Lymph node completely replaced by metastasis from invasive ductal carcinoma. No hilar fat remains. (B) The reniform shape and normal size are retained. (Copyright by Ellen B. Mendelson, MD, FACR. A, From Mendelson EB, Böhm-Vélez M, Berg WA, et al: ACR BI-RADS® Ultrasound. In *ACR BI-RADS® atlas, breast imaging reporting and data system.* Reston, VA, 2013, American College of Radiology.)

The next standard step is US evaluation of the palpable abnormality. US is unique because it allows direct correlation of the clinical and imaging findings. To guide the examiner to the palpable finding, the patient is asked to find the abnormality and point it out to the sonographer. The US probe is then placed directly over the palpable area of concern. If the abnormality is palpated by the referring physician and the patient cannot feel it, then the quadrant of the area specified should be scanned.

Palpable Mass in Pregnant, Lactating, or Young Women

US is the modality of choice in evaluating a breast abnormality in pregnant women because it has no ionizing radiation and is unaffected by breast density, which limits the sensitivity of mammography. US is also the initial examination for evaluating palpable abnormalities in women who are breast feeding and those under 40 years of age.

Although the age criterion for "young" women has historically been considered under 30 years, the ACR Appropriateness Criteria recommends US as the initial imaging modality for women under 40 years of age, with a low threshold for using mammography. The rationale is that the risk of breast cancer is relatively low for women in the fourth decade and that US may be more sensitive than mammography for women under age 40.

If the clinical examination, sonography, or risk factors are suspicious for carcinoma, it is important to note that bilateral mammography should be performed in young, pregnant, or lactating women before an imaging-guided biopsy. As suspicious microcalcifications and subtle architectural distortion may be difficult to detect on US, mammography (a collimated examination during which the patient is shielded with a lead apron) imparts no radiation to the pelvis. Mammography can be safely performed even in early pregnancy when malignancy is suspected.

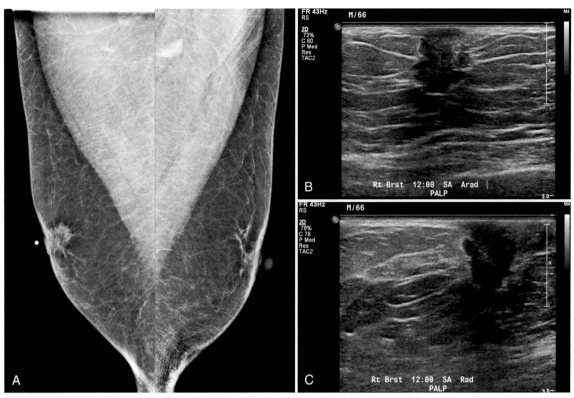

FIG. 5.66 Male breast cancer. Bilateral mediolateral oblique views (A) show an irregular mass behind the right nipple, suspicious for malignancy. Ultrasound (B and C) of the palpable abnormality confirms an irregular, spiculated mass, consistent with biopsy-proven malignancy. (From Mendelson EB, Böhm-Vélez M, Berg WA, et al: ACR BI-RADS® Ultrasound. In *ACR BI-RADS® atlas, breast imaging reporting and data system.* Reston, VA, 2013, American College of Radiology. Copyright by Dipti Gupta, MD.)

Palpable Findings in Men

Gynecomastia and breast cancer are the main differential considerations in a male patient with a palpable mass. It is the most common cause of a palpable mass or pain in the male breast. Male breast cancer is rare, comprising 1% of all breast cancers. Although gynecomastia is not a risk factor for breast cancer, gynecomastia and breast cancer can coexist 50% of the time.

Bilateral diagnostic mammography is the initial examination for evaluation of palpable masses in men 25 years or older. Mammography has a very high sensitivity and specificity in the male breast and is helpful in distinguishing gynecomastia from breast cancer. As only 6% of male breast cancers occur before the age of 40, and only 1% before age 30, US is the modality of choice in men younger than 25 years with a palpable finding. US comparison with the contralateral side is helpful as gynecomastia is frequently bilateral, although often asymmetric, and bilateral synchronous male breast cancer is extremely rare. When there is a suspicious or indeterminate mammographic finding, US can help further evaluation as well as guide intervention.

Sonographic features of male breast cancer are similar to cancers in women. Suspicious masses in men are irregular, hypoechoic, and antiparallel (Fig. 5.66). US is also helpful in assessing the relationship of the mass to the nipple. A discrete mass, which is not subareolar in men, is suspicious because gynecomastia occurs directly behind the nipple.

US features of gynecomastia can be variable. It typically presents as a hypoechoic, vague, or flame-shaped region in the retroareolar breast (Fig. 5.67). Nodular gynecomastia may appear as a more discrete mass directly behind the nipple. Because men do not have breast lobules, they do not develop "probably benign"

masses of lobular origin like fibroadenomas or complicated cysts. Exceptions are Klinefelter males and men who receive estrogenic compounds for treatment of prostate cancer. Lipomas (Fig. 5.68), hemangiomas, and epidermal inclusion cysts are the benign masses seen in the male breast.

Although mammography is the primary modality in evaluation of a palpable mass in the male breast, familiarity with US findings is important when the mammography findings are equivocal for problem solving and avoiding unnecessary biopsies.

Mammography and Magnetic Resonance Imaging–Detected Nonpalpable Masses

Targeted breast US is routinely performed for evaluation of mammographically detected masses by both sonographers and radiologists. The correlation of the US findings with the mammogram is of the utmost importance in these cases. The size of the mass and the quadrant in which it is located should be specified if the scan is performed by the technologist. When the scan is performed for an asymmetry, the hemisphere of the breast, instead of the quadrant, may be scanned. The radiologist must confirm that the depth and relationship of the lesion to the adjacent fibroglandular parenchyma correlate on both modalities (Fig. 5.69). If there is an irregular 7-mm mass on mammogram in the right upper quadrant, and the US shows only a 7-mm lymph node at the right 10 o'clock position, the lymph node is likely not the correlate for the mammographic finding and further investigation is necessary. When an US is performed to evaluate for a mammographic finding, the mammogram should be up in the US room so it can be referred to at the time of the scan.

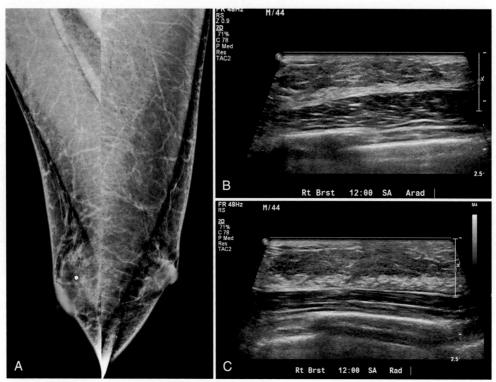

FIG. 5.67 Gynecomastia. Bilateral mediolateral oblique views (A) show fan-shaped subareolar densities, right greater than left, consistent with gynecomastia. Ultrasound (B and C) was performed of the right palpable abnormality, just behind the nipple, which confirms a vague flame-shaped hypoechoic region. (From Mendelson EB, Böhm-Vélez M, Berg WA, et al: ACR BI-RADS® Ultrasound. In *ACR BI-RADS® atlas, breast imaging reporting and data system.* Reston, VA, 2013, American College of Radiology. Copyright by Dipti Gupta, MD.)

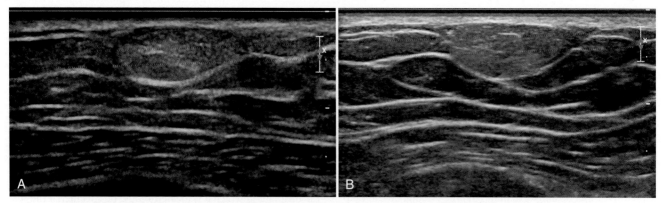

FIG. 5.68 Lipoma in a male patient. Within a superficial fat lobule in a 67-year-old man seen in orthogonal views (A and B) is an echogenic circumscribed mass, which is a lipoma. Increased echogenicity in a circumscribed mass is characteristic of lipomas, and in women, mammography can differentiate the fat density of a lipoma from the soft tissue or water density of a fibroadenoma. Fibroadenomas and other lobular lesions are not ordinarily found in men. (From Mendelson EB, Böhm-Vélez M, Berg WA, et al: ACR BI-RADS® Ultrasound. In *ACR BI-RADS® atlas, breast imaging reporting and data system.* Reston, VA, 2013, American College of Radiology. Copyright by Ellen B. Mendelson, MD, FACR.)

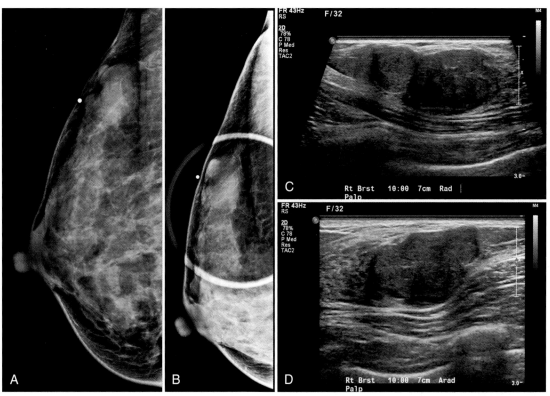

FIG. 5.69 Correlation of mammographically detected mass to ultrasound (US) findings. Small radiopaque pellet placed on the skin on the craniocaudal view (A) marks the palpable area of concern. The spot tangential view in B allows for better evaluation of the anterior aspect of the mass because it is surrounded by subcutaneous fat. Radial (C) and antiradial (D) US images show an oval, hypoechoic mass, which has a similar size, shape, location, and depth as the mass on mammography. (From Mendelson EB, Böhm-Vélez M, Berg WA, et al: ACR BI-RADS® Ultrasound. In *ACR BI-RADS® atlas, breast imaging reporting and data system.* Reston, VA, 2013, American College of Radiology. Copyright by Dipti Gupta, MD.)

Similarly, US can help further evaluate as well as biopsy masses detected on MRI. US-guided biopsy is cheaper, faster, and more comfortable for the patient compared with an MRI-guided biopsy. Because US cannot usually identify areas of nonmass enhancement and foci because they are too small, so-called "second-look US" after MRI should be reserved for masses. Similar to mammography, the size and morphology of the mass as well as the location and depth should all correlate on both modalities (Fig. 5.70). Because MRI is the most sensitive tool for detection of breast cancer, masses may be seen on MRI that cannot be found on a second-look US. In such cases, further management of the mass is based on the MRI features. Generally, if the MRI-detected lesion cannot be found with US or a lesion is found, biopsied, and does not correlate with the MRI finding, MRI-guided biopsy should be performed instead of a 6-month short-interval MRI follow-up.

SPECIAL INDICATIONS

Posttreatment Breast

Postsurgical scars can have a confounding appearance on US and share many of the sonographic features of breast carcinomas. The greatest diagnostic difficulty is encountered in women who have had breast conservation surgery. At the time of lumpectomy, the surgeon excises the tumor and closes only the subcutaneous tissues and the skin above the cavity. The lumpectomy cavity

fills with fluid that is not drained because the slow resorption is thought to improve cosmesis. Breast radiation causes breast edema and skin thickening and prolongs the time it takes for the changes to resolve. Although women who undergo benign excisional biopsies usually have near resolution of postsurgical findings on imaging at 12 to 18 months, those receiving radiation after a lumpectomy have treatment changes for 2 years or more, with some women never returning to a pretreatment appearance.

Immediately post lumpectomy, US shows a fluid-filled pocket in the surgical bed that ranges from hypoechoic to anechoic and may have a sharp or ill-defined edematous rim with or without shadowing (Fig. 5.71). Gradually, fluid in the biopsy cavity may contain solid debris or fibrous septa that move during real-time scanning (Fig. 5.72). Subsequently, the biopsy scar fills in with granulation tissue and becomes fibrotic, forming a hypoechoic mass with indistinct margins with or without acoustic shadowing (Fig. 5.73). This appearance of an intramammary scar can mimic breast cancer. Pressure from the transducer can flatten the compressible fibers in the scar, causing the hypoechoic lesion and shadowing to resolve, which helps in differentiating a scar from cancer. It is also important to examine the lesion in two planes, because a scar will look very different in the two projections. A scar often looks elongated in one view and more masslike in the orthogonal view. Last, as the transducer is moved along the course of a scar, it appears as a linear defect that can be seen extending from the skin to the lumpectomy site.

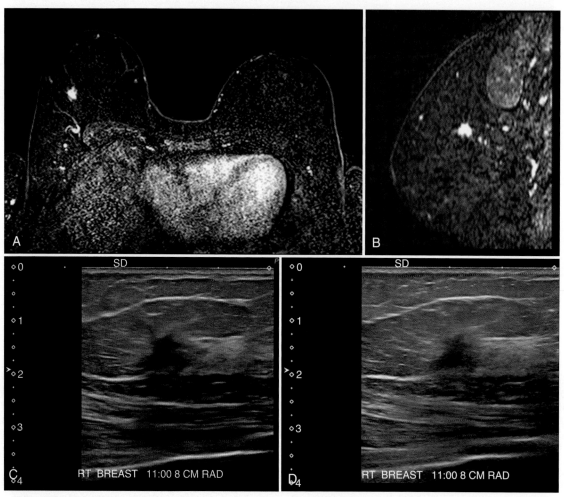

FIG. 5.70 Second-look ultrasound (US). Axial (A) and sagittal (B) post-contrast–subtracted magnetic resonance (MR) images demonstrate an irregular enhancing mass in the right, upper outer breast. Targeted breast US of this region was performed and demonstrates an irregular mass at the right 11 o'clock position (C and D), with the shape, location, and depth correlating with the MR imaging, which is consistent with biopsy-proven invasive ductal carcinoma. (Copyright by Dipti Gupta, MD.)

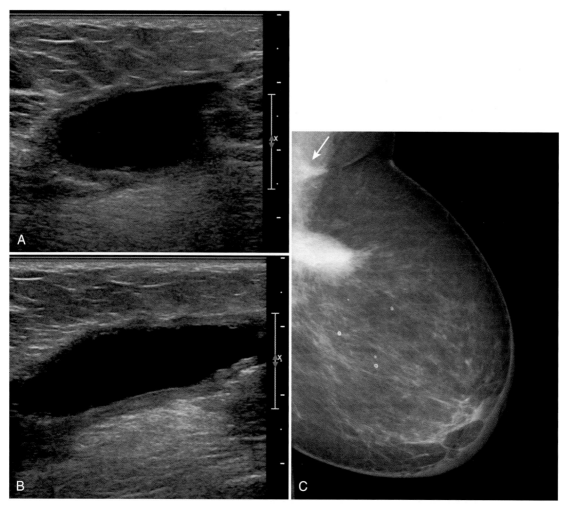

FIG. 5.71 Postsurgical breast. Six months after lumpectomy and radiation therapy for invasive and intraductal carcinoma, grade 2, baseline posttreatment imaging of a 79-year-old patient shows elliptical fluid collection on orthogonal ultrasound (US) views (A and B) as well as mediolateral oblique view of the left breast (C). The thickened wall of the seroma on the US images is of no significance. The mammographic view also shows mild edema and skin thickening, which are common findings after breast conservation. A smaller triangular collection (*arrow*) can be seen projecting over the pectoral muscle at the site of lymphadenectomy. (Copyright by Ellen B. Mendelson, MD, FACR. A and B, From Mendelson EB, Böhm-Vélez M, Berg WA, et al: ACR BI-RADS® Ultrasound. In *ACR BI-RADS® atlas, breast imaging reporting and data system.* Reston, VA, 2013, American College of Radiology.)

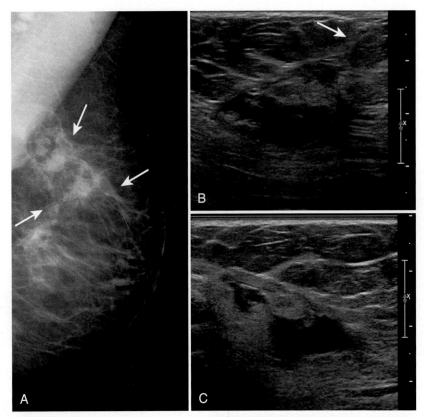

FIG. 5.72 Postsurgical breast. This is a 55-year-old patient in for follow-up imaging 1 year after conservation therapy for invasive ductal carcinoma of the left breast. A triangular scar containing an area of fat necrosis centrally (on mammography [A, *arrows*], radial [B], and antiradial [C] ultrasound view) is identified, with the scalpel's path extending from a V-shaped scar at the skin diagonally to the lumpectomy site (B, *arrow*). Although the scar is complex, mammography–ultrasound correlation helps to exclude recurrence. BI-RADS assessment here can be BI-RADS category 2, Benign. (Copyright by Marcela Böhm-Vélez, MD.)

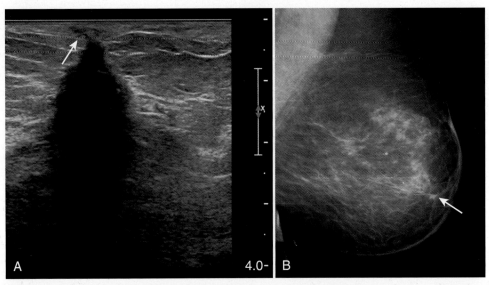

FIG. 5.73 Postsurgical breast. Mature scar 4 years after lumpectomy and radiation therapy. Note the typical V-shaped focal thickening (*arrow*) and hypoechogenicity of the skin at the site of incision on radial ultrasound (US) image (A). It is also seen on the mediolateral oblique mammogram (B; *arrow*). The scar on the US image is markedly hypoechoic and extends from the skin to the pectoral muscle with a margin that shows short spicules consistent with fibrosis and acoustic shadowing. (Copyright by Ellen Mendelson, MD, FACR.)

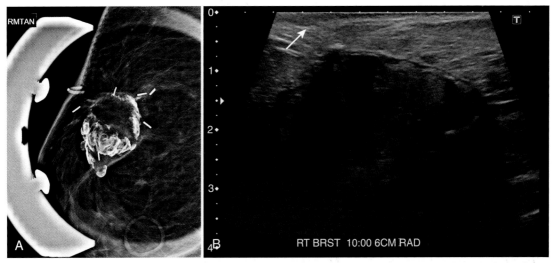

FIG. 5.74 Postsurgical breast with fat necrosis. This 77-year-old patient had undergone lumpectomy 5 years earlier for invasive and intraductal carcinoma, grade 1. Follow-up imaging showed no sign of recurrence on tangential mammographic spot compression view (A). The rim and internal calcifications of the area of fat necrosis cause posterior shadowing on ultrasound (B), and the V-shaped incision at the skin is seen (*arrow*). (Copyright by Ellen Mendelson, MD, FACR.)

There is considerable overlap between the sonographic features of a postsurgical scar, fat necrosis, and recurrence. Thus the initial evaluation of the lumpectomy bed should be performed with mammography. If there are dystrophic fat necrosis calcifications in the lumpectomy bed, they can erroneously appear suspicious on US, but can be accurately characterized as benign on mammography (Fig. 5.74). If the lumpectomy bed is larger and denser on mammography, which may be caused by technique, or if there is a palpable area of concern, US should be performed. US of a breast cancer recurrence will have the same malignant characteristics and appearance of other breast cancers on US, but recurrences are separated from the scar by normal breast parenchyma. The separation of a mass from the scar can help distinguish breast cancer from the biopsy scar. Despite all these techniques and careful sequential imaging studies, in a few cases it may be hard to distinguish breast cancer recurrences in the lumpectomy bed from the scar itself, in which case a biopsy would be warranted.

Many surgeons are now doing oncoplastic surgery. An ellipse of skin is removed and the tumor excised with closure or apposition of the sides of the resection cavity, which does not fill with fluid. On occasion the breast surgeon may perform minor plastic surgical procedures at the time of lumpectomy to promote cosmesis.

Cancers Undergoing Neoadjuvant Chemotherapy

The term locally advanced breast cancer (LABC) includes tumors larger than 5 cm, breast cancers that involve the skin or underlying chest muscles, and those with multiple axillary lymph node involvement. Inflammatory breast cancer, clinically distinct, is also an LABC. In the past, women with LABC usually underwent mastectomy with poor local control and poor 5-year survival rates.

Preoperative neoadjuvant chemotherapy is defined as combination chemotherapy given before definitive surgical treatment (lumpectomy and mastectomy). It is usually given to breast cancer patients who have large tumor masses (stage T3 or T4) or regional lymph node involvement. Neoadjuvant chemotherapy, by shrinking the tumor to decrease tumor burden, may allow

some patients to undergo lumpectomy and radiation for local control instead of mastectomy.

In the setting of neoadjuvant chemotherapy, US can guide percutaneous biopsy to establish a histologic diagnosis as needed, determine initial tumor size and extent, document treatment response, and evaluate for residual tumor after chemotherapy (Fig. 5.75). As neoadjuvant chemotherapy can create a Swiss cheese or moth-eaten appearance in the primary malignancy, the residual tumor becomes less distinct and can be difficult to identify with US. Thus MRI is a more sensitive tool used for detecting both disease extent and chemotherapy response.

After neoadjuvant chemotherapy, the original tumor site is resected to establish absence of residual tumor, and, if present, its histology and extent. This information is important for predicting prognosis. A complete pathologic response (no residual cancer in the original tumor bed by histology) is a good prognostic indicator. When neoadjuvant chemotherapy elicits a complete clinical response and the tumor is undetectable by both physical examination and imaging, the clip placed at the time of US-guided biopsy marks the area to be localized preoperatively and excised at the time of surgery.

Screening Breast Ultrasound

There has been a growing call to inform women about their breast density and educate them about the role of supplemental screening in detection of early breast cancer. As of December 2015, 24 states have passed breast density laws, which vary considerably from some requiring only that women be informed of their density to others requiring that supplemental screening be offered to women with dense breasts. In addition to being an independent risk factor for breast cancer, dense breast tissue can lower the sensitivity of mammography by masking a breast cancer.

The most relevant data on bilateral whole-breast screening US comes from the ACR Imaging Network (ACRIN) 6666 trial (Berg et al., 2008). This was a prospective randomized multiinstitutional trial enrolling 2809 women who had heterogeneously or extremely dense breast tissue and one additional risk factor for breast malignancy. Women underwent physician-performed and interpreted US screening as well as bilateral mammography interpreted by another physician investigator blinded to the results of

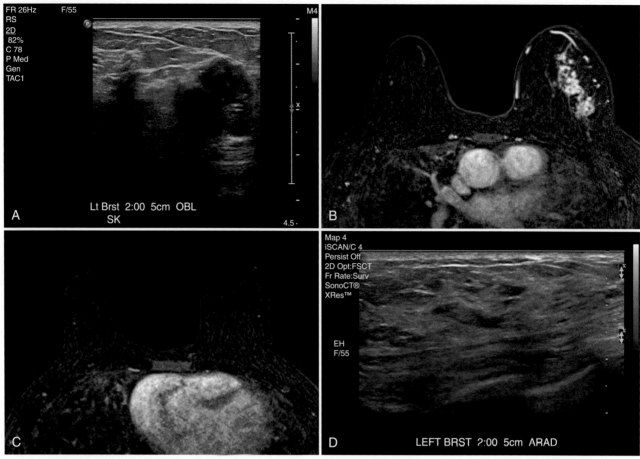

FIG. 5.75 Neoadjuvant chemotherapy. This is a 55-year-old woman with a palpable left breast abnormality who underwent ultrasound-guided core biopsy of a mass at 2 o'clock with a histology of invasive ductal carcinoma, grade 3 (A). Magnetic resonance imaging (MRI) showed 9 cm of nonmass enhancement (B). The MRI after neoadjuvant chemotherapy shows marked response with no residual enhancement (C). Ultrasound of the previously biopsied area shows a moth-eaten appearance with no discrete residual mass (D). (Copyright by Dipti Gupta, MD.)

the US screen. The cancer detection rate of screening US was 4.2 cancers per 1000 women screened, in addition to the mammography-detected cancers. Over 90% of the cancers detected were invasive and most were node negative. The biopsy rates were 4.4% for mammography, 8.1% for US alone, and 10.4% for both. The positive predictive value of breast biopsy decreased from 22.6% for mammography alone to 11.2% for mammography plus handheld screening US. These data are supported by multiple studies that show an increase in cancer detection with screening US, which comes at the cost of a high false-positive rate.

The average time for a physician to perform an US scan in the first year of the ACRIN 6666 trial was 19 minutes. Given the lengthy performance time and inherent operator dependence of handheld US, whole-breast automated US systems have gained popularity for screening (Fig. 5.76). In contrast to a technologist performed scan, in which only specific images are obtained for review by the radiologist, automated US allows for an objective assessment of both breasts by the physician (Fig. 5.77). Automated US allows reproducibility of the examination, reduces operator dependence, and allows the US screen to be interpreted either at the same time as the examination or batch read, which is done for screening mammography.

Ultrasound-Guided Interventions

Ultrasound-guided procedures are useful not just for tissue sampling of suspicious masses but also for aspiration of symptomatic cysts and abscesses as well as preoperative needle localization (see Chapter 6).

Although mastitis and abscesses can occur at any age, they are seen most often during lactation and after surgery. Lactation-related mastitis occurs when microorganisms enter through a fissured nipple, and the patient presents with redness, edema, pain, and fever. Early antibiotics may prevent the formation of an abscess; however, once an abscess has occurred it must be drained (Fig. 5.78). The drained aspirate is sent for cytology to assess for inflammatory cells and microorganisms. Culture and sensitivity of the purulent material is standard. US-guided aspirations may be repeated every few days until the abscess resolves; US-guided catheter placement is an option for larger abscesses. Surgical incision and drainage may be considered for complex, multiloculated collections or those not resolving after numerous US-guided aspirations. In the absence of an appropriate clinical history, it is important to rule out a necrotic malignancy. If there is concern, core biopsy should be performed with samples through the wall of the abscess cavity.

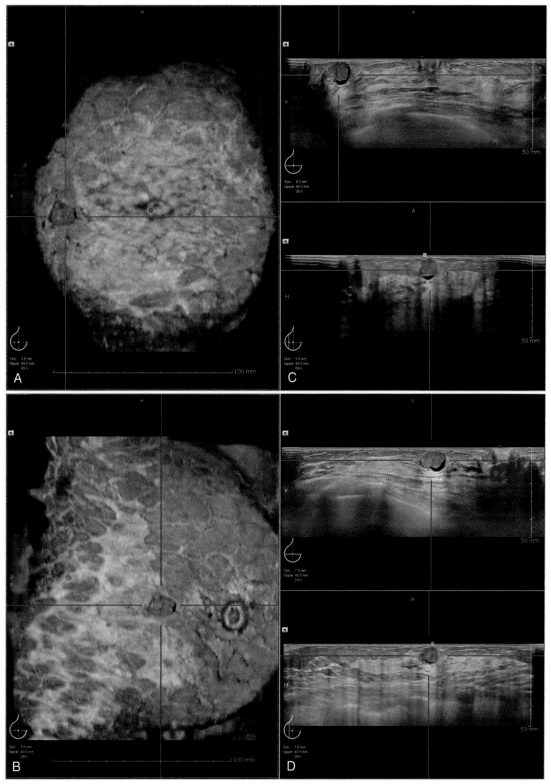

FIG. 5.76 Automated whole-breast ultrasound (US). Anteroposterior (A) and lateral (B) views from an automated whole-breast US demonstrate a complex solid and cystic mass, which can also be confirmed on the axial images (C and D) consistent with biopsy-proven papilloma. (Copyright by Ellen Mendelson, MD, FACR.)

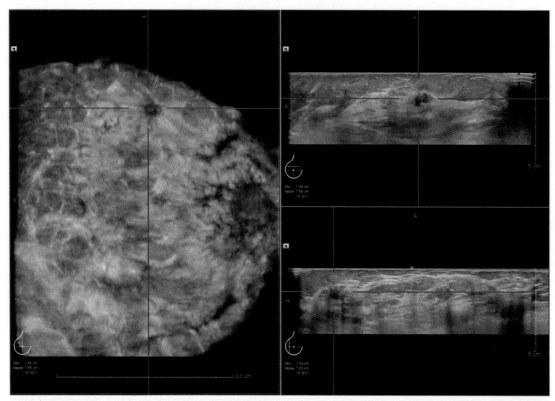

FIG. 5.77 Automated whole-breast ultrasound (US). Coronal plane (*left*), axial plane (*upper right*), and saggital plane (*lower right*) images from an automated whole-breast US demonstrate an irregular hypoechoic mass at the intersection of the lines, consistent with invasive ductal carcinoma on biopsy. (Copyright by Ellen Mendelson, MD, FACR.)

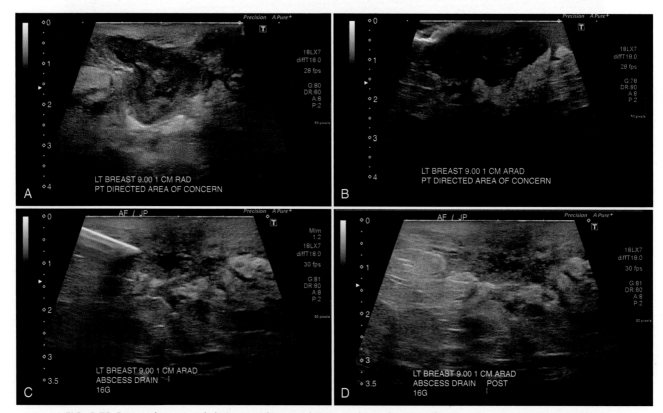

FIG. 5.78 Breast abscess and drainage. Ultrasound (US; A) shows breast edema surrounding an irregular fluid collection with enhanced transmission of sound characteristic of a retroareolar abscess. Note the needle used to drain the abscess (B and C). After drainage of the pus, a postaspiration US (D) shows skin thickening and persistent edema with less fluid in the abscess cavity. (Copyright by Dipti Gupta, MD.)

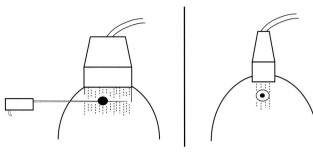

Schematic drawing

FIG. 5.79 Schematics of ultrasound (US)-guided biopsy. To optimally visualize the needle under US, the needle must be parallel to the transducer and perpendicular to the US beam.

To optimally visualize the needle under US, the needle must be parallel to the transducer and perpendicular to the US beam (Fig. 5.79). If the beam encounters the needle at an oblique angle, the needle is only partially visualized. The type and gauge of the needle are less important than the angle at which it is advanced. Before advancing any needles, the lesion to be biopsied should be placed at the center of the US image. The best technique is to insert the needle from the periphery at a shallow angle and advance the needle parallel to the transducer and the chest wall. The needle should never be advanced perpendicular to the chest wall because it makes the needle harder to visualize and increases the risk of complications.

US-guided core biopsies may be performed with spring-activated or vacuum-assisted devices. The spring-activated core biopsy devices are much less expensive and allow for sampling of different areas within the mass. In contrast, vacuum-assisted devices are more expensive, and with only one insertion multiple different samples can be collected. The vacuum-assisted devices are preferred when calcifications are targeted under US, and they increase the likelihood of obtaining a sufficient number of calcifications. If the biopsy is performed for calcifications, radiography of the cores is suggested to confirm accuracy of sampling. Biopsy samples are placed in formalin and sent for pathology interpretation. If more than one biopsy is performed on a patient, a separate labeled jar should be used for specimens from each of the sites. In the United States, marker clips are commonly placed in the lesion that has been biopsied; if more than one site is biopsied, clips of different shapes should be placed if possible.

Key Elements

Ultrasound (US) is useful to differentiate between cysts and solid breast masses, as well as to characterize masses as benign, probably benign, or suspicious based on their sonographic features.

When investigating color flow, it is important to use only modest compression of the probe and to select a sensitive frequency.

The three most important feature categories taken together for assessment of likelihood of malignancy are shape, orientation, and margin.

The entire margin must be circumscribed on US to classify a mass as circumscribed. If any portion of the margin is not circumscribed, the margin of the mass should be reported as not circumscribed.

It is also important to scan masses in orthogonal planes and at multiple angles, preferably in real time, to assess the entire margin of a mass.

Echogenicity of a mass is described relative to the subcutaneous fat.

Echogenicity of most benign and malignant masses is hypoechoic relative to the subcutaneous fat.

A solitary complicated cyst can be characterized as Breast Imaging Reporting and Data System (BI-RADS) category 3, but several or multiple benign-appearing complicated cysts or complicated cysts in combination with simple cysts should receive a BI-RADS category 2 assessment.

An oval, circumscribed, and parallel mass with no suspicious sonographic features can safely be assessed as probably benign, unless it is new on imaging that has shown the area previously.

There is considerable overlap between the sonographic features of a postsurgical scar, fat necrosis, and malignancy.

Screening breast US results in an increase in cancer detection rates at the cost of high false-positive rates.

Mastitis and abscesses are seen most often during lactation and present with redness, edema, pain, and fever

---

SUGGESTED READINGS

American College of Radiology: ACR appropriateness criteria®, 2012. https://acsearch.acr.org/docs/69495/Narrative/. Accessed June 29, 2016.

American College of Radiology: *ACR practice parameter for the performance of a breast ultrasound examination*, Reston, VA, 2014, American College of Radiology.

Barr RG, Zhang Z, Cormack JB, et al.: Probably benign lesions at screening breast US in a population with elevated risk: relevance and risk of malignancy in the ACRIN 6666 trial, *Radiology* 269:701–712, 2013.

Berg WA: Rationale for a trial of screening breast ultrasound: American College of Radiology Imaging Network (ACRIN) 6666, *AJR Am J Roentgenol* 180:1225–1228, 2003.

Berg WA: Sonographically depicted breast clustered microcysts: is follow-up appropriate? *AJR Am J Roentgenol* 185:952–959, 2005.

Berg WA, Blume JD, Cormack JB, et al.: Combined screening with ultrasound and mammography vs mammography alone in women at elevated risk of breast cancer, *JAMA* 299(18):2151–2163, 2008.

Berg WA, Setchin AG, Maques H, et al.: Cystic breast lesions and the ACRIN 6666 experience, *Radiol Clin North Am* 48:931–987, 2010.

Berg WA, Zhang Z, Cormack JB, et al.: Multiple bilateral circumscribed masses at screening breast US: consider annual follow-up, *Radiology* 268(3):6/3-683, 2013.

Gordon PB, Gagnon FA, Lanzkowsky L: Solid breast masses diagnosed as fibroadenoma at fine-needle aspiration biopsy: acceptable rates of growth at long-term follow-up, *Radiology* 229:233–238, 2003.

Graf O, Helbich TH, Hopf G, et al.: Probably benign breast masses at US: is follow-up an acceptable alternative to biopsy? *Radiology* 244:87–93, 2007.

Harvey JA, Nicholson BT, Lorusso AP, et al.: Short-term follow-up of palpable breast lesions with benign imaging features: evaluation of 375 lesions in 320 women, *AJR Am J Roentgenol* 193:1723–1730, 2009.

Kaplan SS: Clinical utility of bilateral whole-breast US in the evaluation of women with dense breast tissue, *Radiology* 221:641–649, 2001.

Kim WH, Chang JM, Moon WK, et al.: Intraductal mass on breast ultrasound: final outcomes and predictors of malignancy, *AJR Am J Roentgenol* 200:932–937, 2013.

Lehman CD, Isaacs C, Schnall MD, et al.: Cancer yield of mammography, MR, and US in high-risk women: prospective multi-institution breast cancer screening study, *Radiology* 244:381–388, 2007.

Mendelson EB, Böhm-Vélez M, Berg WA, et al.: *ACR BI-RADS®—Ultrasound. ACR BI-RADS® atlas, breast imaging reporting and data system*, Reston, VA, 2013, American College of Radiology.

Moon WK, Myung JS, Lee YJ, et al.: US of ductal carcinoma in situ, *Radiographics* 22:269–280, 2002.

Stavros AT, Thickman D, Rapp CL, et al.: Solid breast nodules: use of sonography to distinguish between benign and malignant lesions, *Radiology* 196:123–134, 1995.

Chapter 6

Mammographic and Ultrasound-Guided Breast Biopsy Procedures

Debra M. Ikeda and Kanae K. Miyake

CHAPTER OUTLINE

Imaging-guided biopsy of nonpalpable breast lesions is an essential component of breast imaging services. Percutaneous biopsy provides a diagnosis with minimal patient trauma. If it is cancer, the patient and her team can decide on lumpectomy versus mastectomy, with definitive excision and axillary lymph node biopsy at the first surgery if breast conservation is chosen. This chapter describes percutaneous ultrasound (US)-guided and stereotactic-guided breast needle biopsy techniques, preoperative needle localization, and imaging–pathology correlation. Magnetic resonance imaging (MRI)-guided breast procedures are described in Chapter 7.

BEFORE PROCEDURE

Prebiopsy Patient Workup

Suspicious nonpalpable, imaging-detected breast lesions can be sampled by either percutaneous needle biopsy or preoperative localization and surgical removal for diagnosis and patient treatment planning. The decision to start with needle biopsy or operation depends on the patient's clinical situation and requires discussions between the patient, the surgeon, and the radiologist. There is a strong trend toward using needle biopsy before surgery for diagnosis, reserving breast surgery for definitive therapy.

Whether planning biopsy on x-ray mammography, stereotactic targeting, or planning to scan by US, the finding must be seen in craniocaudal (CC) and mediolateral (ML) orthogonal views (Box 6.1). If not seen definitively on CC and ML views, the radiologist triangulates the lesion with the fine-detail mammographic views described in Chapter 2. Alternatively, stereotactic targeting, tomosynthesis, MRI, and US methods may help determine whether the lesion is real and find its location in the breast.

Nothing substitutes for thorough imaging workups when targeting nonpalpable findings for biopsy. The radiologist must have the lesion's location firmly entrenched in his or her mind to successfully and safely plan a biopsy. Do not attempt to biopsy a breast lesion if you do not know if the lesion is real or if the location of the lesion is unknown.

BOX 6.1 Requirements for Nonpalpable Breast Lesion Biopsy

Lesion is real
Lesion is seen in orthogonal views on mammography or is seen by ultrasound or magnetic resonance imaging
Lesion can be accessed with safety and accuracy
Patient can cooperate and hold still during the procedure
Patient is not allergic to medications used in the biopsy procedure
Blood-thinning medications have been avoided if possible (biopsy may still be done with patient on anticoagulants if the need is urgent)
Patient can follow postbiopsy instructions to diminish bleeding and other complications
Patient will comply with postbiopsy imaging or surgical follow-up

---

Suboptimal workup results in procedure cancellation. Philpotts et al. (1997) reported that stereotactic biopsy cancellation in 16% of cases examined (89/572) occurred mostly because of incomplete workup or inaccurate clinical history. Jackman and Marzoni (2003) reported cancellation of stereotactic biopsy in only 2% (29/1809) of cases; their low cancellation rates were caused by both improved workups and using advanced stereotactic biopsy techniques. An example of a workup preventing biopsy is skin calcifications. Their peripheral location and radiolucent centers are clues to their location in the skin, and tangential views could identify them as dermal calcifications, avoiding the recommendation for biopsy in the first place.

Aside from a visible and correctly localized target, a checklist of prerequisites for safe and accurate biopsies follows: a patient's ability to cooperate and hold still during the procedure, blood-thinning medications have been avoided if possible, no allergies to procedure medications, an ability to follow postbiopsy instructions to diminish bleeding and other complications, and the patient's likelihood to be compliant with postbiopsy follow-up imaging regimens or instructions (see Box 6.1).

Informed Consent

Informed consent is an important part of any procedure (Box 6.2). For percutaneous needle biopsy, the radiologist informs the patient of the risks, benefits, and alternatives to percutaneous biopsy (eg, surgical biopsy), as well as the risks and benefits of any alternatives, and that occasionally the target may not be removed or sampled. The most common complication after core or vacuum needle biopsy is hematoma formation, but it is rarely significant. Other rare complications include untoward bleeding (very rarely requiring surgical intervention), infection (with mastitis it is a very rare complication), pneumothorax, pseudoaneurysm formation, implant rupture, milk fistula (if the patient is pregnant or nursing), and vasovagal reactions (see Box 6.2). The patient is informed that surgical excision may be needed if the biopsy reveals a malignancy, high-risk lesion, or discordant benign lesion, or if the needle biopsy cannot be completed because of technical limitations (see Box 6.2). The patient is informed that a postbiopsy metallic marker will be placed in the biopsy site to guide further surgery and to correlate with other imaging, and that the marker occasionally moves to another location. Last, the patient is given postbiopsy wound management instructions, what to expect and how to manage pain or bleeding, phone numbers to call for untoward complications, and when and how to obtain biopsy results.

For preoperative needle localization, the surgeon obtains informed consent for preoperative needle localization and surgical excision. The radiologist confirms that the patient is properly informed about the needle localization portion of the procedure.

Skin Sterilization, Local Anesthesia, and Skin Incisions

The breast skin is sterilized with a cleansing agent before anesthetic needle insertion. These agents are usually alcohol or iodine based. Most facilities routinely use local anesthesia for percutaneous needle biopsy and preoperative needle localization. A common local anesthetic for breast biopsies is 1% lidocaine in a 10:1 ratio. The lidocaine is given without epinephrine in the skin and subcutaneous tissue (to avoid skin necrosis) and with 1:100,000 epinephrine in the deeper tissue (to increase hemostasis and prolong the anesthetic effect). To avoid mix-ups, the two solutions may be drawn up in different-sized syringes, with a 25-gauge skin injection needle placed only on the syringe containing plain lidocaine, and a longer needle placed only on the syringe containing the lidocaine with 1:100,000 epinephrine. Each syringe is labeled with its contents. The maximum dose of 1% lidocaine with epinephrine is 7 mg/kg (3.5 mg/lb) body weight, not to exceed 500 mg. This translates to 50 mL in a 70-kg patient. The maximum dose of 1% lidocaine without epinephrine is 4.5 mg/kg (2 mg/lb), not to exceed 300 mg. This translates to 30 mL in a 70-kg patient.

A small skin incision made with a scalpel facilitates insertion of the larger needles used for core needle biopsy. Some large-bore needles are extremely sharp and do not need a separate skin incision. Skin incisions usually are not needed for fine-needle aspirations (FNAs) or preoperative localizing needles.

PERCUTANEOUS NEEDLE BIOPSY OF CYSTS, SOLID MASSES, OR CALCIFICATIONS

Breast lesions can be classified as cysts: solid masses, masslike lesions (including true masses, asymmetries, and areas of architectural distortion), and calcifications. Needle types and differences between core and vacuum needle biopsies and cyst aspirations are discussed here, followed by needle biopsies guided by palpation, US, and stereotactic techniques. Needle biopsies guided by MRI are discussed in Chapter 7. This section discusses core specimen radiography; marker placement; carbon and tattoo ink marking; patient safety and comfort after biopsy; complete lesion removal; calcification and epithelial displacement; pathology correlation; high-risk lesions; follow-up of benign lesions; complications; and Mammography Quality Standards Act (MQSA) patient follow-up, outcome monitoring, and noncompliance.

Biopsy Needle Types

Biopsy needle types used for specific breast lesions and guidance methods vary around the world. A trend toward progressively larger needles and more tissue samples per biopsy site has been noted, especially in the United States. Three main types of needles are used for percutaneous biopsies (Table 6.1).

Fine-needle aspiration (FNA) needles are usually 25- to 20-gauge, and are used for cyst aspirations and for solid breast masses. The aspirated material requires interpretation by expert cytopathologists. FNA is usually done with US or palpation guidance with at least four needle passes. It is less commonly done in the United States compared with Europe and Asia.

Automated 18- to 14-gauge large-core (core) needles (Fig. 6.1 A–B) are used most often to biopsy masses with US or palpation

---

BOX 6.2 Informed Consent and Possible Complications

Risks and benefits
Alternatives to procedure, including risks and benefits
Possible complications
- Hematoma (common but rarely significant)
- Untoward bleeding (very rarely needing surgical intervention)
- Infection (with rare mastitis)
- Pneumothorax
- Pseudoaneurysm formation
- Implant rupture
- Milk fistula (if the patient is pregnant or nursing)
Vasovagal reaction (mainly if the procedure is done with the patient upright)
Inability to complete the needle biopsy for technical reasons
Not obtaining the target even if the biopsy is done
Postbiopsy metal marker ends up in suboptimal position or does not deploy
Possible surgical excision after needle biopsy for the following reasons:
- Malignancy
- High-risk lesion
- Benign discordant lesion
Postbiopsy wound management
How and where to get results
If benign, follow-up protocol

TABLE 6.1   Needles Used for Percutaneous Breast Biopsies

Needle Type	Gauge	Biopsy Use
Fine-needle aspiration	25- to 20-gauge	Cyst aspiration; solid mass if highly likely to be either specific benign or malignant diagnosis
Automated large core	18- to 14-gauge	Ultrasound (US)-guided biopsy; uncommon for stereotactic biopsy in the United States, commonly used elsewhere in the world
Directional vacuum assisted	14- to 7-gauge	Stereotactic biopsy and magnetic resonance imaging US-guided biopsy if target is small or as needed

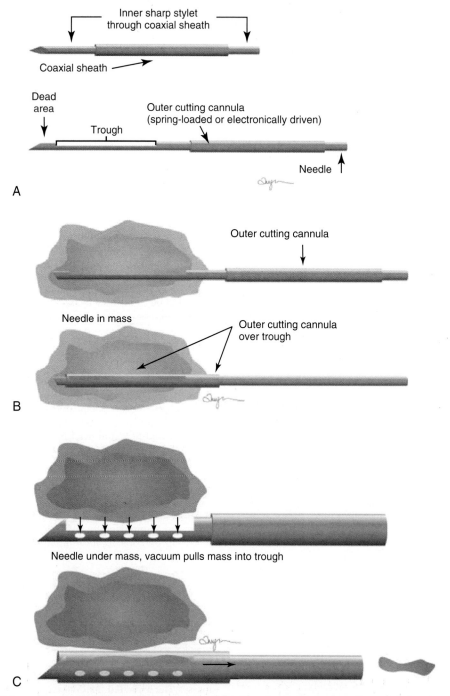

FIG. 6.1 Schematics of needle biopsy systems. (A) Schematic of core biopsy needle parts, showing the inner stylet, coaxial sheath, and needle. (B) Schematic of how to use a multifire core biopsy needle for breast biopsies. The outer cutting cannula shoots over the trough and cuts the mass. The entire needle is removed each time. (C) Schematic of a vacuum-assisted probe for needle core biopsy. The outer cutting cannula shoots over the trough and cuts the mass. The vacuum transports the specimen to the needle end for removal. There may be one or multiple insertions, depending on the vendor.

guidance, with the 14-gauge automated core biopsy needle first introduced by Parker et al. for stereotactic (1991) and US (1993). Many facilities, especially outside the United States, use automated core needles to biopsy masses or calcifications with stereotactic guidance as well. An automated large-core biopsy needle obtains a single tissue biopsy specimen with each pass of the needle. Because separate, repetitive insertions are required for each sample, a coaxial device (trocar and sheath) to gain repeat access to the lesion (especially with US) is often used. Each specimen measures between 15 and 22 mm long depending on the needle, and the width depends on the needle gauge (width). The radiologist obtains samples by firing the needle into the lesion and removing the needle/sample each time to obtain between 2 and 12 specimens. Pathologists who are comfortable interpreting surgically excised breast biopsy tissue also can interpret the core biopsy histologic material.

Directional 7- to 14-gauge vacuum-assisted (vacuum) needles (Fig. 6.1C) are used for stereotactic, US-guided, and MRI-guided biopsies. The vacuum needle was first introduced by Burbank et al. in 1996. Depending on the manufacturer, vacuum biopsy can be done with just one needle pass, with samples measuring up to approximately 2 cm in length and a 4 mm in diameter depending on the gauge of the needle. Specimens are obtained by placing the needle collection aperture of the needle at or in the target by imaging guidance. Specimen collection occurs with the external part of the needle remaining stationary outside of the breast while the cutting part of the needle extracts the samples inside the breast and then vacuums them out to an external collecting chamber. The radiologist points the vacuuming aperture at the target or rotates the aperture within the lesion. Vacuum-assisted devices have the advantage of obtaining larger samples than automated core biopsy sample devices, leading to greater confidence in the diagnosis. For stereotactic guidance, between 6 and 18 specimens are usually obtained, whereas fewer samples may be obtained with US because real-time imaging guides the biopsy. In some facilities, single insertion vacuum biopsies are used to excise benign lesions, such as fibroadenomas previously diagnosed by core needle biopsy, to avoid the need for surgical excision or imaging follow-up.

Other directional vacuum-assisted needles obtain single vacuum specimens with each pass, requiring multiple insertions, similar to the automated large-core needles. These single-insertion vacuum devices have the advantage of obtaining larger samples than automated needles, use smaller handpieces, and may be used with coaxial devices to access the lesion.

Both single-insertion and multiinsertion needles can be used with or without a coaxial guide. Coaxial guides are usually used with US or MRI guidance. The coaxial guide provides a needle path to the target without retraumatizing the breast tissue and consists of an inner sharp stylet and an outer sheath. The radiologist places the coaxial device through the tissue so that the stylet tip/sheath edge is at or in the lesion. Then the radiologist removes the stylet, leaving a sheath that provides a "tunnel" through the breast tissue directly to the lesion. This means the biopsy needle probe may be placed in the lesion to take samples (through the sheath) without having to disturb the surrounding breast tissue. Coaxial biopsies can be done with the sheath placed next to the mass so the needle can fire through the mass (Fig. 6.2A) or with

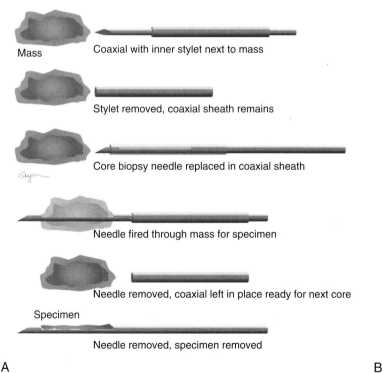

Mass

Coaxial with inner stylet next to mass

Stylet removed, coaxial sheath remains

Core biopsy needle replaced in coaxial sheath

Needle fired through mass for specimen

Needle removed, coaxial left in place ready for next core

Specimen

Needle removed, specimen removed

A

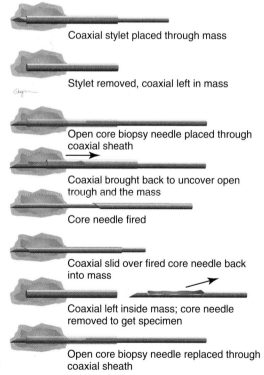

Coaxial stylet placed through mass

Stylet removed, coaxial left in mass

Open core biopsy needle placed through coaxial sheath

Coaxial brought back to uncover open trough and the mass

Core needle fired

Coaxial slid over fired core needle back into mass

Coaxial left inside mass; core needle removed to get specimen

Open core biopsy needle replaced through coaxial sheath

B

FIG. 6.2 Schematics of how to use a coaxial sheath. (A) Schematic of how to use a coaxial sheath next to a mass for ultrasound (US)-guided core biopsies. The radiologist places a coaxial containing a sharp inner stylet through the breast tissue next to a mass. Next he or she removes the stylet, places a core biopsy needle through the co-axial sheath, fires the needle through the mass, and withdraws the needle. The coaxial sheath is left adjacent to the mass, providing a tunnel through the breast tissue. The radiologist removes the specimen from the needle and can replace the needle through the coaxial sheath for the next core. (B) Schematic of how to use a coaxial sheath inside a mass for US-guided core biopsies. The radiologist places a coaxial containing a sharp, inner stylet into a mass. Next he or she removes the stylet, places an open core biopsy needle through the coaxial sheath, withdraws the coaxial to expose the biopsy trough inside the mass, and fires the needle to take the sample. Before withdrawing the biopsy needle, the radiologist threads the coaxial sheath over the fired needle and leaves the sheath inside the mass. The core biopsy needle can now be replaced into the sheath to take the next sample.

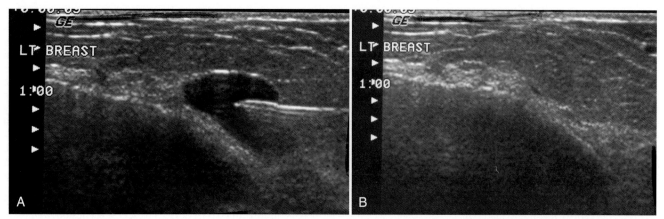

FIG. 6.3 Cyst aspiration. (A) Ultrasound (US) shows a needle in a cyst near an implant. (B) The follow-up US shows that the cyst is gone.

the sheath placed through the mass so that the open trough of the needle may be uncovered while already in the mass to sample it (Fig. 6.2B).

Cyst Aspiration

Masses on mammograms often prompt requests for breast US and aspiration to see if the mass is a cyst. To do a cyst aspiration, the radiologist advances a fine needle into the cyst by palpation or imaging guidance. If the cyst is tense, fluid immediately wells up into the needle hub. If no fluid is seen, the radiologist attaches a syringe to the needle and draws fluid into the syringe until no more fluid can be obtained. If cyst aspiration is done by US, the cyst will disappear in real time (Fig. 6.3). Alternatively, and less commonly, cyst aspiration can be done by x-ray guidance using a fenestrated compression plate and mammography. If the cyst fluid is clear, yellow, blue, or green, it is normal and is discarded.

Aspirated fluid is sent for cytologic evaluation only if there is an intracystic mass or if the fluid is bloody. A large series of cyst aspirations by Tabar et al. (1981) showed that cyst fluid cytology is often falsely negative, even in the presence of an intracystic mass. In these cases, the pneumocystogram was enough to diagnose an intracystic mass and prompt biopsy of the rare intracystic cancer. Currently, an intracystic mass should be evident on US, and one can decide to do a core biopsy instead of fine-needle biopsy.

If the cyst fluid is bloody, a marker may be placed into the biopsy cavity so that the location of the biopsy can be identified (National Comprehensive Cancer Network [NCCN], 2015, version 1). If cytology is positive, biopsy or surgical excision can be obtained with the marker used as guidance. If the cytology is negative, surgical consultation and follow-up with US and diagnostic mammography 1 to 2 years for stability may be obtained.

A *pneumocystogram* is a mammogram obtained after a radiologist injects air into a cyst cavity following cyst aspiration. The pneumocystogram of an air-filled cyst cavity on the mammogram proves that a mass prompting biopsy on the mammogram corresponds to an aspirated cyst, excludes an intracystic mass, and is thought to be therapeutic in preventing cyst recurrence (Fig. 6.4). To do a pneumocystogram, the radiologist aspirates the cyst completely first, then disengages the syringe while carefully holding the needle tip in the decompressed, flattened cyst cavity. The radiologist attaches an air-filled syringe to the needle, injects a small amount of air into the cyst cavity, removes the needle, and immediately obtains CC and ML mammograms. A normal pneumocystogram should show an

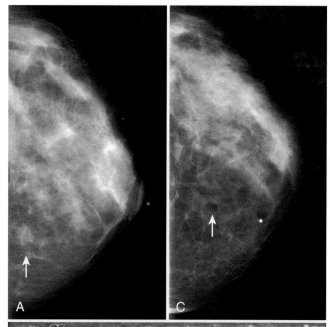

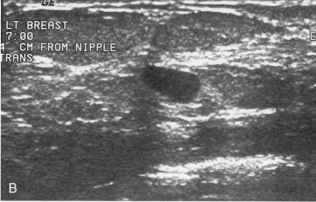

FIG. 6.4 Pneumocystogram. (A) Craniocaudal (CC) mammogram shows an oval breast mass in the inner portion of the breast. (B) Ultrasound (US) shows a complicated cyst versus a solid oval mass. After cyst aspiration under US guidance, air was placed in the cyst cavity. (C) A CC pneumocystogram mammogram shows air (*arrow*) replacing fluid in the mass, which confirms that the finding on the mammogram represents a cyst that was aspirated.

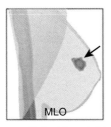
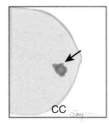
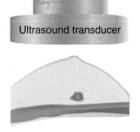
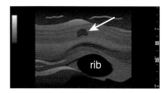

A

Patient is upright on mammogram, mass compressed away from chest wall

Supine patient, the mass drops down toward the chest wall

Ultrasound shows mass near chest wall

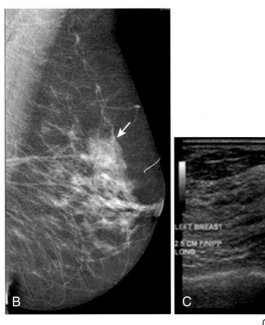
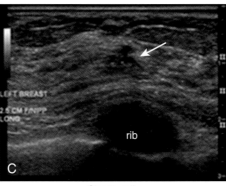

Chest wall

FIG. 6.5 Masses appearing to be far away from the chest wall on mammography may be found near the chest wall on ultrasound (US). (A) Schematic mammograms show a mass in the upper inner quadrant that appears to be far from the chest wall. However, mammograms are obtained with compression; when the patient lies supine, the mass falls dependently against the chest wall. On US, the mass may be closer to the chest wall than expected from the mammogram. (B and C) A representative case. Left mediolateral oblique (MLO) mammogram (B) shows a mass (*arrow*) appearing to be far away from the chest wall, but the corresponding US (C) shows the mass (*arrow*) near the chest wall.

air-filled, thin-walled, round, or oval cavity without intracystic solid masses or mural nodules.

Usually, postaspiration mammograms are done to see if the cyst disappears, whether it is injected with air or not. The mass prompting the cyst aspiration should resolve after aspiration. If the mass persists on the postaspiration mammogram, the mammographic mass is separate from the aspirated cyst and needs further investigation.

Palpation Guidance

Both FNA or core biopsy can be performed on palpable masses. With this method, the radiologist or surgeon reviews the CC and ML mammograms and other imaging studies, but there is no visualization of the lesion or needle during the procedure. Palpation-guided procedures are similar to US-guided procedures. The lesion must be discretely palpable and held well away from the chest wall for the biopsy to be done with accuracy and safety. This procedure is usually reserved for cysts and solid masses that are almost definitely malignant or benign by imaging and palpation criteria.

Ultrasound Guidance

Compared with stereotactic biopsy, US-guided biopsy has the advantage of using readily available equipment and is fast and cost-effective. In the clinic, US is often used on palpable masses to see if they are cysts. If the mass is solid, US determines whether the mass is far enough from the chest wall or other important structures for image-guided or palpation-guided biopsy.

Nonpalpable mammographic masses often prompt US studies to target them for biopsy. When correlating a mammographic mass to the US, the mass may move quite a bit from the upright mammogram to the supine US because the breast falls dependently onto the chest wall when the patient lies down. Thus one can understand why the mass can be far away from the chest wall on the mammogram and lie next to the pectoralis muscle on the US (Fig. 6.5).

Pneumothorax is an important but preventable complication when planning US-guided needle biopsies. Unlike preoperative x-ray–guided needle localization or prone stereotactic localization, the supine US-guided position may not have a needle

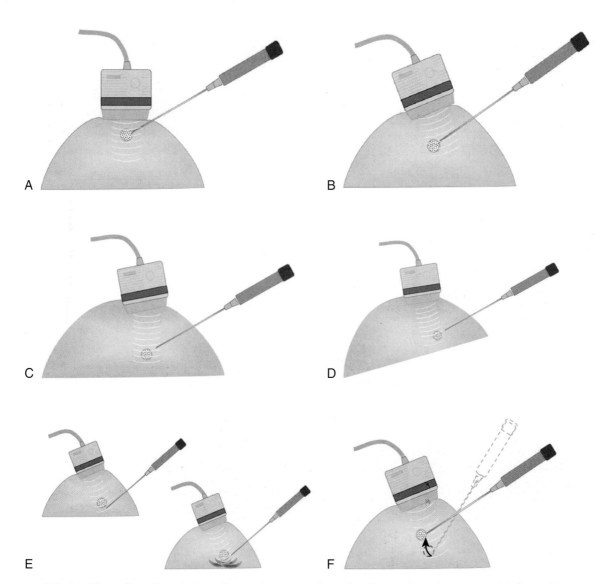

FIG. 6.6 Schematics of how to keep the needle tip away from the chest wall on ultrasound-guided core biopsy. (A) With superficial lesions, the needle tip and throw are usually far away from the chest wall. (B) With deeper lesions, the needle angle is steeper, and the radiologist judges whether the needle throw will penetrate the lung. (C) When the patient is flat and the lesion is even deeper, the needle trajectory can point toward the chest wall. (D) To change the needle trajectory, the patient can be angled so that the chest wall parallels the needle track/ throw. (E) Injecting anesthetic underneath the lesion can lift it away from the chest wall for biopsy. (F) Inserting the needle tip into the lesion and redirecting the throw of the needle avoids placing the needle tip into the chest wall. (Courtesy of Dr. Sunita Pal, Stanford Radiology, Stanford, Calif.)

trajectory parallel to the chest wall. Further complicating matters, some core biopsy needles throw the cutting trough and needle tip 2.5 cm further into the tissue from their initial position. Thus, planning a safe US needle biopsy trajectory must take into account the needle tip, the needle throw trajectory, and the tissue beyond the tip.

To perform a safe procedure, the radiologist rolls the patient on the table so that the chest wall is as parallel to the floor as possible, so that a needle trajectory will traverse safely through the mass into normal tissue and not angle steeply aiming toward the lungs. Patient positioning may take some time, but it is worth the few minutes to position the patient accurately and avoid pneumothorax. Another way to keep the needle away from the chest wall is to inject anesthetic underneath the targeted mass to lift it away from the pectoralis muscle. Alternatively, in some cases, the radiologist may insert the biopsy needle tip into the mass to lift it into a safer

trajectory before firing the needle (Fig. 6.6). Yet another technique is to use a needle that does not use a throw at all, but opens the trough inside the mass to sample it. In any case, the first thing to do is to safely insert the needle into the mass. If the needle cannot be inserted into the mass safely for biopsy, then the mass should be localized and excised instead of sampled percutaneously.

For US-guided FNA, the radiologist introduces a needle in the plane of the transducer axis to show the entire shaft of the needle, its tip, and the lesion. Once the needle is within the lesion, the radiologist aspirates the mass with a vigorous to-and-fro movement to obtain material for cytologic evaluation and then withdraws the needle (Fig. 6.7). At least four passes should be performed; optimally, the material should be analyzed immediately by a cytotechnologist to ensure that adequate cellular material has been obtained for diagnosis. After aspiration, direct pressure is applied to the site.

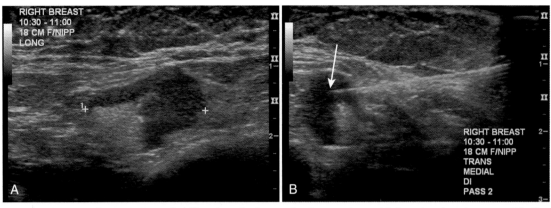

FIG. 6.7 Fine-needle aspiration of axillary lymphadenopathy in a patient with invasive ductal cancer. (A) The right axillary lymph node has an irregular, thickened cortex and a compressed fatty hilum. (B) Ultrasound shows the fine-needle tip (*arrow*) in the lymph node. Cytology showed metastatic disease from invasive ductal cancer.

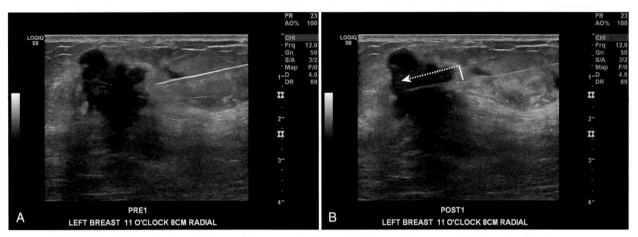

FIG. 6.8 Illustration of automated core biopsy needle throw. A 53-year-old woman with invasive ductal cancer. (A) Ultrasound (US) in the prefire position shows automated core biopsy needle with the tip adjacent to the mass. (B) Postfire US shows the needle through the mass. Note that the needle tip has traversed through the mass (*dashed arrow*), the automated trough had already opened, and the cutter fired over the trough and cut the sample; thus the trough is not seen.

To perform an automated core biopsy under US guidance, the radiologist localizes the lesion by US and chooses the course of needle insertion that offers the most accuracy and safety. While anesthetizing the core biopsy track under direct US guidance, the radiologist uses the anesthesia needle to get an idea of how dense the breast feels and to see the needle trajectory. The radiologist also calculates the core needle throw to determine where to place the core needle tip "prefire" so the core trough will be in the middle of the lesion "postfire" (Fig. 6.8).

Then, under direct US visualization, the radiologist introduces the automated core biopsy needle into the breast. If the lesion is large enough, the radiologist introduces the needle into the edge of the lesion to hold it in place. Otherwise, the radiologist may choose to fire the needle through the mass with or without a coaxial system (Fig. 6.9). In any case, the radiologist fires the biopsy core needle under direct visualization and removes the needle each time to harvest the cores. Optimally, three to six tissue specimens are obtained from different parts of the mass. After sampling, the radiologist places a metallic marker into the mass, and the technologist holds direct pressure on the breast to establish hemostasis. After hemostasis is established, the technologist bandages the wound and takes orthogonal mammograms to show the marker and any residual mass.

A vacuum biopsy is similar to an automated multifire core biopsy, but the vacuum needle is usually placed under or inside the lesion. The probe "vacuums" tissue into the trough, cuts the sample, and carries it into a container outside the breast. Multiple samples can be obtained with one insertion. During a needle biopsy using vacuum technique, the radiologist obtains several samples, concentrating on aiming the trough at the mass (Figs. 6.10 and 6.11; Video 6.1). Afterward, the radiologist may place a marker in the mass either through the probe or by using a marker that is inserted via its own separate needle. This vacuum technique carries a special caveat regarding the skin. If the probe is too close to the skin, the skin can be "vacuumed" into the trough and sampled, causing skin injury, requiring a suture or, in extreme cases, a skin graft.

To do US-guided preoperative needle localization, the radiologist places a 20-gauge needle into the mass or marker under US (similar to the FNA procedure), places a hooked wire through the needle, then removes the needle, takes orthogonal mammograms to show the wire tip and mass/marker, and waits for the excised tissue specimen.

Stereotactic Guidance

This method uses a compression device with a small aperture and an x-ray tube that has the ability to take two stereotactic views about 15 degrees off perpendicular. The patient is in a prone, upright, or decubitus position with the breast compressed

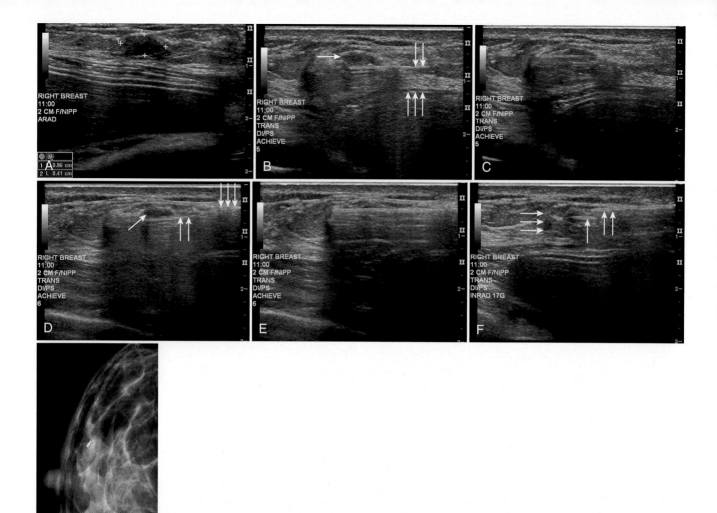

FIG. 6.9 Use of the coaxial to core a mass adjacent to an implant. (A) Ultrasound (US) shows an oval mass on top of a breast implant, for which core biopsy was recommended. (B) The US-guided core biopsy shows the trough of the needle (*double arrows*) traversing an oval mass (*single arrow*) on top of an implant (*triple arrows*). (C) Postfire US shows the needle traversing the mass. At this point, a coaxial was placed over the needle, securing the needle's original position within the mass. (D) The needle was replaced in the coaxial sheath and the coaxial (*triple arrows*) was withdrawn to expose the trough (*double arrows*) and allow the mass (*single arrow*) to fall within it. (E) Postfire US with the coaxial sheath extended over the needle shows both the needle and coaxial traversing the mass. (F) This is a US showing a needle threaded through the coaxial sheath (*double arrows*) placing a marker (*single arrow*) in the mass (*triple arrows*). (G) Cropped implant-displaced digital lateral mammogram shows dense tissue and the marker. Histology showed fibroadenoma.

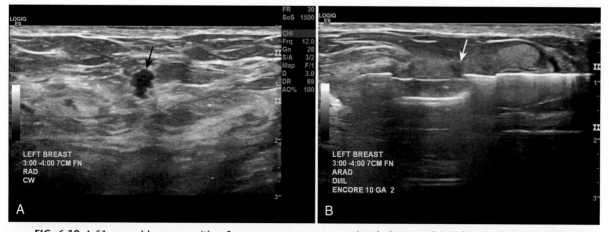

FIG. 6.10 A 51-year-old woman with a 5-mm mass on vacuum-assisted ultrasound (US) biopsy. (A) A US shows 5-mm irregular hypoechoic mass (*arrow*) in the 5 o'clock position of the breast. (B) Single US image from Video 6.1 shows the mass (*arrow*) in the biopsy trough. Vacuum-assisted needle has been placed adjacent to the mass and is shown drawing the mass into the vacuum-needle biopsy trough. Then the outer cutting cannula is fired, obtaining the sample into the trough as the vacuum continues to draw in tissue (not shown). Pathology shows usual ductal hyperplasia columnar change and apocrine metaplasia.

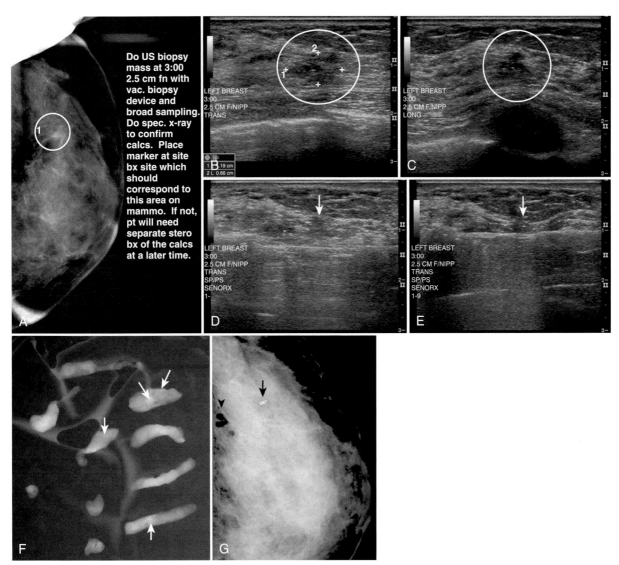

FIG. 6.11 Ultrasound (US)-guided core biopsy of calcifications with core specimen radiography. (A) Craniocaudal mammogram shows calcifications (*circle*) in the outer left breast. Note the radiologist has annotated the mammogram with instructions on how to manage this patient. (B and C) Ultrasound later showed a mass and calcifications in this location. Transverse (B) and longitudinal (C) US show a 1.1-cm hypoechoic mass containing calcifications (*circles*). (D) The US shows the vacuum-assisted core needle trough below the mass and calcifications (*arrow*). (E) Nine samples were obtained by vacuum-assisted core biopsy, and the US shows less of the mass and calcifications (*arrow*) above the trough. (F) Core specimen radiographs of samples show the calcifications (*arrows*) first seen on the mammogram. (G) Postbiopsy mammogram shows the marker (*arrow*) on the outer breast, absence of the calcifications, and air (*arrowhead*) near the chest wall from the biopsy. Biopsy showed ductal carcinoma in situ.

by a fenestrated compression paddle for stereotactic needle biopsy (Fig. 6.12). The radiologist reviews prebiopsy CC and ML mammograms to determine the lesion's location on orthogonal views. The breast is then firmly compressed with the compression paddle aperture placed on the skin surface closest to the breast lesion.

After taking a straight-on scout view that visualizes the lesion, the stereotactic technologist takes two stereotactic views of the lesion (Fig. 6.13). The radiologist locates the lesion on the stereotactic views and targets the finding. A computer calculates the X-, Y- and Z-coordinates of the finding in the breast from the stereotactic views and directs a computer connected to a needle on the stereotactic table to these coordinates. After cleaning the skin, the radiologist anesthetizes the skin and the deeper breast tissue at the coordinates and may take repeat stereotactic images to make sure the target was not moved by the anesthesia.

If the target is in the same place, the radiologist passes a needle into the breast to the calculated depth. The technologist takes two prefire stereotactic images (see Fig. 6.13), which should show the tip of the biopsy needle at the edge of the lesion (Fig. 6.14). The radiologist then fires the needle deeper into the breast and takes two postfire stereotactic images to ensure that the trough of the needle is within the breast lesion.

Not all targeting in stereotactic core biopsy goes so smoothly. After firing, the needle may be in a wrong position, for example, to the left or the right, above or below, or too deep or too shallow to the target. Figure 6.15 shows errors in needle positioning on stereotactic biopsy and how to correct the sampling trough direction or needle position to obtain a sample from the target. For example, if the target is to the side of the needle, and a vacuum device is being used, then the vacuum-sampling trough may be directed toward the target to successfully biopsy the lesion.

PRONE LATERAL UPRIGHT

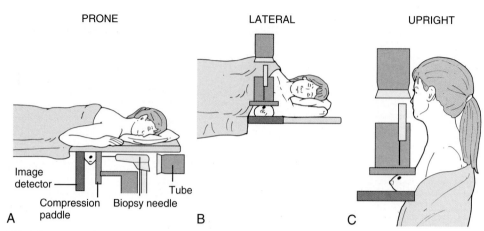

Image detector
Compression paddle
Biopsy needle
Tube

A B C

FIG. 6.12 Schematics of stereotactic biopsy unit and positioning. (A) Prone position. The patient lies prone on the table with the unilateral breast hanging dependently though a hole, compressed against the detector underneath the table with a compression paddle containing an open aperture, through which radiologists perform stereotactic-guided biopsy. This is the conventional stereotactic biopsy table. (B and C) Add-on stereotactic device to upright conventional mammographic units. In this scenario, the stereotactic views are obtained from a conventional mammography unit that has the biopsy needle added on with the patient in the lateral decubitus position with the breast compressed from the side (B) or with the patient sitting in the upright position in a chair with compression in the craniocaudal direction (C) or lateral projection (not shown).

The radiologist collects multiple specimens from the lesion, and if using a multifire automated core biopsy needle, biopsies are taken from different parts of the lesion and the needle is reinserted each time. If a vacuum needle is used, the collection trough of the vacuum needle is rotated 360 degrees to acquire tissue from different parts of the lesion if the finding is targeted centrally; otherwise, the trough is aimed at the finding and the lesion is sampled. In either case, the core samples are radiographed while the needle or probe is still at the target site in case more biopsy samples are needed (see Fig. 6.13). If the core specimen radiographs show the calcifications or mass, the technologist labels the tissue specimens to be sent to the pathology laboratory. The radiologist deploys a metallic marker into the biopsy cavity through the biopsy probe, pulls the probe back slightly, and the technologist takes additional stereotactic images to confirm marker deployment. The technologist then removes the probe, releases the patient from compression, and maintains direct pressure on the biopsy site to achieve hemostasis.

Subsequently, postbiopsy upright CC and ML mammograms are obtained immediately to show the biopsy cavity, confirm removal of all or a portion of the calcifications or mass, and show the location of the marker and its position relative to the targeted findings (see Fig. 6.13). Usually, the marker is located in or near the biopsy site. If the marker is some distance away from the site (ie, inaccurate initial deployment), there is no practical way to insert a second marker. Then, the radiologist should report the marker's location with respect to the original target; for example: "The marker is displaced 3 cm lateral to the original location of the calcifications after stereotactic biopsy." Landmarks from the prebiopsy mammogram and the displaced marker can then guide localization of the original biopsy site. If the patient with an inaccurately placed marker needs surgical excision of the biopsy site, sometimes a postbiopsy hematoma can be visualized by US or mammography to help guide the needle localization.

Jackman and Marzoni (2003) discussed various techniques used to successfully stereotactically biopsy lesions in technically challenging situations with success rates of 98%. A few methods used by Dr. Jackman include taking a standard scout mammogram with skin markers on the breast for the technologist to use as fiducials to target calcifications. The technologist places skin markers on the planned entry side of the breast, closest to the expected location of the calcifications. By looking at the scout mammogram, the technologist uses the skin marker closest to the calcifications to target the calcifications in the biopsy grid.

A second method described by Jackman et al. (2003) is to overcome a thin breast by using a second open grid taped onto the detector. Using this technique, the technologist tapes an open grid onto the detector so that the back paddle allows the posterior breast tissue to puff out of the grid aperture during compression (Fig. 6.16). The technologist sterilizes the anterior and posterior breast skin in case the needle traverses through the entire breast depth. The breast is placed into compression, and the target is localized in the usual manner; however, care is taken to ensure that the needle does not traverse the entire breast or hit the detector. Usually, manual advancement of the probe is wise, as well as watching the needle enter the breast from the side.

Core Specimen Radiography

Core biopsy specimen radiography is mandatory to ensure calcifications are adequately sampled or removed, and this also can be used for masses (see Figs. 6.11 and 6.13). The radiologist usually obtains more specimens if the target has not been sampled. Core specimen radiographs are not usually done after US-guided cores unless the biopsy targets are radiographically detectable calcifications.

Occasionally, the radiologist may be uncertain if the specimen radiograph shows the target, especially if the target was a mass. Then, the radiologist compares the specimen radiograph to the mammogram and immediate postbiopsy mammograms, determining whether the lesion was sampled or removed and where the postbiopsy marker is located.

Calcifications from a biopsied calcific cluster must be evident on the core specimen radiograph for the imaging and histologic findings to be concordant. Most, but not all, calcifications seen on a specimen radiograph are also seen on histologic slides. If the radiologist was targeting calcifications and no calcifications are seen on the specimen radiograph, the ensuing pathology report will not be representative of the calcifications prompting biopsy (which are probably still inside the breast). However, the pathology report may still report calcifications even if they are absent on the core specimen radiograph because pathologists can see tiny calcifications on breast specimen slides that cannot be seen by core specimen radiography. These calcifications are usually smaller than 100 microns and are seen on the slides by

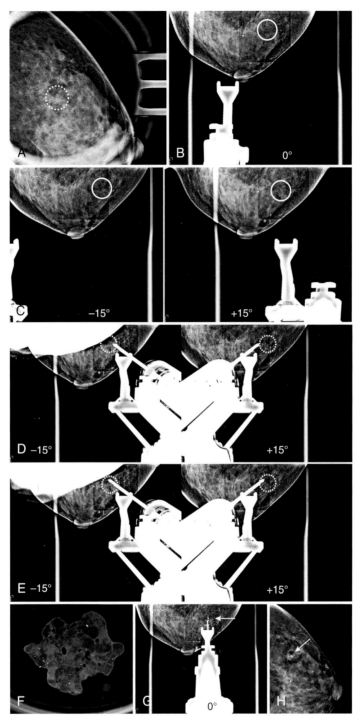

FIG. 6.13 A 50 year-old woman. Images from stereotactic core biopsy. (A) Magnification craniocaudal (CC) mammograms shows pleomorphic calcifications (*dashed circle*). (B and C) Straight-on (B) and 15-degree stereotactic views (C) show the target (*circles*) in the middle of the compression plate aperture. (D) Prefire stereotactic views show the needle pointing at the calcifications (*dashed circles*). (E) Postfire stereotactic views show the needle traversing the calcifications (*dashed circles*). (F) Specimen radiography shows the calcifications in the sample. (G) Postmarker placement views show the marker (*arrow*) in the biopsy site. (H) Photographically magnified postbiopsy CC mammogram shows air in the biopsy site and biopsy marker (*arrow*). Pathology shows invasive ductal cancer.

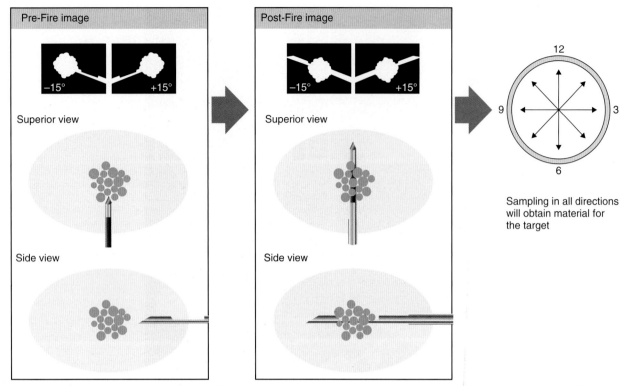

FIG. 6.14 Schematic of perfect positioning on stereotactic biopsy. Two prefire stereotactic images 15 degrees off perpendicular show the tip of the biopsy needle at the edge of the lesion aiming toward its middle. Two postfire stereotactic images show that the trough of the needle is within the breast lesion middle. Because the needle is perfectly placed centrally in the target, samples may be obtained 360 degrees around the needle trough.

serendipity. Thus patients undergoing biopsy for calcifications that have no calcifications on specimen radiographs need rebiopsy, even if the pathology report describes calcifications. Correlation between the specimen radiograph and the pathology is critical to make sure that patient management is correct.

Postbiopsy Markers and Placement, Movement, and Marker Compatibility with Ultrasound and Magnetic Resonance Imaging

Radiologists place metallic markers into the mass or biopsy site immediately after image-guided biopsies in case the biopsy reveals pathology that needs surgical excision. Markers are placed in the residual mass, calcifications, enhancement, or in the biopsy site if the finding is removed, whether the biopsy is guided by stereotaxy, US, or MRI. These markers help correlate US, MRI, and mammogram findings. After US-guided or MRI-guided biopsies, two-view orthogonal mammograms with the postbiopsy markers achieve this goal. If there are two biopsy targets in the same breast, a unique marker shape is used for each target to differentiate the two sites of removal (Fig. 6.17). Also, it is quite helpful to use only one specific marker shape for a specific imaging guidance (stereo, MRI, and US) to specify which marker represents a specific biopsy result (for example, M-shaped markers used only for stereotaxis, circle shapes used only for MRI, and omega shapes used only for US). Last, specifying the marker shape placed in a specific biopsy location for a specific lesion in the report ("ribbon-shaped marker placed in the US-biopsied mass 3:00 position 4.5 cm from the nipple left breast") leaves no questions regarding the meaning of biopsy markers on the postbiopsy mammograms. Rarely, patients request removal of biopsy markers for benign findings, which have been reported to be possible with vacuum-assisted biopsy devices (Brenner, 2001).

The radiologist must determine that the marker has deployed in the correct place after any imaging-guided biopsy. After stereotactic marker placement, the radiologist reviews stereotactic images to be sure the marker is at or near the biopsy site and may deploy a second marker if the first marker is not seen. For US-guided biopsies, US-visible markers are used to be sure the marker has deployed accurately. After MRI-guided biopsy it is hard to be sure that the marker has deployed accurately, but usually signal void from the metallic marker will show the biopsy marker location with respect to the biopsied area. A post-MRI procedure mammogram will show the immediate postbiopsy location of the marker but cannot ensure it is accurately placed.

There are various markers composed of stainless steel, titanium, or other metals either alone or embedded in plugs of Gelfoam, bovine or porcine collagen, suture-type material, or other materials. If markers containing bovine or porcine collagen are used, the patient should be asked about allergies to either beef or pork before deploying the markers.

A variety of problems are associated with markers (Box 6.3). Nondeployment is uncommon, but can occur in stereotaxis with vacuum-assisted probes when the marker deployment sheath is placed through the probe. It was anecdotally noted that some plugs may get stuck during deployment once through the probe, making it impossible to push the plunger in to deploy the plug and making it difficult to withdraw the sheath or close the vacuum trough. This problem is possibly caused by the plugs filling with fluid, expanding in the deployment device, and getting stuck in the trough. For vacuum-assisted needles, the deployment device can get stuck on a retained tissue fragment in the vacuum needle; thus it is important to vacuum the needle before deploying the marker and also important to check that the marker has deployed before removing the probe.

Under US, a US echogenic marker can be seen during deployment, and if the marker does not deploy or deploys in

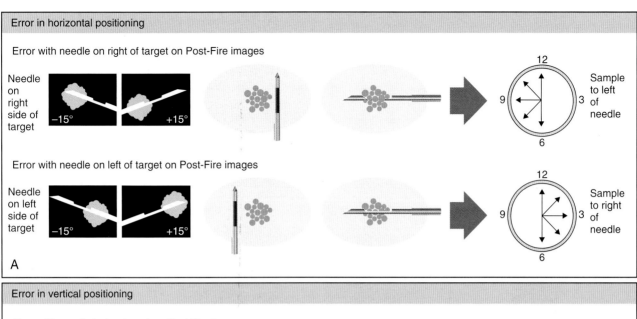

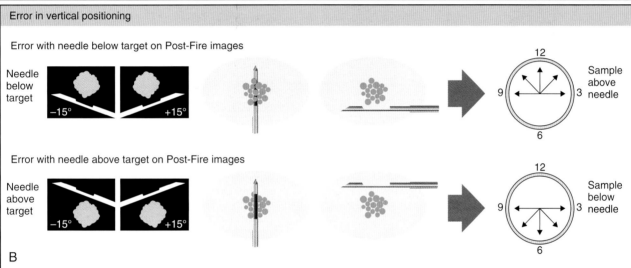

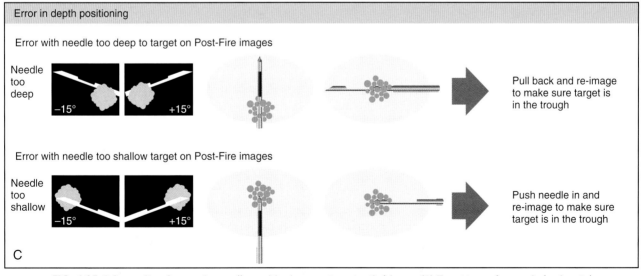

FIG. 6.15 Schematics of errors in needle positioning on stereotactic biopsy. (A) Two types of errors in horizontal positioning, one with needle to the right of target, one to the left of target. (B) Two types of errors in vertical positioning, one with needle below target, one with needle above target. (C) Two types of errors in depth positioning, one with needle too deep to the target, one with needle too shallow to the target. In each situation, the correction in biopsy needle sampling or placement is different to biopsy the target.

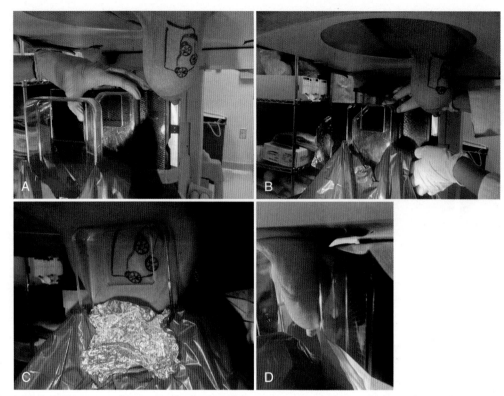

FIG. 6.16 Use of a reversed compression back paddle to increase the breast thickness in thin breasts. (A) The technologist tapes a back paddle with an aperture directly on the stereotactic image detector so that the aperture matches the stereotactic biopsy aperture. Picture illustrates the technologist placing the back paddle on the detector so that the open apertures align. The breast hangs dependently to the side with three skin markers showing the location of calcifications and black skin ink markings showing where the compression paddle aperture should be placed. (B) After sterilizing the breast skin, both front and back, the technologist will place the breast in the compression paddle so that the open apertures will align, as shown. (C) Breast in compression, repositioned after resterilization with skin BBs showing location of faint calcifications and aluminum foil to help with exposure. (D) Seen from the side, the compressed breast tissue extends both forward and backward from the apertures, increasing the breast thickness (Jackman and Marzoni, 2003).

an inaccurate location, a second marker can be placed immediately in the biopsy site or in the mass. These US-visible markers are becoming increasingly important in breast imaging because facilities may use US to localize these US-visible plugs for subsequent needle localization or in the operating room by surgeons. Thus more and more facilities are placing US-visible markers after biopsy of any type of guidance (stereotactic, US, MRI, and palpation biopsy before neoadjuvant chemotherapy) because of the possibility of using US to guide surgery subsequently. Common marker problems are initial inaccurate marker placement or later marker movement, particularly with stereotactic biopsies. Both inaccurate initial placement and delayed migration usually occur along the Z-axis or axis of the needle insertion. Delayed marker movement is uncommon and describes marker migration from its initial placement to a different site in the breast, and can occur with either accurate or inaccurate initial marker placement.

Delayed marker movement and inaccurate marker placement affect preoperative localization planning. Because there is no way to predict delayed marker migration, it is advised that radiologists review the CC and ML mammogram views immediately before x-ray–guided needle localization of findings marked by markers. If the marker was initially inaccurately deployed or moved away from an original biopsy site, the radiologist determines the original targeted lesion's location by using breast architecture and landmarks. The goal of localization is to target the biopsy site, including any residual

cancer, and not just the marker. Using the mammogram, the radiologist then determines whether the marker has moved and whether the marker or the original site, or both, need to be localized for surgery.

Whether it is necessary to also localize and remove an inaccurately positioned marker is controversial, but it could be considered if the needle biopsy revealed cancer. If the needle biopsy revealed a high-risk lesion or a discordant benign lesion, the inaccurately positioned marker presumably does not need to be removed.

MRI is increasingly being used to stage the breast for cancer and to plan patient management. Biopsy site markers placed by stereotaxis, US, or MRI may be imaged by subsequent MRI studies. Thus marker MRI compatibility, safety, and MRI marker signal void artifact is becoming increasingly important. Accordingly, all facilities should use MRI-compatible metallic markers when markers are placed with any modality because MRI might be performed later. Metallic markers cause a signal void on MRI, and the size of the signal void varies according to the marker type and pulse sequence (Fig. 6.18). There is a difference between MRI marker compatibility and safety. MRI *compatibility* means that the marker can be used in the MRI magnet and will cause little artifact. *Marker safety* means that the marker will produce no harm to the patient in the magnet. Some markers are MRI compatible but still cause large artifacts of up to 2 cm, rendering the MRI less readable than when using other markers. MRI testing of markers for artifact by using phantoms on the facility's pulse sequences is a simple way

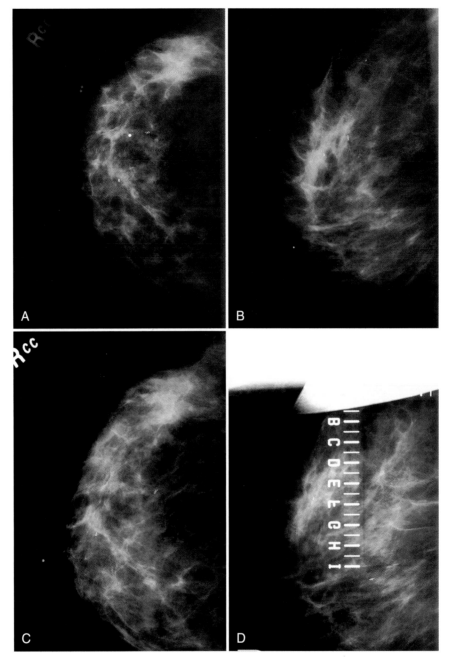

FIG. 6.17 Value of two different types of markers for two stereotactic biopsy sites and marker migration. Because this patient had two suspicious microcalcification clusters, two different markers were placed at stereotactic biopsy. (A and B) Craniocaudal (CC; A) and mediolateral (B) mammograms show the difference in marker configuration, which clearly identifies the biopsy site. If the same type of marker had been placed in both sites, it would be difficult to determine the location of each biopsy site on subsequent mammograms. Cancer was found in the upper biopsy site, and the lower biopsy site was benign. (C and D) Two months later, preoperative CC (C) and lateral (D) views show that the upper marker has migrated to the inferior portion of the breast. Because cancer was taken from the upper biopsy site, breast architecture was used to target the original upper biopsy site for excision because the marker is now in a different quadrant. This case shows the importance of correlation of the prestereotactic biopsy scout mammogram; the immediate postmarker placement mammogram, which documents orientation of the marker to the biopsy site; and scout mammograms before preoperative needle localization.

to determine the marker artifact and the size of the signal void. This should be done before inserting metallic markers for marking tumors or biopsy sites. However, correlation between MRI, US, and mammography can be challenging when markers or even wires are placed for preoperative localization.

Carbon Marking and Tattoo Ink Marking

This method uses activated charcoal USP (Mallinckrodt, Phillipsburg, New Jersey) sterilized and suspended as a 4% weight/weight aqueous suspension to mark breast lesions for excisional biopsy. It is mixed with 0.3-mL sterile saline or water and injected in a to-and-fro motion after core biopsy along the stereotactic or US needle track to yield a dark line of carbon particles in the breast. This line

---

> ### BOX 6.3   Possible Post Needle Biopsy Marker Problems
>
> Nondeployment (rare and recognized on stereo views while the breast is still in compression, occasionally during ultrasound-guided marker placement during real-time scanning)
> Inaccurate initial deployment (common, recognized on postbiopsy views on the biopsy day)
> Delayed migration from initial deployment site (rare, recognized on views taken days to months after biopsy)

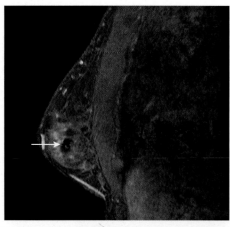

FIG. 6.18 Signal void on breast magnetic resonance imaging (MRI) caused by metallic markers placed from stereotactic core biopsy. Postcontrast 3D spectral-spatial excitation magnetization transfer breast MRI shows a signal void from a metal marker as a dark area (*arrow*) in a patient after stereotactic core biopsy.

of carbon particles can be used as a guide for excisional biopsy days to weeks after the percutaneous biopsy. It is used as an alternative to a postbiopsy metallic marker for intraparenchymal breast lesions, mainly in Europe, and also reported in Korea (Ko K et al., 2007).

Tattoo ink marking of axillary intramammary lymph nodes is an imaging-guided method to mark positive biopsied lymph nodes for subsequent surgical excision during axillary node dissection (Choy et al., 2015). This method marks a positive node to ensure its removal with sentinel lymph nodes so it will not be missed at surgery. With this method, the node to be marked is injected with 0.2 mL to 0.5 mL of sterile ink in the cortex and in the immediate breast parenchyma adjacent to the node on the axillary side where the surgeon will make the incision (Fig. 6.19). This is so the surgeon may see the stained breast tissue and lymph node tattoo at the time of axillary dissection and remove it. The surgeon will also remove any palpable, radioactive, or blue sentinel lymph nodes at this time.

There is a hypothetical problem with tattoo ink from extensive tattoos on the arm migrating to and staining the ipsilateral axillary lymph nodes, which could interfere with this technique. Datrice et al. (2013) reported a case in which a high-risk woman undergoing prophylactic mastectomy had extensive arm tattoos whose ink migrated to nonsentinel lymph nodes, stained the lymph nodes dark, and were identified at surgery. Matsika (2013) reported tattoo ink deposition in an axillary lymph node that calcified, simulating breast cancer. This phenomenon should be recognized if the patient has extensive arm and neck skin tattoos to avoid false-positive node identification.

Patient Safety and Comfort after Biopsy

After needle biopsy, hemostasis is achieved by direct pressure. In some institutions, after hemostasis is confirmed, the patient is taught how to hold pressure on the biopsy site so that she knows what to do if the wound starts to bleed. After adequate hemostasis is achieved, some institutions close the wound with Steri-Strips and cover the Steri-Strips with Opsite, a self-adhesive polyurethane film sterile material used to cover operative wounds. Opsite prevents the Steri-Strips from getting wet and keeps the wound clean and dry. The patient can take a shower with the Opsite on but is instructed not to scrub the Opsite, take a bath, swim, or engage in other activities that might immerse the wound and get it wet and cause infection. The patient is told to expect a quarter-sized spot of blood on the Steri-Strips and that it will feel bigger because of a blood clot in the biopsy site, and to expect a bruise at the biopsy site that may travel to dependent sites. The patient is told to put direct pressure on the biopsy site if oozing or unexpected bleeding occurs and to remove the Opsite and Steri-Strips after 4 to 7 days. Some facilities also bind the breast with wraparound bandages or commercially available binders (commonly used after mastectomy) to hold the breasts tight to the chest wall. These

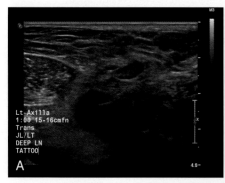
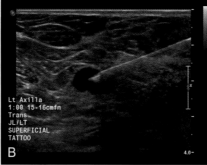
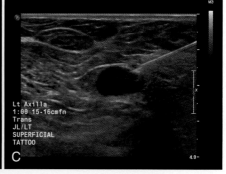

FIG. 6.19 Fine-needle aspiration (FNA) of abnormal lymph node and tattoo marking. A 51-year-old woman with invasive ductal cancer and metastatic lymphadenopathy. (A) Ultrasound shows FNA of an abnormal left lymph node, which showed metastatic breast cancer. (B) Tattoo dye placed in the superficial cortex of the lymph node. (C) Tattoo dye place at the surface of abnormal lymph node.

bandages restrict breast motion while the patient is awake and limit breast motion during the night.

After the biopsy, the technologist places gauze on the skin and an ice pack on the biopsy site, which the patient is told to leave on for 60 minutes initially and then to ice for 10 minutes every hour until bedtime as needed. She is advised *not* to keep it on longer because of the possibility of frostbite. The ice helps decrease postbiopsy discomfort and bleeding. To keep the ice pack in place, the patient may put the ice pack inside a brassiere or use a commercially available breast binder. Each time the 10-minute ice pack is removed, the patient is asked to look at the bandage (which may require using a mirror). If the amount of blood has increased since the last inspection, the patient is told to again firmly compress the biopsy site for 10 more minutes. Afterward, patients are given verbal and written postbiopsy wound care instructions and a phone number to call for problems. Patients are instructed on where and how to obtain their biopsy result. Most patients do well with these instructions. The biopsy personnel call the patient later in the afternoon, early evening, or the next day as a courtesy call to see how the patient is doing and to answer any questions.

Pain control is part of recovery. If the patient is not allergic to acetaminophen and has no liver problems, acetaminophen may be taken initially and then every 6 hours as needed, up to 4 g/day. Stronger medication such as Tylenol No. 3 (acetaminophen with codeine) or Vicodin (acetaminophen with hydrocodone) also may be prescribed for pain. Aspirin or nonsteroidal antiinflammatory drugs (NSAIDs) are withheld for 7 days before biopsy and avoided for 3 days after biopsy to decrease the risk of bleeding.

Complete Lesion Removal

Core biopsy samples showing cancer routinely undergo subsequent excisional biopsy to remove residual cancer at the biopsy location. Even if the entire radiographic finding has been removed by percutaneous biopsy, occult residual cancer has been demonstrated in the needle biopsy site in 73% (15/23) of cases at subsequent surgery.

How is the core biopsy site localized when the entire lesion has been removed and no marker was placed in the biopsy site, or if a marker was placed but is not at the biopsy site (either from inaccurate initial placement or delayed migration)? Because air can move along the biopsy track, air alone is not enough to identify the biopsy site. Although a hematoma may sometimes be mammographically seen in the immediate postbiopsy period, it usually persists for just a few days or weeks. Studies have shown no mammographically detectable findings some months after a stereotactic core or vacuum needle biopsy.

Brenner (2000) suggests using landmarks within the breast to localize the approximate stereotactic biopsy site. Others have suggested localizing the fluid collection in the biopsy site by US. Although this may work in the immediate postbiopsy period, fluid can be reabsorbed if the excisional biopsy is delayed by several weeks, and using the fluid alone may not be reliable. The best option is to use landmarks within the breast to find the approximate biopsy site, using any imaging guidance.

Calcification and Epithelial Displacement

Percutaneous biopsy needles rarely displace calcifications to locations distant from the original biopsy site. It is controversial whether displaced metallic markers or displaced calcifications far from the biopsy site require surgical excision when the percutaneous biopsy specimen shows cancer.

Epithelial displacement of breast cancer cells into benign tissue along the needle track may occur with any gauge biopsy needle. These displaced tumor cells may simulate breast cancer

invasion or a second focus of tumor unless the pathologist knows there was a prior core biopsy. Pathologists should be informed that a needle biopsy has been performed so that they do not mistakenly diagnose displaced epithelium as invasive cancer in a ductal carcinoma in situ (DCIS) lesion or erroneously stage a tumor as multifocal when only one cancerous site is present. Epithelial displacement is more common with FNA or core biopsy (where the needle is removed from the breast with each needle pass) than with vacuum biopsy (where the external part of the needle stays in the breast until the rotational biopsy is finished). A 2009 systematic review by Liebens et al. of nine studies assessing the rate of epithelial cell displacement after core needle biopsy and six studies on the impact on outcome endpoints concluded "although data are limited, [there is] no increased morbidity associated with iatrogenic seeding after core needle biopsy."

Imaging/Pathology Correlation, Invasive Cancer, and Ductal Carcinoma in Situ on Core Biopsy

Imaging/pathology correlation of image-guided biopsies is a critical part of the breast imaging service to avoid falsely negative biopsy results and a delayed diagnosis of cancer. Imaging-pathology discordance is defined as suspicious imaging findings (Breast Imaging Reporting and Data System [BI-RADS] 4 or 5) that are not explained by the pathology or as imaging findings that were not adequately sampled. Liberman et al. (2000a) reported that an imaging/pathology discordance at percutaneous biopsy had a malignancy rate of 24.4%, indicating a need for excisional biopsy. A *false-negative biopsy* is a biopsy that, at the outset, is benign but later shows cancer at the same site. Immediate imaging/pathology correlation helps identify false-negative biopsies when the radiologist recognizes discordant findings, immediately recalls and rebiopsies the patient, and diagnoses the cancer. Other false-negative biopsies occur when the biopsy is mistakenly declared concordant and the cancer grows and is diagnosed at a later date. Both core needle automated multifire and vacuum-assisted core needle biopsy have had false-negative rates reported as low as 0.45% for 11-gauge stereotactic vacuum-assisted core biopsy, and 4.4% for 14-gauge stereotactic automated core biopsy by Jackman et al. (2009). Even if vacuum-assisted core needle biopsies have very high accuracy, there is still potential for false-negative samples. In most of the studies, false-negative rates in the vacuum-assisted needle biopsy were closer to 2% or lower (Lieberman et al., 2000a; Ames and Britton, 2011; Kettritz et al., 2004; Jackman et al., 2009). However, a large series by Poole et al. (2014) that evaluated 8081 core biopsies showed 4 (6.3%) of 63 discordant initially benign lesions biopsied by vacuum-assisted biopsy were proved to be malignant, compared with 2 of 17 (11.8%) originally biopsied by core needle biopsy. This means that discordant biopsies occur even with larger samples obtained by vacuum-assisted core biopsy needles, requiring excisional biopsy or rebiopsy.

All biopsies in which the target has been missed are considered discordant, because the target has not been sampled. One can determine whether the target has not been sampled if the target is either (1) not in the specimen or (2) still in the breast on subsequent imaging. Another example of discordance is if not enough of the target has been included in the sample (for example, if too few calcifications within a calcification group have been included in the biopsy sample to be considered representative of the finding). In the latter instance, too few calcifications in the sample would lead one to be unsure if pathology was truly representative of the entire calcification group, leading to a discordant result.

Concordant imaging/pathology result examples include simple cysts (which resolve completely with benign cyst fluid in the syringe), circumscribed oval masses that are fibroadenomas, spiculated masses that are postbiopsy scars in the right clinical setting, and lymph nodes that have a typical appearance. Concordant or discordant pathology correlations are harder to

TABLE 6.2 Ductal Carcinoma in Situ at Biopsy; Underestimate Ratio of Invasive Cancer

Author	Year	Number	Guidance	Needle Type	Gold Standard	Invasive Cancer (%)	Histology of Invasive Cancer
Burak W. et al.	2000	89 les	Stereo	11-gauge VAB	Surgery	11.2% (10/89)	10 IDC
Jackman et al.	2001	1326 les	Stereo	11- and 14-gauge VAB, 14-gauge CNB	Surgery	13.8% (183/1326); 20.4% (76/373) for CNB; 11.2% (107/953) for VAB	183 IC
Goyal et al.[a]	2006	587 pts	US, Stereo	11- and 14-gauge	Surgery	37.5% (220/587)	220 IC
O'Flynn et al.[a]	2009	402 pts	Stereo	11-gauge VAB, 14-gauge CNB	Surgery	29.4% (118/402)	118 DCIS with IC
Kurniawan et al.[a]	2010	375 pts	US	14-gauge CNB	Surgery	17.3% (65/373)	65 IC
Houssami et al.[a]	2011	442 pts	Stereo	11-gauge VAB	Surgery	17.4% (77/442)	77 IC
Diepstraten et al.[a]	2013	348 pts	Stereo	14-gauge CNB	Surgery	28.7% (100/348)	100 IDC
Ohsumi et al.	2014	103 les	Upright stereo	11- and 14-gauge VAB	Surgery	26.2% (27/103)	14 IC, 13 MIC
Sim et al.[a]	2015	1252 pts	US, Stereo	14-gauge CNB, large-volume VAB	Surgery	23.6% (296/1252)	296 IC

[a]Indicates studies that performed a patient-based analysis; otherwise, a lesion-based analysis was used.
CNB, core needle biopsy; *DCIS,* ductal carcinoma in situ; *IC,* invasive cancer; *IDC,* invasive ductal carcinoma; *les,* lesions; *MIC,* microinvasive cancer; *pts,* patients; *US,* ultrasound; *VAB,* vacuum-assisted biopsy.

determine with other mass lesions, nonmass lesions, and focal or global asymmetries, which may have a more nonspecific pathology. In these cases, one must rely on the accuracy and the volume of the needle biopsy and the pathology result. Correlating these items with the clinical history and medical knowledge are the only way to determine whether there is concordance.

Women with core biopsies showing invasive cancer undergo surgical excision of the biopsy site, usually with axillary lymph node sampling, unless they have neoadjuvant chemotherapy first. The needle biopsy site is excised even if the entire imaging finding was removed because there may still be cancer in and around the biopsy site seen only by pathology. This means that the relative location of a postbiopsy metallic marker should be clearly stated in relationship to the cancer biopsy site (in the biopsy site or displaced) and documented on postbiopsy mammograms for surgical planning.

Women with core biopsies showing noninvasive DCIS undergo surgical excision of the biopsy site, even if all the calcifications are removed, because residual DCIS or even invasive breast cancer may be found at surgical excision. The DCIS core biopsies later showing invasive cancer at surgical excision are called *DCIS underestimates.* Table 6.2 shows publications of core and vacuum-assisted needle biopsies with US or stereotactic guidance showing DCIS initially and later showing invasive cancer at surgical excision. This shows that DCIS underestimates a range from 11.2% to 37.5%, with an average of 22.8% for DCIS underestimates in this literature series. A meta-analysis of 52 studies (Brennan et al., 2011) showed that there were 1736 underestimates (invasive cancer at excision) in 7350 cases with core biopsy-proven DCIS; the random-effects pooled estimate was 25.9% (95% confidence interval: 22.5%, 29.5%). Because women with DCIS usually do not undergo axillary node biopsy, this means about one-fifth of women with core needle biopsies showing DCIS may have invasive cancer at surgery and later need a second surgery for an axillary lymph node sampling.

High-Risk Lesions, Including Controversies

High-risk lesions account for between 3% and 9% of all breast core needle biopsies, and there is controversy regarding whether these lesions require subsequent surgical excisional biopsy

TABLE 6.3 High-Risk Lesions Diagnosed at Needle Biopsy and Need for Surgical Excision

Agreement	Histology
Almost universal agreement about need to excise	Atypical ductal hyperplasia Phyllodes tumor
Majority agreement about need to excise[a]	Lobular carcinoma in situ Atypical lobular hyperplasia Papillary lesion with atypia Radial scar with atypia Flat epithelial atypia Other lesions with atypia
Consider excision[a]	Papillary lesion without atypia Radial scar without atypia Mucin-producing lesions Pseudoangiomatous stromal hyperplasia with features of angiosarcoma

[a]National Comprehensive Cancer Network Guidelines Version 1, 2014, Breast Cancer Screening and Diagnosis states "Select patients may be suitable for monitoring in lieu of surgical excision" (e.g., ALH, LCIS, papillomas, fibroepithelial lesions, radial scars). Other histologies that may require additional tissue: mucin-producing lesions, potential phyllodes tumor, papillary lesions, radial scar or histologies of concern to pathologist."

(Table 6.3). These pathologies include atypical ductal hyperplasia (ADH), lobular proliferative lesions of lobular carcinoma in situ (LCIS), atypical lobular hyperplasia (ALH), flat epithelial atypia (FEA), radial sclerosing lesions or radial scars, papillary lesions including papillomas, papillomas with atypia, papillomas with mixed histology, and "mucocele-like lesions."

In the United States a follow-up recommendation for mammography is 2% or less for BI-RADS category 3 lesions, and biopsy is recommended for a suspicious finding for BI-RADS category 4 lesions with a >2% to <95% suspicion for cancer. This section discusses patient management after core needle biopsy shows a high-risk lesion and the controversies surrounding patient management.

ADH is a proliferative ductal lesion of the breast that usually presents with microcalcifications on mammography and has an associated four- to five-fold increased risk of malignancy (Dupont

TABLE 6.4   Atypical Ductal Hyperplasia at Biopsy; Underestimation Ratio of Malignancy

Author	Year	Number	Guidance	Needle Type	Gold Standard	Malignancy (%)	Histology of Malignancy
Burak et al.	2000	40 les	Stereo	11-gauge VAB	Surgery	12.5% (5/40)	1 DCIS, 4 IC
Jackman et al.	2002	104 les	Stereo	11-gauge VAB	Surgery	21.2% (22/104)	3 IDC (including two associated with DCIS), 19 DCIS
Winchester et al.	2003	65 les	Stereo	11-gauge VAB	Surgery	16.9% (11/65)	2 ILC, 3 IDC, 6 DCIS
Sohn et al.	2007	78 les	Stereo	11-gauge VAB	Surgery	18.0% (14/78)	5 IDC, 9 DCIS
Chae et al.	2009	45 les	US	14-gauge CNB, 11-gauge VAB	Surgery	22.2% (10/45)	8 DCIS, 2 IC
Chivukula et al.	2009	45 les	US, Stereo, MRI	12- and 14-gauge CNB, 14-gauge VAB for US Stereo, 9-gauge VAB for MRI	Surgery	11.1% (5/45)	5 DCIS
Graesslin et al.	2010	26 les	Stereo	8-, 10-, and 11-gauge VAB	Surgery	19.2% (5/26)	4 DCIS, 1 IDC
Deshaies et al.	2011	422 les	US, Stereo	14-gauge CNB, 11-gauge VAB	Surgery	31.3% (132/422)	96 DCIS, 36 IC
Londero et al.	2011	15 les	US, Stereo	14-gauge CNB for US, 11-gauge VAB for Stereo	Surgery or f/u (>1 year)	26.7% (4/15)	1 IDC, 3 DCIS
Polat et al.	2012	330 les	US, Stereo, MRI	12–18 gauge for US, 9–11 gauge for Stereo or MRI	Surgery	11.5% (38/330)	38 DCIS or IC
Gruber et al.	2013	13 les	US, Stereo	11-gauge VAB, 14-gauge CNB/VAB	Surgery or f/u (≥1 year)	15.4% (2/13)	2 DCIS
McLaughlin et al.	2014	101 les	Stereo	8- and 11-gauge VAB	Surgery	12.9% (13/101)	11 DCIS, 2 IC
Youn et al.[a]	2014	27 pts	Stereo	8- and 11-gauge VAB	Surgery	33.3% (9/27)	9 DCIS

[a]Indicates studies that performed a patient-based analysis; otherwise, a lesion-based analysis was used.

ADH, atypical ductal hyperplasia; *CNB*, core needle biopsy; *DCIS*, ductal carcinoma in situ; *f/u*, follow-up; *IC*, invasive cancer; *IDC*, invasive ductal carcinoma; *les*, lesions; *MRI*, magnetic resonance imaging; *pts*, patients; *US*, ultrasound; *VAB*, vacuum-assisted biopsy.

and Page, 1985). ADH has an upgrade rate to DCIS or invasive cancer of at least 11.1% to 33.3% in a recent series (Table 6.4) and up to 56% in an older series (Jackman et al., 1994). Some postulate that ADH is a nonobligate precursor to DCIS (Sinn et al., 2010). Further, pathologists show interobserver and intraobserver variability and reproducibility in distinguishing between ADH and low-grade DCIS (Schnitt et al., 1992; Jain et al., 2011) rendering ADH underestimates an even more significant problem. For these reasons, and supported by the 2015 NCCN guidelines, needle core biopsies showing ADH should undergo subsequent surgical excision, even if all the calcifications are removed. In 2014 Youn et al. showed an upgrade rate to DCIS of 33% (9/33) of women undergoing vacuum-assisted needle biopsy, with 30% upgraded to DCIS when all the calcifications were removed.

Flat epithelial atypia is an emerging pathologic entity that has uncertain clinicopathologic implications; it is part of a series of columnar cell lesions but has no architectural atypia, unlike ADH and DCIS (Schnitt and Vincent-Salomon, 2003). However, in its presence, pathologists search carefully for ADH or low-grade DCIS (Chivukula et al., 2009). It is suggested that FEA, because of its association with lobular neoplasia, low-grade DCIS, and tubular carcinoma, may be a DCIS precursor (Chivukula et al., 2009; Abdel-Fatah et al., 2007; Leibl et al., 2007; Kunju et al., 2008). Table 6.5 shows the FEA underestimates, ranging from 3.5% to 14.3% upgrades for pure FEA. Consideration for surgical excisional biopsy should be done based on these numbers. On the other hand, columnar lesions without atypia, including columnar alterations with prominent apical snouts and secretions, are usually considered benign and do not need excision.

LCIS and ALH on core needle biopsy are high-risk lesions. The LCIS was previously thought to be an incidental finding discovered on biopsies done for other findings (Beute et al.,

1991), but LCIS and ALH are now been shown to be associated with calcifications in 8% to 53% in one series (Hussain and Cunnick, 2011) and in 40.9% (61/149) of cases in another (Bianchi et al., 2013). Table 6.6 shows the incidence of lobular neoplasia underestimates. Although controversial, the upgrade rate to malignancy is over 2%, indicating that surgery is indicated if lobular neoplasia is found on core needle biopsy.

Radial scars are proliferative breast lesions with a fibroelastic core with radiating duct lobules extending outward from the core (Kennedy, 2003) that give it a spiculated appearance mimicking invasive breast cancer on mammography (Adler, 1990). Radial scars associated with atypia need excision because cancer is often found at surgical excision. Brenner et al. (2002), Resetkova et al. (2011), and Becker et al. (2006) suggested that radial scars without atypia do not need excision if the biopsy was done with a vacuum-assisted device with removal of at least 12 specimens. Linda et al. (2010), however, showed that the malignancy underestimation rate was 8% (5/62) for biopsies of radial scars without atypia using vacuum-assisted probes in a later study, contradicting the prior investigators. The underestimation rate of radial scars is shown in Table 6.7. Because mammographic and sonographic features do not predict which radial scars will have malignancy at excision, surgery should be considered in patients with radial scar.

Papillary lesions cover a wide range of lesions from benign papillomas to papillomas with atypia or carcinoma in situ to papillary carcinoma, all of which may be very hard to distinguish from one another on core needle biopsy (Tavassoli, 1992; Renshaw et al., 2004). Tables 6.8–6.10 show the underestimation rates for papillary lesions with and without atypia on core needle biopsy using multiple needle types and imaging guidance systems. In each table, malignancy upgrades are seen, particularly with papillomas containing atypia, with Youk et al. (2010) showing a higher

TABLE 6.5 FEA at Biopsy; Underestimation Ratio of Malignancy

Author	Year	Diagnosis at Biopsy	Number	Guidance	Needle Type	Gold Standard	Malignancy (%)	Histology of Malignancy	High Grade (%)	Histology of High Grade
Chivukula et al.	2009	Pure FEA	35 les	US, Stereo, MRI	12- and 14-gauge CNB, 14-gauge VAB for US and Stereo, 9-gauge VAB for MRI	Surgery	14.2% (5/35)	2 IC, 3 DCIS		
Bianchi et al.	2011	FEA	245 les	Stereo	11-gauge VAB	Surgery	12.7% (31/245)	NA		
Lavoue et al.	2011	Pure FEA	60 les	Stereo, US	8, 10, 11, and 14-gauge CNB, VAB	Surgery	13.3% (8/60)	2 IC, 6 DCIS		
Solorzano et al.	2011	Pure FEA	28 les	Stereo, US	9- and 11-gauge VAB for Stereo, 14-gauge CNB for US	Surgery	14.3% (4/28)	4 DCIS	32.1% (9/28)	6 ADH, 3 LCIS
Becker et al.	2013	Pure FEA	239 les	Stereo	8–12 and 14-gauge CNB, VAB	Surgery or f/u	4.2% (10/239)	8 DCIS, 2 IC		
Khoumais et al.[a]	2013	Pure FEA	104 pts	Stereo, US	10-gauge VAB, 14-gauge CNB	Surgery or f/u	9.6% (10/104)	5 IC, 5 DCIS		
Villa et al.[a]	2013	Pure FEA	57 pts	Stereo	9-gauge VAB	Surgery	3.5% (2/57)	2 DCIS or IC		
Villa et al.[a]	2013	Pure FEA	64 pts	Stereo	11-gauge VAB	Surgery	7.8% (5/64)	5 DCIS or IC		
Calhoun et al.	2014	Pure FEA	73 les	Stereo, US, MRI	NA	Surgery	6.8% (5/73)	2 IC, 3 DCIS	23.3% (17/73)	14 ADH, 3 ALH

[a]Indicates studies that performed a patient-based analysis; otherwise, a lesion-based analysis was used.

ADH, atypical ductal hyperplasia; *ALH,* atypical lobular hyperplasia; *CNB,* core needle biopsy; *DCIS,* ductal carcinoma in situ; *FEA,* flat epithelial atypia; *f/u,* follow-up; *IC,* invasive carcinoma; *LCIS,* lobular carcinoma in situ; *les,* lesions; *MRI,* magnetic resonance imaging; *pts,* patients; *US,* ultrasound; *VAB,* vacuum-assisted biopsy;

TABLE 6.6 Lobular Carcinoma In Situ/Carcinoma In Situ/Atypical Lobular Hyperplasia at Biopsy; Underestimation Ratio of Malignancy

Author	Year	Diagnosis at Biopsy	Number	Guidance	Needle Type	Gold Standard	Malignancy (%)	Histology of Malignancy
Burak et al.	2000	ALH	6 les	Stereo	11-gauge VAB	Surgery	16.7% (1/6)	1 DCIS
Renshaw et al.[a]	2006	LCIS/ALH	92 pts	US, Stereo	11- and 14-gauge CNB	Surgery	7.6% (7/92)	6 IC, 1 DCIS
Karabakhtsian et al.	2007	LCIS/ALH	92 les (63 ALH, 10 ALH/LCIS, 19 LCIS)	US, Stereo	11-gauge VAB, 14-gauge CNB	Surgery	10.9% (10/92); 7.9% (5/63) for ALH; 10.0% (1/10) for ALH/LCIS; 21.1% (4/19) for LCIS	5 DCIS, 3 ILC, 1 TC, 1 ILC and TC
Brem et al.	2008	LCIS/ALH	164 les (67 LCIS, 97 ALH)	US, Stereo	8-, 11-, and 14-gauge VAB, 12- and 14-gauge CNB	Surgery	23.2% (38/164); 25.4 % (17/67) for LCIS, 22.3% (21/94) for ALH	For initial LCIS: 7 DCIS, 6 ILC, 2 IDC, 2 IC; for initial ALH, 15 DCIS, 3 ILC, 3 IDC
Londero et al.	2008	LCIS/ALH	35 les (14 ALH, 21 LCIS)	US, Stereo	14-gauge CNB for US, 11-gauge VAB for Stereo	Surgery and f/u	37.1% (13/35); 7.1% (1/14) for ALH; 57.1% (12/21) for LCIS	6 DCIS, 7 IC
Mulheron et al.[a]	2009	LCIS/ALH	25 pts	US, Stereo	9- and 11-gauge VAB	Surgery and f/u	20.0% (5/25)	3 IDC, 1 ILC, 1 DCIS
Subhawong et al.[a]	2010	ALH	56 pts	US, Stereo	11- and 14-gauge VAB for Stereo, 14-gauge CNB for US	Surgery	0% (0/56)	
Bianchi et al.	2011	LCIS/ALH	377 les	Stereo	11-gauge VAB	Surgery	22.0% (83/377)	
Destounis et al.	2011	LCIS	63 les	Stereo, US, MRI	9, 11, 12, and 14-gauge VAB, 14-gauge CNB	Surgery	33.3% (21/63)	2 IDC, 4 ILC, 15 DCIS
Londero et al.	2011	LCIS/ALH	46 les	US, Stereo	14-gauge CNB, 11-gauge VAB	Surgery	30.4% (14/46)	7 DCIS, 6 ILC, 1 ITLC
Rendi et al.[a]	2012	LCIS/ALH	76 pts (53 ALH, 23 LCIS)	Stereo, US, MRI	9- and 11-gauge VAB, 14-gauge CNB	Surgery	4.4% (3/76); 4.1% (2/52) for ALH; 4.3% (1/23) for LCIS	NA
Shah-Khan et al.	2012	LCIS/ALH	101 les (81 ALH, 20 LCIS)	Stereo, US, MRI	9, 11, 14, 16, and 18-gauge CNB	Surgery	2.0% (2/101); 1.2% (1/81) for ALH, 5.0% (1/20) for LCIS	1 DCIS, 1 IDC
Murray et al.	2013	LCIS/ALH	80 les	Stereo, US, MRI	14-gauge CNB for US, 11-gauge VAB for Stereo, 9-gauge VAB for MRI	Surgery	6.3% (5/80)	2 IDC, 3 DCIS
Meroni et al.[a]	2014	LCIS/ALH/PLICS	76 pts	Stereo, US	11-gauge CNB, 8-gauge VAB	Surgery within 2 years	17.1% (13/76)	7 ILC, 2 IDC, 4 DCIS

[a]Indicates studies that performed a patient-based analysis; otherwise, a lesion-based analysis was used.

ALH, atypical lobular hyperplasia; *CNB,* core needle biopsy; *DCIS,* ductal carcinoma in situ; *f/u,* follow-up; *IC,* invasive cancer; *IDC,* invasive ductal carcinoma; *ILC,* invasive lobular carcinoma; *ITLC,* invasive tubulolobular carcinoma; *LCIS,* lobular carcinoma in situ; *les,* lesions; *MRI,* magnetic resonance imaging; *PLICS,* pleomorphic lobular carcinoma in situ; *pts,* patients; *TC,* tubular cancer; *US,* ultrasound; *VAB,* vacuum-assisted biopsy.

TABLE 6.7 Radial Scar at Biopsy: Underestimation Ratio of Malignancy

Author	Year	Number	Guidance	Needle Type	Gold Standard	Malignancy (%)	Histology of Malignancy	Atypia (%)	Histology of Atypia
Linda et al.	2010	62 les	US, Stereo	14-gauge CNB for US, 11-gauge VAB for Stereo	Surgery	8.1% (5/62)	3 DCIS, 1 ILC, 1 IDC;		
Bianchi et al.	2011	132 les	Stereo	11-gauge VAB	Surgery	10.6% (14/132)	NA		
Londero et al.	2011	88 les	US, Stereo	14-gauge CNB for US, 11-gauge VAB for Stereo	Surgery or f/u (≥1 year)	6.3% (5/80)	1 IDC, 1 ILC, 3 DCIS	13.6% (12/88)	12 high-risk lesions with atypia
Lee et al.[a]	2012	18 pts	Stereo, US, MRI	9-gauge VAB for Stereo; 12- and 14-gauge VAB, 14-gauge CNB for US; 9-gauge VAB for MRI	Surgery	0% (0/18 pts)		38.9% (7/18)	6 ADH, 1 atypical apocrine adenosis
Matrai et al.	2015	77 les	Stereo, MRI	7-11-gauge VAB; 14, 16, 18, and 22-gauge CNB	Surgery	0% (0/77)		11.7% (9/77)	6 LCIS, 2 ADH, 1 ALH
Nassar et al.	2015	38 les	Stereo, US, MRI	9, 11, 14, and 16-gauge	Surgery	10.5% (4/38)	2 IC, 2 DCIS	18.4% (7/38)	5 ALH, 1 LCIS, 1 ADH

[a]Indicates studies that performed a patient-based analysis; otherwise, a lesion based analysis was used.
ADH, atypical ductal hyperplasia; *ALH*, atypical lobular hyperplasia; *CNB*, core needle biopsy; *DCIS*, ductal carcinoma in situ; *f/u*, follow-up; *IC*, invasive carcinoma; *IDC*, invasive ductal carcinoma; *ILC*, invasive lobular carcinoma; *LCIS*, lobular carcinoma in situ; *les*, lesions; *MRI*, magnetic resonance imaging; *pts*, patients; *US*, ultrasound; *VAB*, vacuum-assisted biopsy.

TABLE 6.8 Atypical Papilloma or Atypical Papillary Lesion at Biopsy; Underestimation Ratio of Malignancy

Author	Year	Diagnosis at Biopsy	Number	Guidance	Needle Type	Gold Standard	Malignancy (%)	Histology of Malignancy	Atypia (%)	Histology of Atypia
Sydnor et al.	2007	Atypical papilloma	15 les	US, Stereo	11- and 14-gauge VAB, 14-gauge CNB	Surgery and f/u	66.7% (10/15)	NA		
Kim et al.	2008	Atypical papilloma	4 les	US	8- and 11-gauge VAB	Surgery	0% (0/4)			
Shin et al.	2008	Atypical papilloma	17 les	US, Stereo	14-gauge CNB, 8- and 11-gauge VAB	Surgery or f/u	5.9% (1/17)	Cancer (DCIS or IC)	17.6% (3/17)	High risk (ADH, LCIS/ALH)
Chang et al.	2011	Atypical papilloma	11 les	US	11-gauge VAB	Surgery	18.2% (2/11)	2 DCIS	54.5% (6/11)	6 atypical
Kim et al.	2011	Atypical papilloma	22 les	US	8- and 11-gauge VAB, 14-gauge CNB	Surgery	22.7% (5/22); 33.3% (5/15) for CNB; 0% (0/7) for VAB	5 carcinoma		
Brennan et al.	2012	Atypical papilloma	23 les	MRI	9-gauge VAB	Surgery	8.7% (2/23)	2 DCIS		
Bianchi et al.[a]	2015	Nonmalignant papillary lesions with atypia	46 pts	US	14-gauge VAB	Surgery	47.8% (22/46)	7 DCIS, 15 IC		

[a]Indicates studies that performed a patient-based analysis; otherwise, a lesion-based analysis was used.
ADH, atypical ductal hyperplasia; *ALH*, atypical lobular hyperplasia; *CNB*, core needle biopsy; *DCIS*, ductal carcinoma in situ; *f/u*, follow-up; *IC*, invasive carcinoma; *LCIS*, lobular carcinoma in situ; *les*, lesions; *MRI*, magnetic resonance imaging; *pts*, patients; *US*, ultrasound; *VAB*, vacuum-assisted biopsy.

Author	Year	Diagnosis at Biopsy	Number	Guidance	Needle Type	Gold Standard	Malignancy (%)	Histology of Malignancy	Atypia (%)	Histology of Atypia
Kim et al.	2008	Benign papillary lesion	35 les (31 benign papilloma, 3 papillomatosis, 1 sclerosing papilloma)	US	8- and 11-gauge VAB	Surgery; f/u	0% (0/35)			
Rizzo et al.[a]	2008	Pure benign intraductal papilloma	101 pts (86 single, 15 multiple)	US, Stereo	11-gauge VAB, 14-gauge CNB	Surgery	8.9% (9/101); 10.5% (9/86) for single; 0% (0/15) for multiple	9 DCIS	18.8% (19/101); 14.0% (12/86) for single; 46.7% (7/15) for multiple	19 ADH
Shin et al.	2008	Solitary benign papilloma	96 les	US	14-gauge CNB, 8- and 11-gauge VAB	Surgery; f/u	12.5% (12/96)	Cancer (DCIS or IC)	4.2% (4/96)	4 high-risk (ADH, LCIS/ALH)
Sydnor et al.	2007	Benign papilloma	38 les	US, Stereo	11- and 14-gauge VAB, 14-gauge CNB	Surgery; f/u	2.6% (1/38)	NA		
Chang et al.[a]	2011	Benign papilloma	64 pts	US	11-gauge VAB, 14-gauge CNB	Surgery	3.1% (2/64)	2 DCIS	10.9% (7/64)	7 atypical papilloma
Chang et al.[a]	2011	Benign papilloma	49 pts	US	11-gauge VAB	Surgery	0% (0/49)		6.1% (3/49)	3 atypical papilloma
Kim et al.	2011	Benign papilloma	211 les	US	8- and 11-gauge VAB 14-gauge CNB	Surgery; f/u	5.7% (12/211)	12 carcinoma	1.9% (4/211)	4 atypical papilloma
Londero et al.	2011	Benign papilloma	151 les	US, Stereo	14-gauge CNB for US, 11-gauge VAB for Stereo	Surgery	9.9% (15/151)	1 IPC, 14 DCIS		
Rozentsvayg et al.	2011	Benign papilloma	67 les	US, Stereo, MRI	11-gauge VAB for Stereo; 14-gauge CNB for US, 10-gauge VAB for MRI	Surgery	7.5% (5/67)	2 DCIS, 3 IDC	11.9% (8/67)	6 ADH, 1 ALH, 1 LCIS
Brennan et al.	2012	Papilloma without atypia	44 les	MRI	9-gauge VAB	Surgery	4.5% (2/44)	2 DCIS		
Lu et al.[a]	2012	Benign papillary lesion	66 pts	US	14-gauge CNB	Surgery	6.1% (4/66)	4 papillary DCIS	12.1% (8/66)	8 ADH
Al Hassan et al.	2013	Benign papillary lesion	103 les	US, Stereo	14- and 18-gauge CNB 10-gauge VAB for US, 9-gauge CNB, 11-gauge VAB for Stereo	Surgery; f/u	9.7% (10/103)	10 cancerous lesion	2.9% (3/103)	3 atypia
Maxwell et al.	2013	Benign papillary	96 les	US, Stereo	14-gauge CNB	VAB, surgery	7.3% (7/96)	4 DCIS, 1 IDC, 2 IDC + DCIS	4.2% (4/96)	2 ADH, 1, LISN, 1 ADH + LISN
Mosier et al.	2013	Benign papillary	86 les	US, Stereo	8- and 11-gauge VAB	f/u	0% (0/86)			
Sohn et al.	2013	Benign papillary	39 les	US	14-gauge CNB	VAB, surgery	0% (0/39)		7.7% (3/39)	Papilloma with atypia
Bianchi et al.	2015	Nonmalignant papillary lesion without atypia	68 les	US	14-gauge VAB	Surgery	13.2% (9/68)	5 DCIS, 4 IC		

[a]indicates studies that performed a patient-based analysis; otherwise, a lesion-based analysis was used.

ADH, atypical ductal hyperplasia; ALH, atypical lobular hyperplasia; CNB, core needle-biopsy; DCIS, ductal carcinoma in situ; f/u, follow-up; IC, invasive cancer; IDC, invasive ductal cancer; IPC, invasive papillary carcinoma; LCIS, lobular carcinoma in situ; les, lesions; LISN, lobular in situ neoplasia; pts, patients; US, ultrasound; VAB, vacuum-assisted biopsy.

TABLE 6.10 Papillary Lesion (Not Specified into Atypical or Benign) at Biopsy; Underestimation Ratio of Malignancy

Author	Year	Diagnosis at Biopsy	Number	Guidance	Needle Type	Gold Standard	Malignancy (%)	Histology of Malignancy	Atypia (%)	Histology of Atypia
Gendler et al.[a]	2004	Papilloma, papillary lesion, papillomatosis, atypical papillary hyperplasia	87 pts	US, Stereo	11-gauge VAB, 14-gauge CNB	Surgery	17.2% (15/87)	12 DCIS, 1 IDC, 1 infiltrating PC	18.4% (16/8)	16 ADH
Renshaw et al.[a]	2004	Papilloma (w/wo ADH) and atypical papilloma	40 pts	US, Stereo	11- and 14-gauge CNB	Surgery	37.5% (15/40)	12 DCIS, 3 IC	20.0% (8/40)	8 ADH
Valdes et al.	2006	Intraductal papilloma, atypical papilloma/ papilloma with ADH, papillary neoplasm, papillomatosis	80 les	US, Stereo	11-gauge VAB, 11- and 14-gauge CNB, 22- or smaller gauge FNA	Surgery	23.8% (19/80)	12 DCIS, 4 IDC, 2 infiltrating PC, 1 intracystic PC		
Lee et al.[a]	2012	Intraductal papilloma	17 pts	Stereo, MRI, US	9-gauge VAB for Stereo, 12- and 14-gauge VAB, 14-gauge CNB for US, 9-gauge VAB for MRI	Surgery	0% (0/17)		29.4% (5/17)	3 ADH, 1 ALH, 1 ADH + ALH

[a]indicates studies that performed a patient-based analysis; otherwise, a lesion-based analysis was used.

ADH, atypical ductal hyperplasia; *ALH*, atypical lobular carcinoma; *CNB*, core needle biopsy; *DCIS*, ductal carcinoma in situ; *IC*, invasive carcinoma; *IDC*, invasive ductal carcinoma; *MRI*, magnetic resonance imaging; *PC*, papillary carcinoma; *pts*, patients; *US*, ultrasound; *VAB*, vacuum-assisted biopsy.

TABLE 6.11   Phyllodes at Biopsy; Underestimation Ratio of Malignancy

Author	Year	Diagnosis at Biopsy	Number of Lesion	Guidance	Needle Type	Gold Standard	Malignancy (%)	Histology of Malignancy
Youk et al.	2015	Benign phyllodes	23	US	8- and 11-gauge VAB	Surgery	8.7% (2/27)	Two malignant phyllodes

US, ultrasound; *VAB*, vacuum-assisted biopsy.

upgrade rate when lesions were multiple, vascular within the lesion, or with a higher BI-RADS final assessment. In addition imaging/pathology correlation with benign papillomas is important to not miss a discordant result (Sydnor et al., 2007).

Excisional biopsy for papilloma is controversial; however, it could be considered, especially for high risk-women who may have cancer or have associated high-risk lesions (atypia) that might be treated with chemoprevention. Excision is recommended for papillomas with atypia because of cancer underestimates.

Phyllodes tumors, although generally benign, have a small percentage of malignant forms that are diagnosed only by complete histologic examination. Phyllodes tumor also tends to recur in the biopsy site and should be completely excised by surgery. Youk et al. (2015) reported that two (8.7%) of 23 benign phyllodes tumors diagnosed at US-guided vacuum-assisted excision were upgraded to malignant phyllodes tumors at surgical excision (Table 6.11). This means all phyllodes tumors should be excised.

Mucocele-like lesions (MLLs) of the breast are rare, but may be encountered in practice shown as calcifications, a mass, or both. In the largest series by D. Ha et al. (2015) of MLLs undergoing core biopsy, 34% (12/35) had atypia and 66% (23/35) were benign; all atypical and 12 out of 23 benign MLLs underwent excision. Of the 35 cases, 1 atypical core yielded 1 DCIS (3%, 1/35) and of 23 benign MLLs, 4 yielded atypia (17%) at surgery. The MLLs yield atypia associated with this lesion in this large series. If the core biopsy shows atypia at the outset, excisional biopsy is warranted to exclude cancer. However, if only MLL is seen, the yield of atypia is high enough on subsequent excisional biopsy that if the patient's clinical situation may warrant a change in management, for example, breast cancer risk reduction by chemoprevention, then consideration for surgery, rather than surveillance, should be considered (Ha D et al., 2015).

Currently individual decisions are made to either excise or follow pseudoangiomatous stromal hyperplasia (PASH), if there is no atypia (Box 6.4). However, PASH or hemangiomas that have possible features of angiosarcoma need surgical excision.

If surveillance is chosen, it is important that the patient complies with imaging follow-up. Imaging follow-up should be done as it is for benign concordant percutaneous biopsies at 12 months after biopsy to be sure a cancer was not missed.

Follow-up of Benign Lesions

Long-term studies of benign concordant lesions diagnosed at core or vacuum biopsy are occasionally falsely negative and emphasize the importance of a good follow-up program to minimize the potential for missing cancer. After a concordant benign biopsy, the NCCN (2015, version 1) recommends follow-up every 6 to 12 months for 1 to 2 years then return to screening. In 1999 Lee et al. recommended a 6-month follow-up for concordant benign core needle biopsies with subsequent follow-up at longer intervals, using the reasoning that if the lesion increases in size at follow-up imaging, the lesion would undergo repeat biopsy by needle or surgical excision at a shorter interval. Shin et al. (2006) suggested postbiopsy follow-up imaging, using the same imaging modality that guided the needle biopsy, at 6, 12, and 24 months postbiopsy for all benign concordant lesions. However, studies

---

BOX 6.4   Surgical Breast Specimen Reporting

Specimen includes lesion and any associated markers
Hookwire included
Hookwire tip included
Lesion is at or away from the specimen edge or is transected

---

by Salkowski et al. (2011), Adams et al. (2014), and Johnson et al. (2014) showed that the 6-month short-interval follow up did not contribute significantly to the cancer detection rate compared with an initial follow-up at 12 months. This led to the conclusion that, because rebiopsy recommendation rates and positive predictive values (PPVs) did not differ between 6- and 12-month follow-up for concordant lesions, an annual or 12-month diagnostic follow-up as the first study after benign breast biopsy may be sufficient (Salkowski et al., 2011; Adams et al., 2014; Johnson et al., 2014).

Complications

Complications were discussed earlier (see section: Informed Consent and see Box 6.2). For all procedures, the patient must be able to respond, to cooperate, and remain motionless for their own safety.

Vasovagal reactions occur occasionally during x-ray–guided presurgical needle localization because they are done with the patient sitting upright. Presurgical patients often are anxious and have been fasting and dehydrated, further predisposing them to vasovagal reactions. Thus all personnel in the x-ray procedure room must be able to recognize and treat a vasovagal reaction and be able to release the breast from mammographic compression. Some mammography procedure chairs can be changed from the upright to the supine position in case of a vasovagal reaction. Otherwise, a stretcher and resuscitation cart should be in close vicinity to the procedure room, and the patient should never be unaccompanied in the room during the procedure in case of a vasovagal reaction.

Bleeding is expected after any biopsy, and a small hematoma is not uncommon. Large hematomas or uncontrollable bleeding needing surgery is quite uncommon. Methods to decrease untoward bleeding include familiarity with any blood thinners and working with the patient's referring physician to determine whether administration of Coumadin (warfarin), heparin, Plavix (clopidogrel), or other blood thinners can be safely curtailed, if at all, and checking an international normalized ratio (INR) the day of the biopsy. Physicians should also be aware of the patient's current prescribed medications and over-the-counter self-prescribed drugs, herbs, and vitamins, and the facility should develop a policy regarding when to stop the medications. Many facilities recommend ceasing all pain medications except for acetaminophen for 1 week before the biopsy because aspirin, NSAIDs, and other medications can inactivate platelets. Other herbal medications (particularly Ginkgo biloba, which potentiates anticoagulants), vitamin E, and fish oils are also discontinued 1 week before the biopsy.

At the other extreme of not stopping medications before needle biopsy, Melotti and Berg (2000) reported needle biopsies in 18 patients undergoing anticoagulation therapy. The patients were taking warfarin ($n = 11$), heparin ($n = 1$), or aspirin ($n = 6$). Hematomas measuring 13 mm to 40 mm occurred in three of eight anticoagulated patients undergoing stereotactic 11-gauge vacuum biopsy. A 10-mm hematoma occurred in 1 of 10 anticoagulated patients undergoing US-guided 14-gauge core biopsy. In 2013, Chetlen et al. (2013) prospectively compared hematoma formation in women taking antithrombotic therapy with those who did not who also were undergoing core needle biopsy, showing a 14.4% (89/617 patients) nonclinically significant hematoma formation in patients taking (21.6%) or not taking (13.0%) antithrombotic therapy. Although the probability of nonclinically significant hematoma formation was statistically higher in women taking antithrombotic therapy or larger needle gauge, they concluded that life-threatening risk to the patients of withholding therapy outweighed the nonsignificant hematoma. These two studies suggest that needle biopsy can be performed in anticoagulated patients if the need for biopsy is urgent, but that hematomas may occur after the biopsy.

For US-guided biopsies, pneumothorax is an unusual but reported complication. The risk of pneumothorax increases if the patient is unable to hold still or is coughing, if the angle needed to biopsy the lesion is very steep, if the lesion is on the chest wall, and particularly if the lesion lies between ribs. Pneumothorax has been reported as a complication of both fine-needle breast aspiration and large-core biopsy. It is imperative that the radiologist identifies the chest wall and pleura before the biopsy to evaluate the trajectory of the needle throw. Taking the extra time to position the patient for a needle trajectory parallel to the chest wall is especially important. When there is a possibility of pneumothorax during the biopsy, the radiologist should obtain informed consent from the patient specifically for the possibility that the needle could puncture the lung and result in the need for an emergency room visit and possible stay in the hospital, which is very unusual. Knowledge of pneumothorax and its consequences, as well as strict instructions to the patient to remain immobile during the biopsy, are important for informed consent. If there are serious concerns about pneumothorax during a procedure, one should consider using a needle that may obtain a sample when the needle tip is inserted to the deepest point without a throw beyond the tip. Another alternative is to refrain from a core needle biopsy and to proceed with either FNA or preoperative needle localization and surgical excision.

Mammography Quality Standards Act Patient Audits, Follow-up, Outcome Monitoring, and Noncompliance

For mammography, a minimal audit of all mammograms are required by the MQSA under the Food and Drug Administration (FDA). An attempt to determine the outcome of all mammographic BI-RADS categories 4, 5, and 0 examinations must be made and recorded. Yearly FDA facility inspections are conducted on these audits. The use of mammography, its audits, and benchmarks have been established for many years, and mammography audit conduct/benchmarks are published in the *American College of Radiology (ACR) BI-RADS Atlas*.

The fifth edition of the *ACR BI-RADS Atlas*, published in 2013, contains a new Follow-up and Outcome Monitoring section detailing expanded auditing procedures of mammography, US, and MRI studies. This was because there were no prior standard US or MRI audits or performance benchmarks published or established previously.

Adapted from ACR BI-RADS 2013 Follow-up and Outcome Monitoring (p. 18) with permission, these are the definitions for true-positive (TP), true-negative (TN), false-negative (FN), and false-positive (FP), to be used in the audit:

True-Positive (TP) studies are BI-RADS category 4 or 5 showing cancer, defined as a tissue diagnosis of ductal carcinoma in situ or primary invasive breast cancer.

True-Negatives (TN) are BI-RADS category 1 or 2 screening or diagnostic studies, or BI-RADS category 3 diagnostic study with no tissue diagnosis of cancer within 1 year.

False-Negatives (FN) are BI-RADS category 1 or 2 screening or diagnostic studies, or BI-RADS category 3 diagnostic study with tissue diagnosis of cancer within 1 year.

False-Positive (FP) studies have three definitions:

1. FP1: Positive screening (includes BI-RADS category 3) with no tissue diagnosis of cancer within 1 year
2. FP2: BI-RADS category 4 or 5 with recommendation for tissue diagnosis or surgical consult and no tissue diagnosis of cancer within 1 year
3. FP3: BI-RADS category 4 or 5 with recommendation for tissue diagnosis or surgical consult and benign concordant tissue diagnosis (or discordant benign tissue diagnosis and no tissue diagnosis of cancer within 1 year)

Adapted from ACR BI-RADS 2013 Follow-up and Outcome Monitoring (p. 18) with permission, these are the definitions of PPV in mammography:

Positive Predictive Value (PPV) is calculated as PPV = TP/(TP + FP).

1. PPV1: The PPV of abnormal screenings, or how often an abnormal screening mammogram results in a cancer diagnosis within 1 year
2. PPV2: The PPV of abnormal diagnostic studies and rare screenings that result in a cancer diagnosis within 1 year.
3. PPV3: The PPV of abnormal diagnostic studies and rare screenings that actually go to biopsy and result in a cancer diagnosis within 1 year. PPV3 is also known as the *positive biopsy rate*.

TP, true-positive; *FP*, false-positive.

Sensitivity and *specificity* measure test performance. Sensitivity measures the proportion of true-positive tests correctly identified as positive, is sometimes called the true-positive rate, and is opposite to the false-negative rate.

$$Sensitivity = TP/(TP = FN)$$

Specificity measures the proportion of true-negative tests correctly identified as negative, is sometimes called the true-negative rate, and is opposite to the false positive rate.

$$Specificity = TN/(TN + FP)$$

The *cancer detection rate* is the number of cancers detected at screening per 1000 women and is a metric often quoted in screening studies for populations and in health care literature. This metric can also be calculated for screening studies and diagnostic examinations in a facility or organization.

Abnormal interpretation rate = (positive examinations)/(all examinations)

ACR BI-RADS 2013 defines BI-RADS category 0 on screening mammography as a positive examination. For auditing purposes, BI-RADS categories 3, 4, and 5 are counted as positive studies for all imaging modalities (mammography, US, and MRI) whether screening or diagnostic. Note that as of the ACR BI-RADS 2013 edition, BI-RADS category 3 is not allowed at screening mammography. The ACR BI-RADS 2013 edition also states that the Recall Rate from Screening Mammography should include BI-RADS category 0 and the rare BI-RADS categories 4 and 5 because the abnormal interpretation rate should include all positive screening

TABLE 6.12   Analysis of Medical Audit Data: Acceptable Ranges of Screening Mammography Performance

Cancer detection rate (per 1000 examinations)	≥2.5
Abnormal interpretation (recall) rate	5–12%
PPV (abnormal interpretation)	3–8%
PPV (recommendation for tissue diagnosis)	20–40%
Sensitivity (if measurable)	≥75%
Specificity (if measurable)	88–95%

PPV, positive predictive value.
From ACR BI-RADS®—Follow-up and Outcome Monitoring, p. 29. In *ACR BI-RADS® atlas, breast imaging reporting and data system*, Reston, VA, 2013, American College of Radiology. Original data from Carney PA, Sickles EA, Monsees BS, et al: Identifying minimally acceptable interpretive performance criteria for screening mammography, *Radiology* 255(2):354–361, 2010.

TABLE 6.13   Analysis of Medical Audit Data: Breast Screening Ultrasound Benchmarks

Cancer detection rate (per 1000 examinations)	3.7
Median size of invasive cancer (in millimeters)	10.0
Percentage of node-negative of invasive cancers	96%
PPV (performed biopsy)	7.4%

PPV, positive predictive value.
Modified from ACR BI-RADS®—Follow-up and Outcome Monitoring, p. 26. In *ACR BI-RADS® atlas, breast imaging reporting and data system*, Reston, VA, 2013, American College of Radiology. Original data from Berg WA, Zhang Z, Lehrer D, et al: Detection of breast cancer with addition of annual screening ultrasound or a single screening MRI to mammography in women with elevated breast cancer risk, *JAMA* 307(13):1394–1404, 2012.

TABLE 6.14   Analysis of Medical Audit Data: Breast Magnetic Resonance Imaging Screening Benchmarks

Cancer detection rate (per 1000 examinations)	20–30
Percentage of node-negative of invasive cancers	>80%
Percentage of minimal cancer	>50%
PPV (recommendation for tissue diagnosis)	15%
PPV (biopsy performed)	20–50%
Sensitivity (if measurable)	>80%
Specificity (if measurable)	85–90%

PPV, positive predictive value.
Modified from ACR BI-RADS®—Follow-up and Outcome Monitoring, p. 27. In *ACR BI-RADS® atlas, breast imaging reporting and data system*, Reston, VA, 2013, American College of Radiology; original data from Kriege M, Brekelmans CT, Boetes C, et al: Efficacy of MRI and mammography for breast-cancer screening in women with a familial or genetic predisposition, *N Engl J Med* 351(5):427–437, 2004; Warner E, Plewes DB, Hill KA, et al: Surveillance of BRCA1 and BRCA2 mutation carriers with magnetic resonance imaging, ultrasound, mammography, and clinical breast examination, *JAMA* 292(11):1317–1325, 2004; Leach MO, Brindle KM, Evelhoch JL, et al: The assessment of antiangiogenic and antivascular therapies in early-stage clinical trials using magnetic resonance imaging: issues and recommendations, *Br J Cancer* 92(9):1599–1610, 2005; Kuhl CK, Schrading S, Leutner CC, et al: Mammography, breast ultrasound, and magnetic resonance imaging for surveillance of women at high familial risk for breast cancer, *J Clin Oncol* 23(33):8469–8476, 2005.

TABLE 6.15   Analysis of Medical Audit Data: Acceptable Ranges of Diagnostic Mammography Performance

	Workup of Abnormal Screening	Palpable Lump
Cancer detection rate (per 1000 examinations)	≥20	≥40
Abnormal interpretation rate	8–25%	10–25%
PPV (recommendation for tissue diagnosis)	15–40%	25–50%
PPV (biopsy performed)	20–45%	30–55%
Sensitivity (if measurable)	≥80%	≥85%
Specificity (if measurable)	80–95%	83–95%

PPV, positive predictive value.
From ACR BI-RADS®—Follow-up and Outcome Monitoring, p. 29. In *ACR BI-RADS® atlas, breast imaging reporting and data system*, Reston, VA, 2013, American College of Radiology; original data from Carney PA, Parikh J, Sickles EA, et al: Diagnostic mammography: identifying minimally acceptable interpretive performance criteria, *Radiology* 267(2):359–367, 2013.

within the next 12 months to allow completion of diagnostic studies and biopsies, outcome data collection and determination of cancer diagnoses. Audits must be conducted every 12 months thereafter for inspection. Data are collected and monitored for the entire facility as an aggregate and monitored for each individual interpreting physician. These data are inspected yearly by FDA inspectors.

The medical audit fulfills FDA requirements for MQSA yearly inspections. Importantly, audits from the results from one's own practice used to compare with the literature and other practices informs the practice about its clinical performance compared with others. To compare the false-negative rate with each imaging modality, a linkage to the state tumor registry and long-term follow-up is required. The calcification lesion miss rate from specimen radiographs or post needle biopsy mammograms, ADH, other high-risk or DCIS underestimation rates are obtained comparing one's own core biopsy data to subsequent excisional surgical pathology.

In addition, standard imaging surveillance after the needle biopsy is essential for diagnosing missed cancers. Follow-up details were defined earlier (see section: Follow-up of Benign Lesions). The initial informed consent should indicate that imaging follow-up is expected and that the patient is to return for imaging surveillance after the biopsy even if the results are benign.

The problem of follow-up and compliance with follow-up is a difficult one even in the best of hands. Pal et al. (1996) showed that as many as 40% of women do not return for all their follow-up mammograms after benign results and 15% do not complete the recommended surgery after an abnormal needle biopsy. This was achieved with a vigorous, time-consuming follow-up protocol that is not practical for routine use.

As a result, the MQSA U.S. federal law mandates follow-up on all abnormal mammograms. However, clinical practice tracking is complicated, time-consuming, and expensive, with additional costs for personnel, computer updates, and mailing. It is a cause of frustration despite computerized follow-up programs. Goodman et al. (1998) showed that women's outcomes after core biopsy by stereotaxis are difficult to track as a result of relocation, changing of insurance, decisions by their referring physicians contrary to recommended follow-up, and so forth. Those same tracking problems occur after benign concordant needle biopsies. Thompson et al. (2013) showed that the same problems in tracking occurred after MRI-guided core biopsy. Accordingly, informed consent before biopsy assumes even more importance so that proper patient management can be implemented.

examinations. Table 6.12 shows Acceptable Ranges of Screening Mammography Performance as detailed in ACR BI-RADS 2013. Table 6.13 shows Breast US Screening Benchmarks as detailed in ACR BI-RADS 2013. Table 6.14 shows Breast MRI Screening Benchmarks as detailed in ACR BI-RADS 2013. Table 6.15 shows Acceptable Ranges of Diagnostic Mammography Performance as detailed in ACR BI-RADS 2013.

The FDA regulations state that the facility audit starts 1 year from the date of facility certification and must be completed

PREOPERATIVE NEEDLE LOCALIZATION

Preoperative needle hookwire localization for nonpalpable breast lesions was developed in the 1970s (Hall, 2013). The intent of preoperative needle localization is to provide the surgeon a "road map" to nonpalpable suspicious breast lesions in the breast so the surgeon may excise them in the operating room. This is because the surgeon cannot see or feel suspicious nonpalpable masses or calcifications inside the breast to remove them. The technique of preoperative needle localization uses a needle percutaneously placed into the breast, guided by imaging, so that its tip is in the breast target. The radiologist threads a metallic wire with a hook on its end through the needle such that the wire hook hooks into, or through and beyond, the suspicious nonpalpable target. The radiologist then removes the needle, leaving the hook inside or through the breast target, and the rest of the metallic wire outside the breast. In the operating room the surgeon follows the wire down to the target. Preoperative needle localization can be guided by two-dimensional (2D) mammography, stereotaxy, tomosynthesis, US, or MRI. The 2D x-ray mammography, tomosynthesis, and US preoperative needle localization are discussed in this section, along with specimen radiography and pathology correlation. The MRI-guided biopsy is discussed in Chapter 7.

Orthogonal Radiographic Guidance (X-Ray–Guided Needle Localization)

Two-dimensional mammography preoperative needle localization uses an upright mammographic unit, a compression paddle with a hole in it surrounded by letters and numbers (*an alphanumeric grid*), and 2D mammograms to guide the needle into the target. The radiologist reviews the original orthogonal mammograms to identify the shortest distance to the target from the skin surface. The technologist takes a mammogram with the alphanumeric grid over the skin closest to the lesion and marks the edges of the aperture with an ink marker at its contact with skin (to detect if the patient moves). A single mammogram image is taken and the breast is left in compression (Fig. 6.20). The mammogram should show the lesion within the open aperture. The radiologist finds the target coordinates on the mammogram, then walks to the patient in compression, marks this location in ink on the patient's skin, cleans the skin, and injects a local anesthetic on the ink mark. The radiologist then injects deep anesthesia into the breast, then passes a needle into the target, making sure the needle is parallel to the chest wall. To ensure that the needle path is straight, the radiologist checks that the needle hub's shadow lies directly over the needle shaft during insertion. The technologist repeats a mammogram with the needle in place, and this mammogram should show that the needle shaft projects over the lesion. Once the radiologist confirms that the needle is through the lesion, he or she holds the needle deep in the breast while the technologist releases compression to make sure the needle does not pull out of the lesion. The technologist takes an orthogonal mammogram with the needle still in place and a marker on the skin entry. The radiologist adjusts the needle depth so that the hook will be deployed at or beyond the target. Some surgeons request a small injection of sterile blue dye through the needle to stain the tissue around the lesion at this point, and they will later find the stain in the operating room. The radiologist then places a hookwire through the needle and removes the needle, leaving the hook in or near the target, and the rest of the wire sticking out of the skin. The radiologist bends the wire at the skin surface so that the wire does not become withdrawn into the breast during patient transportation. After any wire placement by imaging guidance (x-ray, US, or MRI) the technologist takes orthogonal mammograms to show the relationship of the target, the hookwire tip, and their location in the breast with respect to the nipple and other breast structures. The radiologist annotates the images for the surgeon and the patient is sent to the operating room, while everyone waits for the breast specimen to be imaged.

The surgeon uses the wire and mammograms as a guide to the target and excises the lesion, any markers, and the hookwire. The excised tissue is called a *breast specimen*. An intraoperative breast specimen radiograph is taken to ensure that the entirety of the hookwire and the target have been removed. The radiologist reviews the specimen radiograph to see if the lesion, any markers, and the entire hookwire (with an intact hook) are included. The radiologist notes if the finding is included in its entirety, if it is transected, and if all markers are present and calls the surgeon in the operating room with these findings. If the findings are not included, the radiologist tries to guide the surgeon to the correct area where the target may still be located inside the breast.

Bracketing wires are used to guide surgeons removing a large area of breast tissue (Fig. 6.21). This happens when the target(s) extend over too wide an area to be localized by one wire. In this situation, the radiologist places two wires in the breast, with one wire at one end of the lesion and the other wire at the other end of the lesion. The brackets help the surgeon remove the lesion between and around the two wires in toto. Breast specimens excised after brackets should include all bracketing wires and the markers, mass, or calcifications between or around them.

Orthogonal Radiographic Guidance (X-Ray–Guided Needle Localization) with Tomosynthesis

With this technique, the radiologist localizes the lesion using an upright mammographic unit capable of tomosynthesis, a compression paddle with an alphanumeric grid, and three-dimensional (3D) mammograms to guide the needle into the target (Fig. 6.22; Video 6.2). The localization technique is the same as for 2D preoperative needle localization except that the orthogonal mammogram does not have to be obtained if the depth is calculated by the tomosynthesis view. Errors in hookwire placement when using tomosynthesis calculations instead of the orthogonal view are usually along the trajectory of the needle (in the Z-axis). If the depth is not calculated by tomosynthesis, the orthogonal view can be obtained with tomosynthesis.

Stereotactic Guidance

With this technique, the radiologist localizes the lesion under stereotactic guidance, as described for stereotactic core biopsy. The radiologist places a needle into the breast, obtains stereotactic views to make sure the needle is in the middle of the lesion, may inject blue dye, and inserts the hookwire. The patient is removed from the stereotactic device and undergoes standard orthogonal mammograms. The usual problem with stereotactic wire placements are errors of the final position of the hookwire along the trajectory of the needle (in the Z-axis), just as in tomosynthesis localizations.

Ultrasound Guidance

To do US localization, the patient is placed supine, rolled, or angled on the table so the needle path is directed safely away from the chest wall to prevent pneumothorax (Fig. 6.23). Using sterile technique and direct US visualization, the radiologist anesthetizes the skin and deep breast tissue, keeping the entire shaft of the needle, the needle tip, and the target in the same plane. The anesthesia needle insertion is a "trial run" to judge the safety of the needle path and the difficulty of needle insertion. Then the radiologist inserts the preoperative localization needle into the lesion under real-time US guidance, injects blue dye, and, if used, a hookwire. A skin BB marker may be placed at the wire skin-entry site. The radiologist may place two skin BBs and an indelible ink X over the skin to mark where the lesion lies when the patient arrives in the operating room. The technologist then takes a mammogram with the US-placed wire within the breast.

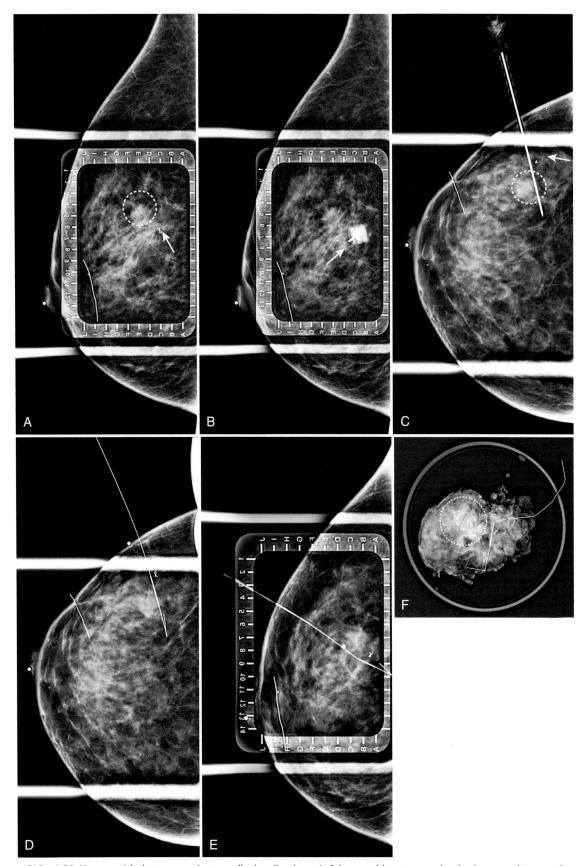

FIG. 6.20 X-ray–guided preoperative needle localization. A 36-year-old woman who had gone ultrasound-guided core biopsy showing invasive ductal cancer with a ribbon marker placed. (A) Lateral mammogram shows an alphanumeric plate with a mass (*dashed circle*) superior to the ribbon marker (*arrow*) at location C.0, 6.5. (B) Lateral mammogram with needle in place shows hub of the needle (*arrow*) directly over the marker and inferior to the mass. (C) Craniocaudal (CC) mammogram with needle in place shows the needle traversing by the marker (*arrow*) and the mass (*dashed circle*). (D and E) The CC view shows the needle has been withdrawn, as well as the marker near the wire stiffener and the hook beyond the mass. The LM mammogram was done with the wire placed through the open aperture of a compression plate so that the wire would not be pushed further into the breast during the mammogram. (F) Breast biopsy specimen radiograph shows the hookwire in its entirety as well as the marker and the mass (*dashed circle*). Pathology shows invasive ductal cancer.

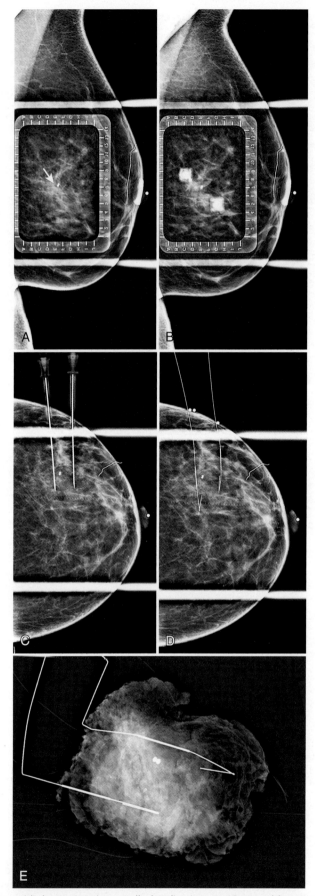

FIG. 6.21 Bracket x-ray–guided preoperative needle localization. A 49-year-old woman who had undergone stereotactic-guided core biopsy showing ductal carcinoma in situ (DCIS) with a dumbbell marker placed. (A) Mediolateral mammogram shows the alphanumeric plate with the dumbbell marker (*arrow*) at location E.5, 7.0. (B) Mediolateral mammogram shows two needles bracketing the marker and residual calcifications. (C) Craniocaudal (CC) mammogram with needles in place shows needles traversing by the marker. (D) The CC mammogram after the needles have been withdrawn shows the wires bracketing the marker and surrounding the residual calcifications. (E) Breast specimen shows the two wires and the marker and residual calcifications. Pathology showed DCIS.

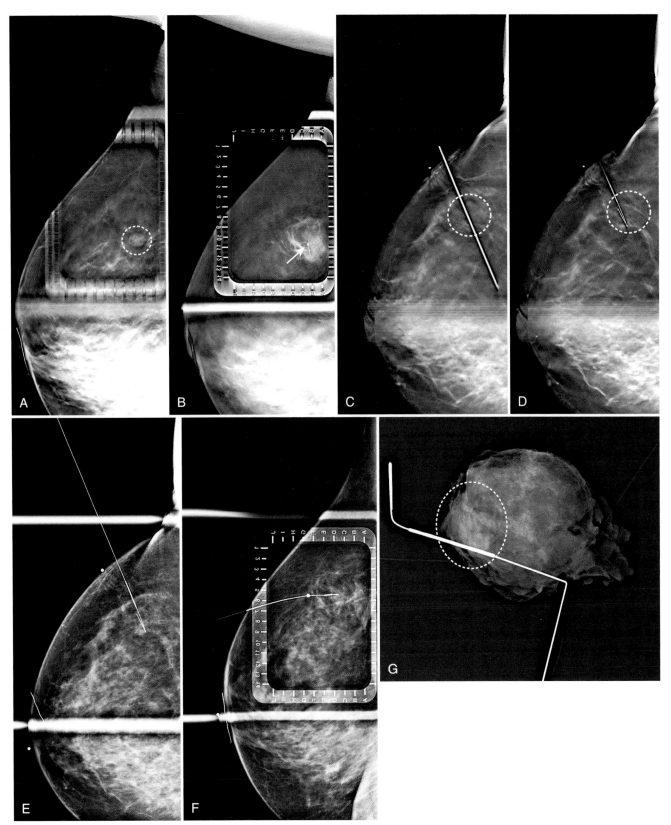

FIG. 6.22 Tomosynthesis needle localization. A 55-year-old woman with a 1.2-cm right upper outer quadrant mass on tomosynthesis not well seen on 2D mammogram or ultrasound. (A) Lateral medial tomosynthesis slice image shows the mass (*dashed circle*) in the localization compression plate aperture. The location was at B.5, 11.0. (B) Tomosynthesis slice image after needle placement shows the needle as a dot en face (*arrow*), but the mass is obscured by adjacent lidocaine. (C) Craniocaudal (CC) tomosynthesis slice shows the mass (*dashed circle*) at the midportion of the needle. (D) The needle was withdrawn and the wire placed showing the mass (*dashed circle*) near the wire tip (seen better on Video 6.2). (E and F) The CC (E) and lateromedial mammograms with an alphanumeric grid (F) after wire placement show the wire tip at the mass. (G) Specimen shows the mass (*dashed circle*) and wire. Pathology showed fibroadenoma with myxoid stromal change.

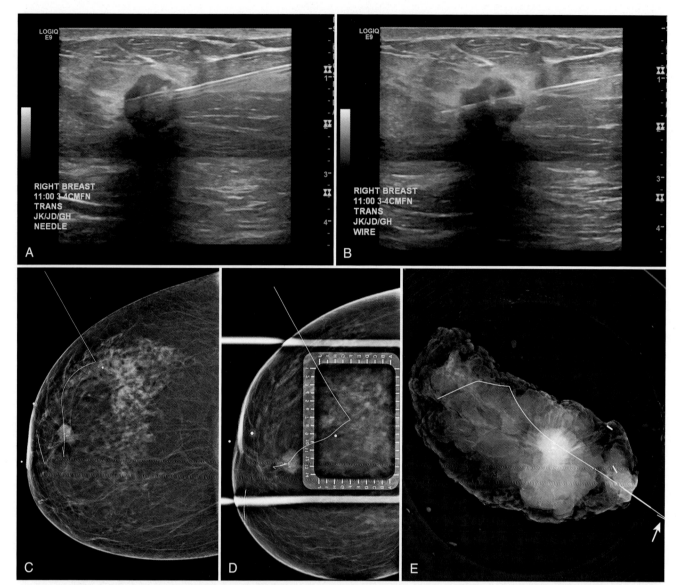

FIG. 6.23 Ultrasound (US)-guided needle localization. A 59-year-old woman with a right upper outer quadrant mass shown to be invasive ductal carcinoma (IDC) by core biopsy with central calcifications. (A) The US image shows a US needle traversing the mass. (B) The US shows the wire traversing the mass after needle removal. (C and D) After wire placement, craniocaudal mammogram (C) and lateromedial mammograms with an alphanumeric grid (D) show the wire traversing the mass. (E) Specimen shows the mass included in its entirety with surgical clips placed at the medial edge, and the hookwire is partly seen but included (*arrow*). Pathology showed IDC.

Radioguided Occult Lesion Localization (ROLL)

Radioguided occult lesion localization, described by Luini et al. in 1998, uses injection of a radio tracer or a depleted radioactive seed into the middle of a nonpalpable breast lesion to guide subsequent surgical removal. Surgeons in the operating room detect the radioactivity with a gamma probe and remove the lesion. Duarte et al. (2016) noted that ROLL showed better median lesion centricity in 64 patients when compared with 65 wire-localized patients. Another type of percutaneously placed preoperative localization device is a reflective marker that can be identified in the operating room using an electromagnetic wave hand piece. This marker can be placed up to 7 days before surgery (Cox et al., 2016). Other potential preoperative localization devices in development include radio frequency identification (RFID) tags (Reicher et al., 2008).

Specimen Radiography

The needle localization procedure is not over until the specimen radiograph results are communicated to the surgeon and made aware if the specimen contains the entire lesion; how far the lesion is away from the specimen edge; if the lesion was transected; and whether the hookwire, hookwire tip, and any markers are included (Box 6.5). The radiologist then calls these findings to the surgeon in the operating room. If the lesion is not in the specimen, the radiologist directs the surgeon to the expected location by using landmarks in the excised tissue and on the mammogram and waits for a second specimen (Fig. 6.24). If subsequent specimen radiographs still do not contain the lesion, the surgeon may close the breast and obtain a mammogram to determine whether the targeted lesion is still in the breast. The mammogram is usually done a few weeks after the biopsy.

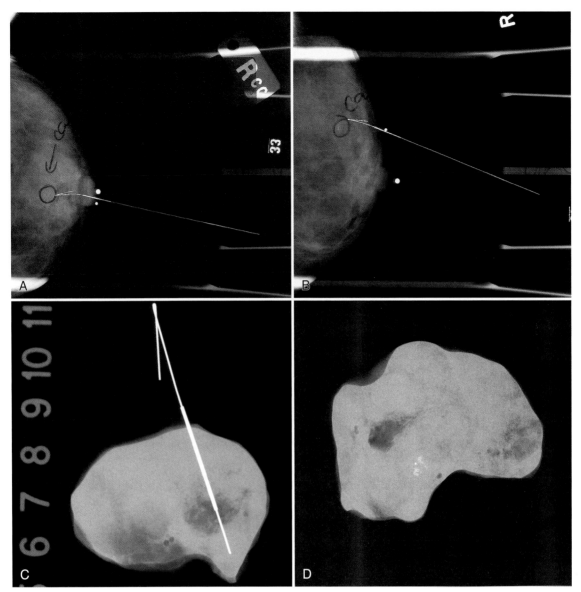

FIG. 6.24 Importance of specimen radiography. (A and B) The hookwire films from a freehand localization show the tip of the hookwire in microcalcifications on the craniocaudal (A) and mediolateral (B) views. (C) The first specimen shows the hookwire but no calcifications. These findings were reported to the surgeon in the operating room. (D) Calcifications are seen in the second specimen.

BOX 6.5 Discordant Needle Biopsy Results

Benign diagnoses can be discordant if
1. There is discordant imaging/pathology
   The histologic diagnosis does not explain the imaging findings
   A BI-RADS category 5 lesion is histologically benign
2. There is inadequate sampling
   An adequate sample of calcifications is not seen on the specimen radiograph from a calcific cluster
   The radiologist is not confident the biopsy was done with accuracy
   The lesion is not smaller on postbiopsy imaging (the finding was not adequately sampled)

Tissue excised at US-guided preoperative localizations also undergoes specimen radiography, even if the finding cannot be seen on mammogram. The specimen radiograph may or may not show the US-localized finding, but will show if the entire hookwire or its tip, as well as any metallic markers, was excised. If the specimen radiograph does not show the US-localized finding, the radiologist can perform specimen US to see if the tissue contains the mass. However, MRI-detected findings shown by enhancement by gadolinium will not be detectable by mammography or US since the contrast is long gone.

Specimen radiography may be obtained by special specimen radiography devices in the operating room. If the findings are not seen on the special device, standard specimen mammography on a mammographic unit with or without compression or even specimen tomosynthesis can be obtained (Fig. 6.25; Video 6.3).

Pathology Correlation

Just as with core needle biopsies and FNAs, the radiologist reviews the pathology report of surgical specimens to see if the pathology reflects what the radiologist expected, based on the lesion's imaging characteristics. Radiologic–pathologic correlation

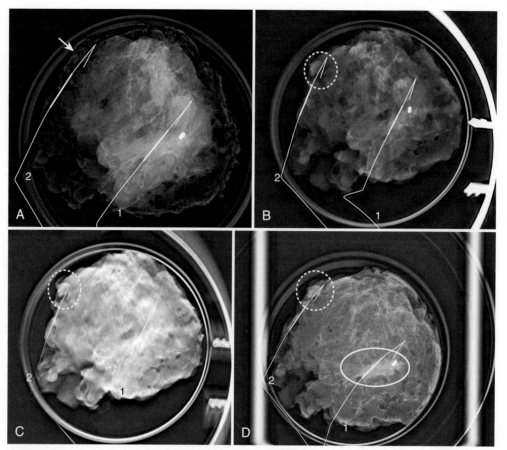

FIG. 6.25 Use of compression in specimen radiography or tomosynthesis when needed. Specimen radiography after two x-ray–guided wire localizations for *(1)* stereotactic biopsy-proven atypical ductal hyperplasia (ADH) with cylinder marker and *(2)* an oval equal density mass in the right breast. (A) Intraoperative specimen radiograph obtained directly in the operating room without compression shows wire 1 with the marker, but the second wire at the edge does not show the targeted mass *(arrow)*, even when the image was windowed and leveled at a workstation. (B) A 2D specimen radiograph on a conventional mammography unit shows the probable mass shadow *(dashed circle)* at the second wire tip. (C) Tomosynthesis through the specimen shows the mass *(dashed circle)* at the second wire tip (see Video 6.3). (D) Compression magnification specimen radiograph on the mammography unit clearly shows the mass *(dashed circle)* around the second wire tip and postbiopsy change *(circle)* near first wire and the marker. Pathology showed a 3-mm focus of ductal carcinoma in situ at the area of ADH localized by the first wire and fibroadenoma representing the mass at the second wire.

ensures that the targeted lesion analyzed at pathologic evaluation is concordant with the imaging finding and, specifically, that the pathology report describes a histologic finding that is known to correlate with the imaging findings. For example, if the targeted lesion shows fine pleomorphic calcifications, a diagnosis of malignancy, high-risk lesion, or benign lesion would all be concordant if the targeted calcifications were definitely seen in the specimen radiograph and preferably also on the pathology slides. If the pathology report showed an uncalcified fibroadenoma when the targeted radiographic finding was fine pleomorphic calcifications, the pathologic–radiologic correlation is discordant, and the case would warrant additional investigation.

Pathologic–radiologic correlation of targeted calcifications is a special subset of breast biopsy correlation. Calcifications from targeted calcifications must be seen on the surgical specimen radiograph for the biopsy to be concordant. Calcifications seen just on histologic slides and not on the specimen radiograph do not represent the calcified lesion being targeted and are not concordant. Calcifications seen on the specimen radiograph are usually seen on pathology slides, but the pathologist may not see them for several reasons.

First, the calcifications may be calcium oxalate and are seen on the slides with polarized light. Unlike calcium phosphate calcifications,

which are easily seen on hematoxylin and eosin (H&E) staining and standard light, calcium oxalate is not visualized with H&E staining and requires a special polarized light to show the calcifications.

Second, the calcifications may be in the paraffin blocks. During specimen processing, thin breast tissue samples are embedded in paraffin blocks, which are then sliced and placed on slides for staining. Each block is several millimeters thick, but each slide contains only micromillimeters of paraffin and tissue. The calcifications may still be in the block and may never have been placed on a slide for review. A radiograph of the blocks may show the calcifications, and resectioning of that particular block will show the calcifications (Fig. 6.26).

Third, other calcifications may be removed from the specimen if the microtome cutting device that slices the tissue/paraffin block for slides pushes large calcifications out of the specimen at the time of sectioning.

If the targeted calcifications seemed to be present in the specimen radiograph but no calcifications are found in the pathology slides or in the paraffin blocks, a repeat mammogram can determine whether the calcifications are still in the breast and were not removed at surgery. Rarely, the calcifications seen in the specimen radiograph may be incidental calcifications and not the ones that were targeted.

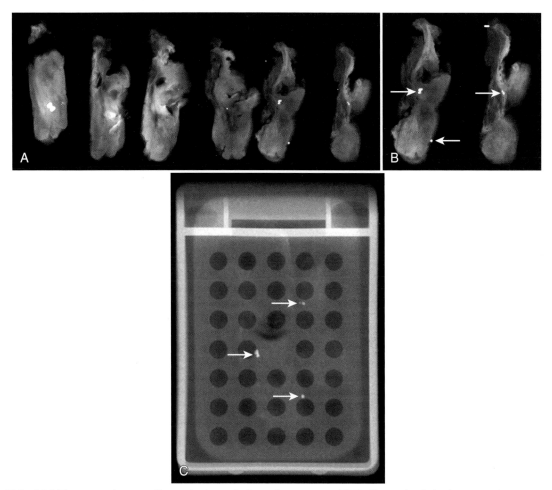

FIG. 6.26 Tissue specimen radiography in pathology department. (A) Radiograph of six tissue specimens sectioned from an excisional breast biopsy performed for calcifications. Calcifications are found in all six specimens. (B) Magnified view of two tissue specimens containing calcifications (*arrows*). (C) Pathology technologists place the tissue pieces in paraffin in a plastic tissue cassette. This paraffin block radiograph shows the calcifications (*arrows*) from the two tissue specimens shown in B. Pathology showed fibrocystic change and calcifications. If the slides from this cassette did not show calcifications, the pathologists would have taken additional samples from this cassette. (Images courtesy of Dr. Gerald Berry, Stanford University, Palo Alto, Calif.)

Key Elements

Know the location of the target lesion in three dimensions. Do not attempt biopsy of a lesion not known to be genuine or one whose location in the breast is not known.

Most nonpalpable lesions are now diagnosed by image-guided percutaneous needle biopsy and not by diagnostic surgical excision.

Specimen radiography of x-ray– or ultrasound (US)–localized surgical specimens should show the lesion, hookwire, hookwire tip, and any associated metallic markers. The findings are called to the surgeon in the operating room.

For US-localized surgical specimens, specimen US can be done if the lesion is not seen on the specimen radiograph.

Reasons that calcifications may not be visualized on the histologic slides include nonremoval, calcium oxalate, location in the paraffin block, or displacement out of the specimen by the microtome.

Risks of core biopsy include hematoma (fairly common but rarely significant) and rarely untoward bleeding, infection, pneumothorax, pseudoaneurysm formation, implant rupture, milk fistula (if the patient is pregnant or nursing), and vasovagal reactions.

Correlation between the pathology results and imaging studies establishes concordance.

If the lesion targeted was calcifications, the specimen radiograph shows no calcifications, and the pathology report describes calcifications, the pathology report has described tiny, serendipitously found 100-micron calcifications that have nothing to do with the target, and the patient needs to undergo rebiopsy.

Markers are fairly often inaccurately deployed in the breast after needle biopsy but rarely migrate significantly after placement.

Surgical excisional biopsy is recommended for core or vacuum biopsy specimens showing invasive cancer, ductal carcinoma in situ, atypical ductal hyperplasia, lobular carcinoma in situ, atypical lobular hyperplasia, any atypical lesions (including flat epithelial atypia, atypical radial scar lesions, and atypical papillary lesions), phyllodes tumors, and discordant benign lesions.

It is controversial whether surgical excisional biopsy should always be performed after obtaining core or vacuum biopsy samples showing radial scar, papillary lesions, and pseudoangiomatous stromal hyperplasia without atypia.

SUGGESTED READINGS

21CFR Part 16 and 900: *Mammography Quality Standards; Final Rule. Federal Register*, Washington, DC, 1997, Government Printing Office, pp 55851-55994. 62:No. 208.

Abdel-Fatah TM, Powe DG, Hodi Z, et al.: High frequency of coexistence of columnar cell lesions, lobular neoplasia, and low grade ductal carcinoma in situ with invasive tubular carcinoma and invasive lobular carcinoma, *Am J Surg Pathol* 31(3):417-426, 2007.

Adams MC, Falcon S, Mooney BP, et al.: Short-term imaging follow-up of patients with concordant benign breast core needle biopsies: is it really worth it? *Diagn Interv Radiol* 20(6):464-469, 2014.

Adler DD, Helvie MA, Oberman HA, et al.: Radial sclerosing lesion of the breast: mammographic features, *Radiology* 176(3):737-740, 1990.

Agoff SN, Lawton TJ: Papillary lesions of the breast with and without atypical ductal hyperplasia: can we accurately predict benign behavior from core needle biopsy? *Am J Clin Pathol* 122(3):440-443, 2004.

Al Hassan T, Delli Fraine P, El-Khoury M, et al.: Accuracy of percutaneous core needle biopsy in diagnosing papillary breast lesions and potential impact of sonographic features on their management, *J Clin Ultrasound* 41(1):1-9, 2013.

American College of Radiology: ACRIN PROTOCOL 6666. http://www.acrin.org/TabID/153/Default.aspx. Accessed November 4, 2013.

Ames V, Britton PD: Stereotactically guided breast biopsy: a review, *Insights Imaging* 2(2):171-176, 2011.

Arora S, Menes TS, Moung C, et al.: Atypical ductal hyperplasia at margin of breast biopsy—is reexcision indicated? *Ann Surg Oncol* 15(3):843-847, 2008.

Arpino G, Allred DC, Mohsin SK, et al.: Lobular neoplasia on core-needle biopsy—clinical significance, *Cancer* 101(2):242-250, 2004.

Arpino G, Laucirica R, Elledge RM: Premalignant and in situ breast disease: biology and clinical implications, *Ann Intern Med* 143(6):446-457, 2005.

Bates T, Davidson T, Mansel RE: Litigation for pneumothorax as a complication of fine-needle aspiration of the breast, *Br J Surg* 89(2):134-137, 2002.

Bazzocchi M, Francescutti GE, Zuiani C, et al.: Breast pseudoaneurysm in a woman after core biopsy: percutaneous treatment with alcohol, *AJR Am J Roentgenol* 179(3):696-698, 2002.

Becker AK, Gordon PB, Harrison DA, et al.: Flat ductal intraepithelial neoplasia 1A diagnosed at stereotactic core needle biopsy: is excisional biopsy indicated? *AJR Am J Roentgenol* 200(3):682-688, 2013.

Becker L, Trop I, David J, et al.: Management of radial scars found at percutaneous breast biopsy, *Can Assoc Radiol J* 57(2):72-78, 2006.

Berg WA: Image-guided breast biopsy and management of high-risk lesions, *Radiol Clin North Am* 42(5):935-946, 2004. vii.

Berg WA, Blume JD, Cormack JB, et al.: Combined screening with ultrasound and mammography vs mammography alone in women at elevated risk of breast cancer, *JAMA* 299(18):215-2163, 2008.

Berg WA, Krebs TL, Campassi C, et al.: Evaluation of 14- and 11-gauge directional, vacuum-assisted biopsy probes and 14-gauge biopsy guns in a breast parenchymal model, *Radiology* 205(1):203-208, 1997.

Berg WA, Zhang Z, Lehrer D, et al.: Detection of breast cancer with addition of annual screening ultrasound or a single screening MRI to mammography in women with elevated breast cancer risk, *JAMA* 307(13):1394-1404, 2012.

Berkowitz JE, Gatewood OM, Donovan GB, et al.: Dermal breast calcifications: localization with template-guided placement of skin marker, *Radiology* 163(1):282, 1987.

Beute BJ, Kalisher L, Hutter RV: Lobular carcinoma in situ of the breast: clinical, pathologic, and mammographic features, *AJR Am J Roentgenol* 157(2):257-265, 1991.

Bianchi S, Bendinelli B, Castellano I, et al.: Morphologic parameters of lobular in situ neoplasia in stereotactic 11-gauge vacuum-assisted needle core biopsy do not predict the presence of malignancy on subsequent surgical excision, *Histopathology* 63(1):83-95, 2013.

Bianchi S, Bendinelli B, Saladino V, et al.: Non-malignant breast papillary lesions—B3 diagnosed on ultrasound-guided 14-gauge needle core biopsy: analysis of 114 cases from a single institution and review of the literature, *Pathol Oncol Res* 21(3):535-546, 2015.

Bianchi S, Caini S, Renne G, et al.: Positive predictive value for malignancy on surgical excision of breast lesions of uncertain malignant potential (B3) diagnosed by stereotactic vacuum-assisted needle core biopsy (VANCB): a large multi-institutional study in Italy, *Breast* 20(3):264-270, 2011.

Birdwell RL, Ikeda DM, Brenner RJ: Methods of compliance with Mammography Quality Standards Act regulations for tracking positive mammograms: survey results, *AJR Am J Roentgenol* 172(3):691-696, 1999.

Birdwell RL, Jackman RJ: Clip or marker migration 5 to 10 weeks after stereotactic 11-gauge vacuum-assisted breast biopsy: report of two cases, *Radiology* 229(2):541-544, 2003.

Bober SE, Russell DG: Increasing breast tissue depth during stereotactic needle biopsy, *AJR Am J Roentgenol* 174(4):1085-1086, 2000.

Bolivar AV, Alonso-Bartolome P, Garcia EO, et al.: Ultrasound-guided core needle biopsy of nonpalpable breast lesions: a prospective analysis in 204 cases, *Acta Radiol* 46(7):690-695, 2005.

Bonnett M, Wallis T, Rossmann M, et al.: Histopathologic analysis of atypical lesions in image-guided core breast biopsies, *Mod Pathol* 16(2):154-160, 2003.

Brem RF, Lechner MC, Jackman RJ, et al.: Lobular neoplasia at percutaneous breast biopsy: variables associated with carcinoma at surgical excision, *AJR Am J Roentgenol* 190(3):637-641, 2008.

Brennan ME, Turner RM, Ciatto S, et al.: Ductal carcinoma in situ at core-needle biopsy: meta-analysis of underestimation and predictors of invasive breast cancer, *Radiology* 260(1):119-128, 2011.

Brennan SB, Corben A, Liberman L, et al.: Papilloma diagnosed at MRI-guided vacuum-assisted breast biopsy: is surgical excision still warranted? *AJR Am J Roentgenol* 199(4):W512-W519, 2012.

Brenner RJ: Lesions entirely removed during stereotactic biopsy: preoperative localization on the basis of mammographic landmarks and feasibility of freehand technique—initial experience, *Radiology* 214(2):585-590, 2000.

Brenner RJ: Needle localization of breast lesions: localizing data, *AJR Am J Roentgenol* 179(6):1643, 2002. author reply 1644.

Brenner RJ: Percutaneous removal of postbiopsy marking clip in the breast using stereotactic technique, *AJR Am J Roentgenol* 176(2):417-419, 2001.

Brenner RJ, Bassett LW, Fajardo LL, et al.: Stereotactic core-needle breast biopsy: a multiinstitutional prospective trial, *Radiology* 218(3):866-872, 2001.

Burak Jr WE, Owens KE, Tighe MB, et al.: Vacuum-assisted stereotactic breast biopsy: histologic underestimation of malignant lesions, *Arch Surg* 135(6):700-703, 2000.

Burbank F: Mammographic findings after 14-gauge automated needle and 14-gauge directional, vacuum-assisted stereotactic breast biopsies, *Radiology* 204(1):153-156, 1997a.

Burbank F: Stereotactic breast biopsy: comparison of 14- and 11-gauge Mammotome probe performance and complication rates, *Am Surg* 63(11):988-995, 1997b.

Burbank F: Stereotactic breast biopsy: its history, its present, and its future, *Am Surg* 62(2):128-150, 1996.

Burbank F, Forcier N: Tissue marking clip for stereotactic breast biopsy: initial placement accuracy, long-term stability, and usefulness as a guide for wire localization, *Radiology* 205(2):407-415, 1997.

Burbank F, Parker SH, Fogarty TJ: Stereotactic breast biopsy: improved tissue harvesting with the Mammotome, *Am Surg* 62(9):738-744, 1996.

Burnside ES, Sohlich RE, Sickles EA: Movement of a biopsy-site marker clip after completion of stereotactic directional vacuum-assisted breast biopsy: case report, *Radiology* 221(2):504-507, 2001.

Calhoun BC, Sobel A, White RL, et al.: Management of flat epithelial atypia on breast core biopsy may be individualized based on correlation with imaging studies, *Mod Pathol* 28(5):670-676, 2014.

Carder PJ, Garvican J, Haigh I, et al.: Needle core biopsy can reliably distinguish between benign and malignant papillary lesions of the breast, *Histopathology* 46(3):320-327, 2005.

Carney PA, Parikh J, Sickles EA, et al.: Diagnostic mammography: identifying minimally acceptable interpretive performance criteria, *Radiology* 267(2):359-367, 2013.

Carney PA, Sickles EA, Monsees BS, et al.: Identifying minimally acceptable interpretive performance criteria for screening mammography, *Radiology* 255(2):354-361, 2010.

Carr JJ, Hemler PF, Halford PW, et al.: Stereotactic localization of breast lesions: how it works and methods to improve accuracy, *Radiographics* 21(2):463-473, 2001.

Cassano E, Urban LA, Pizzamiglio M, et al.: Ultrasound-guided vacuum-assisted core breast biopsy: experience with 406 cases, *Breast Cancer Res Treat* 102(1):103-110, 2007.

Chae BJ, Lee A, Song BJ, et al.: Predictive factors for breast cancer in patients diagnosed atypical ductal hyperplasia at core needle biopsy, *World J Surg Oncol* 7:77, 2009.

Chang JM, Han W, Moon WK, et al.: Papillary lesions initially diagnosed at ultrasound-guided vacuum-assisted breast biopsy: rate of malignancy based on subsequent surgical excision, *Ann Surg Oncol* 18(9):2506-2514, 2011.

Charles M, Edge SB, Winston JS, et al.: Effect of stereotactic core needle biopsy on pathologic measurement of tumor size of T1 invasive breast carcinomas presenting as mammographic masses, *Cancer* 97(9):2137-2141, 2003.

Chetlen AL, Kasales C, Mack J, et al.: Hematoma formation during breast core needle biopsy in women taking antithrombotic therapy, *AJR Am J Roentgenol* 201(1):215-222, 2013.

Chivukula M, Bhargava R, Tseng G, et al.: Clinicopathologic implications of "flat epithelial atypia" in core needle biopsy specimens of the breast, *Am J Clin Pathol* 131(6):802-808, 2009.

Cho N, Moon WK, Cha JH, et al.: Sonographically guided core biopsy of the breast: comparison of 14-gauge automated gun and 11-gauge directional vacuum-assisted biopsy methods, *Korean J Radiol* 6(2):102-109, 2005.

Choy N, Lipson J, Porter C, et al.: Initial results with preoperative tattooing of biopsied axillary lymph nodes and correlation to sentinel lymph nodes in breast cancer patients, *Ann Surg Oncol* 22(2):377-382, 2015.

Cohen MA: Cancer upgrades at excisional biopsy after diagnosis of atypical lobular hyperplasia or lobular carcinoma in situ at core-needle biopsy: some reasons why, *Radiology* 231(3):617-621, 2004.

Collins LC, Connolly JL, Page DL, et al.: Diagnostic agreement in the evaluation of image-guided breast core needle biopsies: results from a randomized clinical trial, *Am J Surg Pathol* 28(1):126-131, 2004.

Cox CE, Garcia-Henriquez N, Glancey MJ, et al.: Pilot study of a new nonradioactive surgical guidance technology for locating non palpable breast lesions, *Ann Surg Oncol* 23:1824-1830, 2016.

Crowe Jr JP, Patrick RJ, Rybicki LA, et al.: Does ultrasound core breast biopsy predict histologic finding on excisional biopsy? *Am J Surg* 186(4):397-399, 2003.

Crystal P, Koretz M, Shcharynsky S, et al.: Accuracy of sonographically guided 14-gauge core-needle biopsy: results of 715 consecutive breast biopsies with at least 2-year follow-up of benign lesions, *J Clin Ultrasound* 33(2):47-52, 2005.

Dahlstrom JE, Sutton S, Jain S: Histologic-radiologic correlation of mammographically detected microcalcification in stereotactic core biopsies, *Am J Surg Pathol* 22(2):256-259, 1998.

Datrice N, Wirth G, Hsiang D, et al.: Can regional tattoos impact sentinel lymph node identification? *Am Surg* 79(3):331–332, 2013.

de Lucena CE, Dos Santos Junior JL, de Lima Resende CA, et al.: Ultrasound-guided core needle biopsy of breast masses: How many cores are necessary to diagnose cancer? *J Clin Ultrasound* 35(7):363–366, 2007.

Dee KE, Sickles EA: Medical audit of diagnostic mammography examinations: comparison with screening outcomes obtained concurrently, *AJR Am J Roentgenol* 176(3):729–733, 2001.

Dengel LT, Van Zee KJ, King TA, et al.: Axillary dissection can be avoided in the majority of clinically node-negative patients undergoing breast-conserving therapy, *Ann Surg Oncol* 21(1):22–27, 2014.

Dershaw DD: Does LCIS or ALH without other high-risk lesions diagnosed on core biopsy require surgical excision? *Breast J* 9(1):1–3, 2003.

Dershaw DD, Morris EA, Liberman L, et al.: Nondiagnostic stereotaxic core breast biopsy: results of rebiopsy, *Radiology* 198(2):323–325, 1996.

Deshaies I, Provencher L, Jacob S, et al.: Factors associated with upgrading to malignancy at surgery of atypical ductal hyperplasia diagnosed on core biopsy, *Breast* 20(1):50–55, 2011.

Destounis SV, Murphy PF, Seifert PJ, et al.: Management of patients diagnosed with lobular carcinoma in situ at needle core biopsy at a community-based outpatient facility, *AJR Am J Roentgenol* 198(2):281–287, 2012.

Deutch BM, Schwartz MR, Fodera T, et al.: Stereotactic core breast biopsy of a minimal carcinoma complicated by a large hematoma: a management dilemma, *Radiology* 202(2):431–433, 1997.

Diaz LK, Wiley EL, Venta LA: Are malignant cells displaced by large-gauge needle core biopsy of the breast? *AJR Am J Roentgenol* 173(5):1303–1313, 1999.

Diepstraten SC, van de Ven SM, Pijnappel RM, et al.: Development and evaluation of a prediction model for underestimated invasive breast cancer in women with ductal carcinoma in situ at stereotactic large core needle biopsy, *PLoS One* 8(10):e77826, 2013.

Dillon MF, Hill AD, Quinn CM, et al.: The accuracy of ultrasound, stereotactic, and clinical core biopsies in the diagnosis of breast cancer, with an analysis of false-negative cases, *Ann Surg* 242(5):701–707, 2005.

Dondalski M, Bernstein JR: Disappearing breast calcifications: mammographic-pathologic discrepancy due to calcium oxalate, *South Med J* 85(12):1252–1254, 1992.

D'Orsi CJSE, Mendelson EB, Morris EA, et al.: *ACR BI-RADS® atlas, breast imaging reporting and data system*, Reston, VA, 2013, American College of Radiology.

Duarte C, Bastidas F, de los Reyes A, et al.: Randomized controlled clinical trial comparing radioguided occult lesion localization with wire-guided lesion localization to evaluate their efficacy and accuracy in the localization of non palpable breast lesions, *Surgery* 159(4):1140–1145, 2016.

Duchesne N, Parker SH, Lechner MC, et al.: Multicenter evaluation of a new ultrasound-guided biopsy device: Improved ergonomics, sampling and rebiopsy rates, *Breast J* 13(1):36–43, 2007.

Dupont WD, Page DL: Risk factors for breast cancer in women with proliferative breast disease, *N Engl J Med* 312(3):146–151, 1985.

Elsheikh TM, Silverman JF: Follow-up surgical excision is indicated when breast core needle biopsies show atypical lobular hyperplasia or lobular carcinoma in situ: a correlative study of 33 patients with review of the literature, *Am J Surg Pathol* 29(4):534–543, 2005.

Fahrbach K, Sledge I, Cella C, et al.: A comparison of the accuracy of two minimally invasive breast biopsy methods: a systematic literature review and meta-analysis, *Arch Gynecol Obstet* 274(2):63–73, 2006.

Fine RE, Boyd BA, Whitworth PW, et al.: Percutaneous removal of benign breast masses using a vacuum-assisted hand-held device with ultrasound guidance, *Am J Surg* 184(4):332–336, 2002.

Frenna TH, Meyer JE, Sonnenfeld MR: US of breast biopsy specimens, *Radiology* 190(2):573, 1994.

Friedman PD, Sanders LM, Menendez C, et al.: Retrieval of lost microcalcifications during stereotactic vacuum-assisted core biopsy, *AJR Am J Roentgenol* 180(1):275–280, 2003.

Gendler LS, Feldman SM, Balassanian R, et al.: Association of breast cancer with papillary lesions identified at percutaneous image-guided breast biopsy, *Am J Surg* 188(4):365–370, 2004.

Golub RM, Bennett CL, Stinson T, et al.: Cost minimization study of image-guided core biopsy versus surgical excisional biopsy for women with abnormal mammograms, *J Clin Oncol* 22(12):2430–2437, 2004.

Goodman KA, Birdwell RL, Ikeda DM: Compliance with recommended follow-up after percutaneous breast core biopsy, *AJR Am J Roentgenol* 170(1):89–92, 1998.

Goyal A, Douglas-Jones A, Monypenny I, et al.: Is there a role of sentinel lymph node biopsy in ductal carcinoma in situ?: analysis of 587 cases, *Breast Cancer Res Treat* 98(3):311–314, 2006.

Grady I, Gorsuch H, Wilburn-Bailey S: Ultrasound-guided, vacuum-assisted, percutaneous excision of breast lesions: an accurate technique in the diagnosis of atypical ductal hyperplasia, *J Am Coll Surg* 201(1):14–17, 2005.

Graesslin O, Antoine M, Chopier J, et al.: Histology after lumpectomy in women with epithelial atypia on stereotactic vacuum-assisted breast biopsy, *Eur J Surg Oncol* 36(2):170–175, 2010.

Grin A, Horne G, Ennis M, et al.: Measuring extent of ductal carcinoma in situ in breast excision specimens: a comparison of 4 methods, *Arch Pathol Laboratory Med* 133(1):31–37, 2009.

Gruber R, Jaromi S, Rudas M, et al.: Histologic workup of nonpalpable breast lesions classified as probably benign at initial mammography and/or ultrasound (BI-RADS category 3), *Eur J Radiol* 82(3):398–403, 2013.

Guerra-Wallace MM, Christensen WN, White Jr RL: A retrospective study of columnar alteration with prominent apical snouts and secretions and the association with cancer, *Am J Surg* 188(4):395–398, 2004.

Ha D, Dialani V, Mehta TS, et al.: Mucocele-like lesions in the breast diagnosed with percutaneous biopsy: is surgical excision necessary? *AJR Am J Roentgenol* 204(1):204–210, 2015.

Ha R, Kim H, Mango V, et al.: Ultrasonographic features and clinical implications of benign palpable breast lesions in young women, *Ultrasonography* 34(1):66–70, 2015.

Hall FM, Kopans DB, Sadowsky NL, et al.: Development of wire localization for occult breast lesions: Boston remembrances, *Radiology* 268(3):622–627, 2013.

Harris AT: Clip migration within 8 days of 11-gauge vacuum-assisted stereotactic breast biopsy: case report, *Radiology* 228(2):552–554, 2003.

Harvey JA, Moran RE, DeAngelis GA: Technique and pitfalls of ultrasound-guided core-needle biopsy of the breast, *Semin Ultrasound CT MR* 21(5):362–374, 2000.

Helvie MA, Ikeda DM, Adler DD: Localization and needle aspiration of breast lesions: complications in 370 cases, *AJR Am J Roentgenol* 157(4):711–714, 1991.

Hoda SA, Rosen PP: Practical considerations in the pathologic diagnosis of needle core biopsies of breast, *Am J Clin Pathol* 118(1):101–108, 2002.

Houssami N, Ambrogetti D, Marinovich ML, et al.: Accuracy of a preoperative model for predicting invasive breast cancer in women with ductal carcinoma-in-situ on vacuum-assisted core needle biopsy, *Ann Surg Oncol* 18(5):1364–1371, 2011.

Huber S, Wagner M, Medl M, et al.: Benign breast lesions: minimally invasive vacuum-assisted biopsy with 11-gauge needles patient acceptance and effect on follow-up imaging findings, *Radiology* 226(3):783–790, 2003.

Husien AM: Stereotactic localization mammography: interpreting the check film, *Clin Radiol* 45(6):387–389, 1992.

Hussain M, Cunnick GH: Management of lobular carcinoma in-situ and atypical lobular hyperplasia of the breast—a review, *Eur J Surg Oncol* 37(4):279–289, 2011.

Ikeda DM, Helvie MA, Adler DD, et al.: The role of fine-needle aspiration and pneumocystography in the treatment of impalpable breast cysts, *AJR Am J Roentgenol* 158(6):1239–1241, 1992.

Irfan K, Brem RF: Surgical and mammographic follow-up of papillary lesions and atypical lobular hyperplasia diagnosed with stereotactic vacuum-assisted biopsy, *Breast J* 8(4):230–233, 2002.

Ivan D, Selinko V, Sahin AA, et al.: Accuracy of core needle biopsy diagnosis in assessing papillary breast lesions: histologic predictors of malignancy, *Mod Pathol* 17(2):165–171, 2004.

Jackman RJ, Birdwell RL, Ikeda DM: Atypical ductal hyperplasia: can some lesions be defined as probably benign after stereotactic 11-gauge vacuum-assisted biopsy, eliminating the recommendation for surgical excision? *Radiology* 224(2):548–554, 2002.

Jackman RJ, Burbank F, Parker SH, et al.: Stereotactic breast biopsy of nonpalpable lesions: determinants of ductal carcinoma in situ underestimation rates, *Radiology* 218(2):497–502, 2001.

Jackman RJ, Lamm RL: Stereotactic histologic biopsy in breasts with implants, *Radiology* 222(1):157–164, 2002.

Jackman RJ, Marzoni Jr FA: Needle-localized breast biopsy: why do we fail? *Radiology* 204(3):677–684, 1997.

Jackman RJ, Marzoni Jr FA: Stereotactic histologic biopsy with patients prone: technical feasibility in 98% of mammographically detected lesions, *AJR Am J Roentgenol* 180(3):785–794, 2003.

Jackman RJ, Marzoni Jr FA, Rosenberg J: False-negative diagnoses at stereotactic vacuum-assisted needle breast biopsy: long-term follow-up of 1280 lesions and review of the literature, *AJR Am J Roentgenol* 192(2):341–351, 2009.

Jackman RJ, Nowels KW, Rodriguez-Soto J, et al.: Stereotactic, automated, large-core needle biopsy of nonpalpable breast lesions: false-negative and histologic underestimation rates after long-term follow-up, *Radiology* 210(3):799–805, 1999.

Jackman RJ, Nowels KW, Shepard MJ, et al.: Stereotaxic large-core needle biopsy of 450 nonpalpable breast lesions with surgical correlation in lesions with cancer or atypical hyperplasia, *Radiology* 193:91–95, 1994.

Jackman RJ, Rodriguez-Soto J: Breast microcalcifications: retrieval failure at prone stereotactic core and vacuum breast biopsy—frequency, causes, and outcome, *Radiology* 239(1):61–70, 2006.

Jacobs TW, Connolly JL, Schnitt SJ: Nonmalignant lesions in breast core needle biopsies: to excise or not to excise? *Am J Surg Pathol* 26(9):1095–1110, 2002.

Jain RK, Mehta R, Dimitrov R, et al.: Atypical ductal hyperplasia: interobserver and intraobserver variability, *Mod Pathol* 24(7):917–923, 2011.

Jang M, Cho N, Moon WK, et al.: Underestimation of atypical ductal hyperplasia at sonographically guided core biopsy of the breast, *AJR Am J Roentgenol* 191(5):1347–1351, 2008.

Johnson JM, Johnson AK, O'Meara ES, et al.: Breast cancer detection with short-interval follow-up compared with return to annual screening in patients with benign stereotactic or US-guided breast biopsy results, *Radiology* 275(1):54–60, 2014. 140036.

Karabakhtsian RG, Johnson R, Sumkin J, et al.: The clinical significance of lobular neoplasia on breast core biopsy, *Am J Surg Pathol* 31(5):717–723, 2007.

Kass R, Kumar G, Klimberg VS, et al.: Clip migration in stereotactic biopsy, *Am J Surg* 184(4):325–331, 2002.

Kennedy M, Masterson AV, Kerin M, et al.: Pathology and clinical relevance of radial scars: a review, *J Clin Pathol* 56(10):721–724, 2003.

Kettritz U, Rotter K, Schreer I, et al.: Stereotactic vacuum-assisted breast biopsy in 2874 patients: a multicenter study, *Cancer* 100(2):245–251, 2004.

Khoumais NA, Scaranelo AM, Moshonov H, et al.: Incidence of breast cancer in patients with pure flat epithelial atypia diagnosed at core-needle biopsy of the breast, *Ann Surg Oncol* 20(1):133–138, 2013.

Kim HS, Kim MJ, Kim EK, et al.: US-guided vacuum-assisted biopsy of microcalcifications in breast lesions and long-term follow-up results, *Korean J Radiol* 9(6):503–509, 2008.

Kim JY, Han BK, Choe YH, et al.: Benign and malignant mucocele-like tumors of the breast: mammographic and sonographic appearances, *AJR Am J Roentgenol* 185(5):1310–1316, 2005.

Kim JY, Kim EK, Kwak JY, et al.: Nonmalignant papillary lesions of the breast at US-guided directional vacuum-assisted removal: a preliminary report, *Eur Radiol* 18(9):1774–1783, 2008.

Kim MJ, Kim SI, Youk JH, et al.: The diagnosis of nonmalignant papillary lesions of the breast: comparison of ultrasound-guided automated gun biopsy and vacuum-assisted removal, *Clin Radiol* 66(6):530–535, 2011.

Ko ES, Cho N, Cha JH, et al.: Sonographically guided 14-gauge core needle biopsy for papillary lesions of the breast, *Korean J Radiol* 8(3):206–211, 2007.

Ko K, Han BK, Jang KM, et al.: The value of ultrasound-guided tattooing localization of nonpalpable breast lesions, *Korean J Radiol* 8(4):295–301, 2007.

Kriege M, Brekelmans CT, Boetes C, et al.: Efficacy of MRI and mammography for breast-cancer screening in women with a familial or genetic predisposition, *N Engl J Med* 351(5):427–437, 2004.

Kuhl CK, Schrading S, Leutner CC, et al.: Mammography, breast ultrasound, and magnetic resonance imaging for surveillance of women at high familial risk for breast cancer, *J Clin Oncol* 23(33):8469–8476, 2005.

Kunju LP, Ding Y, Kleer CG: Tubular carcinoma and grade 1 (well-differentiated) invasive ductal carcinoma: comparison of flat epithelial atypia and other intraepithelial lesions, *Pathol Int* 58(10):620–625, 2008.

Kurniawan ED, Rose A, Mou A, et al.: Risk factors for invasive breast cancer when core needle biopsy shows ductal carcinoma in situ, *Arch Surg* 145(11):1098–1104, 2010.

Lagios MD: Prognostic features of breast carcinoma from stereotactic biopsy material, *Semin Breast Dis* 1:101–111, 1998.

Lai JT, Burrowes P, MacGregor JH: Diagnostic accuracy of a stereotaxically guided vacuum-assisted large-core breast biopsy program in Canada, *Can Assoc Radiol J* 52(4):223–227, 2001.

Lamm RL, Jackman RJ: Mammographic abnormalities caused by percutaneous stereotactic biopsy of histologically benign lesions evident on follow-up mammograms, *AJR Am J Roentgenol* 174(3):753–756, 2000.

Lannin DR, Ponn T, Andrejeva L, et al.: Should all breast cancers be diagnosed by needle biopsy? *Am J Surg* 192(4):450–454, 2006.

Lavoue V, Roger CM, Poilblanc M, et al.: Pure flat epithelial atypia (DIN 1a) on core needle biopsy: study of 60 biopsies with follow-up surgical excision, *Breast Cancer Res Treat* 125(1):121–126, 2011.

Leach MO, Brindle KM, Evelhoch JL, et al.: The assessment of antiangiogenic and antivascular therapies in early-stage clinical trials using magnetic resonance imaging: issues and recommendations, *Br J Cancer* 92(9):1599–1610, 2005.

Lee CH, Carter D, Philpotts LE, et al.: Ductal carcinoma in situ diagnosed with stereotactic core needle biopsy: can invasion be predicted? *Radiology* 217(2):466–470, 2000.

Lee CH, Egglin TK, Philpotts L, et al.: Cost-effectiveness of stereotactic core needle biopsy: analysis by means of mammographic findings, *Radiology* 202(3):849–854, 1997.

Lee CH, Philpotts LE, Horvath LJ, et al.: Follow-up of breast lesions diagnosed as benign with stereotactic core-needle biopsy: frequency of mammographic change and false-negative rate, *Radiology* 212(1):189–194, 1999.

Lee KA, Zuley ML, Chivukula M, et al.: Risk of malignancy when microscopic radial scars and microscopic papillomas are found at percutaneous biopsy, *AJR Am J Roentgenol* 198(2):W141–145, 2012.

Lee KE, Kim HH, Shin HJ, et al.: Stereotactic biopsy of the breast using a decubitus table: comparison of histologic underestimation rates between 11- and 8-gauge vacuum-assisted breast biopsy, *Springerplus* 2:551, 2013.

Lee SG, Piccoli CW, Hughes JS: Displacement of microcalcifications during stereotactic 11-gauge directional vacuum-assisted biopsy with marking clip placement: case report, *Radiology* 219(2):495–497, 2001.

Leibl S, Regitnig P, Moinfar F: Flat epithelia atypia (DIN 1a, atypical columnar change): an underdiagnosed entity very frequently coexisting with lobular neoplasia, *Histopathology* 50:859–865, 2007.

Lehman CD, Shook JE: Position of clip placement after vacuum-assisted breast biopsy: is a unilateral two-view postbiopsy mammogram necessary? *Breast J* 9(4):272–276, 2003.

Liberman L: Percutaneous image-guided core breast biopsy, *Radiol Clin North Am* 40(3):483–500, 2002. vi.

Liberman L, Benton CL, Dershaw DD, et al.: Learning curve for stereotactic breast biopsy: how many cases are enough? *AJR Am J Roentgenol* 176(3):721–727, 2001a.

Liberman L, Bracero N, Vuolo MA, et al.: Percutaneous large-core biopsy of papillary breast lesions, *AJR Am J Roentgenol* 172(2):331–337, 1999a.

Liberman L, Dershaw DD, Glassman JR, et al.: Analysis of cancers not diagnosed at stereotactic core breast biopsy, *Radiology* 203(1):151–157, 1997.

Liberman L, Dershaw DD, Rosen PP, et al.: Percutaneous removal of malignant mammographic lesions at stereotactic vacuum-assisted biopsy, *Radiology* 206(3):711–715, 1998a.

Liberman L, Drotman M, Morris EA, et al.: Imaging-histologic discordance at percutaneous breast biopsy, *Cancer* 89(12):2538–2546, 2000a.

Liberman L, Ernberg LA, Heerdt A, et al.: Palpable breast masses: is there a role for percutaneous imaging-guided core biopsy? *AJR Am J Roentgenol* 175(3):779–787, 2000b.

Liberman L, Feng TL, Dershaw DD, et al.: US-guided core breast biopsy: use and cost-effectiveness, *Radiology* 208(3):717–723, 1998b.

Liberman L, Kaplan J, Van Zee KJ, et al.: Bracketing wires for preoperative breast needle localization, *AJR Am J Roentgenol* 177(3):565–572, 2001b.

Liberman L, Kaplan JB, Morris EA, et al.: To excise or to sample the mammographic target: what is the goal of stereotactic 11-gauge vacuum-assisted breast biopsy? *AJR Am J Roentgenol* 179(3):679–683, 2002.

Liberman L, Sama M, Susnik B, et al.: Lobular carcinoma in situ at percutaneous breast biopsy: surgical biopsy findings, *AJR Am J Roentgenol* 173(2):291–299, 1999b.

Liberman L, Smolkin JH, Dershaw DD, et al.: Calcification retrieval at stereotactic, 11-gauge, directional, vacuum-assisted breast biopsy, *Radiology* 208(1):251–260, 1998c.

Liberman L, Tornos C, Huzjan R, et al.: Is surgical excision warranted after benign, concordant diagnosis of papilloma at percutaneous breast biopsy? *AJR Am J Roentgenol* 186(5):1328–1334, 2006.

Liberman L, Vuolo M, Dershaw DD, et al.: Epithelial displacement after stereotactic 11-gauge directional vacuum-assisted breast biopsy, *AJR Am J Roentgenol* 172(3):677–681, 1999c.

Liberman L, Zakowski MF, Avery S, et al.: Complete percutaneous excision of infiltrating carcinoma at stereotactic breast biopsy: how can tumor size be assessed? *AJR Am J Roentgenol* 173(5):1315–1322, 1999d.

Liebens F, Carly B, Cusumano P, et al.: Breast cancer seeding associated with core needle biopsies: a systematic review, *Maturitas* 62(2):113–123, 2009.

Linda A, Zuiani C, Furlan A, et al.: Radial scars without atypia diagnosed at imaging-guided needle biopsy: how often is associated malignancy found at subsequent surgical excision, and do mammography and sonography predict which lesions are malignant? *AJR Am J Roentgenol* 194(4):1146–1151, 2010.

Lomoschitz FM, Helbich TH, Rudas M, et al.: Stereotactic 11-gauge vacuum-assisted breast biopsy: influence of number of specimens on diagnostic accuracy, *Radiology* 232(3):897–903, 2004.

Londero V, Zuiani C, Linda A, et al.: Borderline breast lesions: comparison of malignancy underestimation rates with 14-gauge core needle biopsy versus 11-gauge vacuum-assisted device, *Eur Radiol* 21(6):1200–1206, 2011.

Londero V, Zuiani C, Linda A, et al.: Lobular neoplasia: core needle breast biopsy underestimation of malignancy in relation to radiologic and pathologic features, *Breast* 17(6):623–630, 2008.

Lourenco AP, Mainiero MB, Lazarus E, et al.: Stereotactic breast biopsy: comparison of histologic underestimation rates with 11- and 9-gauge vacuum-assisted breast biopsy, *AJR Am J Roentgenol* 189(5):W275–W279, 2007.

Lu Q, Tan EY, Ho B, et al.: Surgical excision of intraductal breast papilloma diagnosed on core biopsy, *ANZ J Surg* 82(3):168–172, 2012.

Luini A, Zurrida S, Galminberti V, et al.: Radioguided surgery of occult breast lesions, *Eur J Cancer* 34:204–205, 1998.

Mahoney MC, Robinson-Smith TM, Shaughnessy EA: Lobular neoplasia at 11-gauge vacuum-assisted stereotactic biopsy: correlation with surgical excisional biopsy and mammographic follow-up, *AJR Am J Roentgenol* 187(4):949–954, 2006.

Mainiero MB, Cinelli CM, Koelliker SL, et al.: Axillary ultrasound and fine-needle aspiration in the preoperative evaluation of the breast cancer patient: an algorithm based on tumor size and lymph node appearance, *AJR Am J Roentgenol* 195(5):1261–1267, 2010.

March DE, Coughlin BF, Barham RB, et al.: Breast masses: removal of all US evidence during biopsy by using a handheld vacuum-assisted device—initial experience, *Radiology* 227(2):549–555, 2003.

Matrai C, D'Alfonso TM, Pharmer L, et al.: Advocating nonsurgical management of patients with small, incidental radial scars at the time of needle core biopsy: a study of 77 cases, *Arch Pathol Lab Med* 139(9):1137–1142, 2015.

Matsika A, Srinivasan B, Gray JM, et al.: Tattoo pigment in axillary lymph node mimicking calcification of breast cancer, *BMJ Case Rep*, 2013. pii: bcr2013200284.

Maxwell AJ, Mataka G, Pearson JM: Benign papilloma diagnosed on image-guided 14 G core biopsy of the breast: effect of lesion type on likelihood of malignancy at excision, *Clin Radiol* 68(4):383–387, 2013.

McLaughlin CT, Neal CH, Helvie MA: Is the upgrade rate of atypical ductal hyperplasia diagnosed by core needle biopsy of calcifications different for digital and film-screen mammography? *AJR Am J Roentgenol* 203(4):917–922, 2014.

McNamara Jr MP, Boden T: Pseudoaneurysm of the breast related to 18-gauge core biopsy: successful repair using sonographically guided thrombin injection, *AJR Am J Roentgenol* 179(4):924–926, 2002.

Meloni GB, Dessole S, Becchere MP, et al.: Ultrasound-guided mammotome vacuum biopsy for the diagnosis of impalpable breast lesions, *Ultrasound Obstet Gynecol* 18(5):520–524, 2001.

Melotti MK, Berg WA: Core needle breast biopsy in patients undergoing anticoagulation therapy: preliminary results, *AJR Am J Roentgenol* 174(1):245–249, 2000.

Mercado CL, Hamele-Bena D, Oken SM, Singer CI, et al.: Papillary lesions of the breast at percutaneous core-needle biopsy, *Radiology* 238(3):801–808, 2006.

Mercado CL, Hamele-Bena D, Singer C, et al.: Papillary lesions of the breast: evaluation with stereotactic directional vacuum-assisted biopsy, *Radiology* 221(3):650–655, 2001.

Meroni S, Bozzini AC, Pruneri G, et al.: Underestimation rate of lobular intraepithelial neoplasia in vacuum-assisted breast biopsy, *Eur Radiol* 24(7):1651–1658, 2014.

Michalopoulos NV, Zagouri F, Sergentanis TN, et al.: Needle tract seeding after vacuum-assisted breast biopsy, *Acta Radiol* 49(3):267–270, 2008.

Morris EA, Liberman L, Trevisan SG, et al.: Histologic heterogeneity of masses at percutaneous breast biopsy, *Breast J* 8(4):187–191, 2002.

Mosier AD, Keylock J, Smith DV: Benign papillomas diagnosed on large-gauge vacuum-assisted core needle biopsy which span <1.5 cm do not need surgical excision, *Breast J* 19(6):611–617, 2013.

Mulheron B, Gray RJ, Pockaj BA, et al.: Is excisional biopsy indicated for patients with lobular neoplasia diagnosed on percutaneous core needle biopsy of the breast? *Am J Surg* 198(6):792–797, 2009.

Mullen DJ, Eisen RN, Newman RD, et al.: The use of carbon marking after stereotactic large-core-needle breast biopsy, *Radiology* 218(1):255–260, 2001.

Murray MP, Luedtke C, Liberman L, et al.: Classic lobular carcinoma in situ and atypical lobular hyperplasia at percutaneous breast core biopsy: outcomes of prospective excision, *Cancer* 119(5):1073–1079, 2013.

Nagi CS, O'Donnell JE, Tismenetsky M, et al.: Lobular neoplasia on core needle biopsy does not require excision, *Cancer* 112(10):2152–2158, 2008.

Nassar A, Conners AL, Celik B, et al.: Radial scar/complex sclerosing lesions: a clinicopathologic correlation study from a single institution, *Ann Diagn Pathol* 19(1):24–28, 2015.

National Comprehensive Cancer Network (NCCN): *NCCN clinical practice guidelines in oncology, breast cancer*, 2015. Version 2.

National Comprehensive Cancer Network (NCCN): *NNCN guidelines: breast cancer screening and diagnosis*, 2015. Version 1.

O'Flynn EA, Morel JC, Gonzalez J, et al.: Prediction of the presence of invasive disease from the measurement of extent of malignant microcalcification on mammography and ductal carcinoma in situ grade at core biopsy, *Clin Radiol* 64(2):178–183, 2009.

Ohsumi S, Taira N, Takabatake D, et al.: Breast biopsy for mammographically detected nonpalpable lesions using a vacuum-assisted biopsy device (mammotome) and upright-type stereotactic mammography unit without a digital imaging system: experience of 500 biopsies, *Breast Cancer* 21(2):123–127, 2014.

Pal S, Ikeda DM, Birdwell RL: Compliance with recommended follow-up after fine-needle aspiration biopsy of nonpalpable breast lesions: a retrospective study, *Radiology* 201(1):71–74, 1996.

Parker SH, Burbank F, Jackman RJ, et al.: Percutaneous large-core breast biopsy: a multiinstitutional study, *Radiology* 193(2):359–364, 1994.

Parker SH, Jobe WE, Dennis MA, et al.: US-guided automated large-core breast biopsy, *Radiology* 187(2):507–511, 1993.

Parker SH, Klaus AJ, McWey PJ, et al.: Sonographically guided directional vacuum-assisted breast biopsy using a handheld device, *AJR Am J Roentgenol* 177(2):405–408, 2001.

Parker SH, Lovin JD, Jobe WE, et al.: Nonpalpable breast lesions: stereotactic automated large-core biopsies, *Radiology* 180(2):403–407, 1991.

Perez-Fuentes JA, Longobardi IR, Acosta VF, et al.: Sonographically guided directional vacuum-assisted breast biopsy: preliminary experience in Venezuela, *AJR Am J Roentgenol* 177(6):1459–1463, 2001.

Pfarl G, Helbich TH, Riedl CC, et al.: Stereotactic 11-gauge vacuum-assisted breast biopsy: a validation study, *AJR Am J Roentgenol* 179(6):1503–1507, 2002.

Philpotts LE, Hooley RJ, Lee CH: Comparison of automated versus vacuum-assisted biopsy methods for sonographically guided core biopsy of the breast, *AJR Am J Roentgenol* 180(2):347–351, 2003.

Philpotts LE, Lee CH, Horvath LJ, et al.: Canceled stereotactic core-needle biopsy of the breast: analysis of 89 cases, *Radiology* 205(2):423–428, 1997.

Philpotts LE, Shaheen NA, Jain KS, et al.: Uncommon high-risk lesions of the breast diagnosed at stereotactic core-needle biopsy: clinical importance, *Radiology* 216(3):831–837, 2000.

Pijnappel RM, Peeters PH, van den Donk M, et al.: Diagnostic strategies in nonpalpable breast lesions, *Eur J Cancer* 38(4):550–555, 2002.

Pijnappel RM, van den Donk M, Holland R, et al.: Diagnostic accuracy for different strategies of image-guided breast intervention in cases of nonpalpable breast lesions, *Br J Cancer* 90(3):595–600, 2004.

Pisano ED, Fajardo LL, Caudry DJ, et al.: Fine-needle aspiration biopsy of nonpalpable breast lesions in a multicenter clinical trial: results from the radiologic diagnostic oncology group V, *Radiology* 219(3):785–792, 2001.

Pisano ED, Fajardo LL, Tsimikas J, et al.: Rate of insufficient samples for fine-needle aspiration for nonpalpable breast lesions in a multicenter clinical trial: The Radiologic Diagnostic Oncology Group 5 Study. The RDOG5 investigators, *Cancer* 82(4):679–688, 1998.

Poellinger A, Bick U, Freund T, et al.: Evaluation of 11-gauge and 9-gauge vacuum-assisted breast biopsy systems in a breast parenchymal model, *Acad Radiol* 14(6):677–684, 2007.

Polat AK, Kanbour-Shakir A, Andacoglu O, et al.: Atypical hyperplasia on core biopsy: is further surgery needed? *Am J Med Sci* 344(1):28–31, 2012.

Ponzone R, Cont NT, Maggiorotto F, et al.: Extensive nodal disease may impair axillary reverse mapping in patients with breast cancer, *J Clin Oncol* 27(33):5547–5551, 2009.

Poole BB, Wecsler JS, Sheth P, et al.: Malignancy rates after surgical excision of discordant breast biopsies, *J Surg Res* 195(1):152–157, 2014.

Rebner M, Helvie MA, Pennes DR, et al.: Paraffin tissue block radiography: adjunct to breast specimen radiography, *Radiology* 173(3):695–696, 1989.

Reicher JJ, Reicher MA, Thomas M, et al.: Radiofrequency identification tags for preopretiave tumor localization: proof of concept, *AJR* 191:1359–1365, 2008.

Rendi MH, Dintzis SM, Lehman CD, et al.: Lobular in-situ neoplasia on breast core needle biopsy: imaging indication and pathologic extent can identify which patients require excisional biopsy, *Ann Surg Oncol* 19(3):914–921, 2012.

Renshaw AA: Can mucinous lesions of the breast be reliably diagnosed by core needle biopsy? *Am J Clin Pathol* 118(1):82–84, 2002.

Renshaw AA, Cartagena N, Derhagopian RP, et al.: Lobular neoplasia in breast core needle biopsy specimens is not associated with an increased risk of ductal carcinoma in situ or invasive carcinoma, *Am J Clin Pathol* 117(5):797–799, 2002.

Renshaw AA, Derhagopian RP, Martinez P, et al.: Lobular neoplasia in breast core biopsy specimens is associated with a low risk of ductal carcinoma in situ or invasive carcinoma on subsequent excision, *Am J Clin Pathol* 126(2):310–313, 2006.

Renshaw AA, Derhagopian RP, Tizol-Blanco DM, et al.: Papillomas and atypical papillomas in breast core needle biopsy specimens: risk of carcinoma in subsequent excision, *Am J Clin Pathol* 122(2):217–221, 2004.

Resetkova E, Edelweiss M, Albarracin CT, et al.: Management of radial sclerosing lesions of the breast diagnosed using percutaneous vacuum-assisted core needle biopsy: recommendations for excision based on seven years' of experience at a single institution, *Breast Cancer Res Treat* 127(2):335–343, 2011.

Rizzo M, Lund MJ, Oprea G, et al.: Surgical follow-up and clinical presentation of 142 breast papillary lesions diagnosed by ultrasound-guided core-needle biopsy, *Ann Surg Oncol* 15(4):1040–1047, 2008.

Rosen EL, Bentley RC, Baker JA, et al.: Imaging-guided core needle biopsy of papillary lesions of the breast, *AJR Am J Roentgenol* 179(5):1185–1192, 2002.

Rosen EL, Vo TT: Metallic clip deployment during stereotactic breast biopsy: retrospective analysis, *Radiology* 218(2):510–516, 2001.

Rosenberg RD, Yankaskas BC, Abraham LA, et al.: Performance benchmarks for screening mammography, *Radiology* 241(1):55–66, 2006.

Ross BA, Ikeda DM, Jackman RJ, et al.: Milk of calcium in the breast: appearance on prone stereotactic imaging, *Breast J* 7(1):53–55, 2001.

Rozentsvayg E, Carver K, Borkar S, et al.: Surgical excision of benign papillomas diagnosed with core biopsy: a community hospital approach, *Radiol Res Pract* 679864, 2011.

Salkowski LR, Fowler AM, Burnside ES, et al.: Utility of 6-month follow-up imaging after a concordant benign breast biopsy result, *Radiology* 258(2):380–387, 2011.

Sardanelli F, Podo F: Breast MR imaging in women at high-risk of breast cancer. Is something changing in early breast cancer detection? *Eur Radiol* 17(4):873–887, 2007.

Sauer G, Deissler H, Strunz K, et al.: Ultrasound-guided large-core needle biopsies of breast lesions: analysis of 962 cases to determine the number of samples for reliable tumor classification, *Br J Cancer* 92(2):231–235, 2005.

Schnitt SJ, Connolly JL, Tavassoli FA, et al.: Interobserver reproducibility in the diagnosis of ductal proliferative breast lesions using standardized criteria, *Am J Surg Pathol* 16(12):1133–1143, 1992.

Schnitt SJ, Vincent-Salomon A: Columnar cell lesions of the breast, *Adv Anat Pathol* 10(3):113–124, 2003.

Schoonjans JM, Brem RF: Fourteen-gauge ultrasonographically guided large-core needle biopsy of breast masses, *J Ultrasound Med* 20(9):967–972, 2001.

Schueller G, Jaromi S, Ponhold L, et al.: US-guided 14-gauge core-needle breast biopsy: results of a validation study in 1352 cases, *Radiology* 248(2):406–413, 2008.

Shah-Khan MG, Geiger XJ, Reynolds C, et al.: Long-term follow-up of lobular neoplasia (atypical lobular hyperplasia/lobular carcinoma in situ) diagnosed on core needle biopsy, *Ann Surg Oncol* 19(10):3131–3138, 2012.

Shin HJ, Kim HH, Kim SM, et al.: Papillary lesions of the breast diagnosed at percutaneous sonographically guided biopsy: comparison of sonographic features and biopsy methods, *AJR Am J Roentgenol* 190(3):630–636, 2008.

Shin S, Schneider HB, Cole Jr FJ, et al.: Follow-up recommendations for benign breast biopsies, *Breast J* 12(5):413–417, 2006.

Shin SJ, Rosen PP: Excisional biopsy should be performed if lobular carcinoma in situ is seen on needle core biopsy, *Arch Pathol Lab Med* 126(6):697–701, 2002.

Sickles EA: Management of probably benign breast lesions, *Radiol Clin North Am* 33(6):1123–1130, 1995.

Sickles EA: Periodic mammographic follow-up of probably benign lesions: results in 3184 consecutive cases, *Radiology* 179(2):463–468, 1991.

Sickles EA, et al.: ACR BI-RADS® Follow-up and outcome monitoring. In *ACR BI-RADS® atlas, breast imaging reporting and data system*, Reston, VA, 2013, American College of Radiology.

Sickles EA, Miglioretti DL, Ballard-Barbash R, et al.: Performance benchmarks for diagnostic mammography, *Radiology* 235(3):775–790, 2005.

Sim YT, Litherland J, Lindsay E, et al.: Upgrade of ductal carcinoma in situ on core biopsies to invasive disease at final surgery: a retrospective review across the Scottish Breast Screening Programme, *Clin Radiol* 70(5):502–506, 2015.

Simon JR, Kalbhen CL, Cooper RA, et al.: Accuracy and complication rates of US-guided vacuum-assisted core breast biopsy: initial results, *Radiology* 215(3):694–697, 2000.

Sinn HP, Elsawaf Z, Helmchen B, et al.: Early breast cancer precursor lesions: lessons learned from molecular and clinical studies, *Breast Care (Basel)* 5(4):218–226, 2010.

Smathers RL: Marking the cavity site after stereotactic core needle breast biopsy, *AJR Am J Roentgenol* 180(2):355–356, 2003.

Smith LF, Henry-Tillman R, Rubio IT, Korourian S, Klimberg VS: Intraoperative localization after stereotactic breast biopsy without a needle, *Am J Surg* 182(6):584–589, 2001.

Sneige N, Lim SC, Whitman GJ, et al.: Atypical ductal hyperplasia diagnosis by directional vacuum-assisted stereotactic biopsy of breast microcalcifications. Considerations for surgical excision, *Am J Clin Pathol* 119(2):248–253, 2003.

Sohlich RE, Sickles EA, Burnside ES, Dee KE: Interpreting data from audits when screening and diagnostic mammography outcomes are combined, *AJR Am J Roentgenol* 178(3):681–686, 2002.

Sohn V, Arthurs Z, Herbert G, et al.: Atypical ductal hyperplasia: improved accuracy with the 11-gauge vacuum-assisted versus the 14-gauge core biopsy needle, *Ann Surg Oncol* 14(9):2497-2501, 2007.

Sohn YM, Park SH: Comparison of sonographically guided core needle biopsy and excision in breast papillomas: clinical and sonographic features predictive of malignancy, *J Ultrasound Med* 32(2):303-311, 2013.

Solorzano S, Mesurolle B, Omeroglu A, et al.: Flat epithelial atypia of the breast: pathologic-radiologic correlation, *AJR Am J Roentgenol* 197(3):740-746, 2011.

Soo MS, Baker JA, Rosen EL: Sonographic detection and sonographically guided biopsy of breast microcalcifications, *AJR Am J Roentgenol* 180(4):941-948, 2003.

Soo MS, Baker JA, Rosen EL, Vo TT: Sonographically guided biopsy of suspicious microcalcifications of the breast: a pilot study, *AJR Am J Roentgenol* 178(4):1007-1015, 2002.

Stomper PC, Davis SP, Weidner N, Meyer JE: Clinically occult, noncalcified breast cancer: serial radiologic-pathologic correlation in 27 cases, *Radiology* 169(3):621-626, 1988.

Subhawong AP, Subhawong TK, Khouri N, Tsangaris T, Nassar H: Incidental minimal atypical lobular hyperplasia on core needle biopsy: correlation with findings on follow-up excision, *Am J Surg Pathol* 34(6):822-828, 2010.

Sydnor MK, Wilson JD, Hijaz TA, Massey HD, Shaw de Paredes ES: Underestimation of the presence of breast carcinoma in papillary lesions initially diagnosed at core-needle biopsy, *Radiology* 242(1):58-62, 2007.

Tabar L, Pentek Z, Dean PB: The diagnostic and therapeutic value of breast cyst puncture and pneumocystography, *Radiology* 141(3):659-663, 1981.

Tartter PI, Bleiweiss IJ, Levchenko S: Factors associated with clear biopsy margins and clear reexcision margins in breast cancer specimens from candidates for breast conservation, *J Am Coll Surg* 185(3):268-273, 1997.

Tavassoli F: *Papillary lesions. Pathology of the breast*, ed 2, Stamford, CT, 1992, Appleton & Lange, pp 325-372.

Teh WL, Wilson AR, Evans AJ, et al.: Ultrasound guided core biopsy of suspicious mammographic calcifications using high frequency and power Doppler ultrasound, *Clin Radiol* 55(5):390-394, 2000.

Thompson M, Korourian S, Henry-Tillman R, et al.: Axillary reverse mapping (ARM): a new concept to identify and enhance lymphatic preservation, *Ann Surg Oncol* 14(6):1890-1895, 2007.

Thompson MO, Lipson J, Daniel B, et al.: Why are patients noncompliant with follow-up recommendations after MRI-guided core needle biopsy of suspicious breast lesions? *AJR Am J Roentgenol* 201(6):1391-1400, 2013.

Thompson WR, Bowen JR, Dorman BA, et al.: Mammographic localization and biopsy of nonpalpable breast lesions. A 5-year study, *Arch Surg* 126(6):730-733, 1991. Discussion 733-734.

Tornos C, Silva E, el-Naggar A, Pritzker KP: Calcium oxalate crystals in breast biopsies. The missing microcalcifications, *Am J Surg Pathol* 14(10):961-968, 1990.

Valdes EK, Tartter PI, Genelus-Dominique E, et al.: Significance of papillary lesions at percutaneous breast biopsy, *Ann Surg Oncol* 13(4):480-482, 2006.

Verkooijen HM: Core Biopsy After Radiologic Localisation Study G: Diagnostic accuracy of stereotactic large-core needle biopsy for nonpalpable breast disease: results of a multicenter prospective study with 95% surgical confirmation, *Int J Cancer* 99(6):853-859, 2002.

Verkooijen HM, Peterse JL, Schipper ME, et al.: Interobserver variability between general and expert pathologists during the histopathological assessment of large-core needle and open biopsies of nonpalpable breast lesions, *Eur J Cancer* 39(15):2187-2191, 2003.

Villa A, Chiesa F, Massa T, et al.: Flat epithelial atypia: comparison between 9-gauge and 11-gauge devices, *Clin Breast Cancer* 13(6):450-454, 2013.

Warner E, Plewes DB, Hill KA, et al.: Surveillance of BRCA1 and BRCA2 mutation carriers with magnetic resonance imaging, ultrasound, mammography, and clinical breast examination, *JAMA* 292(11):1317-1325, 2004.

Whaley DH, Adamczyk DL, Jensen EA: Sonographically guided needle localization after stereotactic breast biopsy, *AJR Am J Roentgenol* 180(2):352-354, 2003.

Winchester DJ, Bernstein JR, Jeske JM, et al.: Upstaging of atypical ductal hyperplasia after vacuum-assisted 11-gauge stereotactic core needle biopsy, *Arch Surg* 138(6):619-622, 2003. Discussion 622 to 613.

Yang JH, Lee WS, Kim SW, et al.: Effect of core-needle biopsy vs fine-needle aspiration on pathologic measurement of tumor size in breast cancer, *Arch Surg* 140(2):125-128, 2005.

Yeh IT, Dimitrov D, Otto P, et al.: Pathologic review of atypical hyperplasia identified by image-guided breast needle core biopsy. Correlation with excision specimen, *Arch Pathol Lab Med* 127(1):49-54, 2003.

Youk JH, Kim EK, Kim MJ: Atypical ductal hyperplasia diagnosed at sonographically guided 14-gauge core needle biopsy of breast mass, *AJR Am J Roentgenol* 192(4):1135-1141, 2009.

Youk JH, Kim EK, Kim MJ, Oh KK: Sonographically guided 14-gauge core needle biopsy of breast masses: a review of 2420 cases with long-term follow-up, *AJR Am J Roentgenol* 190(1):202-207, 2008.

Youk JH, Kim EK, Kwak JY, Son EJ: Atypical papilloma diagnosed by sonographically guided 14-gauge core needle biopsy of breast mass, *AJR Am J Roentgenol* 194(5):1397-1402, 2010.

Youk JH, Kim H, Kim EK, et al.: Phyllodes tumor diagnosed after ultrasound-guided vacuum-assisted excision: should it be followed by surgical excision? *Ultrasound Med Biol* 41(3):741-747, 2015.

Youn I, Kim MJ, Moon HJ, Kim EK: Absence of residual microcalcifications in atypical ductal hyperplasia diagnosed via stereotactic vacuum-assisted breast biopsy: is surgical excision obviated? *J Breast Cancer* 17(3):265-269, 2014.

Zografos GC, Zagouri F, Sergentanis TN, et al.: Diagnosing papillary lesions using vacuum-assisted breast biopsy: should conservative or surgical management follow? *Onkologie* 31(12):653-656, 2008.

Chapter 7

Magnetic Resonance Imaging of Breast Cancer and Magnetic Resonance Imaging–Guided Breast Biopsy

Kanae K. Miyake, Debra M. Ikeda, and Bruce L. Daniel

CHAPTER OUTLINE

Magnetic resonance imaging (MRI) is more sensitive for breast cancer than standard x-ray mammography or ultrasound, when using dynamic contrast-enhancement (DCE) methods after administration of intravenous (IV) gadolinium-based contrast agents. Breast MRI both detects breast cancer and distinguishes it from benign breast with high-resolution scanning using breast lesion morphology and enhancement characteristics. Noncontrast MRI methods are in development, but currently they are not as sensitive for cancer detection. Both the National Comprehensive Cancer Network (NCCN) and the American Cancer Society recommend breast MRI screening for women if they have a ≥20% lifetime risk for breast cancer based on family history of breast cancer or if they have a genetic predisposition for breast cancer. This chapter reviews MRI techniques, how to interpret breast MRI, and MRI indications and MRI-guided procedures. Evaluation of breast implants by MRI is discussed in Chapter 9.

MAGNETIC RESONANCE IMAGING TECHNIQUES

Basic Principles

MRI uses repeated radiofrequency pulses in concert with precise spatial modulation of a strong magnetic field to image the distribution and nuclear magnetic resonance characteristics of hydrogen atoms within human tissue. MRI provides either two-dimensional (2D) thin slices or three-dimensional (3D) volumetric tomographic images without ionizing radiation. Like mammography, MRI is comprehensive, reproducible, and operator independent. Like sonography, MRI is not limited by dense breast tissue in detecting breast cancer.

Various MRI pulse sequences create images that reflect different tissue properties, such as T1, T2, or T2* relaxation times; proton density; apparent diffusion coefficient (ADC);

and others. Pulse sequences can also be made to specifically image particular tissues, such as fat, water, or silicone, by a variety of techniques. Because MRI is exquisitely sensitive to paramagnetic substances, such as intravenously injected gadolinium chelate contrast agents, even minimal concentrations of these agents in tissues substantially shorten the T1 relaxation time, resulting in a high signal for enhancing breast lesions on T1-weighted images and improving differentiation of cancers from benign breast entities.

Invasive breast tumors are characterized by an ingrowth of neovascularity at their periphery. Tumor angiogenesis is associated with increased perfusion and abnormal leaky endothelium, leading to preferential tumor enhancement compared with normal breast tissue (Box 7.1). After a bolus administration of an IV contrast agent, the increased vascular flow and the rapid exchange rate of contrast between blood and the

extracellular compartments of invasive breast tumors cause a more rapid, avid enhancement of tumors compared with normal fibroglandular tissue (FGT), even in patients with dense breasts. Thus after injection of IV contrast, invasive breast cancers have high signal intensity and are brighter than the surrounding normal tissue on the first postcontrast scan, which ideally should be obtained about 90 seconds after injection. As a result, MRI exquisitely reveals invasive tumors that are occult on mammography (Fig. 7.1). The sensitivity of MRI for invasive breast cancer is extremely high—over 90%. However, as discussed in detail in this chapter, contrast enhancement on MRI is seen in many benign conditions as well; the specificity of MRI is around 80% to 90%. As also detailed in this chapter, morphology, T1 and T2 characteristics, and the time course of contrast enhancement, or kinetics, help differentiate benign from malignant lesion.

BOX 7.1   Principles of Breast Cancer Magnetic Resonance Imaging

Contrast-enhanced magnetic resonance imaging is extremely sensitive for tumor angiogenesis, regardless of radiographic breast density.

Tumor angiogenesis leads to preferential enhancement of cancers with intravenous contrast.

Lesion morphology helps distinguish cancer from benign conditions.

The time course of contrast enhancement helps distinguish invasive cancer from other conditions:

Most cancers initially enhance rapidly (*fast*) in early phase (*fast washin*).

Most cancers have late-phase stable signal intensity (*plateau*) or declining signal intensity (*washout*).

Benign conditions enhance usually gradually in early phase (*slow*) and continuously in late phase (*persistent*).

Patient Preparation

Benign hormone-related enhancement of normal breast tissue, called *background enhancement,* occurs before the onset of menses and can lead to false-positive studies. When possible, patients should be imaged 7 to 14 days after the onset of their menstrual cycle, when spurious contrast enhancement of normal tissue is at its nadir (Box 7.2). The American College of Radiology (ACR) recommends that breast MRI scans be performed during the second week of the menstrual cycle for women undergoing screening studies (ACR standard amended 2014).

Before MRI scanning, the patient fills out an MRI safety form to exclude contraindications of entering the strong magnetic field, such as ferromagnetic vascular clips, metallic ocular fragments, pacemakers, and implanted electromechanical devices (Fig. 7.2). The ACR has a document on recommendations for MRI safe practices (Expert Panel on MR Safety et al., 2013) and safety of gadolinium contrast injection (ACR Committee on Drugs and Contrast Media, 2015). Patients are cleared for

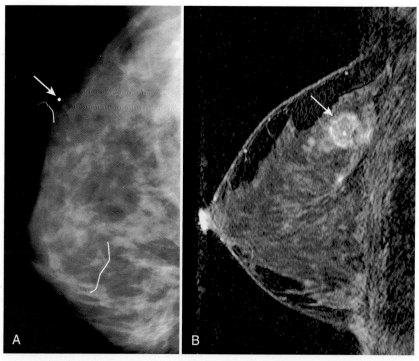

FIG. 7.1 Mammographically occult breast cancer. (A) Mediolateral oblique mammogram in a woman with a palpable mass in the upper portion of the breast indicated by a metallic skin marker (*arrow*) revealed only dense tissue. (B) Contrast-enhanced water-specific 3D magnetic resonance image demonstrated a 1-cm rim-enhancing lesion (*arrow*). Lumpectomy revealed a 1-cm invasive ductal carcinoma.

gadolinium contrast injection to assure that they can excrete the contrast, and most facilities have a protocol and policy for gadolinium contrast injection safety (ie, renal function, age). A qualified person reviews the standardized MRI safety form with the patient before scanning.

As with mammography, an MRI-specific breast history form is helpful to detail patient breast risk factors, family history, breast lumps, scars, or other areas of patient complaints. The technologist places MRI-compatible markers on the patient's breast to indicate lumps or areas of concern and annotates them on the history form. The patient details the location, date, and results of previous breast biopsies. The patient also documents any use of exogenous hormone therapy and the phase of the menstrual cycle or menopause, because those factors may cause spurious background enhancement of normal tissue, which can produce false-positive results. The patient notes if they have undergone prior MRI or other breast-related imaging studies, so they can be compared with the current examination. The patient is then instructed that, for the MRI study to work well, she must remain still during the examination and that motion artifact can cause spurious results.

Equipment, Quality Control, and Safety

The ACR Breast MRI Accreditation Program provides guidance and recommendations on personnel qualifications, equipment, quality control, quality assurance, MR safety policies, and image quality for facilities performing breast MRI and breast MRI-guided procedures (http://www.acr.org/Quality-Safety/Accreditation/BreastMRI). This program also provides feedback to facilities on image quality and minimum requirements to obtain high-quality studies and is a good resource for information on current ACR recommendations on equipment and scanning techniques. The following paragraphs will cover the authors' experience with breast MRI equipment.

Although the ACR does not have a minimum MRI field strength requirement, all MRI equipment is required to meet all state and U.S. Food and Drug Administration (FDA) or a similar regulating agency to meet performance requirements for maximum static magnetic field strength, maximum rate of change of magnetic field strength (dB/dt), maximum radiofrequency power deposition (specific absorption rate [SAR]), and maximum auditory noise levels to pass ACR accreditation.

The authors advise that a high-performance MRI scanner with high-performance gradient systems should be used to ensure adequate rates of dynamic imaging and the spatial resolution; scan quality should be limited by intrinsic signal-to-noise ratio (SNR) and FDA limits on scan parameters, not by the quality of the MRI system. A field strength of at least 1.5 T increases SNR by providing more available magnetization than lower field strengths. To further increase SNR, breast MRI is increasingly performed at 3 T, but is more complicated.

Coverage, spatial resolution, temporal resolution, and SNR are all important for breast MRI, but as with all MRI studies, they are a compromise. For coverage of breast tissue and axillae, most women can be imaged within a 20-cm field of view (FOV) in

the superoinferior and anteroposterior directions and a 36-cm FOV in the left–right direction. The reason for high spatial resolution during the first volumetric acquisition (obtained between 1.0 and 1.5 minutes after contrast injection) is to capture the morphologic features of malignancies when they are brightest and most sharply defined against normal breast tissue. The ACR Breast MRI Accreditation Program states the precontrast and postcontrast T1-weighted scan series sequence acquisition may be sagittal, axial, coronal, and/or slightly oblique. To ensure high resolution, they also recommend a slice thickness of ≤3 mm with a 0-mm gap and ≤1 mm maximum in-plane pixel dimension for phase and frequency. After the initial contrast injection, repeated dynamic postcontrast scans throughout the period of contrast uptake are obtained to capture the change in signal intensity of breast tumors by measuring initial washin and subsequent washout of contrast material over at least 5 minutes and up to 10 minutes. The reason for a high SNR is to provide the highest quality and nongrainy images to display the most subtle signs of breast cancer on the MRI images.

Major safety concerns in MRI studies, including breast MRI, are as follows: (1) force and torque on magnetic materials caused by static magnetic field, (2) tissue heating caused by radiofrequency magnetic field used to flip spins, (3) nerve stimulation caused by gradient magnetic field, and (4) implanted medical devices. To estimate temperature increase caused by radiofrequency-induced tissue heating, the SAR, which is defined as power deposited by a radiofrequency field in a given mass of tissue, can be used. A higher SAR indicates higher risk of tissue heating. The doubling of field from 1.5 T to 3 T leads to a quadrupling of SAR; however, most manufacturers have modified pulse sequences to reduce SAR at 3 T.

Patient Positioning for Magnetic Resonance Imaging Scanning

Before scanning, the technologist places an IV catheter, usually in the patient's antecubital fossa contralateral to any known, previous, or suspected malignancy. The IV is connected to an MRI-compatible remote power injector to allow standard contrast injection, continuous flushing of the IV by using the keep vein open (KVO) setting, the ability to inject contrast without moving the patient, and the ability to flush the contrast through with a 20-mL saline flush.

The patient is then placed prone on the MRI table with her breasts placed within a dedicated breast coil, which is a box-like structure with two holes through which the breasts hang dependently (Fig. 7.3). Many facilities scan with the patient's arms up by her head to minimize artifacts from the arm tissue on axial images. The technologist makes sure that all the breast tissue, including the axillary tail, is included in the FOV, and that she is comfortable. The ACR states that all MRI equipment must have a dedicated bilateral breast coil and be capable of simultaneous bilateral imaging. Dedicated commercial breast coils image the breast in the prone position to minimize respiratory motion, contain an array of four or more elements in close proximity to the breasts to maximize SNR, and may or may not allow gentle breast stabilization by external compression paddles or coil elements. Those breast coils used for interventional procedures contain grids or open apertures in the compression plate for biopsies and localizations. In either diagnostic or interventional breast MRI, one avoids firm breast compression commonly used for x-ray mammography because of the theoretical decrease in breast perfusion, which could reduce the enhancement of cancers.

The phased-array breast coils maximize SNR of the image. Patient discomfort is the primary cause of motion; keeping the patient still during scanning is important to ensure high-quality MR images. The technologist spends considerable time discussing the importance of holding still with the patient to obtain the best scan. The patient then works with the technologist to obtain a comfortable position within the breast coil. Optional mild breast stabilization, or compression, may be used to reduce

---

BOX 7.2 Patient Selection and Preparation

Magnetic resonance imaging (MRI) should be performed 7 to 14 days after onset of menses, which minimizes false-positive enhancement.

Patients should be screened for MRI safety, including pacemakers or other implanted devices.

Patient should be cleared for gadolinium MRI contrast injection.

Patients should document previous and current breast problems on a breast history form.

MAGNETIC RESONANCE (MR) PROCEDURE SCREENING FORM FOR PATIENTS

Date _____/_____/_____   Patient Number _____

Name _____   Age _____   Height _____   Weight _____
　　　Last name　　　First name　　　Middle Initial

Date of Birth _____/_____/_____   Male ☐   Female ☐   Body Part to be Examined _____
　　　　　month day year

Address _____   Telephone (home) (_____) _____-_____

City _____   Telephone (work) (_____) _____-_____

State _____ Zip Code _____

Reason for MRI and/or Symptoms _____

Referring Physician _____   Telephone (_____) _____-_____

---

1. Have you had prior surgery or an operation (e.g., arthroscopy, endoscopy, etc.) of any kind?　　　　☐ No　　☐ Yes
   If yes, please indicate the date and type of surgery:
   Date _____/_____/_____   Type of surgery _____
   Date _____/_____/_____   Type of surgery _____
2. Have you had a prior diagnostic imaging study or examination (MRI, CT, Ultrasound, X-ray, etc.)?　　☐No　　☐ Yes
   If yes, please list:　　　Body part　　　　　　　　　Date　　　　　　　Facility

	Body part	Date	Facility
MRI	_____	_____/_____/_____	_____
CT/CAT Scan	_____	_____/_____/_____	_____
X-Ray	_____	_____/_____/_____	_____
Ultrasound	_____	_____/_____/_____	_____
Nuclear Medicine	_____	_____/_____/_____	_____
Other_____	_____	_____/_____/_____	_____

3. Have you experienced any problem related to a previous MRI examination or MR procedure?　　☐ No　　☐ Yes
   If yes, please describe: _____
4. Have you had an injury to the eye involving a metallic object or fragment (e.g., metallic slivers,
   shavings, foreign body, etc.)?　　　　　　　　　　　　　　　　　　　　　　　　　　☐ No　　☐ Yes
   If yes, please describe: _____
5. Have you ever been injured by a metallic object or foreign body (e.g., BB, bullet, shrapnel, etc.)?　☐ No　　☐ Yes
   If yes, please describe: _____
6. Are you currently taking or have you recently taken any medication or drug?　　　　　　　　☐ No　　☐ Yes
   If yes, please list:_____
7. Are you allergic to any medication?　　　　　　　　　　　　　　　　　　　　　　　　☐ No　　☐ Yes
   If yes, please list:_____
8. Do you have a history of asthma, allergic reaction, respiratory disease, or reaction to a contrast
   medium or dye used for an MRI, CT, or X-ray examination?　　　　　　　　　　　　　　☐ No　　☐ Yes
9. Do you have anemia or any disease(s) that affects your blood, a history of renal (kidney)
   disease, or seizures?　　　　　　　　　　　　　　　　　　　　　　　　　　　　　　☐ No　　☐ Yes
   If yes, please describe: _____

For female patients:
10. Date of last menstrual period: _____/_____/_____　　　　Post menopausal?　　☐ No　　☐ Yes
11. Are you pregnant or experiencing a late menstrual period?　　　　　　　　　　　☐ No　　☐ Yes
12. Are you taking oral contraceptives or receiving hormonal treatment?　　　　　　☐ No　　☐ Yes
13. Are you taking any type of fertility medication or having fertility treatments?　　☐ No　　☐ Yes
    If yes, please describe: _____
14. Are you currently breastfeeding?　　　　　　　　　　　　　　　　　　　　　　☐ No　　☐ Yes

© F.G. Shellock, 2002   www.IMRSER.org

FIG. 7.2 Magnetic resonance imaging (MRI) safety form. As part of routine safety interview procedures before MRI, patients fill out a history form to screen for implanted devices or other conditions that might affect the safety of the MRI. (Courtesy of Dr. Frank Shellock, www.MRI-Safety.com. Reprinted by permission.)

WARNING: Certain implants, devices, or objects may be hazardous to you and/or may interfere with the MR procedure (i.e., MRI, MR angiography, functional MRI, MR spectroscopy). **Do not enter** the MR system room or MR environment if you have any question or concern regarding an implant, device, or object. Consult the MRI Technologist or Radiologist BEFORE entering the MR system room. **The MR system magnet is ALWAYS on.**

Please indicate if you have any of the following:

❒ Yes ❒ No Aneurysm clip(s)
❒ Yes ❒ No Cardiac pacemaker
❒ Yes ❒ No Implanted cardioverter defibrillator (ICD)
❒ Yes ❒ No Electronic implant or device
❒ Yes ❒ No Magnetically-activated implant or device
❒ Yes ❒ No Neurostimulation system
❒ Yes ❒ No Spinal cord stimulator
❒ Yes ❒ No Internal electrodes or wires
❒ Yes ❒ No Bone growth/bone fusion stimulator
❒ Yes ❒ No Cochlear, otologic, or other ear implant
❒ Yes ❒ No Insulin or other infusion pump
❒ Yes ❒ No Implanted drug infusion device
❒ Yes ❒ No Any type of prosthesis (eye, penile, etc.)
❒ Yes ❒ No Heart valve prosthesis
❒ Yes ❒ No Eyelid spring or wire
❒ Yes ❒ No Artificial or prosthetic limb
❒ Yes ❒ No Metallic stent, filter, or coil
❒ Yes ❒ No Shunt (spinal or intraventricular)
❒ Yes ❒ No Vascular access port and/or catheter
❒ Yes ❒ No Radiation seeds or implants
❒ Yes ❒ No Swan-Ganz or thermodilution catheter
❒ Yes ❒ No Medication patch (Nicotine, Nitroglycerine)
❒ Yes ❒ No Any metallic fragment or foreign body
❒ Yes ❒ No Wire mesh implant
❒ Yes ❒ No Tissue expander (e.g., breast)
❒ Yes ❒ No Surgical staples, clips, or metallic sutures
❒ Yes ❒ No Joint replacement (hip, knee, etc.)
❒ Yes ❒ No Bone/joint pin, screw, nail, wire, plate, etc.
❒ Yes ❒ No IUD, diaphragm, or pessary
❒ Yes ❒ No Dentures or partial plates
❒ Yes ❒ No Tattoo or permanent makeup
❒ Yes ❒ No Body piercing jewelry
❒ Yes ❒ No Hearing aid
　　　　　　　(Remove before entering MR system room)
❒ Yes ❒ No Other implant _____
❒ Yes ❒ No Breathing problem or motion disorder
❒ Yes ❒ No Claustrophobia

Please mark on the figure(s) below the location of any implant or metal inside of or on your body.

RIGHT　　　　LEFT　　LEFT　　　　RIGHT

⚠ | **IMPORTANT INSTRUCTIONS**

Before entering the MR environment or MR system room, you must remove all metallic objects including hearing aids, dentures, partial plates, keys, beeper, cell phone, eyeglasses, hair pins, barrettes, jewelry, body piercing jewelry, watch, safety pins, paperclips, money clip, credit cards, bank cards, magnetic strip cards, coins, pens, pocket knife, nail clipper, tools, clothing with metal fasteners, & clothing with metallic threads.

Please consult the MRI Technologist or Radiologist if you have any question or concern BEFORE you enter the MR system room.

NOTE: You may be advised or required to wear earplugs or other hearing protection during the MR procedure to prevent possible problems or hazards related to acoustic noise.

I attest that the above information is correct to the best of my knowledge. I read and understand the contents of this form and had the opportunity to ask questions regarding the information on this form and regarding the MR procedure that I am about to undergo.

Signature of Person Completing Form: _____   Date _____/_____/_____
　　　　　　　　　　　　　　　　　　　　　　Signature

Form Completed By: ❒ Patient ❒ Relative ❒ Nurse_____   _____
　　　　　　　　　　　　　　　　　　　　　　Print name　　　　　　　　　　　　Relationship to patient

Form Information Reviewed By: _____   _____
　　　　　　　　　　　　　　　　　　Print name　　　　　　　　　　　　　　Signature

❒ MRI Technologist　　❒ Nurse　　❒ Radiologist　　❒ Other_____

FIG. 7.2, cont'd

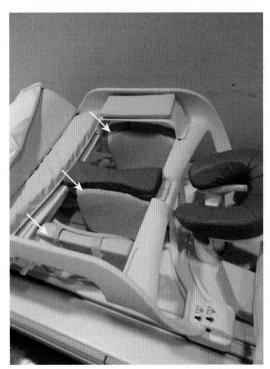

FIG. 7.3 Dedicated breast coil for breast magnetic resonance imaging. This dedicated, 16-channel, phased-array breast coil has medial and lateral immobilization plates (*arrows*) that can be adjusted depending on the breast size to bring coil elements as close as possible to the breasts. The patient will be studied in prone position with the breasts in the apertures of the coil.

BOX 7.3 Equipment and Practice Guidelines for Breast Magnetic Resonance Imaging

Remote-controlled power injector connected to the antecubital IV line on keep vein open setting
Dedicated breast coil
    Prone position minimizes respiratory motion
    Small volume maximizes signal-to-noise ratio (SNR)
    Multiple receiver channels enable parallel imaging acceleration
    Mild stabilization or no compression used; firm compression
      may alter contrast enhancement.
1.5 T magnet with high-performance gradient system
    3.0 T magnets may increase SNR but are limited by tissue heating and radiofrequency transmit field inhomogeneity
Contrast dose: 0.1 mmol/kg followed by saline flush ≥10 mL
Bilateral simultaneous breast imaging
Spatial resolution: ≤1 mm in-plane; ≤3 mm slice thickness fat suppression chemical suppression preferred over sole reliance on subtraction.
Scan time: every 4 minutes or less for kinetic information

---

breast motion and decrease the volume of tissue to be scanned so that the whole breast is included. However, marked compression is discouraged so there is free inflow of contrast material into the breast. Scanners with a magnetic field strength of 1.5 T or 3.0 T provide the best SNR. Magnets with high-performance gradients enable the fastest, highest resolution scans (Box 7.3).

Protocols and Image Processing

The ACR Breast MRI Accreditation Program recommends at minimum a T2-weighted/bright fluid series and at least a

TABLE 7.1 American College of Radiology–Based Minimal Standard Protocol and Requirements for Breast Magnetic Resonance Imaging

	Series	Requirements
1	Localizer	
2	T2-weighted/bright fluid series	Sufficient bright fluid contrast
3	Multiphase T1-weighted series Precontrast Early-phase postcontrast Delayed-phase postcontrast	Slice thickness ≤3 mm Gap 0 mm In-plane resolution ≤1 mm Bilateral breasts must be included Early-phase postcontrast imaging must be completed within 4 minutes after contrast injection Fat suppression or subtraction of precontrast from postcontrast series may be used bright signal from fat

All sequences must demonstrate sufficient signal-to-noise ratio and not appear too grainy.
From The ACR Breast MRI Accreditation Program. http://www.acr.org/~/media/ACR/Documents/Accreditation/BreastMRI/Requirements.pdf. Accessed October 2015.

three multiphase T1-weighted series including precontrast T1-weighted series, early-phase (first) postcontrast T1-weighted scan, and delayed-phase (last) postcontrast T1-weighted scans (http://www.acr.org/~/media/ACR/Documents/Accreditation/BreastMRI/Requirements.pdf; Table 7.1). Diffusion-weighted series are optional, and not yet standard of care.

Precontrast T1- and T2-Weighted Imaging

Conventional breast MRI begins with T1-weighted images, a so-called localizer or scout, to define the position and anatomy of the breast. T1-weighted images using the signal from the "body coil" rather than the breast coil enable basic evaluation of the axillae, anterior mediastinum, chest wall, and supraclavicular fossa for enlarged regional lymph nodes. Thereafter, the dedicated breast coil should be used to perform all subsequent sequences.

T2-weighted noncontrast fast spin-echo (FSE) images, or other sequences that shows fluid as high signal, are then obtained to characterize the breast and any lesions. T2-weighted scans using an FSE, turbo spin-echo (TSE), or rapid acquisition with relaxation inhibition technique, with effective echo time (TE) 80 to 100 ms and repetition time (TR) at least 3000 ms, produce high quality images within reasonable scan times of 5 to 6 minutes using 3- to 4-mm-thick slices and 256 × 192 matrix or higher for small FOV sagittal images.

High fat signal on T2-weighted FSE images can be prevented with fat suppression. Proper shimming of the magnetic field and choice of center frequency are essential to ensure adequate fat suppression. Bilateral high-spatial resolution imaging is possible on most scanners because of the development of hardware and software required for bilateral shimming and because coverage is possible with reasonable scan times. However, despite optimal shimming, the breast anatomy near the nipple, axilla, chest wall, and interior breast may cause unavoidable variations in B0 field homogeneity and fat suppression failures, resulting in artifacts. Evaluation of T1-weighted scan allows the radiologist to evaluate shimming of the magnetic field and helps determine whether any abnormally bright areas on fat-suppressed T2-weighted images are caused by poor fat signal suppression.

Dixon imaging (also known as two-point Dixon, three-point Dixon, IDEAL, or Flex) is another approach to water-specific imaging that uses the differential evolution of water and fat spin phase on nonfat-suppressed images obtained with different echo times to generate water- and fat-specific images, but may take longer than fat suppression, unless performed with high acceleration factors.

Diffusion-Weighted Imaging

Diffusion-weighted imaging (DWI) is an unenhanced breast MRI image sequence sensitive to the variability of water molecule mobility in vivo. The amount of movement or diffusion of a water molecule depends on the random molecule mobility called *Brownian motion*. In vivo, it is also affected by structural or biological factors, such as cell density, membrane integrity, vascular structures, and extracellular matrix composition. Higher signal intensity on DWI indicates increased restriction of diffusion. However, high DWI signal is occasionally seen in regions in which diffusion is not restricted; this is known as T2 shine-through phenomenon. *B*-values have not been standardized yet, but most investigators use 500 to 1000 with good results. Parallel imaging may reduce distortions in echo planar imaging.

ADC is a measure of the magnitude of diffusion, and is calculated from two or more DWI scans obtained at different *b*-values. A lower ADC value represents increased restriction of diffusion. The ADC map is more accurate in visualizing the diffusion variability than DWI, without misleading artifacts from the T2 shine-through phenomenon. A reliable estimation of the ADC requires perfect registration of high-quality source images at different *b*-values without motion artifacts.

Dynamic Contrast-Enhancement Study

Significant variation exists worldwide in methods used for the contrast-enhanced portion of the examination. Most investigators agree that both the time course of enhancement provided by dynamic contrast-enhancement (DCE) scanning and lesion morphology on high-spatial resolution scanning provide distinct and useful information about the risk of malignancy in enhancing lesions. However, commercially available MRI pulse sequences necessitate a compromise between the dynamic and high-spatial resolution approaches. Currently, most scans are done with repeated T1-weighted, fat-saturated, 3D spoiled gradient-echo (SPGR) scans (TR ≤6 ms; flip angle [FA] 10°–15° for T1 weighting). SPGRs provide adequate T1-weighted images with faster scanning than spin-echo sequences, but must be used with optimized flip or tip angles, depending on field strength and repetition time, for proper T1 weighting. Three-dimensional imaging is most often used to avoid interslice gaps, to image faster than 2D multislice imaging, to provide improved reformatted images caused by reconstruction of overlapping slice locations, and to avoid SAR limits at 3 T. Slice thickness and resolution are selected to give maximum resolution and bilateral whole-breast coverage within a 60- to 90-second scan duration. Parallel imaging, fractional *k*-space (1/2 NEX, etc.), and intermittent/partial fat saturation substantially speed up imaging, allowing much higher resolution within the same scan time. This sequence is repeated as rapidly as possible before, during, and for approximately 5 to 7 minutes after administration of a rapid IV bolus of gadolinium contrast agent. Most investigators use axial or coronal images with a rectangular FOV to maximize efficiency.

According to ACR guidelines (http://www.acr.org/~/media/ACR/Documents/PGTS/guidelines/MRI_Breast.pdf), dynamic images should be obtained at intervals separated by 4 minutes or less. In the authors' experience, a shorter time interval than 4 minutes is advised to capture the features of the dynamic curves. Contrast material should be administered as an IV bolus dose of 0.1 mmol/kg bodyweight, followed by a flush of at least 10 mL of saline, so that the entire bolus rapidly reaches the systemic circulation. A poor bolus may result in poor image quality or false-negative DCE curves. Although the ACR does not specifically recommend a specific rate for contrast injection, many studies achieve satisfactory results with 2 mL/s. All standard low molecular weight gadolinium-based contrast materials (gadoteridol, gadopentetate dimeglumine, gadobutrol, etc.) have been used by the vast majority of studies with very high-quality results, without clear differences in performance. Gadobutrol (Gadavist) is specifically labeled for use for breast MRI in the United States.

Subtraction images describes the images of contrast enhancement derived from a subtraction of precontrast images from postcontrast images so that only brightly enhancing findings are seen, such as cancer. Subtraction processing suppresses signal from bright fat because adipose tissue does not enhance significantly. However, motion artifact may plague subtraction images, resulting in grainy or noisy images with altered shapes or kinetics. Some software packages allow spatial smoothing of adjacent voxels, reducing noise and artifacts in color mapping, but at the risk of obscuring some intrinsic spatial heterogeneity and features within tumors. For this reason fat suppression is more often used so that high spatial resolution scans may reveal subtle features of cancer such as spiculated margins, and fat suppression can also reduce motion artifacts during subtraction processing. Fat suppression pulses applied intermittently can achieve good fat suppression with little effect on scan time; adiabatic spectrally selective inversion recovery fat suppression is the most efficient method that yields robust, rapid, high-quality images regardless of field strength from 1 T to 3 T.

Maximum intensity projections (MIPs) present the entire breast in a 3D display rather than a single slice to show the entire extent of enhancing findings from the first postcontrast scan. Kuhl et al. (2014) recently showed that a rapid 3-minute breast MRI first postcontrast subtracted T1-weighted image (FAST) scan displayed as an MIP showed 11 breast cancers (7 invasive and 4 ductal carcinoma in situ [DCIS]) in 443 women undergoing 603 screening rounds. MIP analysis showed a sensitivity of 98.9% increasing to 100% with the FAST images; this is a very promising technique for breast cancer screening. MIPs may be reconstructed to sagittal and axial projections resembling x-ray mammograms or may be manipulated to show either volume renderings or thin slabs to display extensive multifocal tumors or extent of nonmass enhancement, while limiting overlapping signal from other regions in the breasts. However, cross-sectional thin-slice MRI planes display fine details of lesions, whereas the MIP may obscure some internal features. Thus the MIP alone should not be used to diagnose tumors. On the other hand, multiplanar MIPs may be reformatted to display tumor distances to the nipple, skin, and chest wall; there are software programs that measure these distances automatically or semiautomatically.

A DCE curve (kinetic curve, or a time intensity curve) shows a lesion's signal intensity as a function of time during the bolus IV administration of contrast material and over the postcontrast scan time periods. This is usually done by using commercially available programs or computer workstations with the user drawing a region of interest (ROI) greater than 3 pixels large over the enhancing finding.

A variety of image-processing techniques have been developed to automate analysis of dynamic images throughout the breast. Most commercially available programs generate color maps and kinetic curves on a pixel-by-pixel basis using the following steps. First, the program calculates the *percentage of enhancement* or *relative enhancement* (*RE*) to the baseline/background signal intensity [SI] value at the operator-defined time point of the early postinjection phase using the formula $(SI1 - SI0)/SI0 \times 100$ (%), where SI0 and SI1 are signal intensities at the baseline and at the operator-defined early postinjection time, respectively. The early postinjection time point is usually defined as between 60 and 90 seconds or at least within the first 2 minutes after a bolus injection. The program then identifies voxels that enhance more than a specified threshold, which can be set by the operator (frequently an RE of 50%–100%, but may vary depending on the intrinsic T1-weighting of the scan protocol, which depends on field strength, FA, and scan repetition rate), at the early postinjection time point, and colorizes these voxels according to the subsequent dynamic kinetics during the delayed phase. The late postinjection time point is usually defined at 4 to 5 minutes after the bolus injection or later, because washout is generally seen at 4 to 5 minutes postinjection. Although no specific color has been set by ACR for the color of the lesion, most vendors determine the color using the following thresholds: (1) increase or decrease by 10% of the early-phase enhancement (Breast Imaging Reporting and Data System [BI-RADS] 2013) or (2) *signal enhancement ratio (SER)* of 0.9 and 1.1 (Hylton, 1999). SER is the ratio of SI at the early postinjection time point relative to SI at the late postinjection time point expressed by (SI1 − SI0)/(SI2 − SI0), where SI0, SI1, and SI2 are signal intensities at the precontrast, the early postinjection, and the late postinjection time points, respectively (Hylton, 1999). For example, voxels with persistent enhancement, characterized by increase of relative SI by at least 10% or defined as SER <0.9, is colored in blue, and those with washout enhancement, defined as decease of relative SI by at least 10% or SER >1.1, in red. The others, which belong to plateau kinetics, are colored in green or yellow. Suspicious lesions, that usually have plateau or washout kinetics, stand out against normally gradually enhancing background parenchymal enhancement (BPE).

Some software packages automatically calculate and segment breast tumor volumes by detecting suspicious enhancement kinetics (visually these would be based on their color). Automated volume measurements are less accurate in malignancies that are heterogeneous, enhance slowly or poorly, and may produce spurious results in the face of uncorrected motion artifact. Strong spatial variations in signal intensity caused by variations in surface coil sensitivity, and B1 + transmit inhomogeneity may also produce inaccurate breast tumor results.

Pharmacokinetic scans or physiologic scans are scans that superimpose physiologic maps, such as enhancement information, on morphologic images, combining both types of information into one format. This type of scan usually shows the morphologic appearance of a lesion with the physiologic image superimposed in color.

MRI Spectroscopy

MRI spectroscopy can be performed as an optional study to obtain information about the chemical content of breast lesions. Several studies have shown that choline-containing compounds (tCho) peak measured with hydrogen (^{1}H)-spectroscopy were more often elevated in malignant breast lesions than in benign lesions or normal breast tissues (Roebuck, 1998; Yeung 2001), suggesting the potential utility of MRI spectroscopy in the diagnosis of breast cancer. For single-voxel choline spectroscopy, a minimum voxel size of $1 \times 1 \times 1$ cm is recommended for adequate signal-to-noise. Localized shimming and high-quality spatial saturation pulses, fat suppression, and partial water suppression improve quality of spectra. It has been recommended to avoid negatively charged gadolinium agents if spectroscopy is performed after contrast enhancement study, because they may reduce choline signal (Lenkinski, 2009).

Common Magnetic Resonance Imaging Artifacts and Pitfalls

Common Artifacts

Common artifacts and pitfalls seen in breast MRI include line(s) of noise, ghosting artifact, blurring, misregistration artifacts, wraparound artifact (*aliasing*), susceptibility artifact, poor fat saturation, and chemical shift artifact (Table 7.2). They can make interpretation of breast MRI challenging and lead to misdiagnosis.

Lines of noise can be generated when there is electronic noise, room shielding is poor, scan room door opens, or there is a failure of MRI equipment.

Physiologic movement, including cardiac pulsation, respiration, or gastrointestinal peristalsis, as well as patient motion, can cause a few types of artifact. Physiologically moving objects, such as blood in the heart and vessels, pleural fluid, or bowel fluid, can become blurred and produce duplicated high signal intensity in the phase-encoding direction. This is called *ghosting* (Fig. 7.4). Ghosting occurs always in the phase-encoding direction, regardless of the direction of the motion. Ghosting can be prevented from obscuring breast tissue by careful selection of phase- and frequency-encoding directions, and by placing a saturation band over the moving structure. Patient motion can result in blurring of the entire image, so it is especially important that the patient hold still and breathe quietly during scanning. Specifically on subtraction images, patient motion can cause alternating bright and dark bands at structure interfaces (such as fat–skin or fat–glandular interfaces) called *misregistration artifact*, when the patient moves between the images to be subtracted (Fig. 7.5).

TABLE 7.2 Common Artifacts and Pitfalls

Artifact	Cause	Solution
Line(s) of noise	Electronic noise/poor room shielding/scan room door open	Close the door, call MRI service technician
Ghosting (eg, ghosting from heart across the breast)	Moving objects that cause wrong frequency-encoding direction, errors in parallel imaging	Change frequency direction to anterior posterior, correct parallel-imaging parameters
Blurring	Patient motion	Keep patient still
Misregistration (bright and dark edges on subtraction)	Patient motion	Keep patient still
Wraparound artifact (eg, wraparound from abdominal fat on sagittal images)	Aliasing from excited tissue outside imaging FOV	Increase the imaging FOV, perform oversampling (eg, change to axial scan plane from sagittal scan plane), decrease parallel imaging acceleration factor
Susceptibility artifact	Metallic objects that cause inhomogeneity in the magnetic field	Remove all metallic objects from breast
Poor fat suppression	Poor shimming, center frequency, non-MRI compatible skin marker left on breast, some anatomies	Repeat shim, remove all MRI compatible objects from breast, volume shimming over just the breasts
Chemical shift artifact	Shift of fat signal in the read-out direction relative to water signal.	
Failure of dynamic contrast enhancement study	Slow or failed contrast injection, delayed contrast injection, late MRI scanning, impaired heart function, etc.	Detect by putting ROI over heart and seeing poor contrast injection, use power injector followed by saline flush bolus, correct the protocol

FOV, field of view; *MRI*, magnetic resonance imaging; *ROI*, region of interest.

One other cause of noise, including unstructured noise or structured ghosting, arises from problems with parallel image reconstruction. Parallel imaging is an image-processing technique that uses spatial information contained in the component coils of an array to partially replace spatial encoding, which would normally be performed using gradients. There have been various parallel imaging techniques developed, such as ASSET, SENSE, mSENSE, GRAPPA, and ARC. The parallel imaging has advantages, including significant reduction in imaging acquisition time and reduction in susceptibility artifacts, but also has disadvantages, including reduction in SNR and increased artifacts caused by the additional imaging processing. These parallel imaging-specific artifacts happen if the acceleration factor and/or coil sensitivity mapping (obtained by the calibration scan) is not correct for the type of breast coil used and are caused by the shape and size of the patient.

Wraparound artifact (also called *aliasing* or *phase wrap*) is caused by aliasing from tissue outside the prescribed imaging FOV that is excited during the image acquisition process. In this artifact, the excited tissue outside the imaging FOV is misregistered and is wrongly superimposed on structures within the FOV in the reconstructed image (Fig. 7.6). Wrapped around artifact is mostly encountered in the phase-encoding direction, because wrapped around artifact in the frequency-encoding direction is usually suppressed by oversampling or the use of a frequency filter. To minimize wrapped around artifact in the phase-encoding direction, increasing the imaging FOV or oversampling in the phase-encoding direction can be used, although these techniques have several disadvantages, such as increasing imaging time and reducing the temporal resolution.

Susceptibility artifact is caused by metallic objects, which induce inhomogeneity in the magnetic field, and is shown as local signal dropout, bright spots, or tissue distortion (Fig. 7.7). Ferromagnetic metals (such as iron, nickel, and cobalt) cause more severe inhomogeneity compared with nonferromagnetic metals (such as titanium). *Susceptibility artifacts* appear more prominent on gradient-echo images than on FSE images, and at higher field strength (on 3 T than on 1.5 T). These are common around marker clips.

Poor or inhomogeneous fat suppression is usually caused by poor shimming or incorrect choice of the excitation center frequency (usually 220 Hz at 1.5 T), especially in patients with silicone implants or non–MRI-compatible objects, such as metallic BB skin markers, magnetic tissue expanders, metallic scar markers, and metal infusion ports, in or near the breast. Even with optimal shimming, the breast anatomy near the nipple, axilla, chest wall, and interior breast may cause unavoidable variations in B0 field homogeneity and fat suppression failures, resulting in artifacts. Poor fat suppression is easily identified as hyperintense fat on fat-suppressed images (Fig. 7.8).

Chemical shift artifact can be common on nonfat suppressed gradient-echo images. It occurs at the interface of fat:water pixels. Because the fat signal is shifted a few pixels in the read-out direction relative to water, there can be a piling up of combined fat:water signal at some interfaces, and lack of signal at others. This may cause artificial appearance of asymmetric skin thickness, and bright/dark signal around biopsy clips especially on spin-echo images.

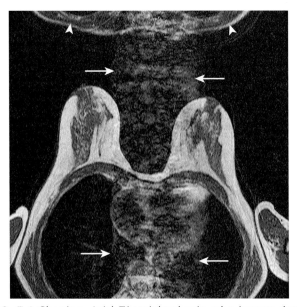

FIG. 7.4 Ghosting. Axial T1-weighted spin-echo images shows *ghosting* (*arrows*) from the heart, which linearly spreads to the phase-encoding direction. Note wraparound artifact (*arrowheads*) seen on the top of the image.

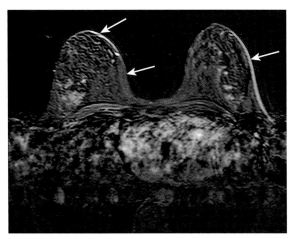

FIG. 7.5 Misregistration artifacts. Poor fat suppression on subtraction images is caused by patient motion, causing misregistration artifacts at fat–skin or fat–glandular interfaces (*arrows*).

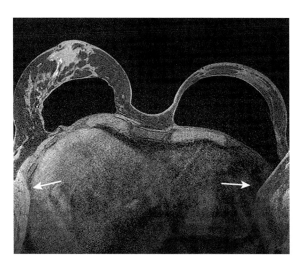

FIG. 7.6 Wraparound artifact. Axial precontrast water-specific T1-weighted image shows lateral sides of chest wall (*arrows*), which are outside of image field of view but are wrongly visualized at the right and left sides of the image. These *wraparound artifacts* are seen in the phase-encoding direction. Note bilateral breast implants, left mastectomy, and linear soft tissue representing postoperative scar in the right lateral chest wall.

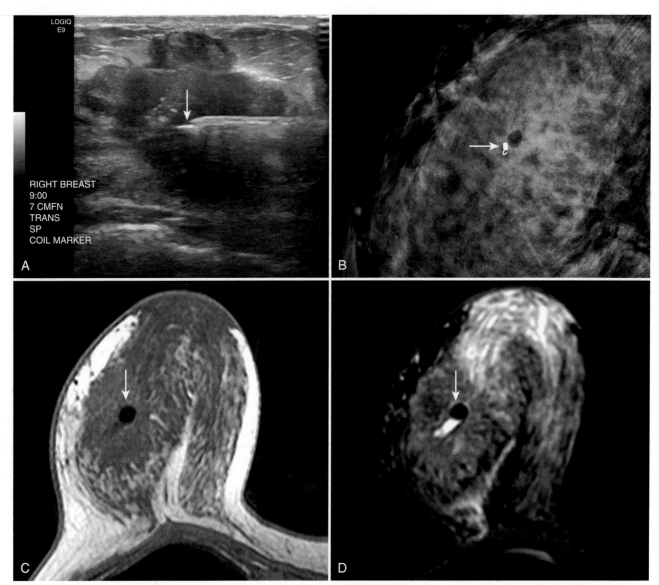

FIG. 7.7 Susceptibility artifact. (A) Ultrasound shows a coil lock–shaped titanium biopsy marker (*arrow*) placed within a mass through a needle after biopsy. Biopsy result was invasive ductal carcinoma. (B) Photographically magnified craniocaudal mammogram of the right breast shows the coil-shaped marker (*arrow*). Note air close to the marker caused by the biopsy. (C and D) Magnetic resonance imaging (MRI) was performed 2 weeks after the biopsy. T1-weighted image (C) and fat-suppressed T2-weighted image (D) show signal void from *susceptibility artifact* of the biopsy marker (*arrows*), associated with linear fluid collection at the biopsy site behind it. Because the marker is an MRI-compatible titanium clip, the susceptibility artifact is relatively small.

Pitfalls in DCE Studies

Only a good bolus of contrast and timely scanning will translate into breast cancer enhancing rapidly on MRI scans. Failure in DCE studies, including slow bolus, delayed bolus, or late scanning, may result in a nondiagnostic examination and may cause misinterpretation of kinetic curves. Before interpreting dynamic curves, it is important to assess if the technical factors producing the dynamic curves were optimal, resulting in dynamic data good enough to be evaluated.

Cardiovascular kinetic curve obtained with a ROI over large vessels (aorta) or the heart is a useful indicator of failure in DCE studies. The healthy heart/aorta usually shows normal rapid, avid (fast) initial enhancement and rapid late washout (Figs. 7.9 and 7.10A). Alternation of the normal cardiovascular dynamic curve pattern tells the radiologist that the DCE study is suboptimal (Fig. 7.10 B–D).

Slow or poor bolus of IV contrast may occur when the IV line is injected slowly or may even become detached from the vein, the connector may leak, the catheter may be kinked, there may be a poor saline flush, or heart function is impaired. The contrast either enters slowly, rather than in a bolus, or never enters the patient. Insufficient delivery of contrast media may cause the decrease or absence of the peak of cardiovascular dynamic curve (Fig. 7.10B), resulting in poor enhancement of breast lesions and leading to misinterpretation of the washout kinetics as plateau or persistent patterns.

Delayed bolus of IV contrast or poor circulation may cause the delay of the cardiovascular enhancement with or without decrease of the peak enhancement (Fig. 7.10C). The first post-contrast scan, which is usually performed to detect rapid peak enhancement, can be obtained earlier than expected, and thus cannot detect a cancer with rapid initial enhancement as different from background.

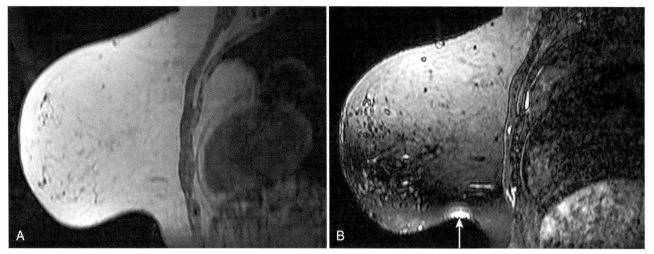

FIG. 7.8 Poor fat suppression. (A) The breast is almost entirely fat, which is bright on a 3D spoiled gradient-echo T1-weighted image without fat suppression. (B) The 3D T2-weighted fast spin-echo (CUBE) image with fat suppression shows variable fat signal. The fat is well suppressed in the lower half of the breast. In the upper half, poor shimming of the magnet field resulted in incomplete and only partial suppression of the fat signal. In addition there is focal fat suppression failure causing abnormal very high signal intensity (*arrow*) at the inferior margin of the breast. The inferior breast is one of the anatomic areas in which unavoidable variations in the B0 field naturally occur, which sometimes result in focal failures of fat suppression.

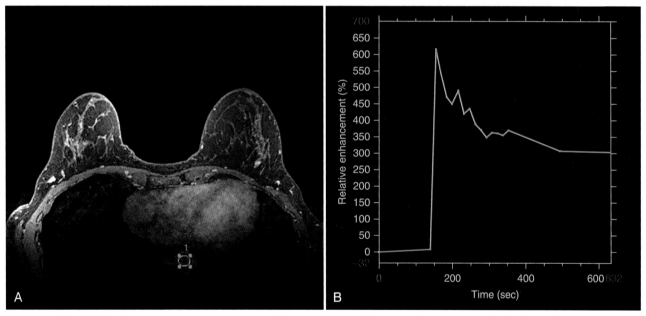

FIG. 7.9 Cardiovascular enhancement after intravenous bolus injection of contrast media. Region of interest (ROI) in the descending aorta (A) and its kinetic curve (B). The kinetic curve show fast initial enhancement followed by a relatively abrupt washout onset, indicating ideal bolus of contrast media and subsequent saline and normal heart function, which is the minimal requirement for the analysis of dynamic kinetics of breast lesions. Either the large vessel or heart ROIs can be checked for ideal cardiovascular enhancement.

In late MRI scanning, the early postcontrast scan can miss the peak enhancement (Fig. 7.10D). If a cancer has been already washed out at the start of MRI scan, a bright signal from the cancer during the early phase will be missed (Fig. 7.11). Late scanning is caused by an operator error and an incorrect protocol, or when a patient interrupts the scan. Cancers may be obscured by BPE with late scans.

When the cardiovascular dynamic curve pattern is altered, these MRI scans cannot be trusted to show cancer in the breast, and further investigation would be needed to determine the causes of the failed bolus or the late scanning. It is sometimes difficult even for trained technologists to notice the failure in contrast enhancement, thus it is important for radiologists to pay attention to the adequacy of contrast enhancement bolus whenever they assess DCE MRI studies.

Motion artifact is another cause that leads spurious results in DCE analysis. Patient motion can generate faulty kinetic curves if the ROI includes different parts of the lesion or if it includes the adjacent breast parenchyma instead of the target between dynamic images (Kuhl et al., 1999b). Particular attention should be paid to identify any patient motion.

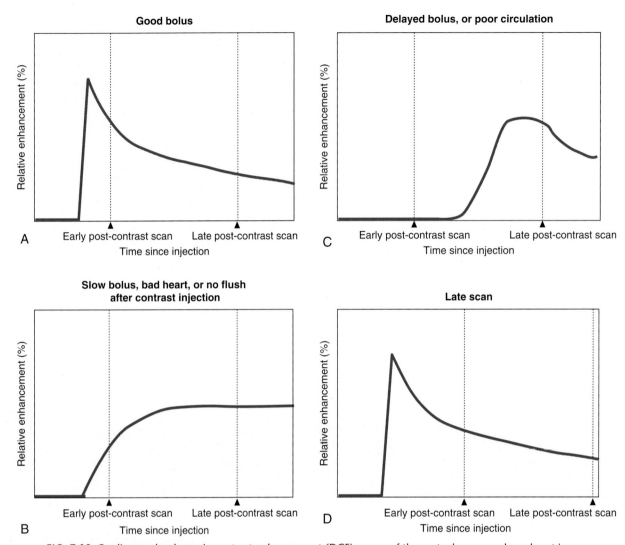

FIG. 7.10 Cardiovascular dynamic contrast-enhancement (DCE) curves of the aorta, large vessels, or heart in optimal and suboptimal DCE studies. (A) Representative study with good bolus. A steep, high peak of enhancement is observed in the aorta, large vessels, or heart immediately after the contrast media reaches them. This peak is followed by a relatively abrupt washout onset caused by the subsequent saline flush bolus and cardiac activity. (B) Slow bolus or bad heart. The cardiovascular enhancement gradually increases without a steep peak, and persists for longer time. Subcutaneous extravasation and absent saline flush also cause similar DCE curves. (C) Delayed bolus or poor circulation. The cardiovascular enhancement is delayed and reaches peak later than expected. The peak can be lower and flatter. (D) Late scan. The cardiovascular DCE kinetics is normal. However, because of the late scanning, the early postcontrast scan can miss the peak. Late scan is caused by an operator error and an incorrect protocol, or when a patient interrupts the scan.

INTERPRETATION OF BREAST MAGNETIC RESONANCE IMAGING

Contrast-enhanced breast MRI has high performance in the detection of breast cancer. Initial studies of contrast-enhanced MRI reported a sensitivity of more than 90% for invasive breast cancer. The sensitivity of contrast enhancement has remained high for invasive breast cancer. However, achieving high specificity remains difficult because some benign breast conditions enhance more avidly than normal breast tissue and may resemble breast cancer. Specifically, benign fibroadenoma, papilloma, and proliferative fibrocystic change (FCC) also enhance to a greater degree than normal surrounding breast tissue. Not surprisingly, the highest sensitivity and specificity of contrast-enhanced MRI arise when dynamic enhancement curves are taken into account.

This section first describes the MRI lexicon (except for breast implants) with optimal reporting defined or recommended by BI-RADS 2013. Then, the section discusses essential features of breast lesions on MRI in terms of morphology, DCE kinetics, and signal intensity, which may serve as clues to characterize the lesions. Then presented is a practical systematic image interpretation approach that achieves full assessment of each single MRI study. Finally, diagnostic limitations are discussed.

Magnetic Resonance Imaging Lexicon and Reporting Based on Breast Imaging Reporting and Data System 2013

The ACR BI-RADS MRI 2013 provides a valuable standard for the terminology used to analyze breast lesions on MRI (Table 7.3) and is recommended for all breast MRI reporting.

Breast composition should be stated in terms of the amount of FGT, the amount of the BPE, and the position of implants if they are present. The descriptors for important findings include size,

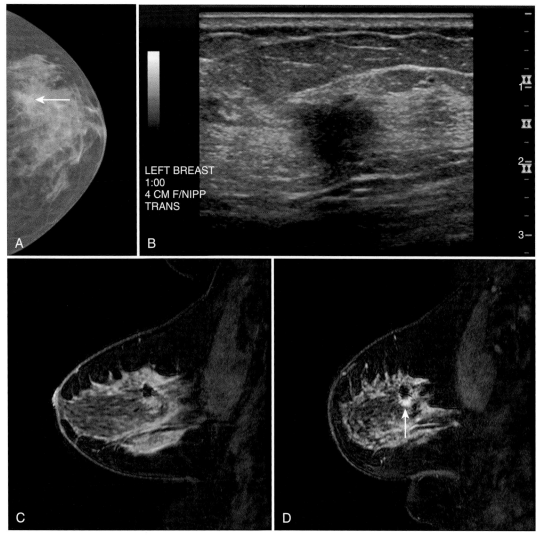

FIG. 7.11 Poor cancer enhancement caused by late scanning. (A) Craniocaudal (CC) mammogram of the left breast shows a focal asymmetry with possible spiculations (*arrow*) within dense fibroglandular tissue in the outer left breast. This was seen only on the CC view. Invasive ductal cancer (IDC) was proven by biopsy, followed by marker placement. (B) Left breast ultrasound shows a very hypoechoic irregular suspicious breast mass corresponding to the density seen in A. (C) Postcontrast sagittal 3D water-specific spoiled gradient-echo T1-weighted magnetic resonance image (MRI) shows heterogeneously dense breast tissue and marked background enhancement in the left breast. There is signal void from the marker placed in the IDC in the upper breast, but the cancer itself is not seen, possibly obscured by the marker or the surrounding background enhancement. However, it was noted the scan start was delayed to approximately 10 minutes after injection when normal breast tissue enhances and breast cancers have washed out. A repeat MRI was performed. (D) Repeat postcontrast sagittal water-specific T1-weighted was done within the first 2 minutes after injection when cancers enhance most brightly and the background tissue signal is least bright. Even though there is marked background enhancement in the left breast, there is a bright signal from the enhancing tumor (*arrow*) at the signal void because the scan was obtained at peak cancer enhancement (within the first 2 minutes of injection).

location, distribution, morphologic characteristics, and dynamic contrast features.

Abnormal enhancement, which is defined as enhancement significantly different and greater than normal BPE, is categorized as a *focus, masses,* and *nonmass enhancement.* Focus is a tiny dot of enhancement (<5 mm) that cannot be characterized otherwise. Masses are 3D space-occupying objects. Mass shapes are categorized as *oval, round,* and *irregular.* Mass margins are described as *circumscribed* or *not circumscribed* (*irregular* or spiculated). Mass internal enhancing characteristics include *homogeneous, heterogeneous, rim enhancement,* or *dark internal septations.* If the finding is a nonmass, its distribution should be further classified using the terms *focal, linear,*

segmental, regional, multiple regions, or *diffuse.* The radiologist further evaluates whether the finding is bilaterally symmetric or if it is asymmetric. Asymmetric findings are more likely to be cancer than are symmetric findings. The internal enhancement pattern of a nonmass should be classified as *homogeneous, heterogeneous, clumped,* or *clustered ring.*

In the kinetic curve assessment, the initial signal curve characteristics are classified as *slow, medium,* or *fast.* The late signal intensity curve characteristics are classified as either continually enhancing (*persistent*), flat (*plateau*), or washout (*washout*). Details of the BI-RADS definition in the kinetic curve assessment are described in the following section: Dynamic Contrast-Enhancement Kinetic Analysis.

TABLE 7.3 American College of Radiology Breast Imaging Reporting and Data System Magnetic Resonance Imaging Lexicon Terms and Classification Scheme

AMOUNT OF FIBROGLANDULAR TISSUE	**INTRAMAMMARY LYMPH NODE**
Almost entirely fat	**SKIN LESION**
Scattered fibroglandular tissue	**NONENHANCING FINDINGS**
Heterogeneous fibroglandular tissue	Ductal precontrast high signal on T1W
Extreme fibroglandular tissue	Cyst
BACKGROUND PARENCHYMAL ENHANCEMENT	Postoperative collections (hematoma/seroma)
Level	Posttherapy skin thickening and trabecular thickening
Minimal	Nonenhancing mass
Mild	Architectural distortion
Moderate	Signal void from foreign bodies, clips, etc.
Marked	**ASSOCIATED FEATURES**
Symmetric or asymmetric	Nipple retraction
Symmetric	Nipple invasion
Asymmetric	Skin retraction
LESION TYPE (SELECT ONE)	Skin thickening
Focus/foci	Skin invasion
Mass	Direct invasion
Nonmass enhancement	Inflammatory cancer
FOCUS	Axillary adenopathy
MASSES	Pectoralis muscle invasion
Shape	Chest wall invasion
Oval	Architectural distortion
Round	**FAT-CONTAINING LESIONS**
Irregular	Lymph nodes
Margin	Normal
Circumscribed	Abnormal
Not circumscribed	Fat necrosis
Irregular	Hamartoma
Spiculated	Postoperative seroma/hematoma with fat
Internal enhancement characteristics	**LOCATION OF LESION**
Homogeneous	Location
Heterogeneous	Depth
Rim enhancement	**KINETIC CURVE ASSESSMENT**
Dark internal septations	*Initial phase*
NONMASS ENHANCEMENT	Slow
Distribution	Medium
Focal	Fast
Linear	*Delayed phase*
Segmental	Persistent
Regional	Plateau
Multiple regions	Washout
Diffuse	
Internal enhancement patterns	
Homogeneous	
Heterogeneous	
Clumped	
Clustered ring	

Note: Focus = dot of enhancement so small (<5 mm) it cannot be otherwise characterized; mass = 3D, space-occupying lesion, convex-outward contour; nonmass enhancement = an area that is neither a mass or a focus; homogeneous = confluent, diffuse enhancement; heterogeneous = confluent and nonconfluent, mixed enhancement; clumped = confluent regions of enhancement, like cobblestones; clustered ring = thin rings of enhancement clustered together around ducts.

Reporting of kinetic data should also include the size of the region of interest used to generate the kinetic data and the location (ie, edge, center, entire lesion), as well as the overall degree of enhancement (ie, mild, moderate, strong).

From *ACR BI-RADS atlas, breast imaging reporting and data system,* ed 5, Reston, VA, 2013, American College of Radiology.

TABLE 7.4 American College of Radiology Breast Imaging Reporting and Data System Code Assessment Categories

BI-RADS Category	Definition	Likelihood of Malignancy	Management Recommendation
0	Incomplete	N/A	Recommend additional imaging
1	Negative	0%	Routine breast MRI screening
2	Benign	0%	Routine breast MRI screening
3	Probably benign	>0% but ≤2%	Short-interval (6-month) follow-up
4	Suspicious	>2% but <95%	Tissue diagnosis
5	Highly suggestive of malignancy	≥95%	Tissue diagnosis
6	Known biopsy-proven malignancy	N/A	Surgical excision when clinically appropriate

BI-RADS, Breast Imaging Reporting and Data System; *MRI,* magnetic resonance imaging.

From *ACR BI-RADS atlas, breast imaging reporting and data system,* ed 5, Reston, VA, 2013, American College of Radiology.

BI-RADS also provides recommendations on the framework of the MRI report and the definition of final category. Reporting should include clinical history, previous imaging examinations, and a brief summary of the scan technique (including the scanner, field strength, pulse sequences used, and the specifics of contrast injection), imaging findings described using the BI-RADS MRI lexicon, final assessment categories, and management recommendations. The radiologists' final impression of the study is sorted into categories numbered BI-RADS category 0 through 6 (Table 7.4), mostly like mammography. The first BI-RADS category, category 0, is used when additional studies, such as mammogram or targeted ultrasound, are needed at the end of a case to make a final assessment. Categories 1 and 2 are used for normal findings requiring no action, with essentially 0% likelihood of cancer. Category 3 is used for probably benign findings thought to have 2% or less chance of malignancy and for which a short-term, 6-month follow-up may be implemented. Category 4 encompasses a wide variety of findings for which biopsy is recommended. In breast MRI, category 4 is not currently subcategorized into 4A, 4B, and 4C, which are adopted from mammography. Category 5 is reserved for MRI findings highly suggestive of cancer, with 95% or greater likelihood of cancer. Category 6 is intended for cancers for which a known diagnosis has been established before definite therapy such as surgery or chemotherapy. At the end of the report, radiologists should provide a combined summary statement, including an overall assessment of suspicion for cancer, correlation with any other imaging studies, and recommendations for patient management.

Morphologic Analysis

The morphologic characteristics of enhancing malignant and benign lesions are summarized in Box 7.4, and are shown in Fig. 7.12. Consistent with mammography, masses with spiculated or very irregular borders are suspicious. Bright enhancement, particularly rim enhancement and enhancing septations, is usually suspicious for tumor angiogenesis. A ductal, linear, or segmental pattern of clumped (cobblestone-like) enhancement is suspicious for DCIS, but it can also be seen in benign duct ectasia or FCC. Clustered ring is worrisome for DCIS. Nonenhancing lesions are benign.

As with mammography, entirely smooth, oval, or lobulated masses oriented parallel to Cooper's ligaments suggest benign lesions, whereas lesions traversing Cooper's ligaments are abnormal and suggest invasive ductal cancer. Nonenhancing dark internal septations in smooth, oval, or lobulated masses are highly specific for a benign fibroadenoma, although they have been reported in mucinous cancers as well. However, it is important to evaluate the dynamic curves of benign-appearing enhancing masses because round or oval homogeneous cancers mimic benign fibroadenomas. Sometimes the suspicious kinetic curves may be the only clue that the morphologically benign mass is a cancer .

When evaluating lesion morphology, including shapes, borders, or internal enhancement patterns, Nunes et al. (2001) showed a sensitivity and a specificity of contrast-enhanced MRI of 96% and 80%, respectively, for cancer. Leong et al. (2000) reported the presence of either skin thickening, or a combination of a spiculated or microlobulated border, with a rim, ductal, linear, or clumped enhancement pattern was 54% sensitive and 94% specific for malignancy.

Dynamic Contrast-Enhancement Kinetic Analysis

Breast malignancies usually enhance rapidly after an IV bolus of gadolinium contrast material on DCE MRI (Fig. 7.13). Inflammation, angiogenesis, and tumor necrosis increases tumor vascularity, causing them to be of high signal intensity on the first postcontrast scan. Then, in the later phase, contrast material spreads into various tissues, including intratumoral fibrotic/necrotic portions and normal FGT, while contrast material is often washed out from dense cellular portions consisting of cancer cells within the tumor. In contrast, typical benign lesions poorly or slowly enhance.

BOX 7.4 Typical Morphologic Features of Benign and Malignant Breast Lesions

FEATURES SUGGESTING BENIGN LESIONS

Minimal enhancement
Circumscribed or gently lobulated margin
Homogeneous enhancement
Nonenhancing internal septations
Oriented along Cooper's ligaments
No enhancement
Center enhances first

FEATURES SUGGESTING MALIGNANCY

Bright enhancement
Spiculated, very irregular margin
Rim enhancement
Heterogeneous enhancement
Linear, linear-branching/segmental enhancement
Clumped or clustered ring enhancement

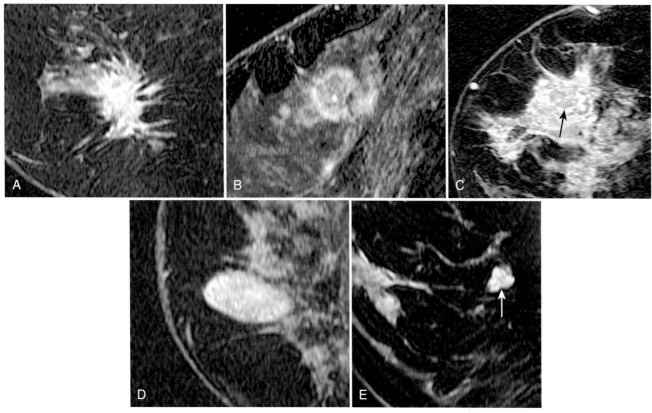

FIG. 7.12 Morphologic features of malignant and benign breast lesions. (A–C) Morphologic features suggesting malignancy include spiculated margin (A), rim enhancement (B), and irregular shape with heterogeneous internal enhancement (C, *arrow*). (D and E) Morphologic features suggesting benignancy include oval-shaped mass with circumscribed margin (D) and circumscribed round mass with dark internal septations (E, *arrow*).

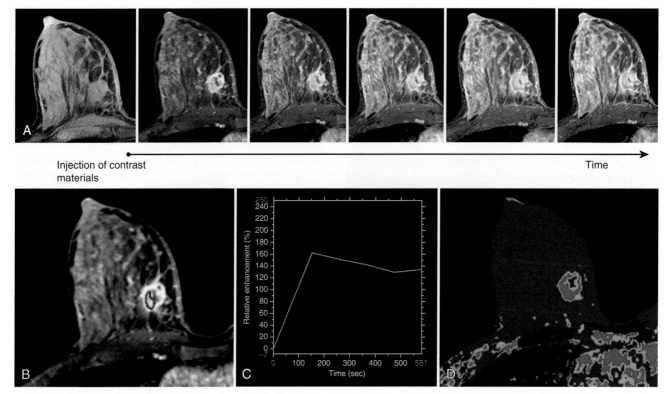

FIG. 7.13 Typical time course of contrast enhancement of breast cancer on dynamic contrast-enhanced magnetic resonance imaging (MRI). (A) Precontrast and five serial postcontrast water-specific T1-weigted images. On the first postcontrast image, breast cancer (histology, invasive breast cancer) enhances at its periphery around a central necrotic area with the brightest part at the mass edge, whereas the background parenchymal enhancement (normal fibroglandular tissue enhancement) is not obvious in the early phase. In the later phases, the early-enhanced area within the tumor is getting darker, representing washout kinetics. In contrast, the surrounding tissue around the mass, the central necrotic area, and the fibroglandular tissue, are getting brighter with time. (B and C) Region of interest is placed at the early-enhanced area within the tumor (B), and its kinetic curve represents the fast initial and late washout kinetics, corresponding to Daniel type V and Kuhl type III curves. (D) Color map (red, washout; green, plateau; blue, persistent) shows the tumor mostly has washout kinetics, shown as a ring-shaped red area, whereas the central area and background breast tissue show persistent kinetics colored in blue.

These dynamic kinetic curves have initial and delayed enhancement phases (Fig. 7.14). The 2013 ACR BI-RADS MRI Lexicon defines initial enhancement as a description of the kinetic curve in the first 2 minutes during the bolus or before the curve shape begins to change. It further defines the *initial-phase enhancement* as either *slow*, an increase of signal intensity less than 50% than baseline; *medium*, an increase of signal intensity 50% to 100% higher than baseline; or *fast*, an increase of signal intensity >100% higher than baseline. The slow initial rise curve usually indicates benign findings, whereas a fast initial curve may indicate suspicious findings. The 2013 ACR BI-RADS MRI Lexicon defines the delayed phase of enhancement as occurring after the first 2 minutes after contrast injection or after the curve shape starts to change. It further defines the *delayed-phase enhancement* as either *persistent* if the signal intensity increases by at least 10% of the initial-phase signal intensity, *plateau* if signal intensity does not change from the initial phase, or *washout* if the signal intensity decreases by at least 10% of the initial-phase signal intensity. A delayed-phase persistent curve usually indicates benign findings, whereas a delayed-phase plateau or washout curve indicates suspicious findings (Box 7.5).

Curve types may be classified by a five-category system suggested by Daniel et al. (1998b) or by a three-category system (Kuhl et al. 1999b; ACR BI-RADS; Fig. 7.15). In the five-category Daniel system—nonenhancing (type I); gradually enhancing (type II); or fast initial enhancement with a sustained gradual

enhancement, plateau, or early washout (types III, IV, and V, respectively)—types I and II typically indicate benignancy and types IV and V indicate a high likelihood of malignancy. Type III curves are indeterminate. Kuhl/ACR type I curves are gradually enhancing with a late persistent plateau. Kuhl/ACR type II curves have a fast initial enhancement with a late plateau. Kuhl/ACR type III curves have a fast initial enhancement with a late washout.

Generally, the most suspicious curve is one that has a fast initial rise and abrupt transition to a late-phase plateau or washout (see Fig. 7.13); the curve shape is also called a *square root sign* or a *cancer corner*. When Kuhl types II and type III are used as criteria to diagnose breast cancer, the three-category curve system had a sensitivity of 91% and a specificity of 83% (Kuhl et al., 1999b). A geographic distribution of dynamic enhancement also appears to be predictive, with tumors usually enhancing most rapidly at their periphery and benign lesions enhancing most rapidly at the center (see Box 7.5).

However, not all cancers or benign findings follow the rules. Not all cancers enhance rapidly, such as invasive lobular carcinoma (ILC). DCIS may exhibit any curve type, including nonenhancing or gradually enhancing curves. Some DCIS lesions may not enhance at all, and are found only as suspicious calcifications on mammography. Benign papillomas may exhibit any kinetic patterns, often initial fast/medium and delayed plateau/washout enhancement, and may mimic cancers. Normal lymph nodes usually enhance fast and wash out like most cancers. Therefore it is

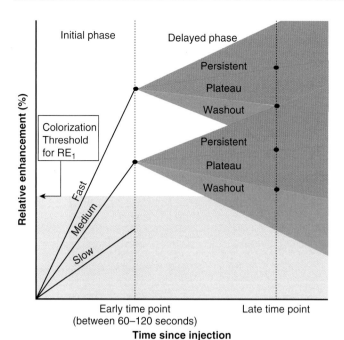

FIG. 7.14 Dynamic contrast-enhancement (DCE) curves. DCE curves consisting of two basis components: initial-phase enhancement and delayed-phase enhancement. ACR BI-RADS 2013 defines initial enhancement as a description of the kinetic curve in the first 2 minutes after bolus injection, and classifies it into three types: *slow* (relative enhancement less than 50%), *medium* (relative enhancement 50%–100%), and *fast* (relative enhancement >100%). The delayed phase of enhancement after the first 2 minutes is classified into three types with comparing the signal to that at the early time point: *persistent* (signal increases by >10%), *plateau* (signal change within ±10%), and *washout* (signal decreases by >10%). On a three-color map, pixels are colorized if their enhancement at the early time point exceeds an operator-defined threshold (frequently a relative enhancement of 50%–100% but may vary depending on the intrinsic T1-weighting of the scan protocol, which depends on field strength, flip angle, and scan repetition rate) when using a color code based on the delayed-phase enhancement. (Modified from Daniel B: Breast cancer. *MR and CT perfusion and pharmacokinetic imaging: clinical applications and theory*, Philadelphia, PA, 2006, LWW.)

Daniel et al. 1998	I	II	III	IV	V
Kuhl et al. 1999		Ia	Ib	II	III
ACR BI-RADS® 2013		I Slow persistent	I Medium persistent	II Fast plateau	III Fast wash-out

FIG. 7.15 Classification of the time course of dynamic contrast enhancement from the most likely benign (type I) through the most likely malignant (type V). No enhancement (Daniel type I) or gradual enhancement (Daniel type II, Kuhl type Ia, and Breast Imaging Reporting and Data System [BI-RADS] type I) suggests a benign lesion. Fast initial enhancement followed by gradual late enhancement (Daniel type III, Kuhl type Ib, and BI-RADS type I) is indeterminate. Fast initial enhancement followed by a plateau signal intensity (Daniel type IV and Kuhl/BI-RADS type II) or early washout of signal intensity (Daniel type V and Kuhl/BI-RADS type III) is suspicious for invasive malignancy. (From Daniel BL, et al: Breast disease: dynamic spiral MR imaging. *Radiology* 209:499–509, 1998b; Kuhl CK, et al: Dynamic breast MR imaging: are signal intensity time course data useful for differential diagnosis of enhancing lesions? *Radiology* 211:101–110, 1999b; ACR BI-RADS®—MRI. In *ACR BI-RADS atlas, breast imaging reporting and data system,* ed 5, Reston, VA, 2013, American College of Radiology; Modified from Daniel B: Breast cancer. *MR and CT perfusion and pharmacokinetic imaging: clinical applications and theory*, Philadelphia, PA, 2006, LWW.)

TABLE 7.5 T2-Weighted Imaging of Breast Lesions

	T2 > Glandular Tissue or Muscle	T2 ≤ Glandular Tissue
Enhances with contrast	Benign (eg, lymph node or hyalinized fibroadenoma)[a]	Possible cancer
Nonenhancing	Benign (eg, cyst or duct)	Benign (eg, sclerotic fibroadenoma or normal glandular tissue)

[a]The exceptions are rare mucinous carcinomas and some invasive ductal cancers, which may enhance and have high T2 signal; irregular, rim-enhancing morphology and dynamic enhancement curves may help with diagnosis.

BOX 7.5 Typical Kinetic Features of Benign and Malignant Breast Lesions

FEATURES SUGGESTING BENIGN LESION

Slow early-phase and persistent late-phase enhancement kinetics

FEATURES SUGGESTING MALIGNANCY

Fast early-phase and plateau or washout late-phase enhancement kinetics
Periphery enhances first

---

important to analyze contrast-enhanced images in combination with morphologic information and T2 signal characteristics.

Kinkel et al. (2000) reported the combined assessment of the dynamic kinetic curves and the margin status improved the diagnostic performance of DCE with a sensitivity of 97% and a specificity of 96%, compared with dynamic kinetic curve assessment alone with a sensitivity of 85% and a specificity of 87%.

Signal Intensity Analysis

T2-weighted imaging also plays an important role in discriminating which enhancing lesions are likely to be benign or malignant (Table 7.5). Generally, invasive breast cancers have a lower T2 signal similar to glandular tissue, higher than muscle but not as high as fluid (Fig. 7.16A). Lesions with very high signal, intrinsically much brighter than glandular tissue and even higher than fat on nonfat-suppressed T2-weighted FSE images, usually suggest benign lesions such as cysts, fluid-filled ducts, lymph nodes, or type I fibroadenomas (Fig. 7.16B–D). In addition, the T2-weighted study easily displays fat within bright lymph nodes, which helps distinguish them from cancer. Low-signal dark septations within very high signal smooth oval or lobulated lesions on T2-weighted imaging suggest benign fibroadenomas.

Exceptions to these rules include mucinous cancers, which can be very bright on T2-weighted images and occasionally contain dark septations like fibroadenomas. Similarly, some invasive ductal cancers may be bright on T2-weighted images. These

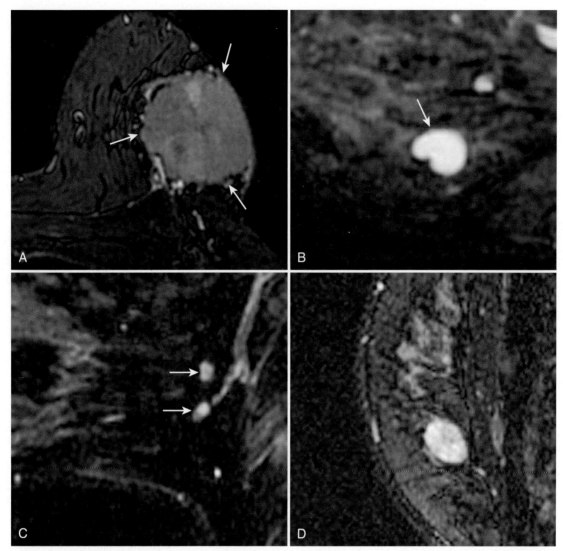

FIG. 7.16 T2-weighted imaging features of malignant and benign lesions. (A) Most malignancies, unless frankly necrotic, have a T2 signal intensity that is similar or slightly higher than that of fibroglandular tissue (*arrows*). (B–D) Benign lesions often have very high signal on T2-weighted images that are brighter than fat (on nonfat-suppressed sequences) and substantially brighter than glandular tissue. Three examples include a cyst (B, *arrow*), intramammary lymph nodes (C, *arrows*), and a fibroadenoma (D). Low-signal internal septations are particularly specific for fibroadenoma (D). The exceptions to high T2 signal occurring in only benign lesions are some invasive ductal cancers or mucinous cancers that have a high T2 signal.

T2-bright cancers often display irregular margins and internal inhomogeneity. However, it is important to check kinetic curves on all masses, because occasionally cancer may be round or oval and have circumscribed borders. Specifically, a benign-appearing oval or round circumscribed mass that looks like a fibroadenoma, T2-weighted bright or not, should be checked for a fast uptake and washout kinetic curve, because it might be cancer mimicking a benign mass.

DWI studies of breast cancers showed that ADC values may help contribute to the differentiation between malignant and benign breast lesions. Malignant lesions usually have lower ADC values than benign lesions and normal breast parenchyma (Fig. 7.17). It was thought that a higher cell density in breast cancer causes an increased restriction of the extracellular matrix, with the resultant increased signal fraction coming from intracellular water. With an optimal threshold used in individual studies, reported sensitivity and specificity range from 80% to 96% and 46% to 94%, respectively (Woodhams, 2005; Rubesova, 2006; Marini, 2007; Hatakenaka, 2008;

Yabuuchi, 2008; Bogner, 2015). A 2009 meta-analysis by Tsushima showed a pooled sensitivity of 89% (95% confidence interval [CI], 85%, 91%) and a pooled specificity of 77% (95% CI, 69%, 84%).

Practical Systemic Interpretation Guide

Practically, to achieve a complete, full assessment of the MRI study using many pulse sequences for each single patient, a systematic interpretation approach described in this section may be helpful (Box 7.6).

First, a radiologist reviews the breast history, clinical symptoms, prior biopsies, and results of other imaging tests. The radiologist then reviews the T1-weighted nonfat-suppressed scout images obtained at the beginning of the MRI scan. Because axial, coronal, or sagittal scout images have the largest FOV among the MR sequences obtained at a single MRI study, the scout images can be helpful to detect any unexpected findings outside the breast not identified by mammography and ultrasound before

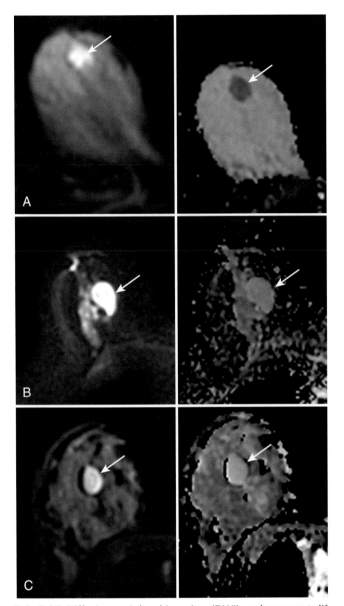

FIG. 7.17 Diffusion-weighted imaging (DWI) and apparent diffusion coefficient (ADC) map of malignant and benign lesions. (A) Breast cancer. DWI (*left*) shows a mass with high signal intensity. ADC map (*right*) demonstrates the mass is darker than the surrounding dense breast tissue, with a relatively low ADC value of 1.24×10^{-3} mm^2/s, indicating the restricted diffusion in the cancer. This was an infiltrating ductal carcinoma. (Case details in Fig. 7.42.) (B) Cyst. The cyst is bright on DWI (*left*) like cancers; however, it has higher signal intensity (ADC value 2.09×10^{-3} mm^2/s) than fibroglandular tissue on the ADC map (*right*), unlike cancers. The high signal on the ADC map indicates that the high signal intensity on DWI was caused by T2-shine through artifact, not by restriction of diffusion. (C) Fibroadenoma. DWI (*left*) shows a mass with high signal intensity, again caused by T2-shine through. The ADC map (*right*) demonstrates higher signal intensity (ADC value 2.78×10^{-3} mm^2/s) than the fibroglandular tissue. (Case details in Fig. 7.32.) Generally, malignant tumors have low ADC values, whereas benign lesions have higher ADC values. All DWI images were obtained with a *b*-value of 600 in the absence of contrast medium administration, and ADC maps were generated from DWI images with *b*-values of 0 and 600.

MRI. Other sequences should also be examined for abnormal findings outside the breast. Abnormal findings can be found elsewhere in the body on the breast MRI, including axillary lymph nodes (Fig. 7.18); lymph nodes within the mediastinum, supraclavicular regions, and other areas not commonly searched; lung (lung cancer, lung metastases; Fig. 7.19); bone (Fig. 7.20); liver (most commonly liver cysts); thyroid gland (Fig. 7.21); and adrenal gland and kidney (Fig. 7.22).

The radiologist then examines the noncontrast T1-weighted and T2-weighted (usually fat-suppressed) images. The T1-weighted precontrast scan provides a source image to let the radiologist know what findings had high signal intensity (sometimes seen in ducts filled with fluid or in blood-filled ducts) on precontrast studies. T2-weighted images allow the radiologist to see findings that are filled with fluid or have fluid-packed cells, such as type I fibroadenomas. In addition, the radiologist can see if fat is present within bright lymph nodes, which may help distinguish them from cancer.

Most breast lesions are best depicted on contrast-enhanced MR images. Specifically, the first postcontrast scan at approximately 90 seconds should have marked enhancement in the heart, blood vessels, and any rapidly enhancing finding, such as cancer or lymph nodes. The radiologist looks for the whitest part of the image, suggesting either BPE or abnormal enhancement. Once the radiologist has identified a possible enhancing lesion, it is classified as a *focus, mass,* or *nonmass enhancement*. Further characterization of the lesion is then done by its morphology, kinetic curves, and T1 and T2 signal intensity, as described earlier in this section. Finally, all lesions would be categorized into BI-RADS categories 0 through 6 based on the likeliness of malignancy and the recommended management following the MRI study.

Diagnostic Limitations

Although the sensitivity of MRI is very high for invasive carcinoma, significantly higher than mammography or sonography in some settings, substantial diagnostic challenges remain. Common false-positives mimicking DCIS include focal FCC, hormone-related enhancement, focal fibrosis, and

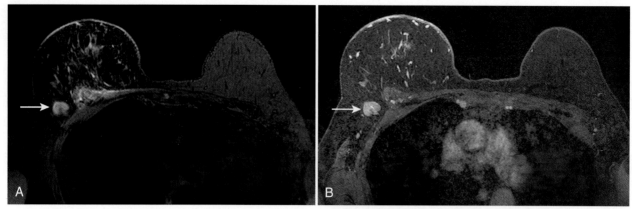

FIG. 7.18 Axillary lymph node metastasis. (A) Fat-suppressed noncontrast T2-weighted image shows an enlarged, hyperintense (but relatively low compared with bright normal nodes) lymph node in the right axilla with a thickened cortex and loss of the fatty hilum (*arrow*). (B) Early-phase postcontrast water-specific T1-weighted image shows that the node enhances (*arrow*). This represents lymph node metastasis from right inflammatory breast cancer. Because axillary nodal metastasis is the most common metastatic form of breast cancer and changes the subsequent patient management, the axilla should be evaluated routinely with breast magnetic resonance imaging as long as it is included in the field of view.

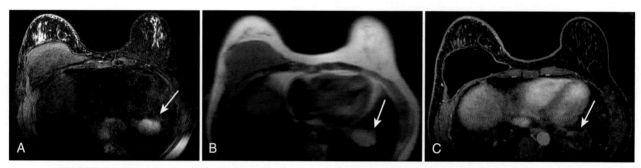

FIG. 7.19 Incidental findings on breast magnetic resonance imaging (MRI) scans: lung metastases. A mass is seen behind the heart in the left lung. This mass is hyperintense on fat-suppressed T2-weighted image (A), mildly hyperintense on T1-weighted image (B), and poorly enhances on postcontrast water-specific T1-weighted image (C). This was lung metastasis from breast invasive ductal carcinoma with mucinous feature and necrosis.

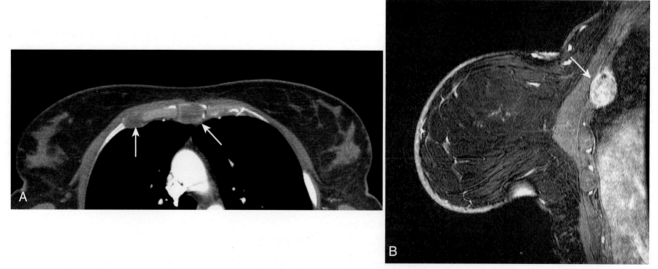

FIG. 7.20 Incidental findings on breast magnetic resonance imaging (MRI) scans: bone metastases. (A) Axial computed tomography (CT) scan shows expansive metastases of the sternum and the right rib (*arrows*). (B) Sagittal contrast-enhanced breast MRI shows the enhancing right rib metastasis demonstrated on the axial CT scan in A.

fibroadenomatous change (Box 7.7). False-positives occasionally mimicking invasive carcinomas include rapidly enhancing intraductal papillomas, avidly enhancing fibroadenomas lacking high T2 signal, intramammary lymph nodes without a fatty hilum, rim-enhancing fat necrosis, radial scar, and enhancing spiculated surgical scars (see Box 7.7). False-negatives remain rare; they are usually caused by nonenhancing DCIS or ILC (Box 7.8). Recent or ongoing chemotherapy may also reduce the sensitivity of contrast-enhanced MRI.

Small incidental enhancing lesions (IELs) are foci that are smaller than 5 mm, too small to characterize, and common. Investigators vary in the level of concern they attribute to these lesions. Regardless of size, an initial attempt should be made to characterize each lesion's morphology, dynamic enhancement, and T2 signal, because invasive carcinomas, fibroadenoma, and papilloma can also be very small. However, biopsy of an IEL frequently reveals no identifiable explanation. A practical approach to management is to use both the character of individual lesions along with their number and distribution, as well as the patient's clinical setting to determine whether biopsy or follow-up MRI should be performed. In patients at very high risk for occult breast malignancy, such as those with known axillary nodal metastases and normal mammograms and physical examination, even a single relatively nonspecific IEL that is the dominant abnormality in the breast may be the index tumor and should prompt biopsy. In patients with lower risk, multiple bilateral, diffusely scattered,

nonspecific small IELs have been successfully managed with serial MRI to document stability.

BREAST MAGNETIC RESONANCE IMAGING ATLAS

Normal Breast

Typical images from a normal patient who underwent both bilateral dynamic and high spatial resolution imaging are provided in Fig. 7.23. On T1-weighted noncontrast-enhanced images, aqueous tissues (including skin, FGT, muscle, and lymph nodes) have moderately low signal intensity compared with the higher signal intensity of fat, which has a short T1 relaxation time. In the absence of previous surgery or pathology, a layer of subcutaneous and retromammary fat completely surrounds the mammary gland tissue except where it enters the nipple-areola complex. The mammary gland itself is composed of a mix of low-signal FGT and high signal fat lobules. The mix and distribution of fat and FGT vary greatly between patients from dense, uniformly glandular tissue with almost no visible fat, to heterogeneous, to predominantly fatty tissue separated by thin strands or septa of FGT. In the ACR BI-RADS MRI 2013 lexicon, the amount of dense glandular tissue by volume is described in the same terms as used in the mammography lexicon. These include *almost all fat, scattered FGT, heterogeneously dense,* or *dense* (Box 7.9; Fig. 7.24).

T2-weighted noncontrast-enhanced images reveal heterogeneous FGT that is usually higher in signal intensity than adjacent muscle but still not as bright as the small subcutaneous blood vessels commonly seen at the periphery of the breast or as pure fluid (ie, cysts, ducts).

After contrast injection, the normal fibroglandular breast tissue enhances to variable degrees, but in generally does not enhance avidly. This normal fibroglandular breast tissue enhancement is called BPE in the 2013 BI-RADS lexicon. The radiologist judges whether enhancing foci in the breast are normal BPE or whether they are abnormal based on their morphology, symmetry, kinetics, and change over time. BPE usually enhances slowly in the initial phase and gradually continues to enhance gradually over time in the late phase (persistent; Fig. 7.25). The degree to which BPE occurs is not correlated with breast density on the mammogram or the amount of FGT on MRI (i.e., a dense extremely fibroglandular breast by volume may have little or marked BPE after IV contrast injection). The amount of enhancement cannot be predicted by how much

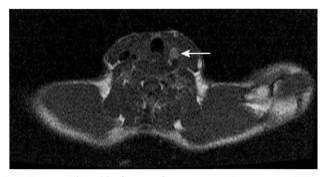

FIG. 7.21 Incidental findings on breast magnetic resonance imaging (MRI) scans: thyroid cyst. Noncontrast T1-weighted MRI to the neck shows a high signal intensity mass in the left thyroid gland (*arrow*). Ultrasound showed colloid cysts in the thyroid.

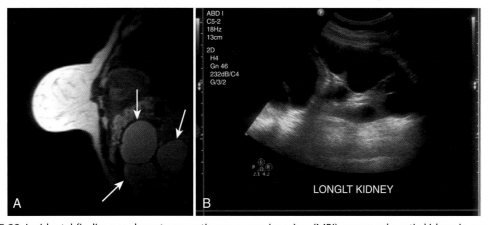

FIG. 7.22 Incidental findings on breast magnetic resonance imaging (MRI) scans: polycystic kidney in a patient with polycystic kidney disease. (A) The sagittal scout image in the patient with polycystic kidney disease shows multiple cysts in the left kidney below the diaphragm (*arrows*). (B) Renal ultrasound showed multiple left kidney cysts.

Fibrocystic change, hormone-related enhancement, or focal fibrosis, especially if unilateral and regional or if in a linear/segmental distribution mimicking ductal carcinoma in situ

Radial scar, especially if spiculated and rapidly enhancing

Surgical scar, especially if spiculated

Fat necrosis, especially if rim enhancing or lacking macroscopic central fat

Intraductal papilloma, especially if irregular, rapidly enhancing, and not associated with symptoms or a dilated duct

Fibroadenoma, especially if rapidly enhancing (hyalinized) and lacking a high T2 signal

Intramammary lymph node, especially if in an unusual location, lacking a visible fatty hilum, and not associated with a feeding vessel

Nonenhancing ductal carcinoma in situ (DCIS)

Nonenhancing invasive lobular carcinoma

Circumscribed mucinous tumor with bright T2 signal mimicking a fibroadenoma

Residual poorly enhancing tumor, especially DCIS during or after chemotherapy

Gradually enhancing tumor surrounded by marked background parenchymal enhancement (e.g., from scanning at the wrong time in the menstrual cycle)

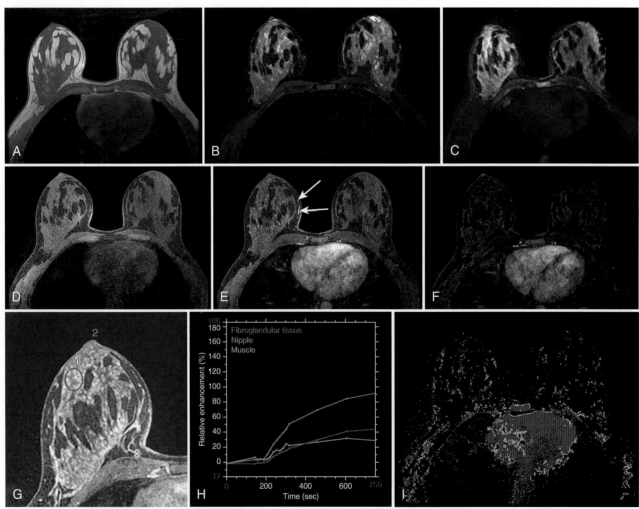

FIG. 7.23 Normal breast on magnetic resonance imaging (MRI). (A) Axial 3D fast spoiled gradient-echo T1-weighted image reveals high-signal fat within the breast and axilla. Soft tissues, including skin, fibroglandular tissue, lymph nodes, and muscles are dark. (B) Fat-saturated, T2-weighted fast spin-echo images reveal dark signal within fat and moderately low signal within the pectoralis muscle. Glandular tissue has mixed T2-weighted signal intensity and is symmetric. (C) Diffusion-weighted image shows moderately high signal within fibroglandular tissue. (D) Precontrast 3D water-specific T1-weighted gradient-echo image reveals dark fat and moderately low fibroglandular and muscle tissue signal. (E) Early postcontrast 3D water-specific T1-weighted image reveals enhancing vascular vessels (*arrows*) and mild nipple enhancement. (F) Subtraction processing of early postcontrast images (E) minus precontrast baseline images (D) reveals diffuse low-level fibroglandular and muscle enhancement. (G and H) Dynamic contrast-enhancement curves obtained using regions of interest shown in G revealed mild (<50%) gradual enhancement in the fibroglandular tissue, mild to moderate (around 50%) gradual enhancement in the nipple, and mild (<50%) fast enhancement in the pectoralis muscle. (I) Three-color map shows the most parts of the fibroglandular tissue, the nipple and the muscle is colored in blue, representing persistent dynamic kinetics (red, washout; green, plateau).

glandular tissue is present. An understanding of normal background enhancement is important because normal BPE can obscure cancers and make the MRI harder to read. BPE has various patterns including stippled enhancement (tiny <5 mm foci of enhancement separated by normal tissue) that can be scattered, diffuse, regional, or within multiple regions of enhancement throughout both breasts. These areas of normal BPE show dotlike enhancements usually separated by nonenhancing normal breast tissue. Occasionally, BPE may be limited to the

---

BOX 7.9   Amount of Fibroglandular Tissue: Assessed on Fat-Saturated T1W Imaging or Nonfat-Saturated T1 Imaging

Almost entirely fatty
Scattered fibroglandular tissue (FGT)
Heterogeneous FGT
Extreme FGT

---

periphery of the FGT away from the nipple, which is called *cortical enhancement*. In the 2013 BI-RADS lexicon, the amount of background enhancement is visually determined (categorizing based on percentages is not recommended currently) usually on the first postcontrast image, and categorized as *minimal, mild, moderate,* and *marked* (Box 7.10; Fig. 7.26) and whether the enhancement is *symmetric or asymmetric*.

The amount of background enhancement depends on the patient's hormonal status, menstrual cycle phase, and whether the patient is premenopausal or postmenopausal. For example, in premenopausal women, normal breast tissue enhances most avidly right before the onset of menses, and may show marked BPE. The normal breast tissue enhances the least 7 to 14 days after the onset of menses, and the same women who showed marked BPE before menses may show minimal or no BPE 7 to 14 days after the onset of menses. Postmenopausal women on exogenous hormone therapy (HRT) may display avid, marked BPE after starting HRT. Women on aromatase inhibitors, who have undergone neoadjuvant chemotherapy or radiation therapy, may show decreased BPE. Of course, cancers can occur in both

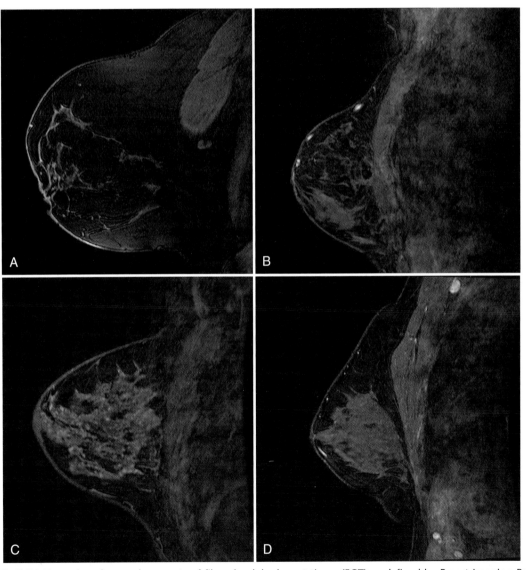

FIG. 7.24 Examples of normal amounts of fibroglandular breast tissue (FGT) as defined by Breast Imaging Reporting and Data System 2013 on magnetic resonance imaging (MRI) by volume on noncontrast sagittal 3D water-specific spoiled gradient-echo T1-weighted scans. (A) Sagittal postcontrast MRI shows mostly fatty tissue defined as "almost entirely fat." (B) "Scattered fibroglandular tissue." (C) "Heterogeneous fibroglandular tissue." (D) "Extreme fibroglandular tissue," previously dense glandular tissue.

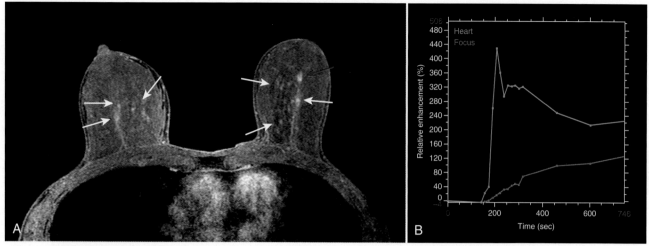

FIG. 7.25 Normal breast magnetic resonance imaging (MRI) with minimal background parenchymal enhancement. (A) On delayed-phase postcontrast 3D water-specific T1-weighted image, there are nonspecific multiple enhancing foci (*arrows*). (B) Kinetic curve of one focus (pink arrow on A) show slow initial and late persistent enhancement, whereas the heart demonstrates fast initial and late washout enhancement, suggesting good bolus.

BOX 7.10   Background Parenchymal Enhancement: Refers to the Normal Enhancement of Fibroglandular Tissue, Occurs on the First Postcontrast Imaging at Approximately 90 Seconds

LEVEL

Minimal
Mild
Moderate
Marked

SYMMETRIC OR ASYMMETRIC

Symmetric
Asymmetric

Note: Background enhancement details how much of the breast tissue is enhancing, which may obscure a breast cancer.

---

the dense or fatty parts of the breast. Some authors have shown that a decrease in BPE after neoadjuvant chemotherapy may predict tumor response to treatment, and others suggest that avidly enhancing BPE may be an independent risk factor for subsequent development of breast cancer.

Reporting normal background enhancement gives a clinician and other radiologists an idea of how likely it would be for the normal enhancing structures to hide a breast cancer and how confident the radiologist is in detecting breast cancer on the MRI.

After contrast injection, peripheral small subcutaneous vessels, the nipple, adjacent retroareolar tissue, and muscle enhances to variable degrees (see Fig. 7.23). The normal nipple enhances along its edge in a thin line; the rest of the nipple is dark, with an occasional dot of enhancement centrally within the nipple itself. The areolar complex is dark on the normal MRI. The normal skin is 2 to 3 mm in thickness and may enhance only slightly, but normally does not enhance. Skin enhancement is abnormal.

Dynamic imaging shows that FGT enhances mildly and slowly (see Fig. 7.23). Nipple enhancement curves are more avid, but still gradual. Muscle enhances rapidly at first, but never enhances very avidly. Subtraction imaging of a normal breast should show mild glandular and muscle enhancement. Normal breast tissue kinetic curves show a slow initial rise and a late persistent plateau. This normal slow initial and late persistent curve helps to distinguish normal breast tissue from cancers.

Variations of Breast Parenchyma

Hormone-Mediated Variations of Background Parenchymal Enhancement

Hormone-related enhancement occurs in premenopausal women and women taking oral contraceptives, and is a cause for normal BPE, which on occasion may be moderate or marked. Usually, diffuse gradual glandular enhancement is seen, and it is commonly bilateral, diffuse, and symmetric. Dynamic enhancement is generally initially slow, gradual with a late persistent phase (Daniel type II, III; Kuhl/ACR type I), and is rarely confused with invasive carcinoma on dynamic imaging. However, because of marked variations throughout the menstrual cycle in premenopausal women, overall BPE is lowest 7 to 14 days after onset of menses, increases thereafter, and peaks at the fourth week after menses onset. Less commonly, hormone-related enhancement may be focal and asymmetric (Fig. 7.27) and may resemble lobular carcinoma or DCIS, requiring short-term follow-up to distinguish it from temporary normal BPE. Hormone-related enhancement is minimized by scanning during the second week of a woman's menstrual cycle.

BPE can be decreased with aromatase inhibitors, after breast conservation and radiation therapy, and in postmenopausal women. Some studies suggest that a decrease in BPE after neoadjuvant chemotherapy may predict tumor response to treatment, and other studies suggest that avidly enhancing BPE may be an independent risk factor for subsequent development of breast cancer.

Lactation

In lactating women, breast volume and density increase as glandular tissue hypertrophies to produce milk. Breast parenchyma often becomes a high T2-weighted signal intensity and associates with dilated central ducts (Espinosa et al., 2005). In the DCE study, fast or medium initial enhancement can be observed from increased perfusion; however, the overall peak level of enhancement is less than many other breast lesions, such as fibroadenomas and cancers. Although diagnostic accuracy of breast cancer among lactating women has not been fully defined, Espinosa et al. (2005) showed invasive carcinomas were readily apparent on both the nonenhanced T2-weighted images and the contrast-enhanced images (Fig. 7.28), against the surrounding lactating tissue with high T2-weighted signal intensity and less enhancement.

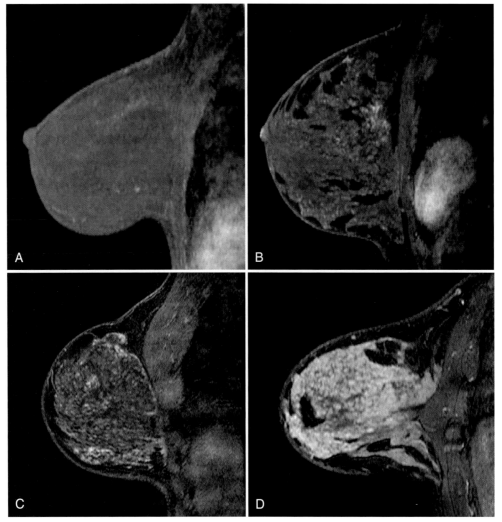

FIG. 7.26 Background parenchymal enhancement (BPE) on contrast-enhanced breast magnetic resonance imaging. (A) Minimal BPE in extreme (dense) fibroglandular tissue. (B) Mild BPE in heterogeneous (dense) fibroglandular breast tissue. (C) Moderate BPE in heterogeneous (dense) fibroglandular tissue. (D) Marked BPE in extreme (dense) fibroglandular tissue with marked BPE.

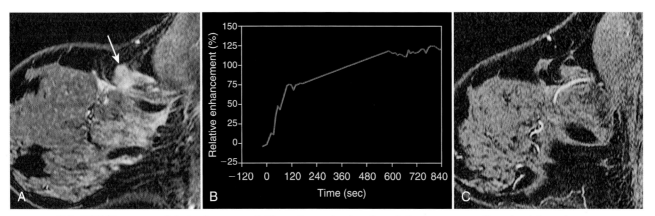

FIG. 7.27 Hormone-related enhancement. Normal menstrual cycle variations may cause fibroglandular enhancement. Although hormone-related enhancement is usually mild and diffuse, it may occasionally cause focal intense enhancement that can simulate disease (A, *arrow*). Even though the persistent late enhancement suggested a benign etiology (B), repeat breast magnetic resonance imaging was performed during the second week of the menstrual cycle (C) and showed that all previous findings had resolved and were presumably related to menstrual cycle variations.

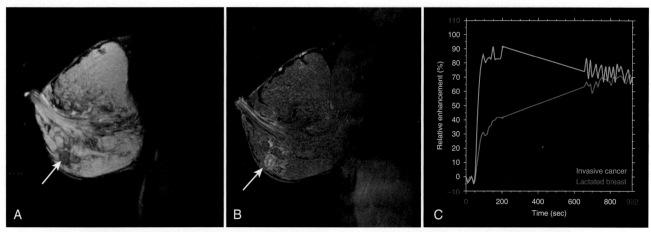

FIG. 7.28 Lactating breast with invasive breast cancer. (A) Sagittal fat-suppressed T2-weighted image shows a very dense (extreme), hyperintense hypertrophic fibroglandular tissue associated with dilated central ducts, representing lactating breast. There is a 1.6-cm mass with relatively low signal intensity in the lower breast. (B) On sagittal early-phase postcontrast water-selective T1-weighted image, the mass is depicted as an oval rim-enhancing mass that enhances more intensely than the surrounding fibroglandular tissue. (C) The kinetic curve of the mass shows fast initial enhancement followed by washout kinetics, which is worrisome for malignancy. This was an invasive ductal cancer. On the other hand, the lactating breast tissue has a fast initial followed by gradual persistent late enhancement kinetic pattern. In this case the cancer during lactation was readily identifiable on both T2-weighted image and contrast-enhanced image. (From Daniel B: Breast cancer. *MR and CT perfusion and pharmacokinetic imaging: clinical applications and theory*, Philadelphia, PA, 2006, LWW.)

The overall amount of gadolinium-based contrast material excreted into breast milk is minimal, and the amount transferred to a nursing infant orally is estimated to be quite low (Kubik-Huch, 2000). The ACR Committee on Drugs and Contrast Media considers that the available data suggest it is safe for the mother and infant to continue breast feeding after receiving such an agent (ACR Committee on Drugs and Contrast Media, 2015). However, they also recommend that, if the mother remains concerned about any potential ill effects to the infant, she may abstain from breast feeding from the time of contrast administration for a period of 12 to 24 hours and discard the breast milk after contrast administration until breast feeding resumes.

Fibrocystic Change

FCC is a common benign breast finding and is often associated with focal (geographic) or regional nonspecific enhancement, especially in premenopausal women, with slow, gradual early enhancement, and with sustained gradual, persistent late enhancement. Occasionally, a specific diagnosis can be made by the presence of tiny associated microcysts. FCC can be associated with stromal fibrosis, adenosis, macrocysts, or apocrine metaplasia. Adjacent cysts do not necessarily exclude carcinoma; however, so careful scrutiny of all enhancing foci remains essential to exclude concurrent malignancy.

Physiologic and Benign Lesions

Table 7.6 summarizes noncontrast signal intensity and the morphologic and kinetic enhancement features of major physiologic and benign lesions, including cyst, papilloma, fibroadenoma, fat necrosis, and old scar, as well as normal lymph node. Notice that papilloma may mimic breast cancer with initial rapid/medium and delayed washout/plateau kinetics. Type I fibroadenomas and cysts are typically bright on noncontrast T2-weighted scans.

Duct Ectasia and Breast Cysts

Fluid-filled cysts and focally dilated fluid-filled ducts are normal and occur frequently. Simple cysts are round or oval with sharp margins (Fig. 7.29). Adjacent cysts may be separated by thin, low-signal septations. Simple cysts have very high T2 signal and display no internal enhancement with contrast, although a faint thin rim of gradual enhancement may be seen on high-resolution images. An inflamed cyst can have a thin rim of enhancement. Occasionally, benign cysts may demonstrate high signal on unenhanced T1-weighted images, with corresponding lower signal on T2-weighted images, presumably because of their protein content or blood products. Fluid-filled galactoceles in the lactating breast are similar to cysts in appearance, and also do not enhance. Dilated fluid-filled ducts are linear, radiate from the nipple, commonly occur in the anterior breast, and may branch (Fig. 7.30).

They appear as nonenhancing tubular structures extending from the nipple and may have high T1-weighted signal if they contain proteinaceous secretions or met-hemoglobin from blood products (especially if there is a patient complaint of bloody nipple discharge). High intrinsic bright T1-weighed signal does not usually indicate malignancy if there is no associated enhancement. However, the intrinsic bright T1-weighed signal may be associated with intraductal mass enhancement and is a limitation of MRI to detect intraductal mass, such as papillomas, in the setting of bloody nipple discharge. Subtraction may be useful to highlight areas of enhancement when there is a background of intrinsically high signal cysts or ducts on unenhanced T1-weighted images.

Intramammary Lymph Nodes

Intramammary lymph nodes are common, especially in the upper outer quadrant and along blood vessels. Typically, intramammary nodes are small (≤5 mm) and have uniform high T2 signal in their cortex (Fig. 7.31). They are sharply circumscribed oval or kidney bean–shaped masses that have a central fatty hilum. On dynamic imaging, they enhance avidly and rapidly, with a fast initial enhancement and a late-phase plateau or washout (Fig. 7.31); hence, cannot be distinguished from malignancy based on dynamic criteria alone. Sometimes a normal fatty hilum can cause a central low signal on fat-suppressed or subtracted images that mimics rim enhancement. However, a

TABLE 7.6   Typical Magnetic Resonance Imaging Features of Physiologic and Benign Lesions

	Signal Intensity		Contrast-Enhanced Imaging			
	T1	T2	Overall Enhancement	Morphology	Initial Dynamic Pattern	Late Dynamic Pattern
Cyst	Dark, occasionally high	Bright	None	Mass with circumscribed margin (may have rim enhancement)	None	None
Lymph node[a]	Dark cortex Bright fat in hilum	Bright cortex Dark fat in hilum	Well	Mass with circumscribed margin with central fatty hilum	Rapid	Washout
Fibroadenoma: myxoid, hyalinized (type I)	Dark	Bright	Well	Mass with circumscribed margin (may have dark internal septations[b])	Variable	Persistent/plateau
Fibroadenoma: old, sclerotic (type II or III)	Dark	Dark	Enhance (type II), not enhanced above background (type III)	Mass with circumscribed margin	Slow or none	Persistent
Papilloma	Dark	Dark or bright	Well	Variable (associated with fluid-filled duct)	Fast/medium	Washout/plateau/persistent
Postsurgical scar	Dark	Bright soon after surgery Dark	Variable None or minimal after 12–18 months	Irregular	Slow	Persistent
Fat necrosis	Dark, bright fat in center	Dark	Variable	Rim (fat in center)	Slow/medium/fast	Persistent/occasionally, washout

[a]Lymph nodes are usually in the upper outer quadrant near blood vessel.
[b]Twenty percent of fibroadenomas have dark internal septations.

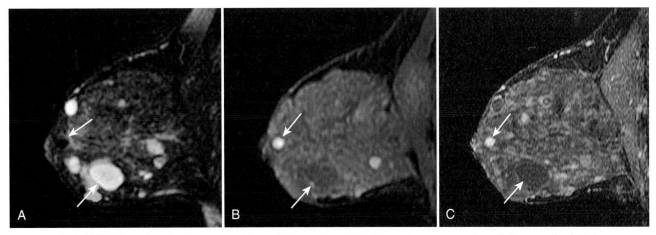

FIG. 7.29 Normal variants: a case with multiple cysts. (A) Benign cysts cause focal, well-circumscribed high signal (*bottom arrow*) on noncontrast T2-weighted images. (B) On unenhanced T1-weighted images, normal cysts appear dark with low signal intensity (*bottom arrow*); however, some benign cysts may appear bright (*top arrow*) because of the signal intensity of internal debris. This precontrast intrinsic high signal should not be mistaken for contrast enhancement on postcontrast scans. Some facilities use subtraction postprocessing to avoid this problem. (C) Postcontrast magnetic resonance imaging. Normal benign cysts do not enhance, but they may be surrounded by a faint rim of gradual enhancement (*bottom arrow*).

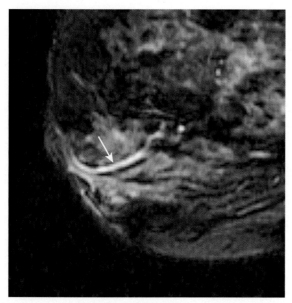

FIG. 7.30 Normal variants: dilated ducts. Dilated milk ducts cause linear high signal extending from the nipple (*arrow*) on fat-suppressed noncontrast T2-weighted fast spin-echo images.

definitive diagnosis is usually possible when lesion morphology shows their fatty hilum (T1-high and T2-low signal), close proximity to blood vessels with a "grapes on a vine" appearance, and uniform high intensity on T2-weighted image. Correlation with sonography may avoid biopsy in cases in which location or morphologic criteria remain inconclusive. MRI is not as reliable as sentinel node sampling in determining the presence or absence of intranodal metastases. Abnormal lymph nodes become rounder, enlarge from prior studies, and lose their fatty hilum. Lymphadenopathy can also be diagnosed when the node becomes completely replaced by metastases and becomes dark (instead of light) on T2-weighted images.

Fibroadenoma

Fibroadenoma is a common benign breast mass often found in young women. Hochman et al. (1997) classified fibroadenomas into three types based on T2-signal intensity and contrast enhancement on MRI: type I (T2-high, intensely enhance), type II (T2-low, enhance), and type III (T2-low, do not enhance). Type I fibroadenoma usually represents hyalinized cellular fibroadenoma containing myxoid stroma, and appears as a T2-bright, sharply marginated, oval, or macrolobulated mass with avid and uniform contrast enhancement (Fig. 7.32). Types II and III fibroadenomas are both dark on T2-weighted scans, but type II enhances with contrast above background (Fig. 7.33), whereas type III does not. More sclerotic stroma and older age in fibroadenomas are associated with low T2-signal intensity and lack of enhancement.

Nonenhancing dark internal septations is a specific sign of fibroadenomas and is seen in about 20% of cellular fibroadenomas (Fig. 7.34). However, dark internal septations may also very rarely be seen in mucinous cancer, so dynamic contrast features on benign-appearing masses should be evaluated to distinguish fibroadenomas from T2-bright mucinous cancers.

On dynamic imaging, most fibroadenomas show early gradual enhancement with sustained late gradual enhancement scans. However, young fibroadenomas may have a fast initial enhancing curve with sustained or persistent late-phase gradual enhancement (see Fig. 7.32) and occasionally demonstrate a late plateau of signal intensity that overlaps with the appearance of some invasive cancers. In these cases, the geographic distribution of

dynamic enhancement can be another clue to distinguish them from invasive cancers. In fibroadenomas, most avid enhancement is frequently central rather than peripheral, whereas cancers enhance most rapidly at their periphery.

The rare, well-differentiated phyllodes tumor has an appearance similar to that of fibroadenomas.

Intraductal Papilloma

Intraductal papillomas occur in the breast ducts as proliferation of ductal epithelium with central fibroglandular stalk that can cause bloody or serous nipple discharge and can expand the breast duct. Clinically, papillomas may present spontaneous bloody or nonbloody nipple discharge, and can be detected as an intraductal filling defect on galactography or an intraductal mass on ultrasound. Intraductal papilloma has a wide variety of appearances on MRI. In many cases, a papilloma is found as a round enhancing mass with a fast or medium initial enhancement and late-phase washout or plateau, mimicking breast cancer (Fig. 7.35), and thus is a common cause of false-positives on MRI. In other cases, a papilloma enhances slowly. In cases with a complaint of nipple discharge, a dilated fluid-filled duct leading to the enhancing mass can be found on T2-weighted images. The analogous classic finding on MRI is an avidly enhancing mass at the posterior end of a fluid-filled duct (Fig. 7.36). Occasionally, high T1-signal precontrast fluid in breast ducts may mask an enhancing intraductal papilloma, unless subtraction images are used, and is a possible cause of false-negative MRI studies. Asymptomatic papillomas are not uncommonly detected on MRI. Multiple papillomas or papillomatosis may be seen but are uncommon, and may require either biopsy or serial MRI follow-up to differentiate them from multifocal DCIS or carcinoma.

Intraductal papilloma is usually considered a high-risk lesion meriting excision if discovered by core biopsy because of underestimation of association of malignancy or other high-risk lesions (see Tables 6.8, 6.9, and 6.10). Brennan et al. (2012) showed that the malignancy underestimation ratio for atypical papilloma and papilloma without atypia proven by MRI-guided vacuum-assisted biopsy was 8.7% (2/23) and 4.5% (2/44), respectively. However, some practitioners suggest that excisional biopsy is unnecessary for small incidental papillomas under 2 mm, for which MRI follow-up may be sufficient in the appropriate clinical circumstances (Jaffer et al., 2013).

Atypical Ductal Hyperplasia

Atypical ductal hyperplasia (ADH) describes mammary ductal epithelium atypia. It may enhance but has no specific appearance on DCE MRI. When found on core biopsy, ADH is considered a high-risk lesion and is usually surgically excised because of its potential upgrade to malignancy on the surgical pathology specimen. Recent studies showed that at least 11.1% to 33.3% of ADH discovered on imaging-guided core biopsy were upgraded to DCIS or invasive cancer (see Table 6.4). Small studies that investigated the performance of MRI-guided vacuum-assisted core biopsy showed the malignancy underestimation rate in MRI-guided biopsy-proven ADH ranges 25% to 50% (Orel et al., 2006; Lourenco et al., 2014; Crystal et al., 2011).

Atypical Lobular Hyperplasia and Lobular Carcinoma in Situ

Lobular neoplasia includes breast lesions with terminal ductal lobular unit (TDLU) epithelium atypia, called atypical lobular hyperplasia (ALH) or the more severe atypia of lobular carcinoma in situ (LCIS). Like ADH, ALH or LCIS may enhance on MRI but have no specific appearance on DCE MRI. Although neither ALH nor LCIS are actual cancers, they have a risk of simultaneous

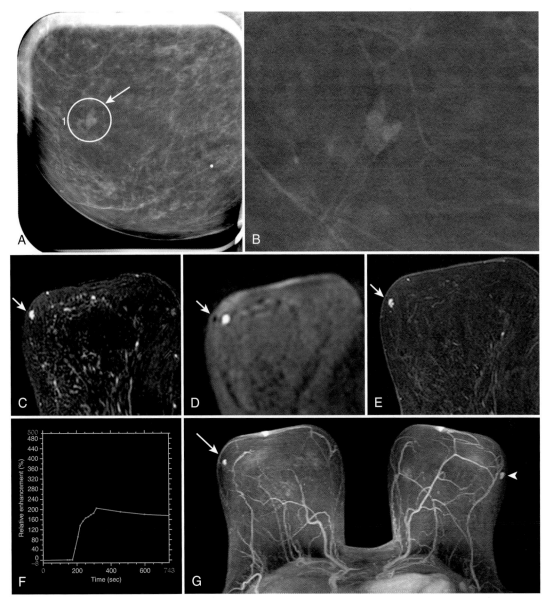

FIG. 7.31 Intramammary lymph node. (A and B) Magnified lateromedial spot mammogram (A) and a to-mosynthesis slice (B) show a small reniform mass with smooth margins in the anterior right breast. (C) On fat-suppressed T2-weighted magnetic resonance (MR) image, this mass demonstrates uniform high signal intensity (*arrow*). (D) Diffusion weighted image (DWI) with a *b*-value of 600 shows high signal intensity (*arrow*) corresponding to the mass, caused by the T2-shine through effect. Apparent diffusion coefficient value was 1.20×10^{-3} mm^2/s. (E) Postcontrast water-specific T1-weighted MR image shows intense enhancement (*arrow*). (F) Kinetic curve demonstrates fast initial and late washout enhancement. (G) Maximum intensity projection image shows the mass (*arrow*) is located near vessels, and that another similar mass (*arrowhead*) presents in a similar place in the contralateral breast. Although the fast initial and plateau kinetics and high signal intensity on DWI are suggestive of breast cancers, very high T2-signal intensity and the morphologic characteristics may allow the diagnosis of intramammary lymph nodes.

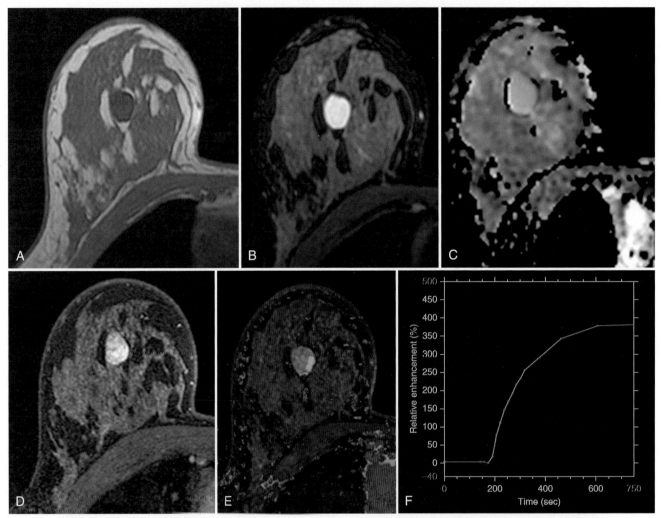

FIG. 7.32 Type I fibroadenoma. Magnetic resonance imaging (MRI) was performed for a 28-year-old woman with right nipple discharge and a family history of *BRCA*, whose ultrasonography detected a nodule in her right breast. Noncontrast MR images show a 19 × 13 × 21 mm oval mass with circumscribed margins that is dark on noncontrast T1-weighted image (A) and uniformly very bright on fat-suppressed noncontrast T2-weighted image (B). On apparent diffusion coefficient (ADC) map (C), the mass exhibits higher signal intensity than fibroglandular tissue, with an ADC value of 2.78×10^{-3} mm²/s. (Note that despite a high ADC value, the diffusion weighted image showed high signal intensity caused by the T2 shine-through effect; see Fig. 7.17C.) Axial contrast-enhanced water-specific postcontrast T1-weighted images (D) show a high signal-enhancing mass associated with dark internal septations. Fusion image (E) of color map (coloring threshold, 50%; red, washout; green, plateau; blue, persistent) and postcontrast image demonstrate that the mass mostly has persistent kinetics except for the small area with plateau late enhancement at the edge. The kinetic curve (F) shows fast initial enhancement followed by persistent late enhancement. Fibroadenoma was suspected. Biopsy was performed because of a family history of *BRCA*-positive and showed fibroadenoma.

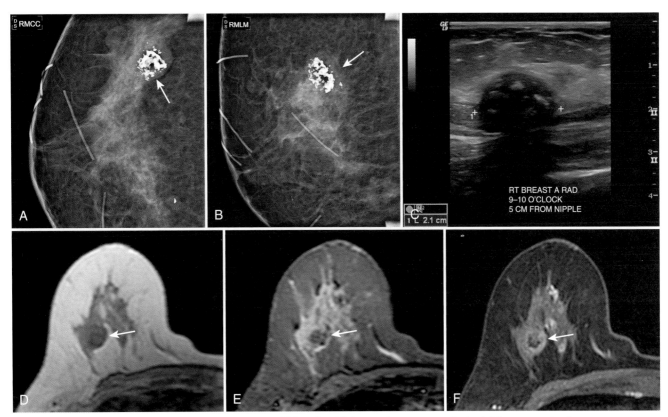

FIG. 7.33 Type II fibroadenoma. A 56-year-old female with known breast cancer in the left breast received screening imaging studies for the right breast. (A and B) Magnified craniocaudal (A) and lateromedial (B) mammograms of the right breast show a well-circumscribed oval mass with popcorn-like calcifications (*arrows*), representing degenerating or involuting fibroadenoma. There are several other smaller masses, also representing fibroadenomas. Note linear scar markers for previous biopsies. (C) Target ultrasonography shows a well-circumscribed hypoechoic mass associated with multiple small hyperechoic foci consistent with the calcified mass. (D–F) Magnetic resonance (MR) images. The signal intensity of the fibroadenoma (*arrow*) is low on noncontrast T1-weighted image (D). On the fat-suppressed T2-weighted image (E), the fibroadenoma (*arrow*) appears as a hypointensity mass surrounded by thin rim with relatively high signal intensity equal to the background fibroglandular tissue. With contrast enhancement the mass (*arrow*) enhances only at its periphery (F). These MR imaging features suggest a type II fibroadenoma.

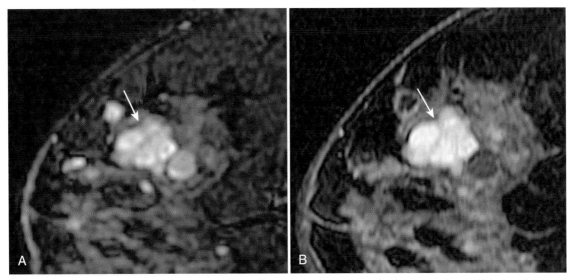

FIG. 7.34 Dark internal septations in type I fibroadenoma. Note the smooth, sharp margins and lobulated shape on precontrast, fat-suppressed T2-weighted images (A) and on contrast-enhanced, water-specific 3D spectral-spatial excitation magnetization transfer gradient-echo images (B). The low-signal septations (A, *arrow*) that do not enhance (B, *arrow*) are particularly specific for fibroadenoma but can occasionally be seen in mucinous carcinoma.

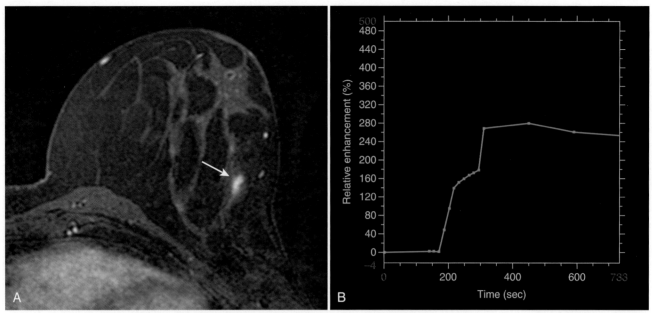

FIG. 7.35 Intraductal papilloma detected with screening magnetic resonance imaging (MRI) in a 56-year-old female with a family history of breast cancer. (A) Axial contrast-enhanced water-specific T1-weighted image shows a 6-mm enhancing mass (*arrow*) deep to the retroareolar region. (B) Kinetic curve shows fast initial and plateau late enhancement. MRI-guided biopsy showed intraductal papilloma.

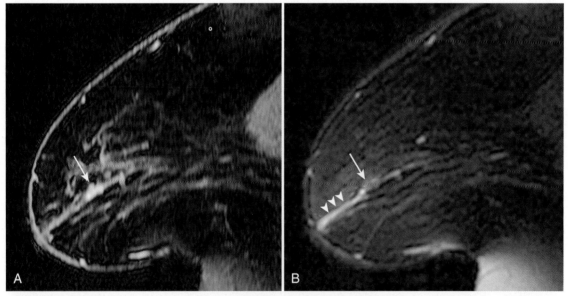

FIG. 7.36 Intraductal papilloma associated with a fluid-filled duct in a 68-year-old female with nipple discharge. (A) Contrast-enhanced water-selective 3D gradient-echo T1-weighted image revealed a small, slightly lobulated, avidly enhancing retroareolar mass with circumscribed margins (*arrow*). (B) A fluid-filled duct (*arrowheads*) extended to the mass (*arrow*) on precontrast, fat-suppressed T2-weighted image. This is the classic appearance of intraductal papilloma, although not all papillomas demonstrate all these features. (From Daniel BL, et al: Magnetic resonance imaging of intraductal papilloma of the breast, *Magn Reson Imaging* 21:887–892, 2003.)

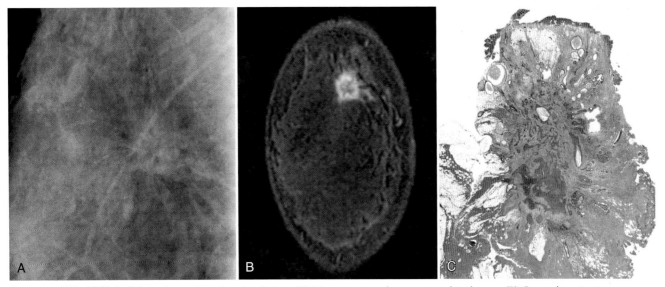

FIG. 7.37 Radial scar/complex sclerosing lesion. (A) Mammogram shows a speculated mass. (B) Coronal contrast-enhanced T1-weighted image shows a spiculated mass with rim enhancement. (C) Surgical specimen (hematoxylin and eosin stain) shows prominent fibrotic change with florid usual ductal hyperplasia, resulting in the formation of a mass-like lesion with spiculated margins. (Courtesy Shotaro Kanao, M.D., Ph.D., Kyoto University, Kyoto, Japan.)

malignancy. Many studies of imaging-guided core biopsy have reported the upgrade rate to malignancy of over 2%, with the highest ratio of approximately 30% (see Table 6.6). In ALH/LCIS discovered by MRI-guided vacuum-assisted core needle biopsy, the upgrade rate to malignancy has been reported to be 50% (4/8; Crystal et al., 2011), 28.6% (2/7; Lourenco et al., 2014), and 0% (0/7; Orel et al., 2006). For this reason, ALH and LCIS are often considered high-risk lesions that merit excision when found on core biopsy.

Radial Scar/Complex Sclerosing Lesion

A radial scar, and its larger variant the complex sclerosing lesion, is histologically characterized by a fibroelastic core with entrapped ducts. Radial scar may have an appearance of a spiculated mass on mammography and can be visible as an enhancing lesion on MRI (Fig. 7.37). Linda et al. (2012) showed that of 29 surgically proven radial scar lesions, 10 manifested as masses, 5 architectural distortions, 4 nonmass lesions, and 1 focus, and 9 were occult on MRI, and that of the 18 lesions with kinetic analysis, 7 (39%) had suspicious dynamic enhancement features. It is often not possible to distinguish benign radial scar from breast cancer with imaging. When diagnosed by core biopsy, radial scar is generally considered as a high-risk lesion because of its association with atypia, DCIS, or even small invasive carcinoma . Lourenco et al. (2014) reported the malignancy underestimation rate of MRI-guided vacuum-assisted core needle biopsy was 23.1% (3/13). Studies of imaging-guided biopsy, including stereotactic- and ultrasound-guided biopsy, consistently demonstrated the upgrade of some radial scars to malignant (0–11%) or high-risk lesions (12–39%) at subsequent excision (see Table 6.7). These data may suggest that excision might be encouraged in patients with biopsy-proven radial scar, although there is controversy as to whether excisional biopsy is necessary because a percentage of the radial scars are not upgraded to malignancy or atypia.

Sclerosing Adenosis

Sclerosing adenosis is a benign proliferative process of the lobules that may have associated dilated ducts and stromal fibrosclerosis

of the TDLU that may be microscopic or confluent (Cucci et al., 2015). Sclerosing adenosis has been reported on MRI as clumped nonmass enhancement (NME), spiculated mass, or round or oval lobulated masses with early rapid and late persistent or washout kinetics, and may mimic breast cancer (Cucci et al., 2015; Oztekin and Kosar, 2014).

Postoperative Seroma and Hematoma

Sterile benign serous fluid may collect in the breast biopsy cavity after surgery, is normal, and may persist for years. Seroma and hematoma resemble cysts with variable intrinsic signal intensity and with circumscribed margins, but they also may have more irregular margins. A thin, uniform rim-like enhancement occurs normally. Peripheral nodular enhancement suggests residual tumor in the setting of pathologically transected margins.

Postoperative Scar Tissue

In the early postbiopsy period, the breast biopsy cavity fills in with fluid, then with granulation tissue as it heals, and is sometimes associated with fat necrosis. On MRI, the scar enhancement is common after surgery and is often slow and persistent. However, an initial fast and late washout dynamic pattern can be seen, particularly in fat necrosis. The enhancement decreases over time as healing occurs and the scar matures. Although rigid criteria have not been established, the scar enhancement usually becomes absent or minimal 12 to 18 months after surgery (Viehweg et al., 1998; Heywang-Köbrunner et al., 1993). On the other hand, scars with enhancement more than 12 to 18 months, with increasing enhancement, or with changes suggestive of tumor growth are suspicious. At a late stage, fibrosis of the scar leads to no enhancement at all.

The differentiation between postoperative scar tissue and local recurrence is a major clinical concern after excisional biopsy, lumpectomy, or breast conservative therapy. According to NCCN Guideline 2015, only annual mammography is recommended as a standard surveillance/follow-up imaging modality after treatment. However, breast MRI has been shown to better perform in the detection of local recurrence compared with conventional diagnostic methods, such as clinical examination, mammography, and ultrasound. According to a systemic review by Quinn (2012), reported sensitivities and specificities of MRI for detection of recurrence ranged 75% to 100% and 67% to 100%, respectively. Some studies have suggested that rapid enhancement on DCE MRI may indicate recurrence rather than postoperative change (Gilles et al., 1993; Kerslake et al., 1994), although false-positives can occur because of postoperative change, such as fat necrosis and a foreign-body reaction (Gilles et al., 1993; Cohen et al., 1996).

Fat Necrosis

Fat necrosis is a benign inflammatory process of adipose tissue caused by infarction, usually because of breast trauma or surgery, and occasionally as an unknown etiology. Fat necrosis occurs commonly in breast biopsy sites and in the reconstructed breast by a reduction mammoplasty or a breast flap reconstructive surgery. Fat necrosis may have hemorrhagic areas but then undergo saponification, calcification, central liquefaction, or fibrosis. The infarcted fat incites a chronic inflammatory response. On MRI, fat necrosis is commonly recognized as rim enhancement surrounding a fatty mass or a lipid cyst (Fig. 7.38). The kinetics of fat necrosis ranges widely from slow, to gradual, to very fast initial enhancement. Occasionally late-phase washout enhancement

can be seen. Enhancement related to fat necrosis may resolve with time; however, it can persist for years because of chronic inflammation. Generally, if the fatty areas of fat necrosis are small, or if the inflammation is intense or produces a nodular or spiculated appearance mimicking cancer, biopsy may be necessary to exclude recurrence of breast cancer.

Radiation Therapy

Soon after radiation therapy, the breast undergoes increased vascular permeability from small vessel damage and inflammation that can lead to transient diffuse contrast enhancement. Commonly, there is diffuse T2-hyperintense breast edema, with skin thickening, usually diminishing gradually over the next 2 to 3 years. Occasionally, breast edema persists for years, and the skin thickening persists and becomes fibrotic. At the late-stage, the radiation therapy treatment will often decrease BPE in the treated breast.

Silicone Granuloma

Silicone breast implant scars do not usually enhance on contrast-enhanced breast MRI. However, extruded silicone from an implant rupture or directly injected silicone to the breast can

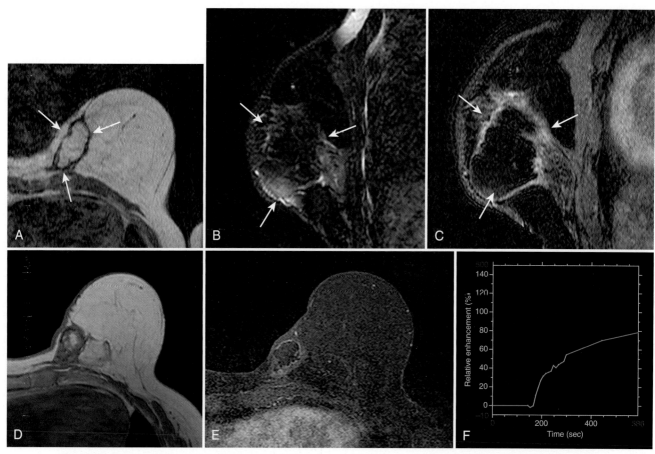

FIG. 7.38 Fat necrosis in a transverse rectus abdominis musculocutaneous (TRAM) flap on magnetic resonance (MR) images. (A–C) MR images obtained 3 years after the reconstruction of the left breast with a TRAM flap. Fat necrosis (*arrows*) in the TRAM flap appears as low signal intensity with central high intensity representing fat on axial T1-weighted image (A) and mildly high intensity on sagittal T2-weighted image (B) and is contrast-enhanced with gadolinium on the edge around the low signal fat (C). Because fat necrosis does not typically enhance 2 years after the surgery, follow-up MRI studies every 6 months were recommended. (D–F) Follow-up MR images 14 years after the reconstruction. The fat necrosis shrank over 10 years on T1-weighted image (D) but still enhances (E). No dominant mass is seen. The dynamic curve shows slow initial and persistent late enhancement (F). Biopsy was performed to exclude recurrence, but pathology showed fat necrosis with chronic inflammation without malignancy.

cause chronic inflammation or fibrosis that occasionally enhances on contrast-enhanced MRI. Direct injections of silicone and paraffin droplets into the breast for augmentation was banned in the United States by the FDA but was still practiced outside of the United States and Europe. Silicone droplets are specifically identified with silicone-specific images as round, high signal intensity masses (see Fig. 9.44). Silicone granulomas may present as hard, nodular masses and architectural distortion, and it is often difficult to diagnose breast cancer in the breast with free silicone with conventional methods, including physical examination, mammography, and ultrasound. However, dynamic contrast MRI has been a more useful method for cancer diagnosis and often allows the identification of cancers with suspicious morphology or dynamic kinetic patterns against the background of silicone or paraffin nodules with gradual enhancement (Po et al., 2006; Youk et al., 2009).

Granulomatous Mastitis

Granulomatous mastitis is an inflammatory process of the breast with unknown origin. A significant relationship between granulomatous mastitis and pregnancy and lactation has been suggested, since this disease entity typically affects younger women, usually within 6 years of pregnancy. Granulomatous mastitis usually presents as a palpable mass with overlying skin erythema, sometimes associated with pain or nipple retraction. Granulomatous mastitis often has multifocal, extensive areas of inflammation and necrosis. Occasionally chronic fistulous tracts draining to the skin can be identified on MRI, which is fairly specific for this disease. Other reported MRI appearance of granulomatous mastitis include either mass or nonmass enhancement, segmental T2-hyperintensity, rim-enhancing collections from microabscesses, various dynamic kinetic patterns (Kuhl/ACR type I, II, and III), skin involvement, and extension to chest wall (Al-Khawari et al., 2011; Yildiz et al., 2015). The diagnosis of granulomatous mastitis is often challenging because it is indistinguishable from breast abscess or inflammatory cancer, and biopsy is required to exclude these etiologies. Treatment includes surgery, steroids, antibiotics, and methotrexate.

Malignant Lesions

Table 7.7 summarizes noncontrast signal intensity and the morphologic and kinetic enhancement features of major malignant lesions, including invasive ductal carcinoma (IDC), ILC, mucinous carcinoma, and DCIS. Cancers are typically dark on both T1 and T2 with an early, fast enhancement rise and a late plateau or washout; however, not all cancers follow the rules. ILC and DCIS have variable kinetic patterns, and occasionally, DCIS may not enhance at all. Mucinous carcinoma is bright on noncontrast T2-weighted scans like fibroadenoma.

Invasive Ductal Carcinoma

Invasive ductal carcinoma (IDC) is the most common breast cancer, comprising up to 80% of all breast malignancies and virtually always manifesting as a focal, avidly enhancing mass. Because it is comprised of abnormal tumor cells arising from ductal epithelium that invade into the adjacent stroma, the mass shape is often irregular but may have any shape, and the mass margins are usually irregular or spiculated (Fig. 7.39). On occasion, IDC may be circumscribed or smooth. The irregularity of mass margins could be underestimated on MRI compared with mammography and tomosynthesis, which have higher spatial resolution (see Fig. 7.39). The IDC T2 signal is similar to that of breast tissue; the lack of high signal distinguishes IDC from benign intramammary lymph nodes and fibroadenomas. However, there are some T2-bright IDCs, so kinetic evaluation of all benign-appearing masses is important.

IDC usually enhances very well because of its high perfusion and permeability. Enhancement may occur heterogeneously throughout the tumor. Rim enhancement (Fig. 7.40) and enhancing internal septations (note this terminology is not used in BI-RADS 2013 anymore; Fig. 7.41) are particularly suspicious. Rim enhancement is enhancement that occurs at a mass periphery, and is usually observed on the early postcontrast scan (Fig. 7.40A). On occasion, rim enhancement is displayed on later postinjection scans (Fig. 7.40B). Similarly, enhancement in the spiculations from the desmoplastic reaction from breast cancers may enhance on later scans, so all postcontrast scans should be reviewed for rim enhancement and spiculation. True nonenhancing central necrosis is rare, but can occur in large locally advanced tumors. Dynamic curve assessment usually reveals fast initial enhancement, followed by a late-phase plateau or washout of signal intensity (Fig. 7.42).

IDC is occasionally associated with DCIS (Fig. 7.43). DCIS may be present close to the IDC, and may extend away from the invasive focus. The coexistence of IDC and DCIS in the same breast field possibly implies a concept known as *field effect* (also called *field cancerization* or *field defect*). The field effect denotes a biologic phenomenon caused by the presence of oncogenic molecular alterations over a certain duct or field of breast tissue, which accumulates over time and eventually leads to the development of DCIS and invasive cancer (Heaphy et al., 2009). DCIS may be identifiable only when clumped or clustered ring nonmass enhancement in linear or segmental distribution is seen on postcontrast images. Kinetic curves and signal intensities on T2-weighted and diffusion-weighted images

TABLE 7.7 Typical MRI Features of Malignant Lesions

| | Signal Intensity | | Contrast-Enhanced Imaging | | | |
	T1	T2	Overall Enhancement	Morphology	Initial Dynamic Pattern	Late Dynamic Pattern
Invasive ductal carcinoma	Dark	Dark[a]	Well	Mass with rim, spiculated or irregular margin	Fast	Plateau or washout
Invasive lobular carcinoma	Dark	Dark	Variable	NME or mass	Variable	Variable
Mucinous cancer	Dark	Bright	Mild to well	Mass with rim or irregular margin	Variable Fast at periphery, slow at center	Variable
Ductal carcinoma in situ	Dark	Dark	Variable	NME, occasionally mass	Variable	Variable

[a]Invasive ductal carcinoma is rarely T2 bright; these are usually dark or isointense compared with glandular tissue.
NME, nonmass enhancement.

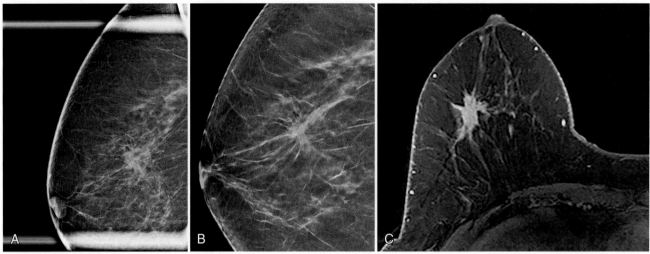

FIG. 7.39 Infiltrating ductal carcinoma visualized as an irregular mass with spiculated margins on magnetic resonance (MR) imaging. (A) Magnified spot craniocaudal mammogram of the right breast shows a mass. The margins are partly spiculated, but largely obscured by overlapping fibroglandular tissue and Cooper's ligaments. (B) Tomosynthesis depicts the spiculated margins in details that radiate from the irregular mass. (C) Axial contrast-enhanced water-specific T1-weighted MR image visualizes the irregular mass with better contrast compared with mammography and tomosynthesis. Spiculated margins are identifiable on the MR image, but look less fine compared with tomosynthesis and mammography. However, MR image shows contrast enhancement not visible on tomosynthesis or mammography.

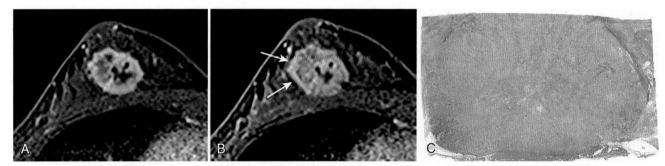

FIG. 7.40 Rim enhancement on early and late postcontrast images seen in an invasive ductal cancer. (A and B) Dynamic contrast-enhanced water-specific T1-weighted images at the early (A) and the late (B) phases. On the early postcontrast image (A), the tumor enhances strongly at its periphery, producing a rim appearance. On the late postcontrast image (B), abnormal enhancement expands toward the outside of the mass (so-called blooming sign) with its margin being more indistinct, and the most bright area is seen outer to the mass, generating another rim appearance around the mass (so-called delayed rim enhancement), which is thinner and wider than the rim at the early phase. The tumor parenchyma inside the delayed rim enhancement, except for the central necrotic region, mostly demonstrates a washout kinetic feature. (C) Surgical specimen (hematoxylin and eosin stain) shows dense viable cancer cells at the periphery (blue/purple) and fibrotic necrosis area (pink) at the center of the tumor. (Courtesy Shotaro Kanao, M.D., Ph.D., Kyoto University, Kyoto, Japan.)

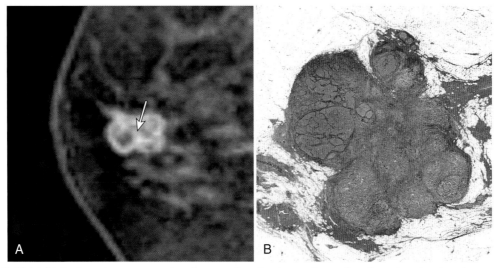

FIG. 7.41 Multiple rim enhancements showing as enhancing internal septations in an invasive ductal cancer. (A) Sagittal early postcontrast water-specific T1-weighted magnetic resonance (MR) image shows a circumscribed, macrolobulated oval mass containing multiple rims displayed as enhancing internal septations (*arrow*). (B) Surgical specimen (hematoxylin and eosin stain) shows a gently lobulated oval mass with partly irregular margins. Between tumor nests consisting of grouped dense cancer cells (blue/purple) within the tumor, there are fibrotic zones (pink), likely corresponding to the enhancing internal septations. Enhancing internal septation is known as one of the MR imaging features usually suggesting malignancy. Although this term is no longer used in Breast Imaging Reporting and Data System 2013, in the authors' clinical experience, it can be a morphologic sign of breast cancer. (Courtesy Shotaro Kanao, M.D., Ph.D., Kyoto University, Kyoto, Japan.)

are unreliable to distinguish DCIS as a malignancy (details are discussed in a later section). Partial maximal intensity projection images or thick-slab images may be helpful to visualize the characteristic distribution of DCIS associated with IDC, as well as the extension of IDC itself.

Direct skin or muscle invasion, growth of the tumor through Cooper's ligaments, and architectural distortion are secondary signs of invasive carcinoma. Large breast cancers with increased blood flow may lead to dilatation of and an increased number of macroscopic blood vessels in the ipsilateral breast, reported as suggestive as a sign of breast cancer. Axillary lymph nodes that have become rounder and lost their fatty hila are worrisome for lymphadenopathy from breast carcinoma metastases.

Inflammatory breast cancer is an uncommon and aggressive form of breast cancer, which is characterized by the inflammatory appearance of the breast. Inflammatory breast cancer is diagnosed based on these clinical findings: the presence of erythema and dermal edema (*peau d'orange*) involving one-third or more of the skin of the breast with a palpable raised border to the erythema. On MRI, inflammatory breast cancer may be associated with substantial T2-hyperintensities around the tumor, skin thickening, abnormal skin enhancement, and swelling of the breast (Fig. 7.44), but it may look similar to noninflammatory breast cancers.

The morphology of enhancement patterns is roughly correlated with a molecular subtype. Luminal A tumors (estrogen receptor [ER]+/progesterone receptor [PR]+, human epidermal growth factor receptor 2 [Her2]–, with low Ki67, a histologic proliferation index) are more commonly spiculated. Luminal B tumors (ER+/PR+, Her2+, with high Ki67) are commonly multifocal. Among ER-negative tumors, Her2-positive tumors (ER–, Her2+) are more likely to have spiculated margins and be associated with calcifications than HER2-negative tumors (ER–, Her2–). Triple negative tumors often have more rounded, smoother margins with "pushing" borders.

Invasive Lobular Carcinoma

ILC is a difficult tumor to diagnose on mammography because of its infiltrating pattern of growing cell by cell without much

mass effect and with rare calcifications (Fig. 7.45). On DCE MRI, ILC has a much more variable appearance than IDC. A particularly unique appearance is enhancement that follows the course of normal fibroglandular elements without a substantial mass effect, which may lead to a missed diagnosis. However, ILC can also appear as a solitary mass (Fig. 7.46), nonmass enhancement, or a combination of multiple masses with or without enhancing intervening FGT, and it is seen to greater advantage on MRI than on mammography. ILC rarely enhances enough to be distinguished from surrounding breast tissue. On dynamic imaging, ILC may have any pattern, including fast initial and late washout or plateau enhancement, and gradual, sustained enhancement (see Fig. 7.45). Thus normal dynamic kinetics patterns do not exclude ILC.

Mucinous Carcinoma

Mucinous carcinoma is a rare breast cancer that includes less than 10% of all breast malignancies, and on MRI it is a round mass with a unique appearance. Mucinous carcinoma is characterized by the presence of mucin that is secreted to the surrounding extracellular matrix from cancer cells, and is histologically classified into two types: pure and mixed. The large central pool of mucin has a very high T2 signal (Fig. 7.47). Thus mucinous carcinoma, particularly the pure type, sometimes resembles a cyst by its high T2 signal, but unlike the cyst, mucinous cancers are usually heterogeneous and have an irregular, thickened, and avidly enhancing rim (see Fig. 7.47). Mucinous cancers also occasionally may have irregular internal enhancement. The dynamic curve of mucinous cancer varies between tumors and even varies within a tumor. Curve types include a fast initial and late plateau or washout curve identical to invasive ductal cancer, or a persistent late curve caused by the hypocellular mucin component, which delays the intratumoral diffusion of contrast material. Centrally, the cancer may not enhance at all. The differential diagnosis includes myxoid/hyalinized fibroadenoma, breast abscess, cyst, intracystic tumor, and necrotic tumor, all of which are very bright on T2-weighted images. If mucinous cancer has fast initial

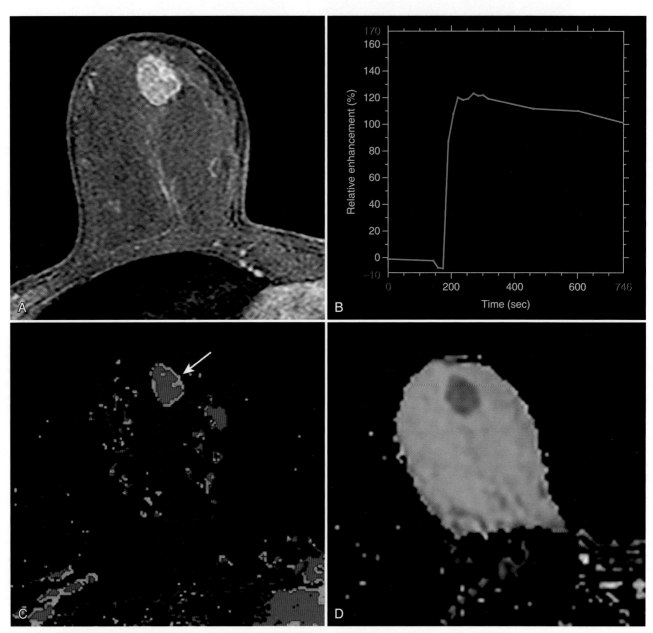

FIG. 7.42 Infiltrating ductal carcinoma in dense breast. (A) Early postcontrast T1-weighted image shows an oval mass with rim enhancement with partly irregular margins. (B) Kinetic curve of the tumor demonstrates fast initial enhancement followed by washout late-phase enhancement, suggestive of malignancy. (C) A color map (coloring threshold, 50%; red, washout; green, plateau; blue, persistent) shows the tumor as a *red* mass (*arrow*) that stands out against the blue background. (D) Apparent diffusion coefficient (ADC) map gener-ated form noncontrast diffusion weighted images with *b*-values of 0 and 600 represents the mass has low ADC values (1.24×10^{-3} mm²/s), suggestive of malignancy (diffusion weighted image shown in Fig. 7.17A). This mass was mammographically occult, because it was obscured by dense fibroglandular tissue, but breast magnetic resonance imaging successfully identified and characterized the tumor.

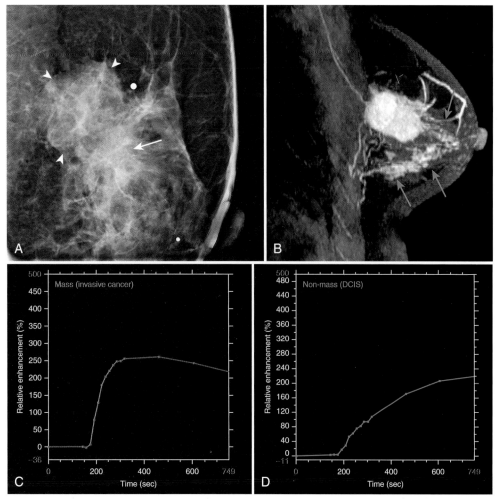

FIG. 7.43 Invasive ductal carcinoma (IDC) associated with ductal carcinoma in situ (DCIS), possibly representing field effect or field cancerization. (A) Magnified spot mediolateral mammogram of the upper left breast shows an irregular dense mass (*arrowheads*) at the palpable area marked with a BB marker. There are a cluster of pleomorphic microcalcifications (*arrow*) anterior to the mass. (B) Magnetic resonance imaging (MRI) was performed to evaluate the extent of disease. Partial maximal intensity projection image of contrast-enhanced water-specific T1-weighted study shows an enhancing irregular mass (the index lesion) and clumped nonmass enhancement (*arrows*) suggestive of DCIS, which is more extensive than the microcalcifications seen on mammography. (C) The dynamic contrast-enhancement curve at the index mass is a fast initial and late washout pattern, suggestive of malignancy. (D) In contrast, the kinetic curve of nonmass enhancement shows nonspecific gradual, persistent enhancement. Based on the pathologic examination, the index mass was proven as IDC, and the nonmass enhancement as DCIS. The morphologic analysis on contrast-enhanced MRI is useful for the identification and diagnosis of DCIS.

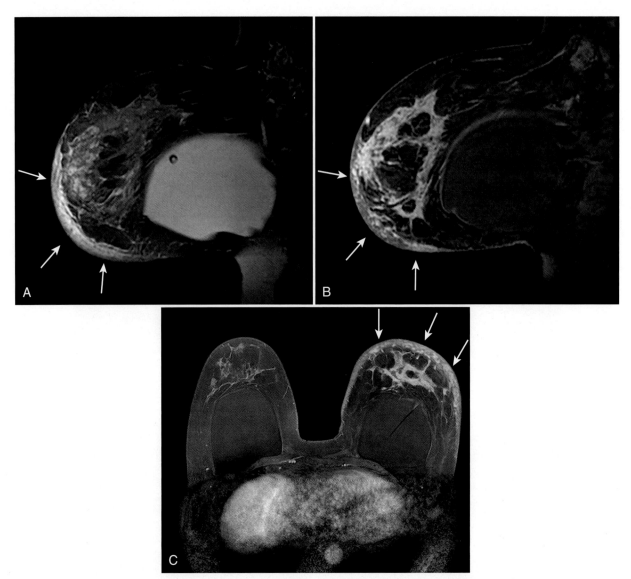

FIG. 7.44 Inflammatory breast cancer patient with raised red skin and a breast mass. (A) Sagittal fat-suppressed T2-weighted image shows marked breast edema and skin thickening (*arrows*) extending anterior to distortion and a mass in the left breast. There is a breast implant behind the mass. (B) Sagittal postcontrast water-specific T1-weighted image shows enhancement in the right breast mass and enhancement in the thickened skin, which is abnormal (*arrows*). (C) Axial image shows the enlarged left breast with the enhancing mass and skin enhancement (*arrows*). Pathology showed invasive ductal carcinoma, and punch biopsy of the raised, reddened skin showed breast cancer in dermal lymphatics, consistent with inflammatory breast cancer on clinical diagnosis.

and late-phase washout enhancement curves, the mucinous cancer can be distinguished from a myxoid fibroadenoma, which has a late-phase persistent enhancement curve. The geographic distribution of enhancement also seems to be useful in differentiating between mucinous cancer and myxoid fibroadenoma, with mucinous cancer showing rim enhancement and myxoid fibroadenoma enhancing centrally. Breast abscess may have a similar appearance, but should have a clinical history suggestive of prior infection, immunosuppression, or diabetes predisposing the patient for an abscess.

Ductal Carcinoma in Situ

DCIS grows within breast ducts that extend from the nipple, expanding them but not extending through the basement membrane or invading into the surrounding stroma. DCIS grade is classified as low, intermediate, or high nuclear grade, with the high-grade DCIS having a higher incidence of invasive disease.

The coexistence of IDC and DCIS in the same breast field can imply a field effect, as described earlier.

DCIS is often seen as NME rather than a mass, and often affects only the ducts of a single lobe, which explains the classic clumped enhancement in a ductal system distribution extending from the nipple on DCE MRI (Figs. 7.48 and 7.49). Medium-sized ducts may produce linear or segmental NME or linear/branching NME emanating from the nipple. One common, but nonspecific sign for DCIS includes clumped NME, representing enhancement of tumor growing within and expanding the duct, simulating a string of pearls or a cobblestone appearance. If the duct is larger, periductal enhancement may cause the "clustered ring" or "tram-track" appearance of DCIS (Fig. 7.48C). Linear (nonclumped or not clustered ring) NME that branches may be sign of either DCIS or of FCC. DCIS can manifest as a focal clumped NME, as segmental enhancement, or even as enhancement indistinguishable from other breast tissue, or, less commonly, as a focal mass. When associated with an invasive tumor, DCIS commonly appears as a

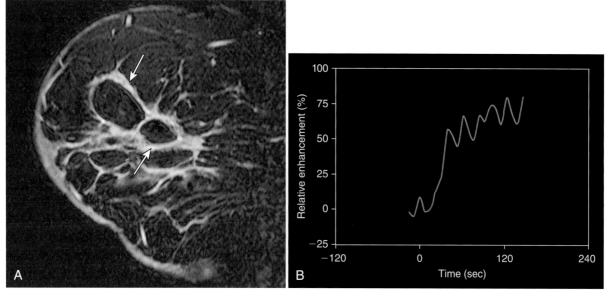

FIG. 7.45 Invasive lobular carcinoma. (A) Contrast-enhanced, water-selective, 3D gradient-echo images reveal nonmass enhancement along the normal fibroglandular elements (*arrows*), without a significant mass effect, and findings corresponding to the infiltrating pattern of spread. (B) Initial enhancement is medium and is followed by persistent late enhancement.

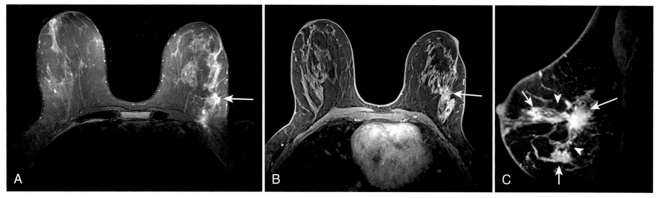

FIG, 7.46 Invasive lobular carcinoma (ILC). (A) T2-weighted axial images shows spiculated masses (*arrow*) in the outer left breast where biopsy had shown ILC with marker placement (signal void). (B) Axial postcontrast water-specific T1-weighted image shows an irregular mass with spiculated margins and heterogeneous internal enhancement in the outer left breast (*arrow*). (C) Sagittal postcontrast views of the left breast show suspicious masses (*arrows*) and streaming enhancement in the tumor that flows along the normal breast parenchyma (*arrowheads*). The biopsy showed ILC.

clumped NME that has a less worrisome dynamic enhancement curve than does the invasive tumor.

Dynamic enhancement curves are unreliable to distinguish DCIS as a malignancy. The enhancement from DCIS varies from nonspecific fast initial enhancement with a late-phase persistent enhancement curve (Fig. 7.49D) or no enhancement, to suspicious fast initial enhancement with a late-phase plateau (Fig. 7.48D) or early washout. Thus DCIS dynamic curves may resemble focal FCC, hormone-related enhancement, intraductal papilloma, or even invasive carcinoma.

Abnormal enhancement on contrast-enhanced MRI may reflect the presence and the extent of DCIS better than microcalcifications on mammography in some cases (see Figs. 7.49 and 3.71). However, in some cases, MRI may fail to visualize DCIS, and it may be better to perform a mammography than an MRI (see Fig. 3.70). Calcifications cannot be reliably assessed with MRI. Up to 25% of cases of DCIS may be diagnosed only by pleomorphic calcifications seen on mammography (eg, some DCIS is invisible

on contrast-enhanced MRI). Therefore the correlation of MRI and mammograms remains essential when attempting to determine the extent or presence of DCIS. It is important to biopsy pleomorphic calcifications if they are of concern for cancer even if the MRI is negative.

Phyllodes Tumor

Phyllodes tumor contains both stromal and glandular tissue, are rare, and are most common in women 30 to 40 years of age. They are usually discovered as a palpable mass, and on histology may range from well-differentiated tumors that resemble benign fibroadenoma to a malignant phyllodes tumor, which is rare (Kraemer et al., 2007). All phyllodes tumors can grow back in the same place if they are not completely excised, even if they are benign. On contrast-enhanced MRI, benign well-differentiated phyllodes tumors are homogeneous, circumscribed masses with intrinsic high T2 signal and slow initial and late

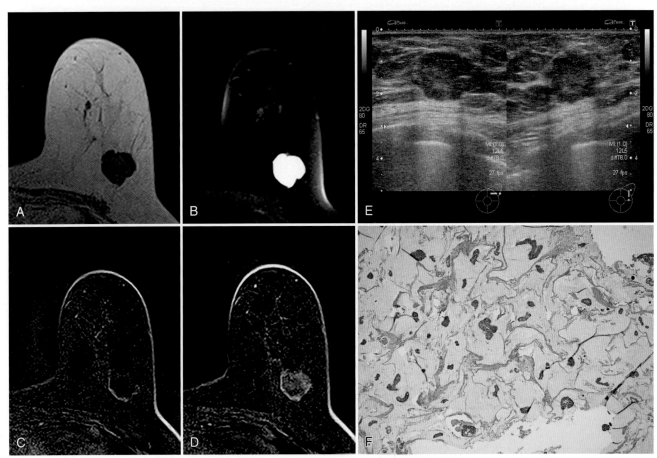

FIG. 7.47 Pure type mucinous carcinoma. (A) T1 weighted image shows a mass with irregular margins. (B) On fat-suppressed T2-weighted image, the mass is remarkably bright. (C and D) Subtraction processing images of early (C) and late (D) postcontrast minus precontrast baseline show predominantly peripheral enhancement (*rim enhancement*), which gradually extends toward central. (E) On ultrasonography, the mass is isoechoic to fat. (F) Photograph of pathologic specimen (hematoxylin and eosin stain) shows sparse cancer cell distribution surrounded by abundant mucin, representing pure type mucinous carcinoma. In addition to the Breast Imaging Reporting and Data System (BI-RADS) lexicon terms describing this mass, it is noted that the mass has angulated, polygonal margins and that the rim is irregular. These additional features, while not part of the formal BI-RADS lexicon, are, in the authors' experience, often suggestive of mucinous carcinoma. (Courtesy Shotaro Kanao, M.D., Ph.D., Kyoto University, Kyoto, Japan.)

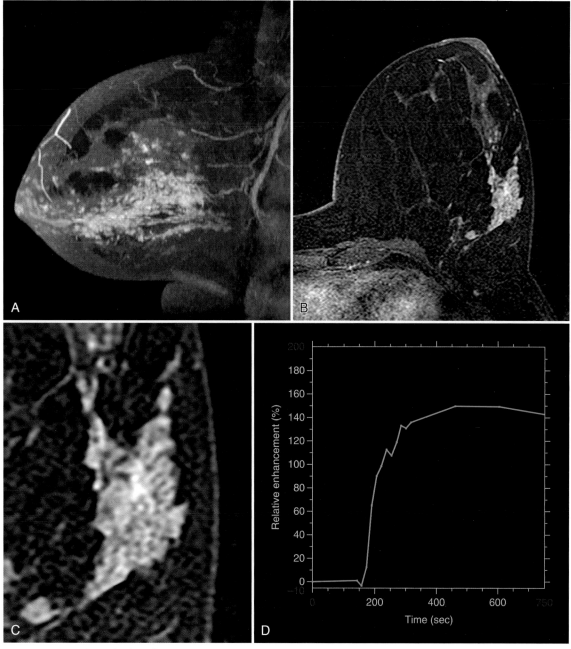

FIG. 7.48 High-grade ductal carcinoma in situ (DCIS). A 44-year-old female with left breast pain and nipple inversion. Mammography (not shown) showed heterogeneously dense breasts but no abnormal findings. (A) Maximal intensity projection image of postcontrast water-specific T1-weighted images shows segmentally distributed nonmass enhancement extending toward the nipple in the lower left breast. (B and C) Axial contrast-enhanced water-specific T1-weighted image of the left breast (B) and its photography magnified image (C) show heterogeneous nonmass enhancement with clustered ring elements. (D) Kinetic curve shows fast initial enhancement followed by late plateau enhancement.

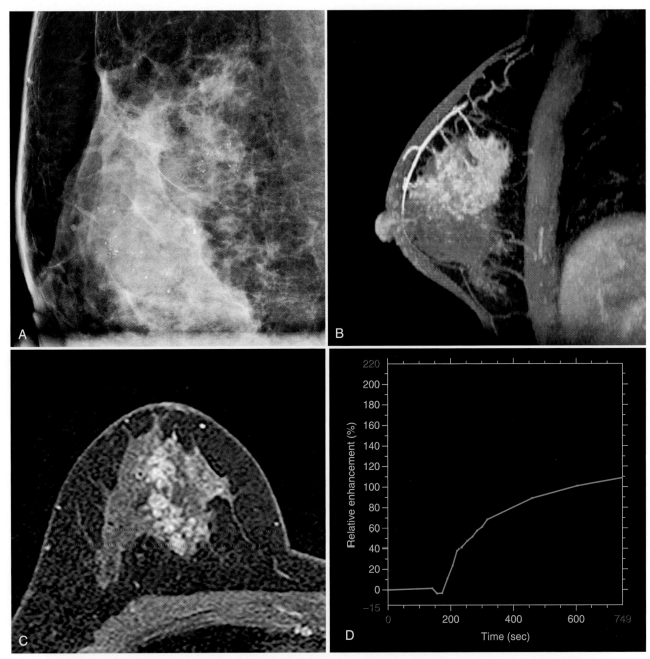

FIG. 7.49 High-grade ductal carcinoma in situ (DCIS). A 37-year-old female with DCIS in the right breast that was found during the screening for additional lesions to a known invasive breast cancer in the left breast. (A) Spot magnified lateromedial mammogram of the right breast shows fine pleomorphic and coarse heterogeneous calcifications in a segmental distribution in the upper breast. (B) Partial maximal intensity projection image of postcontrast water-specific T1-weighted images shows segmental nonmass enhancement in the upper central right breast, corresponding to the microcalcifications on the mammography. Enlarged vessels connecting to the lesion are observed. (C) Axial contrast-enhanced water-specific T1-weighted image shows clumped nonmass enhancement. (D) Kinetic curve is a medium initial and late persistent enhancement pattern.

TABLE 7.8 Diagnostic Performance of Breast Magnetic Resonance Imaging in Screening of High-Risk Women in Comparison with Mammography and Ultrasound: Evidence from Major Prospective Studies

Author	Year	Number of Women	Screening Method	Detected Malignancy	Mammography		US		MRI	
					Sen	Spe	Sen	Spe	Sen	Spe
Kriege et al.	2004	1909	Annual screening including MRI (4169 MRI scans)	44 IC, 6 DCIS, 1 lymphoma	40	95	—	—	71	90
Warner et al.	2004	236	1–3 annual screening including MRI	16 IC, 6 DCIS	36	99.8	33	96	77	95
Kuhl et al.	2005	529	2–7 annual screening including MRI (1452 rounds)	34 IC, 9 DCIS	33	97	40	91	91	97
Leach et al.	2005	649	2–7 annual screening including MRI	29 IC (18 w/ DCIS), 6 DCIS	40	93	—	—	77	81
Kuhl et al.	2010	687	Annual screening including MRI (1679 MRI scans)	11 DCIS, 16 IC	33	99	37	98	93	98
Sardanelli et al.	2011	501	1–4 annual screening including MRI (1592 rounds, 1045 MRI scans)	44 IC, 8 DCIS	50	99	52	98	91	97
Berg et al.	2012	612	Single MRI scan after 3 annual mammography and US	12 IC, 4 others	31	92	—	—	88	76

DCIS, ductal carcinoma in situ; *IC,* invasive carcinoma; *MRI,* magnetic resonance imaging; *Sen,* sensitivity; *Spe,* specificity; *US,* ultrasound.

persistent kinetic curves that mimic benign fibroadenomas, but more often than fibroadenoma may contain cystic components or lobulated borders (Kamitani et al., 2014). Malignant phyllodes tumors may appear as irregularly marginated masses with areas of necrosis.

Angiosarcoma

Angiosarcomas are rare malignancies of endovascular origin accounting for 0.04% to 1% of all breast cancers (O'Neill et al., 2014). Primary angiosarcoma occurs in young women and secondary angiosarcomas occur in older women as late sequelae 5 to 6 years after surgery for breast cancer and radiation therapy, sometimes presenting with skin thickening and skin nodules or discoloration. On MRI, high-grade angiosarcomas present as large heterogeneous, rapidly enhancing masses with washout (Yang et al., 2007). Because skin thickening is common after radiation therapy, but dermal enhancement is abnormal, angiosarcoma should be suspected on MRI if there is dermal enhancement and associated underlying enhancing mass (Marchant et al., 1997).

INDICATIONS

Large-scale randomized, controlled trials, similar to the early mammography studies, have not been reported to support the widespread use of contrast-enhanced breast MRI in the general normal-risk population at this time. However, MRI's utility has been demonstrated by smaller studies in many specific situations.

Screening

Genetic testing and counseling identify women who are at high risk for breast cancer development. Current screening options include routine clinical and imaging screening with mammography or ultrasound and prophylactic mastectomy. MRI has recently been investigated as an adjunct to conventional imaging. In 2003 Morris et al. performed a large retrospective study consisting of 367 asymptomatic women at high risk of

BOX 7.11 Accepted Indications for Breast Magnetic Resonance Imaging in Screening

BRCA mutation (*BRCA1* or *BRCA2*)[a]
First-degree relative of *BRCA* carrier, but untested
Lifetime risk of approximately 20% to 25% or greater, as defined by BRCAPRO or other models[a]
Obscured breast tissue (eg, previous free silicone injection)
Radiographically dense breast
Radiation to chest between ages 10 and 30 (eg, for Hodgkin disease)[a]
Li-Fraumeni, Cowden, and Bannayan–Riley–Ruvalcaba syndromes, or first-degree relatives[a]

[a] ACS recommendations. (Data from Saslow D, Boetes C, Burke W, et al: American Cancer Society guidelines for breast screening with MRI as an adjunct to mammography, *CA Cancer J Clin* 57:75–89, 2007;Table 1.)

developing breast cancer (based on personal or family history, *BRCA* status, etc.) with negative mammograms, and showed breast MRI contributed to detect 14 mammographically occult breast cancers. Subsequent large prospective studies consistently revealed breast MRI had much higher sensitivity (sensitivity range, 71%–93%) compared with mammography (sensitivity range, 31%–50%) and ultrasound (sensitivity range, 33%–52%) in screening of high-risk women (Table 7.8).This evidence led to the 2007 recommendation by the American Cancer Society for cancer screening with MRI in the United States in women with a greater than 20% lifetime risk of breast cancer (such as *BRCA1/2* mutation carriers or women undergoing risk assessment based on validated family history models) and in patients who have a history of radiation therapy to chest for Hodgkin disease (Box 7.11; Saslow, 2007). Optimal MRI screening intervals are varied. For young women with Hodgkin disease, the NCCN recommends that the age at which MRI screening should be initiated is 8 to 10 years after radiation therapy or at 40 years of age, whichever comes first. In patients with a personal history of breast cancer, there are higher rates of breast cancer in the opposite breast as well.Viehweg et al. (2004) reported that breast MRI screening for patients with a personal history of breast cancer treated with breast-conserving therapy detected contralateral breast cancers in 10 (8%) of 119 patients, including 4 invasive cancers, 3 DCIS with microinvasion, and 3 pure DCIS.

Women at average risk for breast cancer benefit less from MRI screening because the rate of false-positive abnormalities may substantially exceed the rate at which cancers are found; further investigation of these false-positive results may subject these women to significant morbidity. Patients with a history of direct free silicone injections of the breast for augmentation, however, cannot undergo any other type of screening (ie, clinical breast examination, mammography, or sonography) with confidence; hence, they may be appropriate screening subjects when counseled accordingly about the risks associated with false-positive lesions. On the other hand, women with dense tissue have an increased risk of breast cancer, although the risk is much smaller than that conferred by a genetic predisposition. To evaluate this population, the DENSE Trial in Utrecht, the Netherlands, is a study evaluating women 50 to 75 years of age with extremely dense breast tissue; this trial started in 2011 an is to be completed in December 2019 to evaluate mammography and MRI versus mammography only in women with dense breast tissue.

Practical issues of breast MRI screening include its high cost, which is partly related to the current time-consuming protocols. To overcome this problem, Kuhl et al. (2014) proposed a new, abbreviated protocol, consisting of only precontrast and one early postcontrast image acquisition with the image reconstruction of subtracted postcontrast and MIP images. In this protocol, radiologists review the MIP image first to look for abnormal enhancement and then review all of the images, including MIP images and subtracted postcontrast images, to make a diagnosis. Kuhl et al. (2014) showed that, compared with the regular full diagnostic protocol, consisting of a full dynamic study and T2-weighted and T1-weighted imaging, this abbreviated protocol significantly reduced the image acquisition time (3 minutes for the abbreviated protocol versus 17 minutes for the full protocol). The time to read an MIP image and the whole images obtained with the abbreviated protocol was only 2.8 and 28 seconds, respectively. The diagnostic performance was equivalent between the abbreviated protocol and the regular full diagnostic protocol. This abbreviated protocol could lead to reducing the cost of current MRI screening programs and increasing access to breast MRI. However, it should be also noted that this approach was developed after the 2013 ACR Protocol Guidelines, and that the impact of not performing a T2-weighted scan has not been evaluated for its impact on diagnostic accuracy. Also, this method relies on high-quality subtraction of precontrast and postcontrast images; hence, it may be limited if there is patient motion.

Diagnosis

MRI is infrequently used to diagnose equivocal findings on mammography, sonography, or physical examination (Box 7.12), because the cost of MRI, including follow-up MRI, approaches the cost of the more traditional minimally invasive core biopsy. However, in rare instances, lesions are found on MRI that are not amenable to conventional biopsy, such as suspicious findings seen on only one mammographic view (Fig. 7.50). MRI is also used to evaluate patients with persistent bloody or cytologically abnormal nipple discharge in whom conventional galactography and ductoscopy were either unrevealing or unsuccessful. In addition, MRI is used to evaluate patients with equivocal findings on physical examination that are mammographically and sonographically occult (Lee, 2004). However, the potential for false-positive and equivocal

---

findings that generate biopsy or follow-up MRI must be balanced against the accuracy of simple palpation-based biopsy in this setting.

Staging

MRI is frequently used preoperatively to image the extent of biopsy-proven breast cancer, especially in patients contemplating breast-conserving therapy. NCCN 2015 guidelines recommended that breast MRI be considered as an optional study for patients with a newly diagnosed breast cancer at any clinical stages, to evaluate the extent of ipsilateral disease and to screen the contralateral breast (Lehman et al., 2009). Controversy exists over whether all patients who have breast cancer should undergo breast MRI as part of the staging process. In fact, several articles indicate that the MRI may cause false-positive biopsies as well as fail to improve the resection rate at the first surgery. However, although not routinely indicated as part of the local staging process in all newly diagnosed carcinomas, MRI is commonly used in selected subgroups, including the following (Box 7.13):

- Patients with biopsy-proven axillary lymph node metastases of breast cancer origin who have normal mammograms and ultrasound (Fig. 7.51); although the primary treatment of these patients remains systemic therapy, MRI may identify an occult primary breast tumor that can be treated with breast-conserving therapy.
- Patients with equivocal chest wall invasion on imaging or physical examination (Fig. 7.52).
- Patients with breast tissue that is suboptimally imaged by mammography, especially those with dense breast tissue, silicone implants, or silicone injections obscuring the breast.
- Patients with tumors that are poorly seen on conventional mammography, including ILC or DCIS, without corresponding microcalcifications.
- Patients with DCIS. Breast MRI may be used to detect occult invasive cancer, not identified by mammography and ultrasound. If invasive foci are discovered and confirmed by biopsy, patient management may be changed because surgeons usually perform sentinel lymph node biopsy with invasive cancer, and not always with DCIS.
- Patients who are candidates for accelerated partial breast irradiation, in which only the breast cancer biopsy cavity and the margins around the cavity are treated with radiation therapy rather than whole-breast radiation.

In these patients, MRI may be used to plan the shape of the lumpectomy in an attempt to minimize the chance of transecting tumor margins.

MRI may also reveal mammographically occult multifocal or multicentric carcinoma (Fig. 7.53), prompting wider local excision. Previous studies indicate breast MRI detects an unsuspected ipsilateral malignancy in approximately 10% to 20% of cases with recent diagnosis of breast cancer, although accurate comparison is challenging because of the difference in the study designs (Table 7.9). In addition, MRI may reveal occult contralateral carcinoma (Fig. 7.54). Research articles indicate that mammographically and clinically occult contralateral carcinoma is detected by

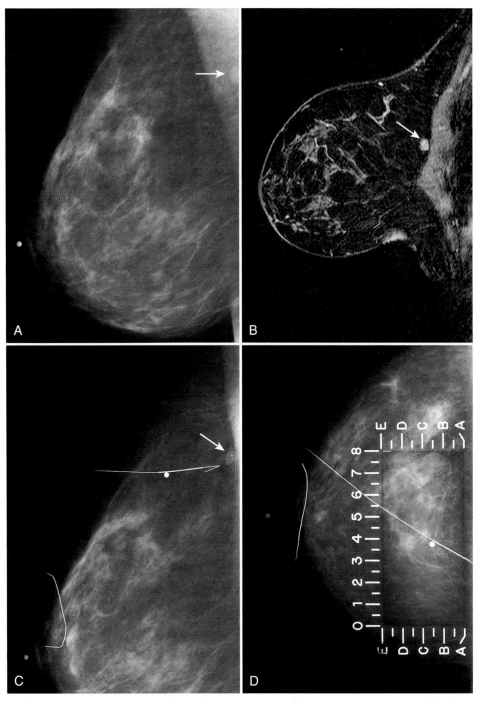

FIG. 7.50 Magnetic resonance imaging (MRI) of a suspicious mass seen on one x-ray mammographic view. (A) A suspicious mass was noted in the superior aspect of the breast, near the chest wall on the mediolateral oblique (MLO) mammogram only (*arrow*). (B) Water-selective 3D gradient-echo MRI revealed a focal enhancing mass (*arrow*). Preoperative MRI-guided wire localization was performed (not shown). (C and D) After localization, an MLO (C) mammogram confirmed that localization was successful and the lesion (*arrow*) was too close to the chest wall to be seen on craniocaudal views (D). Pathologic evaluation revealed a small fibroadenoma. (From Offodile RS, Daniel BL, Jeffrey SS, et al: Magnetic resonance imaging of suspicious breast masses seen on one mammographic view, *Breast J* 10(5):416–422, 2004.)

breast MRI in 3.8% to 18.6% of patients with unilateral carcinoma (Table 7.10). In these circumstances, preoperative biopsy is critical to pathologically confirm multicentric carcinoma or bilateral carcinoma, because MRI findings can be nonspecific and may even lead to more extensive surgery than necessary in occasional patients.

Although MRI is most easily interpreted when performed in the absence of recent surgery because of the potential overlap of postsurgical healing scars and imaging findings of tumor, it has been successfully used to map the extent of residual disease in patients with transected tumor detected at the margins of an initial excisional biopsy specimen. Asymmetric and nodular enhancement or enhancement that is noncontiguous with the biopsy site is suspicious.

Formal outcome studies demonstrating the benefit of staging MRI as an adjunct to conventional breast-conserving therapy are tempered by controversy regarding the exact role and benefit of staging breast cancer by MRI given the high success rate of traditional breast-conserving therapy without MRI.

BOX 7.13   Indications for Breast Magnetic Resonance Imaging in Staging

Locate the breast primary in patients with axillary metastases
Detect chest wall invasion
Evaluate ipsilateral tumor extent in the breasts suboptimally imaged on mammography (eg, dense breast, implants or free silicone injection)
Evaluate ipsilateral extent of tumors poorly seen on mammography (eg, infiltrating lobular carcinoma, ductal carcinoma in situ [DCIS] without microcalcifications)[a]
Detect occult invasive foci within DCIS
Detect occult multifocal or multicentric cancer
Detect occult contralateral cancer

---

[a]Some indications are more controversial.
Data from Lehman CD, DeMartini W, Anderson BO, Edge SB: Indications for breast MRI in the patient with newly diagnosed breast cancer, *J Natl Compr Canc Netw* 7:193-201, 2009.

Management of Patients Undergoing Neoadjuvant Chemotherapy

Patients undergoing neoadjuvant chemotherapy are frequently imaged with breast MRI (Box 7.14). Pretreatment scans provide the most accurate nonsurgical 3D measurements of the extent of tumor. Scans performed after the first one or two chemotherapy cycles showing treatment response that may possibly predict whether chemotherapy will be successful; however, interim MRI examinations are often not reimbursed in the United States. In patients who do respond, MRI after completion of chemotherapy may be used to identify and localize residual tumor, even in patients who have had a complete clinical response (Fig. 7.55). It is important to note that in these circumstances, the robustly angiogenic abnormal tumor vascularity may have been treated, and dynamic enhancement of tumors may even resemble benign disease with a slow initial rise and late persistent kinetic phase. Thus any residual enhancement at the site of a previously known tumor is suspicious, even if its kinetics are benign appearing. Because of the poor specificity of MRI findings after chemotherapy, pretreatment MRI is essential as a baseline for comparison.

MRI has also been investigated for its ability to detect local breast cancer recurrence. Debate persists regarding the duration of enhancement in benign postsurgical scars, although enhancement clearly decreases substantially over the first 2 years. Nevertheless, interpretation is best performed on serial MRI scans to assess whether enhancement is normally decreasing over time or suspiciously increasing over time.

MAGNETIC RESONANCE IMAGING–DIRECTED INTERVENTION

Magnetic Resonance Imaging–Directed "Second-Look" Ultrasound

Lesions detected by MRI must frequently be biopsied (Box 7.15). The easiest way to biopsy an MRI-detected finding is to perform a second-look or targeted ultrasound examination directed toward the specific area of abnormality noted on MRI and biopsy it under

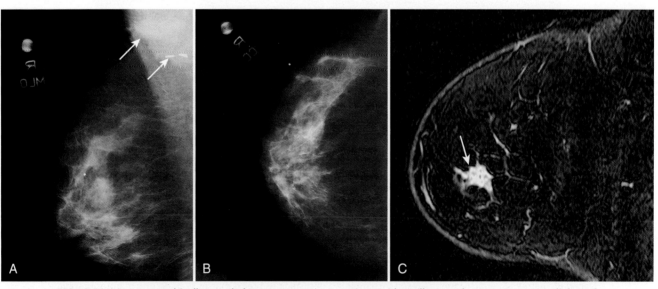

FIG. 7.51 Mammographically occult breast cancer in a patient with axillary node metastases. Mediolateral oblique (A) and craniocaudal (B) mammograms revealed only postoperative changes in the right axilla (A, *arrows*) in this patient with a history of metastatic breast cancer discovered on recent excision of a palpable axillary node. (C) Sagittal water-selective contrast-enhanced magnetic resonance imaging (MRI) revealed an 11-mm focal mass in the lateral portion of the breast (*arrow*). MRI-guided, wire-localized excision revealed a 9-mm invasive ductal carcinoma that was excised with tumor-free margins.

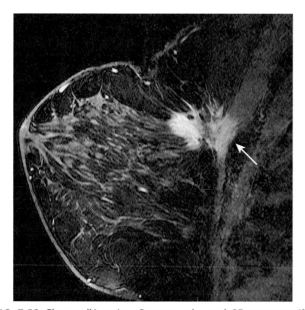

FIG. 7.52 Chest wall invasion. Contrast-enhanced, 3D water-specific breast magnetic resonance imaging reveals a large spiculated mass in the posterior of the breast. The enhancing tissue traverses the normal retromammary fat plane to abut the chest wall. The focal enhancement of the pectoralis muscle (*arrow*) is consistent with invasion and indicates locally advanced disease. (From American College of Radiology: ACR BI-RADS®—MRI. In *ACR BI-RADS atlas, breast imaging reporting and data system*, ed 4, Reston, VA, 2003, American College of Radiology.)

ultrasound guidance. Careful attention to the finding's position in the breast is essential to ensure that the MRI abnormality corresponds to the sonographic lesion, given the difference in patient position and breast configuration between the prone MRI and the supine ultrasound.

Studies evaluating MRI-detected findings with sonography show that ultrasound demonstrates a finding in between 46% and 82% (Table 7.11) A 2010 study by Abe et al. showed that 57% (115/202) of MRI-detected findings were seen by ultrasound. Of the remaining 87 lesions undetected by ultrasound, 13% (11/87) were cancer. Other studies by Linda et al. (2008) and Destounis et al. (2009) showed that 82% and 70% of 173, and 182 MRI-detected findings, respectively, were seen on second-look ultrasound. A meta-analysis (Spick et al., 2014a) that reviewed 17 studies showed a general lesion detection rate of second-look ultrasound was 58% (95% CI: 50%, 64%), and pooled positive and negative predictive values (positive or negative second-look ultrasound correlates of MRI-detected malignant or benign lesions) calculated by using random-effects models were 31% (95% CI: 25%, 36%) and 88% (95% CI: 82%, 93%), respectively. Malignant and mass lesions were more likely to be detected at second-look ultrasound.

In the largest study designed to evaluate which MRI lesion should undergo targeted ultrasound for purposes of biopsy, Meissnitzer et al. showed in 2009 that 290 of 519 MRI-detected lesions (56%) were seen with second-look ultrasound, with masses more likely to be seen compared with nonmass lesions (62% of masses versus 31% of nonmass lesions). This study showed that MRI-detected lesions were most likely to be ultrasound detected if the MRI finding was a mass, large, BI-RADS category 5, had rim enhancement, or if it was a nonmass with a

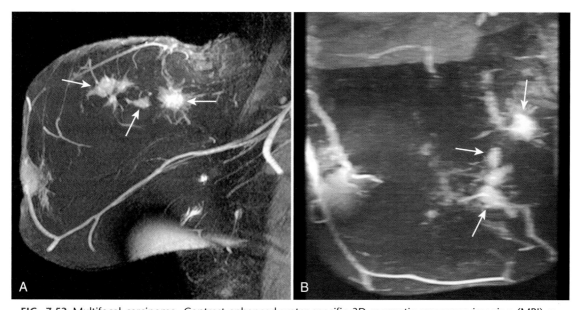

FIG. 7.53 Multifocal carcinoma. Contrast-enhanced water-specific 3D magnetic resonance imaging (MRI) revealed multiple suspicious enhancing masses in the upper outer quadrant (*arrows*), as shown on these 2-cm-thick slab, maximum intensity projections in the sagittal (A) and axial (B) planes. MRI-guided lumpectomy confirmed multifocal invasive carcinoma.

TABLE 7.9 Detection of Unsuspected Ipsilateral Breast Cancer on Magnetic Resonance Imaging in Patients with a Recent Diagnosis of Breast Cancer

Author	Year	Number of Patients	Unsuspected Ipsilateral Cancer Detection Yield, % (N/Total)
Fischer et al.	1998	336	16.1% (54/336)
Bedrosian et al.	2003	267	18.4% (49/267)
Schelfout et al.	2004	170	19.4% (33/170)
Schnall et al.	2005	423	9.7% (41/423)

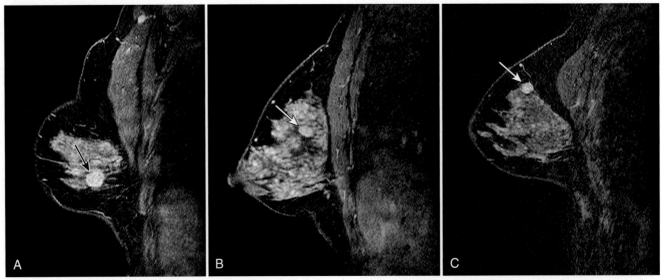

FIG. 7.54 Multicentric and contralateral breast lesions. (A) Water-selective magnetic resonance imaging (MRI) confirmed a 1.5-cm palpable invasive ductal carcinoma in the lower outer portion of the right breast (*arrow*) of a patient with normal bilateral mammograms. (B) In addition, a suspicious upper inner quadrant enhancing focus (*arrow*) was shown to be stromal fibrosis and fibrocystic changes by MRI-guided, wire-localized biopsy. (C) MRI of the asymptomatic left breast also demonstrated a brightly enhancing focus (*arrow*) that proved to be an 8-mm invasive ductal carcinoma at MRI-guided biopsy.

TABLE 7.10 Detection of Unsuspected Synchronous Contralateral Breast Cancer on Magnetic Resonance Imaging in Patients with a Recent Diagnosis of Breast Cancer

Author	Year	Number of Patients	Contralateral Cancer Detection Yield, % (N/Total)	PPV % (TP/MRI+)	Pathology
Fischer et al.	1999	336	4.5% (15/336)	—	3 DCIS, 12 IC
Lee et al.	2003	182	3.8% (7/182)	47% (7/15)	4 DCIS, 3 IDC (2 w/DCIS)
Liberman et al.	2003	223	5.4% (12/223)	17% (12/72)	6 DCIS, 6 IC
Lehman et al.	2007	969	3.1% (30/969)	22% (30/135)	12 DCIS, 12 IDC, 4 ILC, 2 TC
Pediconi et al.	2007	118[a]	18.6% (22/118)	79% (22/28)	10 DCIS, 6 IDC, 4 LCIS[b], 2 ILC

[a]This study included not only patients with known cancer but also those with high-risk lesion.
[b]Note that LCIS was categorized as malignant in this study.
DCIS, ductal carcinoma in situ; *IC,* invasive cancer; *IDC,* invasive ductal cancer; *ILC,* invasive lobular carcinoma; *LCIS,* lobular carcinoma in situ; *MRI,* magnetic resonance imaging; *PPV,* positive predictive value; *TC,* tubular carcinoma; *TP,* true-positive.

BOX 7.14 Indications for Breast Magnetic Resonance Imaging in Management of Patients Undergoing Neoadjuvant Chemotherapy

Measure disease before initiating neoadjuvant chemotherapy (NAC)
Assess response to treatment after NAC
Localize potential residual tumor after a complete clinical response
(Magnetic resonance imaging during NAC not reimbursed in the
    United States.)

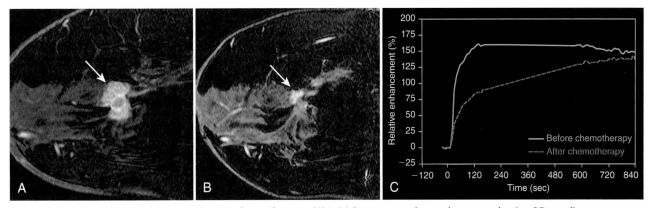

FIG. 7.55 Response to neoadjuvant chemotherapy. (A) Initial contrast-enhanced, water-selective 3D gradient-echo magnetic resonance imaging (MRI) confirmed a discrete, central avidly enhancing mass approximately 2.5 cm in diameter consistent with biopsy-proven invasive ductal carcinoma (*arrow*). (B) Follow-up MRI after a complete clinical response to neoadjuvant chemotherapy revealed a small residual mass (*arrow*). (C) Note that after chemotherapy, the time course of contrast enhancement of the residual tumor had a benign kinetic curve, a marked change in comparison to the suspicious pretreatment curve caused by changes in tumor angiogenesis and posttreatment blood supply. Despite the presence of viable tumor, postneoadjuvant chemotherapy enhancement curves may resemble benign disease and should not be trusted to diagnose residual cancer.

BOX 7.15 Options for Biopsy of Magnetic Resonance Imaging Abnormalities

Second-look ultrasound-guided biopsy
Magnetic resonance imaging (MRI)-guided needle localization
MRI-guided core needle biopsy

---

clumped enhancement. Furthermore, Meissnitzer's study showed that 10 of 80 findings were discordant on a follow-up MRI after ultrasound-guided biopsy for second-look sonographic findings thought to represent the MRI target. This means that the concordant second-look ultrasound biopsy did not sample the MRI-detected abnormality. Of the 9 out of 10 patients who underwent subsequent MRI-guided core biopsy, 5 had cancers. For patients with persistent unbiopsied masses by ultrasound, biopsy must be pursued by direct MRI guidance.

Percutaneous Magnetic Resonance Imaging–Guided Core Biopsy

MRI-guided core biopsy can be especially helpful after a breast cancer diagnosis if MRI detects a possible second cancer that is nonpalpable and is not seen on any other modality (Fig. 7.56). This is particularly true in the postbiopsy surgical patient who has already undergone one operation and now seeks definitive surgical therapy (Fig. 7.57).

MRI-guided percutaneous core needle biopsy can be performed by both MRI grid and freehand methods. Biopsy devices include MRI-compatible 9- to 14-gauge titanium needles and vacuum-assisted biopsy devices. The imaging artifacts associated with core biopsy needles and the potential for breast motion remain limitations to reliable biopsy of subcentimeter lesions given the current technology. MRI-guided core biopsy must be performed rapidly because the signal intensity of the tumor may be indistinguishable from surrounding enhancing breast tissue within 10 minutes.

MRI-compatible clips may be deployed after MRI-guided core needle biopsy to mark the site of biopsy. When benign results are obtained that do not specifically correspond to the expected appearance of the MRI lesion, repeat MRI-guided needle-localized surgical biopsy or follow-up MRI must be performed. The use of the MRI-guided markers or markers placed under ultrasound that are later imaged by MRI or mammography can help guide the surgeon to excise the entire tumor and tumor bed.

The results of several major studies of MRI-guided core needle biopsy are shown in Table 7.12. MRI-guided biopsy was primarily performed for lesions that were visible or able to be localized on MRI alone. Of lesions biopsied under MRI guidance, approximately 10% to 60% were proven as breast cancer at the biopsy. However, approximately 15% to 25% of high-risk lesions at the biopsy were upgraded to cancer at subsequent surgical excision. Hematoma is a common complication, but sampling error was rare and reported in ≤2% of biopsies.

Preoperative Magnetic Resonance Imaging–Guided Needle Localization

Preoperative MRI-guided needle localization, followed by lumpectomy, is also useful to remove nonpalpable suspicious lesions detected on MRI but not seen on any other modality. This technique avoids issues that arise from clip migration that can be experienced at core biopsy.

MRI-guided needle localization and hookwire marking is done through an open breast coil using an 18- to 21-gauge MRI-compatible needle directed toward the abnormality after contrast enhancement, just before the surgery. A single hookwire may be placed to locate an area of interest for surgery (Fig. 7.58), or two or more hookwires may be used to bracket the extent of disease (Fig. 7.59). Grid-positioning devices and freehand methods can be used to direct the needle into the breast. Procedure speed is important because suspicious enhancing lesions commonly do not enhance preferentially over normal breast tissue more than 5 to 10 minutes after injection, and the target can fade into the normal BPE over time.

After MRI-guided preoperative wire placement, a mammogram is recommended for four reasons. First, most breast surgeons are familiar with mammograms showing hookwires to plan their surgical approach. Second, mammography may show a mass or calcifications at the MRI-guided wire tip not previously appreciated; these may be looked for on intraoperative specimen radiographs, maximizing the chance for accurate surgical

TABLE 7.11 Second-Look Ultrasonography for Magnetic Resonance Imaging-Detected Findings: Detection Rate and Positive and Negative Predictive Values

Author	Year	Number of Lesions	MRI PPV % (TP/MRI+)	Second-Look US Positive			Second-Look US Negative		
				% (US+/MRI+)	Malignancy % (TP/US+)	Pathology of TP	% (US−/MRI+)	Malignancy % (FN/US−)	Pathology of FN
Linda et al.	2008	173 (BI-RADS-2/3/4/5)	28% (49/173)	82% (142/173)	32% (46/142)	46 BC	18% (31/173)	10% (3/31)	3 BC
DeMartini et al.	2009	167 suspicious (BI-RADS-4/5)	28% (47/167)	46% (76/167)	36% (27/76)	27 BC	54% (91/167)	22% (20/91)	20 BC
Destounis et al.	2009	182 suspicious[a]	26% (47/182)	70% (128/182)	32% (39/121)	24 IDC (9 w/DCIS), 8 ILC (1 w/DCIS), 6 DCIS, 2 mucinous C, 2 metastatic C, 1 TC, 1 biopsy-proven malignancy	30% (54/182)	16% (8/50)	5 IDC (4 w/ DCIS), 1 ILC, 2 not specified
Meissnitzer et al.	2009	519 suspicious (BI-RADS-4/5); 422 biopsied	29% (121/422 biopsied)	56% (290/519)	34% (87/253 biopsied)	10 DCIS, 55 IDC, 13 ILC, 2 invasive mixed C, 7 not specified	44% (229/519)	20% (34/169 biopsied)	17 DCIS, 10 IDC, 6 ILC, 1 invasive mixed C
Abe et al.	2010	202 suspicious (BI-RADS-0)	22% (44/202)	57% (115/202)	29% (33/115)	25 IDC (2 w/DCIS), 4 ILC, 4 DCIS	43% (87/202)	13% (11/87)	4 IDC (2 w/ DCIS), 3 ILC, 4 DCIS
Candelaria et al.	2011	131 suspicious (BIRADS-4/5)	34% (44/131)	67% (88/131)	31% (27/88)	11 IDC, 3 DCIS, 11 ILC, 1 mucinous C, 1 metastatic node	33% (43/131)	2% (1/41)	1 BC
Fiaschetti et al.	2012	84 unclear (BI-RADS-3)	11% (9/84)	51% (43/84)	16% (7/43)	3 IDC, 3 DCIS, 1 ADH[b]	49% (4/84)	13% (121/935)	1 DCIS, 1 ADH[b]
Lourenco et al.	2012	118 unclear (BI-RADS-3)	1.7% (2/118)	46% (54/118)	4% (2/54)	2 BC	54% (64/118)	10% (3/31)	3 BC
Plecha et al.[c]	2014	96 suspicious (BI-RADS-4/5)	30% (29/96)	52% (50/96)	44% (22/50)	13 IDC, 4 ILC, 2 DCIS, 2 IC, 1 epithelioid myxofibrosarcoma	48% (46/96)	22% (20/91)	4 IDC, 3 DCIS
Spick et al. (meta-analysis)	2014a	2201 suspicious/unclear (from 17 studies)	23% (501/2201)	58% (1266/2201); 95% CI, 50%, 64%	30% (380/1266)	380 BC	43% (935/2201)	16% (8/50)	8 BC

[a]Only lesions that were additionally detected on presurgical MRI in patients with known BC were included. The other studies have various MRI indications, such as high-risk screening, postsurgical follow-up, suspicious mammographic or ultrasonographic findings, and diagnostic problem solving.

[b]Note that ADH was categorized as a malignant lesion in this study.

[c]Shear-wave elastography (SWE) was added to second-look US study. Five of 50 US-detected lesions were identified by SWE alone.

ADH, atypical ductal hyperplasia; *BC,* breast cancer (further histopathologic details were not available); *BI-RADS,* Breast Imaging-Reporting And Data System; *CI,* confidence interval; *DCIS,* ductal carcinoma in situ; *FN,* false-negative; *IC,* invasive carcinoma; *IDC,* invasive ductal carcinoma; *ILC,* invasive lobular carcinoma; *MRI,* magnetic resonance imaging; *PPV,* positive predictive value; *TC,* tubular carcinoma; *TP,* true-positive; *US,* ultrasonography.

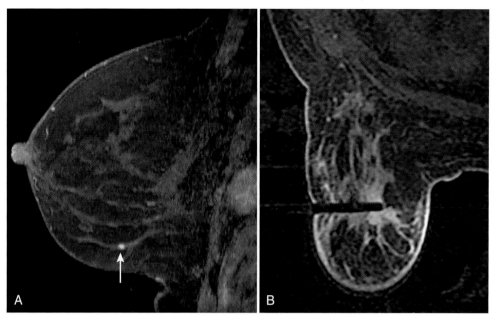

FIG. 7.56 Magnetic resonance imaging (MRI)-guided core biopsy for incidental enhancing lesion (IEL) in a patient with recently diagnosed right invasive lobular carcinoma. (A) Axial contrast-enhanced water-specific T1-weighted image of the left breast shows a 4-mm rounded, homogenously enhancing mass with circumscribed margins (*arrow*) that was incidentally found in the contralateral breast. (B) MRI-guided biopsy was performed. An axial, water-specific, T1-weighted MRI shows an introducer of a 9-gauge biopsy system advanced toward the IEL. High signal around the tip indicates a small hematoma. Pathologic evaluation of IEL revealed synchronous contralateral invasive ductal carcinoma.

excision. Third, mammograms show previously placed markers that might confuse specimen interpretation should they be removed. Last, mammograms document the location of the MRI-guided needle tip, providing a critical baseline for future postoperative mammograms.

Correlating the MRI, mammographic, and ultrasound finding can be challenging. Use of and reporting of specific marker shapes placed in findings biopsied under ultrasound, MRI, or stereotactic guidance can be extremely helpful to determine the location of each biopsied finding, especially if the patient is to undergo excision of cancer seen on more than one modality.

On occasion, the target may not enhance during the MRI-guided preoperative needle localization procedure. Nonvisualization may be caused by vigorous breast compression impeding contrast material inflow to enhance the lesion, resolution of spurious enhancement of a lesion caused by hormonal influences, or nonvisualization for unknown reasons. In most cases, definite

localization can proceed based on surrounding breast architecture rather than targeting the enhanced lesion if such architecture exists. Otherwise, a 1-month follow-up contrast-enhanced MRI study will confirm or exclude whether the enhancing lesion still exists. On occasion, breast cancers may not enhance on the day of preoperative needle localization. In these cases, the short-term MRI follow-up may be helpful to confirm if the lesion is still present and that the need for biopsy still exists.

Based on published data, contrast-enhanced breast MRI preoperative needle localization positive predictive values range between approximately 30% and 60%, similar to mammographically detected breast lesion needle-localization data (Table 7.13). MRI-guided bracket wire localization is often performed in some institutions for patients who have extensive disease but are possible candidates for breast conservative therapy; however, the evidence of the performance of this procedure is currently limited.

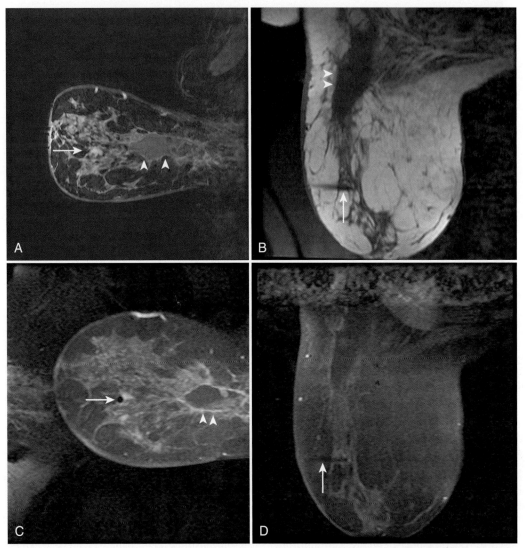

FIG. 7.57 Magnetic resonance imaging (MRI)-guided core biopsy for incidental enhancing lesion (IEL) after lumpectomy for invasive ductal cancer (IDC). This patient had a lumpectomy for IDC, resulting in a seroma in the posterior breast. The MRI was performed to look for extent of disease. (A) Postcontrast sagittal 3D water-specific gradient-echo T1-weighted MRI scan shows the postsurgical seroma (*arrowheads*) and a nonspecific IEL (*arrow*) with fast initial enhancement and late plateau enhancement 3.5 cm anterior to the seroma. To determine whether the IEL was cancer, MRI-guided core biopsy was performed. (B) Axial noncontrast T1-weighted MRI shows the needle (*arrow*) adjacent to the expected location of the IEL. Note the seroma (*arrowhead*) in the posterior aspect of the breast. (C) Sagittal three-point Dixon postcontrast MRI-guided vacuum-assisted core biopsy scan shows signal void of needle biopsy trough (*arrow*) adjacent to the IEL in the anterior breast. Note that the seroma (*arrowhead*) demonstrates rim enhancement and has the fluid/fluid level and the fibrin ball in the superior aspect of the cavity. (D) Axial three-point Dixon postcontrast MRI shows the needle (*arrow*) adjacent to the IEL. Core needle biopsy showed a second focus of IDC.

TABLE 7.12 Magnetic Resonance Imaging–Guided Core Needle Biopsy: Cancer Yield and Underestimation Rate

| Author | Year | Number of Lesions | Technique | MRI-Guided Core Needle Biopsy | | | | | Upgrade to Cancer at Subsequent Excision | |
| | | | | Diagnosis at Biopsy | | | | Sampling Failure | High Risk at Biopsy | Benign at Biopsy |
				Cancer % (N/Total)	High Risk[a] % (N/Total)	Pathology	Benign % (N/Total)	% (N/Total)	Upgrade % (N/Resection)	Upgrade % (N/Resection)
Daniel et al.[b]	2001	27	1.5 T, 14-gauge CNB, free hand	30% (8/27)	—	—	70% (19/27)	0% (0/27)	—	9% (1/11)
Kuhl et al.[b]	2001	78[c]	1.5 T, 14- or 13-gauge CNB	35% (27/78)	—	—	64% (50/78)	1% (1/78)	—	NA
Perlet et al.	2002	341[c]	10 or 1.5 T, 11-gauge VAB	25% (84/341)	5% (17/341)	17 ADH	68% (233/341)	2% (7/341)	18% (3/17)	NA
Orel et al.	2006	85	9-gauge VAB	61% (52/85)	21% (18/85)	8 ADH, 7 LCIS/ALH, 3 RS	18% (15/85)	0% (0/85)	25% (2/8)	13% (2/15)
Meeuwis et al.	2012	55[d]	3 T, 14-gauge CNB	13% (7/55)	5% (3/55)	3 LCIS	82% (45/55)	0% (0/55)	NA	NA
		64[d]	3 T, 9-gauge VAB	28% (18/64)	5% (3/64)	3 LCIS	67% (43/64)	0% (0/64)	NA	NA
Myers et al.	2015	200[c]	1.5 T, 10-gauge VAB	8% (16/200)	20% (39/200)	10 papilloma, 7 ADH, 7 ALH, 5 CSL, 10 other	73% (145/200)	0% (0/200)	17% (4/23)	0% (0/3)

[a]The definitions of high-risk lesions are different between articles.
[b]Lesions were classified as malignant or benign. There was no category of high risk.
[c]All lesions were visible or able to be localized by breast MRI alone.
[d]All lesions were ultrasonographically occult, and were BI-RADS 3, 4, or 5 on breast MRI.
ADH, atypical ductal carcinoma; *ALH*, atypical lobular hyperplasia; *CNB*, core needle biopsy; *CSL*, complex sclerosing lesion; *LCIS*, lobular carcinoma in situ; *MRI*, magnetic resonance imaging; *RS*, radial scar; *VAB*, vacuum-assisted biopsy.

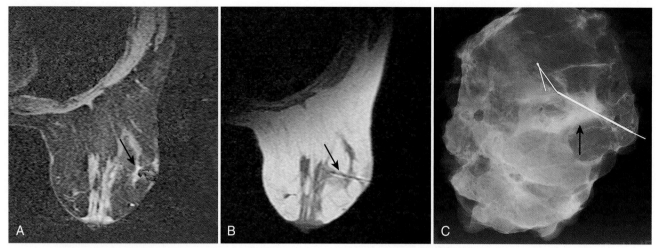

FIG. 7.58 Magnetic resonance imaging (MRI)-guided needle localization. (A) Axial, contrast-enhanced, water-selective 2D gradient-echo MRI reveals an MRI-compatible localizing needle abutting the suspicious focus of contrast enhancement (*arrow*). (B) An axial T1-weighted fast spin-echo image after hookwire deployment reveals the mass centered on the stiffener of the hookwire (*arrow*). (C) Radiography of the excised specimen demonstrated nonspecific glandular tissue adjacent to the hookwire (*arrow*). Pathologic examination revealed invasive ductal carcinoma.

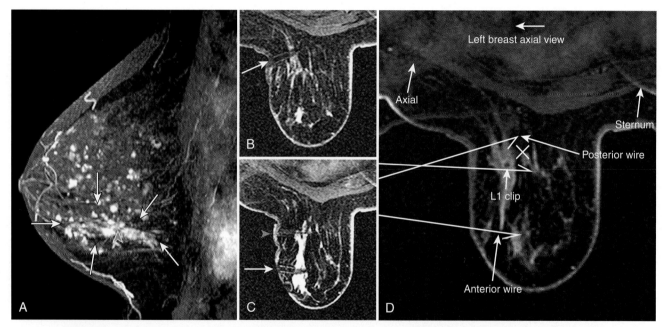

FIG. 7.59 Magnetic resonance imaging (MRI)-guided bracket needle localization in a patient with biopsy-proven invasive ductal cancer (IDC). (A) Maximal intensity projection image of sagittal contrast-enhanced MRI of the left breast shows clumped nonmass enhancement (NME; *arrows*), suggestive for ductal carcinoma in situ (DCIS), extending linearly anterior and posterior to the biopsy-proven IDC (*arrowhead*) in the lower outer left breast. (B and C) Bracket needle localization for NME and a single needle wire localization at the known invasive focus was performed under MRI guidance in the free-hand approach. Axial water-selective gradient-echo MR images show a total of three 20-gauge MRI-compatible titanium biopsy needles: two at the anterior and posterior margins of NME (B and C, *arrows*), and one at the biopsy-proven invasive focus (C, *arrowhead*). (D) Then, hookwires were inserted along the needles and left in the breast. Final locations of hookwires are illustrated on an MRI image. These wires served as guides for subsequent lumpectomy of the bracketed area including the localized invasive focus. Histologic sections of the lumpectomy specimen revealed DCIS (2 cm) surrounding a single area of invasion (0.6 cm). Margin status was negative with the minimum negative margin width of 2 mm to the superior/medial margin.

TABLE 7.13   **Magnetic Resonance Imaging–Guided Needle/Wire Localization: Cancer Yield**

Author	Year	Number of Lesions	Technique	Malignancy % (N/Total)	Malignancy Pathology	High Risk % (N/Total)	High Risk Pathology
Orel et al.	1994	11	1.5 T, grid compression or stereotactic	45% (5/11)	1 IC, 2 IDC, 2 DCIS,	9% (1/11)	1 ADH
Kuhl et al.	1997b	97[a]	0.5 or 1.5 T, stereotactic	55% (53/97)	11 DCIS, 42 IDC	23% (22/97)	5 LCIS, 9 proliferative dysplasia with atypias, 8 papilloma
Daniel et al.	1998	19	0.5 or 1.5 T, free hand, 20- or 21-gauge	63% (8/19)	4 IDC, 1 ILC, 3 DCIS	11% (2/19)	1 ADH, 1 LCIS
Morris et al.	2002	101[b]	1.5 T, grid compression, 18- or 20-gauge	31% (31/101)	16 IC , 15 DCIS	9% (9/101)	9 ADH or LCIS
Van den Bosch et al.	2006	304	0.5 T, free hand, 20- or 21-gauge	34% (104/304)	22 IDC, 8 ILC, 5 TC, 3 lymphoma, 36 DCIS, 30 IC w/DCIS	17% (51/304)	22 papilloma, 14 ADH, 11 RS, 4 LCIS

[a]All lesions were mammographically, ultrasonographically, and clinically occult.
[b]All lesions were mammographically and ultrasonographically occult.
ADH, atypical ductal carcinoma; *DCIS,* ductal carcinoma in situ; *IC,* invasive carcinoma; *IDC,* invasive ductal carcinoma; *ILC,* invasive lobular carcinoma; *LCIS,* lobular carcinoma in situ; *RS,* radial scar; *TC,* tubular carcinoma.

Key Elements

Contrast enhancement in breast cancers is due to angiogenesis.

Indications for breast MRI are breast cancer screening in high-risk patients (BRCA1, BRCA2, or equivalent); breast cancer staging to detect mammographically occult bilateral, multicentric, multifocal, or locally extensive disease; poorly visualized tumors on mammography; diagnosis of suspicious findings that cannot be fully evaluated with conventional imaging; and before and after neoadjuvant chemotherapy.

Chemotherapy produces a potential pitfall in interpretation because it can decrease tumor conspicuity and change suspicious enhancement curves to benign persistent curves despite the persistence of viable, residual cancer.

Proper technique includes a dedicated breast coil, a contrast bolus followed by a saline flush, fat suppression, or subtraction.

Both morphology and enhancement curves are important in the interpretation of MRI.

Abnormal enhancement is defined as enhancement brighter than normal surrounding glandular tissue on the first post-contrast scan or early in the initial enhancement phase.

According to ACR BI-RADS, abnormal enhancement is classified as *focus, masses,* and *nonmass enhancement.*

Suspicious morphologic findings on MRI include an irregular shape, irregular or spiculated margins, rim enhancement, and enhancing internal septations.

Associated findings of focal skin thickening, satellite lesions, lymphadenopathy, and skin or chest wall invasion are suspicious for cancer in the appropriate clinical setting.

Suspicious enhancement curves include a fast initial rise and abrupt transition to a late-phase plateau or washout.

Benign enhancement curves include a slow initial rise and a late persistent enhancement phase.

Fibroadenomas are usually bright on T2-weighted images if myxoid and dark on T2-weighted images if sclerotic and may have dark internal septations and a persistent late enhancement phase.

DCIS may be difficult to distinguish from fibrocystic changes.

Classic patterns for DCIS include clumped enhancement in a ductal, linear, or segmental distribution, particularly if it is asymmetric.

DCIS does not always display rapid initial enhancement with a plateau or washout.

Pitfalls in interpreting rim enhancement include fat necrosis and inflamed cysts; precontrast T2-weighted images can reduce false-positives.

Pitfalls in interpreting benign-appearing masses include cancers with a benign morphology and a suspicious enhancement curve.

Mastitis and inflammatory cancer both produce breast edema and abnormal enhancement.

Papillomas and lymph nodes may have rapid initial rise and plateau or washout patterns and can thus be a cause of false-positive findings that generate biopsy.

MRI-guided preoperative needle localization and MRI-guided core biopsy must be performed rapidly because the signal intensity of the tumor may be indistinguishable from surrounding enhancing breast tissue within 10 minutes.

SUGGESTED READINGS

Abe H, Schmidt RA, Shah RN, et al.: MRI-directed ("second-look") ultrasound examination for breast lesions detected initially on MRI: MR and sonographic findings, *AJR Am J Roentgenol* 194(2):370–377, 2010.

Agoston AT, Daniel BL, Herfkens RJ, et al.: Intensity-modulated parametric mapping for simultaneous display of rapid dynamic and high-spatial resolution breast MR imaging data, *Radiographics* 21:217–226, 2001.

Akbari H, Macyszyn L, Da X, et al.: Pattern analysis of dynamic susceptibility contrast-enhanced MR imaging demonstrates peritumoral tissue heterogeneity, *Radiology* 273(2):502–510, 2014.

Al-Khawari HA, Al-Manfouhi HA, Madda JP, et al.: Radiologic features of granulomatous mastitis, *Breast J* 17:645-650, 2011.

Allen SD, Wallis MG, Cooke R, Swerdlow AJ: Radiologic features of breast cancer after mantle radiation therapy for Hodgkin disease: a study of 230 cases, *Radiology* 272(1):73-78, 2014.

American College of Radiology: ACR practice parameter for the performance of contrast-enhanced magnetic resonance imaging (MRI) of the breast. http://www.acr.org/Quality-Safety/Standards-Guidelines. Accessed July 1, 2015.

American College of Radiology Committee on Drugs and Contrast Media: *ACR manual on contrast media*, 2015. version 10.1.

Appleton DC, Hackney L, Narayanan S: Ultrasonography alone for diagnosis of breast cancer in women under 40, *Ann R Coll Surg Engl* 96(3):202-206, 2014.

Aracava MM, Chojniak R, Souza JA, Bitencourt AG, Marques EF: Identification of occult breast lesions detected by magnetic resonance imaging with targeted ultrasound: a prospective study, *Eur J Radiol* 83(3):516-519, 2014.

Baltzer PA, Dietzel M, Burmeister HP, et al.: Application of MR mammography beyond local staging: is there a potential to accurately assess axillary lymph nodes? evaluation of an extended protocol in an initial prospective study, *AJR Am J Roentgenol* 196(5):W641-W647, 2011.

Balu-Maestro C, Chapellier C, Bleuse A, et al.: Imaging in evaluation of response to neoadjuvant breast cancer treatment benefits of MRI, *Breast Cancer Res Treat* 72:145-152, 2002.

Bedrosian I, Mick R, Orel SG, et al.: Changes in the surgical management of patients with breast carcinoma based on preoperative magnetic resonance imaging, *Cancer* 98:468-473, 2003.

Bedrosian I, Schlencker J, Spitz FR, et al.: Magnetic resonance imaging-guided biopsy of mammographically and clinically occult breast lesions, *Ann Surg Oncol* 9:457-461, 2002.

Beran L, Liang W, Nims T, et al.: Correlation of targeted ultrasound with magnetic resonance imaging abnormalities of the breast, *Am J Surg* 190:592-594, 2005.

Berg WA, Blume JD, Cormack JB, Mendelson EB: Operator dependence of physician-performed whole-breast US: lesion detection and characterization, *Radiology* 241:355-365, 2006.

Berg WA, Blume JD, Adams AM, et al.: Reasons women at elevated risk of breast cancer refuse breast MR imaging screening: ACRIN 6666, *Radiology* 254(1):79-87, 2010.

Berg WA, Zhang Z, Lehrer D: Detection of breast cancer with addition of annual screening ultrasound or a single screening MRI to mammography in women with elevated breast cancer risk, *JAMA* 307:1394-1404, 2012.

Boetes C, Mus RD, Holland R, et al.: Breast tumors: comparative accuracy of MR imaging relative to mammography and US for demonstrating extent, *Radiology* 197:743-747, 1995.

Bogner W, Pinker K, Zaric O, et al.: Bilateral diffusion-weighted MR imaging of breast tumors with submillimeter resolution using readout-segmented echo-planar imaging at 7 T, *Radiology* 274(1):74-84, 2015.

Brennan SB, Corben A, Liberman L, et al.: Papilloma diagnosed at MRI-guided vacuum-assisted breast biopsy: is surgical excision still warranted? *AJR Am J Roentgenol* 199:512-519, 2012.

Brenner RJ: Needle localization of breast lesions: localizing data, *AJR Am J Roentgenol* 179:1643-1644, 2002.

Brinck U, Fischer U, Korabiowska M, et al.: The variability of fibroadenoma in contrast-enhanced dynamic MR mammography, *AJR Am J Roentgenol* 168:1331-1334, 1997.

Brown J, Buckley D, Coulthard A, et al.: Magnetic resonance imaging screening in women at genetic risk of breast cancer: imaging and analysis protocol for the UK Multicentre Study. UK MRI Breast Screening Study Advisory Group, *Magn Reson Imaging* 18:765-776, 2000.

Brown J, Smith RC, Lee CH: Incidental enhancing lesions found on MR imaging of the breast, *AJR Am J Roentgenol* 176:1249-1254, 2001.

Buadu LD, Murakami J, Murayama S, et al.: Breast lesions: correlation of contrast medium enhancement patterns on MR images with histopathologic findings and tumor angiogenesis, *Radiology* 200:639-649, 1996.

Bulte JW: Science to practice: can decreased lymph node MR imaging signal intensity be used as a biomarker for the efficacy of cancer vaccination? *Radiology* 274(1):1-3, 2015.

Candelaria R, Fornage BD: Second-look US examination of MR-detected breast lesions, *J Clin Ultrasound* 39:115-121, 2011.

Carbognin G, Girardi V, Calciolari C, et al.: Utility of second-look ultrasound in the management of incidental enhancing lesions detected by breast MR imaging, *Radiol Med* 115:1234-1245, 2010.

Chadashvili T, Ghosh E, Fein-Zachary V, et al.: Nonmass enhancement on breast MRI: review of patterns with radiologic-pathologic correlation and discussion of management, *AJR Am J Roentgenol* 204(1):219-227, 2015.

Chen X, Lehman CD, Dee KE: MRI-guided breast biopsy: clinical experience with 14-gauge stainless steel core biopsy needle, *AJR Am J Roentgenol* 182:1075-1080, 2004.

Chenevert TL, Helvie MA, Aisen AM, et al.: Dynamic three-dimensional imaging with partial k-space sampling: initial application for gadolinium-enhanced rate characterization of breast lesions, *Radiology* 196:135-142, 1995.

Cheung JY, Moon JH: Follow-up design of unexpected enhancing lesions on preoperative MRI of breast cancer patients, *Diagn Interv Radiol* 21(1):16-21, 2015.

Cho N, Im SA, Park IA, et al.: Breast cancer: early prediction of response to neoadjuvant chemotherapy using parametric response maps for MR imaging, *Radiology* 272(2):385-396, 2014.

Cohen EK, Leonhardt CM, Shumak RS, et al.: Magnetic resonance imaging in potential postsurgical recurrence of breast cancer: pitfalls and limitations, *Can Assoc Radiol J* 47:171-176, 1996.

Crystal P, Sadaf A, Bukhanov K, McCready D, O'Malley F, Helbich TH: High-risk lesions diagnosed at MRI-guided vacuum-assisted breast biopsy: can underestimation be predicted? *Eur Radiol* 21:582-589, 2011.

Cucci E, Santoro A, Di Gesu C, Di Cerce R, Sallustio G: Sclerosing adenosis of the breast: report of two cases and review of the literature, *Pol J Radiol* 80:122-127, 2015.

Daniel B: *Breast cancer. MR and CT perfusion and pharmacokinetic imaging: clinical applications and theory*, Philadelphia, PA, 2006, LWW.

Daniel B, Herfkens R: Intraoperative MR imaging: can image guidance improve therapy? *Acad Radiol* 9:875-877, 2002.

Daniel BL, Birdwell RL, Black JW, et al.: Interactive MR-guided, 14-gauge core-needle biopsy of enhancing lesions in a breast phantom mode, *Acad Radiol* 4:508-512, 1997.

Daniel BL, Birdwell RL, Butts K, et al.: Freehand iMRI-guided large-gauge core needle biopsy: a new minimally invasive technique for diagnosis of enhancing breast lesions, *J Magn Reson Imaging* 13:896-902, 2001.

Daniel BL, Birdwell RL, Ikeda DM, et al.: Breast lesion localization: a freehand, interactive MR imaging-guided technique, *Radiology* 207:455-463, 1998a.

Daniel BL, Yen YF, Glover GH, et al.: Breast disease: dynamic spiral MR imaging, *Radiology* 209:499-509, 1998b.

Davenport MS, Khalatbari S, Cohan RH, Dillman JR, Myles JD, Ellis JH: Contrast material-induced nephrotoxicity and intravenous low-osmolality iodinated contrast material: risk stratification by using estimated glomerular filtration rate, *Radiology* 268(3):719-728, 2013.

Degani H, Chetrit-Dadiani M, Bogin L, Furman-Haran E: Magnetic resonance imaging of tumor vasculature, *Thromb Haemost* 89:25-33, 2003.

Degani H, Gusis V, Weinstein D, et al.: Mapping pathophysiological features of breast tumors by MRI at high spatial resolution, *Nat Med* 3:780-782, 1997.

Demartini WB, Eby PR, Peacock S, Lehman CD: Utility of targeted sonography for breast lesions that were suspicious on MRI, *AJR Am J Roentgenol* 192:1128-1134, 2009.

DeMartini WB, Hanna L, Gatsonis C, Mahoney MC, Lehman CD: Evaluation of tissue sampling methods used for MRI-detected contralateral breast lesions in the American College of Radiology Imaging Network 6667 trial, *AJR Am J Roentgenol* 199(3):W386-W391, 2012.

Destounis S, Arieno A, Somerville PA, et al.: Community-based practice experience of unsuspected breast magnetic resonance imaging abnormalities evaluated with second-look sonography, *J Ultrasound Med* 28:1337-1346, 2009.

Dietzel M, Kaiser C, Baltzer PA: Magnetic resonance imaging of intraductal papillomas: typical findings and differential diagnosis, *J Comput Assist Tomogr* 39(2):176-184, 2015.

Dogan BE, Le-Petross CH, Stafford JR, Atkinson N, Whitman GJ: MRI-guided vacuum-assisted breast biopsy performed at 3 T with a 9-gauge needle: preliminary experience, *AJR Am J Roentgenol* 199(5):W651-W653, 2012.

Dula AN, Dewey BE, Arlinghaus LR, et al.: Optimization of 7-T chemical exchange saturation transfer parameters for validation of glycosaminoglycan and amide proton transfer of fibroglandular breast tissue, *Radiology* 275(1):255-261, 2015.

Ebner L, Bonel HM, Huber A, et al.: Diagnostic performance and additional value of elastosonography in focal breast lesions: statistical correlation between size-dependent strain index measurements, multimodality-BI-RADS score, and histopathology in a clinical routine setting, *ISRN Radiol* 396368, 2014.

El Khouli RH, Macura KJ, Jacobs MA, et al.: Dynamic contrast-enhanced MRI of the breast: quantitative method for kinetic curve type assessment, *AJR Am J Roentgenol* 193:W295-W300, 2009.

El Khouli RH, Macura KJ, Kamel IR, et al.: The effects of applying breast compression in dynamic contrast material-enhanced MR imaging, *Radiology* 272(1):79-90, 2014.

El Khouli RH, Macura KJ, Jacobs MA, et al.: Dynamic contrast-enhanced MRI of the breast: quantitative method for kinetic curve type assessment, *AJR Am J Roentgenol* 193(4):W295-W300, 2009.

Elmore JG, Armstrong K, Lehman CD, Fletcher SW: Screening for breast cancer, *JAMA* 293:1245-1256, 2005.

Espinosa LA, Daniel BL, Vidarsson L, et al.: The lactating breast: contrast-enhanced MR imaging of normal tissue and cancer, *Radiology* 237:429-436, 2005.

Esserman L, Hylton N, Yassa L, et al.: Utility of magnetic resonance imaging in the management of breast cancer: evidence for improved preoperative staging, *J Clin Oncol* 17:110-119, 1999.

Evans DG, Kesavan N, Lim Y, et al.: MRI breast screening in high-risk women: cancer detection and survival analysis, *Breast Cancer Res Treat* 145(3):663-672, 2014.

Expert Panel on MR Safety, Kanal E, Barkovich AJ, et al.: ACR guidance document on MR safe practices: 2013, *J Magn Reson Imaging* 37(3):501-530, 2013.

Fallenberg EM, Dromain C, Diekmann F, et al.: Contrast-enhanced spectral mammography: does mammography provide additional clinical benefits or can some radiation exposure be avoided? *Breast Cancer Res Treat* 146(2):371-381, 2014.

Fiaschetti V, Salimbeni C, Gaspari E, et al.: The role of second-look ultrasound of BI-RADS-3 mammary lesions detected by breast MR imaging, *Eur J Radiol* 81:3178-3184, 2012.

Fischer U, Kopka L, Grabbe E: Magnetic resonance guided localization and biopsy of suspicious breast lesions, *Top Magn Reson Imaging* 9:44-59, 1998.

Giess CS, Yeh ED, Raza S, Birdwell RL: Background parenchymal enhancement at breast MR imaging: normal patterns, diagnostic challenges, and potential for false-positive and false-negative interpretation, *Radiographics* 34(1):234-247, 2014.

Giess CS, Raza S, Birdwell RL: Patterns of nonmasslike enhancement at screening breast MR imaging of high-risk premenopausal women, *Radiographics* 33(5):1343-1360, 2013.

Gilbert FJ, van den Bosch HC, Petrillo A, et al.: Comparison of gadobenate dimeglumine-enhanced breast MRI and gadopentetate dimeglumine-enhanced breast MRI with mammography and ultrasound for the detection of breast cancer, *J Magn Reson Imaging* 39(5):1272-1286, 2014.

Gilles R, Guinebretiere JM, Shapeero LG, et al.: Assessment of breast cancer recurrence with contrast-enhanced subtraction MR imaging: preliminary results in 26 patients, *Radiology* 177:473-478, 1993.

Ginter PS, Winant AJ, Hoda SA: Cystic apocrine hyperplasia is the most common finding in MRI detected breast lesions, *J Clin Pathol* 67(2):182-186, 2014.

Guo Y, Cai YQ, Cai ZL, et al.: Differentiation of clinically benign and malignant breast lesions using diffusion-weighted imaging, *J Magn Reson Imaging* 16:172-178, 2002.

Gutierrez RL, DeMartini WB, Eby PR, et al.: BI-RADS lesion characteristics predict likelihood of malignancy in breast MRI for masses but not for nonmasslike enhancement, *AJR Am J Roentgenol* 193:994-1000, 2009.

Gutierrez RL, DeMartini WB, Eby PR, Kurland BF, Peacock S, Lehman CD: BI-RADS lesion characteristics predict likelihood of malignancy in breast MRI for masses but not for nonmasslike enhancement, *AJR Am J Roentgenol* 193(4):994-1000, 2009.

Gweon HM, Cho N, Han W: Breast MR imaging screening in women with a history of breast conservation therapy, *Radiology* 272(2):366-373, 2014.

Haakma W, Steuten LM, Bojke L: MJ IJ: Belief elicitation to populate health economic models of medical diagnostic devices in development, *Appl Health Econ Health Policy* 12(3):327-334, 2014.

Harms SE, Flamig DP, Hesley KL, et al.: MR imaging of the breast with rotating delivery of excitation off resonance: clinical experience with pathologic correlation, *Radiology* 187:493-501, 1993.

Hartman AR, Daniel BL, Kurian AW, et al.: Breast magnetic resonance image screening and ductal lavage in women at high genetic risk for breast carcinoma, *Cancer* 100:479-489, 2004.

Harvey JA, Hendrick RE, Coll JM, Nicholson BT, Burkholder BT, Cohen MA: Breast MR imaging artifacts: how to recognize and fix them, *Radiographics* (Suppl 1) S131-S145, 2007.

Hashimoto BE, Morgan GN, Kramer DJ, Lee M: Systematic approach to difficult problems in breast sonography, *Ultrasound Q* 24:31-38, 2008.

Hashimoto BE: Sonographic assessment of breast calcifications, *Curr Probl Diagn Radiol* 35:213-218, 2006.

Hatakenaka M, Soeda H, Yabuuchi H, et al.: Apparent diffusion coefficients of breast tumors: clinical application, *Magn Reson Med Sci* 7:23-29, 2008.

Heaphy CM, Griffith JK, Bisoffi M: Mammary field cancerization: molecular evidence and clinical importance, *Breast Cancer Res Treat* 118:229-239, 2009.

Hegenscheid K, Schmidt CO, Seipel R, et al.: Normal breast parenchyma: contrast enhancement kinetics at dynamic MR mammography—influence of anthropometric measures and menopausal status, *Radiology* 266(1):72-80, 2013.

Helbich TH, Wunderbaldinger P, Plenk H, Deutinger M, Breitenseher M, Mostbeck GH: The value of MRI in silicone granuloma of the breast, *Eur J Radiol* 24:155-158, 1997.

Heywang SH, Wolf A, Pruss E, et al.: MR imaging of the breast with Gd-DTPA: use and limitations, *Radiology* 171:95-103, 1989.

Heywang-Köbrunner SH, Schlegel A, Beck R, et al.: Contrast-enhanced MRI of the breast after limited surgery and radiation therapy, *J Comput Assist Tomogr* 17:891-900, 1993.

Hochman MG, Orel SG, Powell CM, et al.: Fibroadenomas: MR imaging appearances with radiologic-histopathologic correlation, *Radiology* 204:123-129, 1997.

Houssami N, Ciatto S, Macaskill P, et al.: Accuracy and surgical impact of magnetic resonance imaging in breast cancer staging: systematic review and meta-analysis in detection of multifocal and multicentric cancer, *J Clin Oncol* 26:3248-3258, 2008.

Hrung JM, Langlotz CP, Orel SG, et al.: Cost-effectiveness of MR imaging and core-needle biopsy in the preoperative work-up of suspicious breast lesions, *Radiology* 213:39-49, 1999.

Hrung JM, Sonnad SS, Schwartz JS, Langlotz CP: Accuracy of MR imaging in the work-up of suspicious breast lesions: a diagnostic meta-analysis, *Acad Radiol* 6:387-397, 1999.

Hwang ES, Kinkel K, Esserman LJ, et al.: Magnetic resonance imaging in patients diagnosed with ductal carcinoma in situ: value in the diagnosis of residual disease, occult invasion, and multicentricity, *Ann Surg Oncol* 10:381-388, 2003.

Hylton NM: Vascularity assessment of breast lesions with gadolinium-enhanced MR imaging, *Magn Reson Imaging Clin N Am* 7:411-420, 1999.

Hylton NM: Suspension of breast-feeding following gadopentetate dimeglumine administration, *Radiology* 216:325-326, 2000.

Ikeda DM, Baker DR, Daniel BL: Magnetic resonance imaging of breast cancer: clinical indications and breast MRI reporting system, *J Magn Reson Imaging* 12:975-983, 2000.

Ikeda DM, Hylton NM, Kinkel K, et al.: Development, standardization, and testing of a lexicon for reporting contrast-enhanced breast magnetic resonance imaging studies, *J Magn Reson Imaging* 13:889-895, 2001.

Jaffer S, Bleiweiss IJ, Nagi C: Incidental intraductal papillomas (<2 mm) of the breast diagnosed on needle core biopsy do not need to be excised, *Breast J* 19:130-133, 2013.

Kamitani T, Matsuo Y, Yabuuchi H, et al.: Differentiation between benign phyllodes tumors and fibroadenomas of the breast on MR imaging, *Eur J Radiol* 83:1344-1349, 2014.

Kelcz F, Santyr GE, Cron GO, Mongin SJ: Application of a quantitative model to differentiate benign from malignant breast lesions detected by dynamic, gadolinium-enhanced MRI, *J Magn Reson Imaging* 6:743-752, 1996.

Kerslake RW, Fox JN, Carleton PJ, et al.: Dynamic contrast-enhanced and fat suppressed magnetic resonance imaging in suspected recurrent carcinoma of the breast: preliminary experience, *Br J Radiol* 67:1158-1168, 1994.

Kikuchi M, Tanino H, Kosaka Y, et al.: Usefulness of MRI of microcalcification lesions to determine the indication for stereotactic mammotome biopsy, *Anticancer Res* 34(11):6749-6753, 2014.

Kim TY, Kim SH, Kang BJ, et al.: Characterization of the enhancing lesions on dynamic contrast enhanced magnetic resonance imaging in patients with interstitial mammoplasty, *Eur J Radiol* 82:2205-2211, 2013.

Kinkel K, Helbich TH, Esserman LJ, et al.: Dynamic high-spatial resolution MR imaging of suspicious breast lesions: diagnostic criteria and interobserver variability, *AJR Am J Roentgenol* 175:35-43, 2000.

Kinner S, Herbrik M, Maderwald S, Umutlu L, Nassenstein K: Preoperative MR-guided wire localization for suspicious breast lesions: comparison of manual and automated software calculated targeting, *Eur J Radiol* 83(2):e80-e83, 2014.

Kinoshita T, Odagiri K, Andoh K, et al.: Evaluation of small internal mammary lymph node metastases in breast cancer by MRI, *Radiat Med* 17:189-193, 1999.

Kinoshita T, Yashiro N, Ihara N, et al.: Diffusion-weighted half-Fourier single-shot turbo spin echo imaging in breast tumors: differentiation of invasive ductal carcinoma from fibroadenoma, *J Comput Assist Tomogr* 26:1042-1046, 2002.

Kinoshita T, Yashiro N, Yoshigi J, et al.: Inflammatory intramammary lymph node mimicking the malignant lesion in dynamic MRI: a case report, *Clin Imaging* 26:258-262, 2002.

Ko EY, Han BK, Shin JH, Kang SS: Breast MRI for evaluating patients with metastatic axillary lymph node and initially negative mammography and sonography, *Korean J Radiol* 8:382-389, 2007.

Kovatcheva R, Guglielmina JN, Abehsera M, Boulanger L, Laurent N, Poncelet E: Ultrasound-guided high-intensity focused ultrasound treatment of breast fibroadenoma-a multicenter experience, *J Ther Ultrasound* 3(1):1, 2015.

Kraemer B, Hoffmann J, Roehm C, Gall C, Wallwiener D, Krainick-Strobel U: Cystosarcoma phyllodes of the breast: a rare diagnosis: case studies and review of literature, *Arch Gynecol Obstet* 276:649-653, 2007.

Kriege M, Brekelmans CT, Boetes C, et al.: Efficacy of MRI and mammography for breast-cancer screening in women with a familial or genetic predisposition, *N Engl J Med* 351:427-437, 2004.

Kubik-Huch RA, Gottstein-Aalame NM, Frenzel T, et al.: Gadopentetate dimeglumine excretion into human breast milk during lactation, *Radiology* 216:555-558, 2000.

Kuhl CK: High-risk screening: multi-modality surveillance of women at high risk for breast cancer (proven or suspected carriers of a breast cancer susceptibility gene), *J Exp Clin Cancer Res* 21(3 Suppl):103-106, 2002a.

Kuhl CK: Interventional breast MRI: needle localisation and core biopsies, *J Exp Clin Cancer Res* 21(3 Suppl):65-68, 2002b.

Kuhl CK, Bieling HB, Gieseke J, et al.: Healthy premenopausal breast parenchyma in dynamic contrast-enhanced MR imaging of the breast: normal contrast medium enhancement and cyclical-phase dependency, *Radiology* 203:137-144, 1997a.

Kuhl CK, Elevelt A, Leutner CC, et al.: Interventional breast MR imaging: clinical use of a stereotactic localization and biopsy device, *Radiology* 204:667-675, 1997b.

Kuhl CK, Klaschik S, Mielcarek P, et al.: Do T2-weighted pulse sequences help with the differential diagnosis of enhancing lesions in dynamic breast MRI? *J Magn Reson Imaging* 9:187-196, 1999a.

Kuhl CK, Mielcareck P, Klaschik S, et al.: Dynamic breast MR imaging: are signal intensity time course data useful for differential diagnosis of enhancing lesions? *Radiology* 211:101-110, 1999b.

Kuhl CK, Morakkabati N, Leutner CC, et al.: MR imaging—guided large-core (14-gauge) needle biopsy of small lesions visible at breast MR imaging alone, *Radiology* 220:31-39, 2001.

Kuhl CK, Schild HH: Dynamic image interpretation of MRI of the breast, *J Magn Reson Imaging* 12:965-974, 2000a.

Kuhl CK, Schmutzler RK, Leutner CC, et al.: Breast MR imaging screening in 192 women proved or suspected to be carriers of a breast cancer susceptibility gene: preliminary results, *Radiology* 215:267-279, 2000b.

Kuhl CK, Schrading S, Leutner CC, et al.: Mammography, breast ultrasound, and magnetic resonance imaging for surveillance of women at high familial risk for breast cancer, *J Clin Oncol* 23:8469-8476, 2005.

Kuhl CK, Schrading S, Strobel K, et al.: Abbreviated breast magnetic resonance imaging (MRI): first postcontrast subtracted images and maximum-intensity projection-a novel approach to breast cancer screening with MRI, *J Clin Oncol* 32:2304-2310, 2014.

Laguna AD, Arranz SJ, Checa VQ, et al.: Sonographic findings of additional malignant lesions in breast carcinoma seen by second look ultrasound, *J Clin Imaging Sci* 1:34, 2011.

Le Bihan D, Turner R, Douek P, Patronas N: Diffusion MR imaging: clinical applications, *AJR Am J Roentgenol* 159:591-599, 1992.

Leach MO, Boggis CR, Dixon AK, et al.: Screening with magnetic resonance imaging and mammography of a UK population at high familial risk of breast cancer: a prospective multicentre cohort study (MARIBS), *Lancet* 365:1769-1778, 2005.

Leach MO, Brindle KM, Evelhoch JL, et al.: The assessment of antiangiogenic and antivascular therapies in early-stage clinical trials using magnetic resonance imaging: issues and recommendations, *Br J Cancer* 92:1599-1610, 2005.

Lee CH: Problem solving MR imaging of the breast, *Radiol Clin North Am* 42:919-934, vii, 2004.

Lee SG, Orel SG, Woo IJ, et al.: MR imaging screening of the contralateral breast in patients with newly diagnosed breast cancer: preliminary results, *Radiology* 226:773–778, 2003.

Lehman CD, Blume JD, Thickman D, et al.: Added cancer yield of MRI in screening the contralateral breast of women recently diagnosed with breast cancer: results from the International Breast Magnetic Resonance Consortium (IBMC) trial, *J Surg Oncol* 92:9–16, 2005.

Lehman CD, Blume JD, Weatherall P, et al.: Screening women at high risk for breast cancer with mammography and magnetic resonance imaging, *Cancer* 103:1898–1905, 2005.

Lehman CD, DeMartini W, Anderson BO, Edge SB: Indications for breast MRI in the patient with newly diagnosed breast cancer, *J Natl Compr Canc Netw* 7:193–201, 2009.

Leong CS, Daniel BL, Herfkens RJ, et al.: Characterization of breast lesion morphology with delayed 3DSSMT: an adjunct to dynamic breast MRI, *J Magn Reson Imaging* 11:87–96, 2000.

Lehman CD, Gatsonis C, Kuhl CK, et al.: MRI evaluation of the contralateral breast in women with recently diagnosed breast cancer, *N Engl J Med* 356:1295–1303, 2007.

Lehman CD, Isaacs C, Schnall MD, et al.: Cancer yield of mammography, MR, and US in high-risk women: prospective multi-institution breast cancer screening study, *Radiology* 244:381–388, 2007.

Lenkinski B, Wang X, Elian M, Goldberg SN: Interaction of gadolinium-based MR contrast agents with choline: implications for MR spectroscopy (MRS) of the breast, *Magn Reson Med* 61:1286–1292, 2009.

Li J, Dershaw DD, Lee CH, et al.: MRI follow-up after concordant, histologically benign diagnosis of breast lesions sampled by MRI-guided biopsy, *AJR Am J Roentgenol* 193:850–855, 2009.

Li E, Li J, Song Y, Xue M, Zhou C: A comparative study of the diagnostic value of contrast-enhanced breast MR imaging and mammography on patients with BI-RADS 3-5 microcalcifications, *PLoS One* 9(11):e111217, 2014.

Liberman L, Morris EA, Benton CL, et al.: Probably benign lesions at breast magnetic resonance imaging: preliminary experience in high-risk women, *Cancer* 98:377–388, 2003.

Liberman L, Morris EA, Dershaw DD, et al.: Ductal enhancement on MR imaging of the breast, *AJR Am J Roentgenol* 181:519–525, 2003.

Liberman L, Morris EA, Dershaw DD, et al.: Fast MRI-guided vacuum-assisted breast biopsy: initial experience, *AJR Am J Roentgenol* 181:1283–1293, 2003.

Liberman L, Morris EA, Dershaw DD, et al.: MR imaging of the ipsilateral breast in women with percutaneously proven breast cancer, *AJR Am J Roentgenol* 180:901–910, 2003.

Liberman L, Morris EA, Kim CM, et al.: MR imaging findings in the contralateral breast of women with recently diagnosed breast cancer, *AJR Am J Roentgenol* 180:333–341, 2003.

Liberman L, Morris EA, Lee MJ, et al.: Breast lesions detected on MR imaging: features and positive predictive value, *AJR Am J Roentgenol* 179:171–178, 2002.

Linda A, Zuiani C, Girometti R, et al.: Unusual malignant tumors of the breast: MRI features and pathologic correlation, *Eur J Radiol* 75:178–184, 2010.

Linda A, Zuiani C, Londero V, Bazzocchi M: Outcome of initially only magnetic resonance mammography-detected findings with and without correlate at second-look sonography: distribution according to patient history of breast cancer and lesion size, *Breast* 17:51–57, 2008.

Linda A, Zuiani C, Londero V: Role of magnetic resonance imaging in probably benign (BI-RADS category 3) microcalcifications of the breast, *Radiol Med* 119(6):393–399, 2014.

Linda A, Zuiani C, Londero V, et al.: Magnetic resonance imaging of radial sclerosing lesions (radial scars) of the breast, *Eur J Radiol* 81:3201–3207, 2012.

Lobbes MB, Lalji U, Houwers J: Contrast-enhanced spectral mammography in patients referred from the breast cancer screening programme, *Eur Radiol* 24(7):1668–1676, 2014.

Lourenco AP, Chung MT, Mainiero MB: Utility of targeted sonography in management of probably benign breast lesions identified on magnetic resonance imaging, *J Ultrasound Med* 31:1033–1040, 2012.

Lourenco AP, Khalil H, Sanford M, Donegan L: High-Risk lesions at MRI-guided breast biopsy: frequency and rate of underestimation, *AJR Am Roentgenol* 203:682–686, 2014.

Lubina N, Schedelbeck U, Roth A: 3.0 Tesla breast magnetic resonance imaging in patients with nipple discharge when mammography and ultrasound fail, *Eur Radiol* 25:1285–1293, 2014.

Luciani ML, Pediconi F, Telesca M, et al.: Incidental enhancing lesions found on preoperative breast MRI: management and role of second-look ultrasound, *Radiol Med* 116:886–904, 2011.

Lyng H, Haraldseth O, Rofstad EK: Measurement of cell density and necrotic fraction in human melanoma xenografts by diffusion weighted magnetic resonance imaging, *Magn Reson Med* 43:828–836, 2000.

Majedah S, Alhabshi I, Salim S: Granulomatous reaction secondary to intramammary silicone injection, *BMJ Case Rep*, pii:bcr2012007961, 2013.

Manion E, Brock JE, Raza S, Reisenbichler ES: MRI-guided breast needle core biopsies: pathologic features of newly diagnosed malignancies, *Breast J* 20(5):453–460, 2014.

Marchant LK, Orel SG, Perez-Jaffev LA, Reynolds C, Schnall MD: Bilateral angiosarcoma of the breast on MR imaging, *AJR Am J Roentgenol* 169:1009–1010, 1997.

Marini C, Iacconi C, Giannelli M, et al.: Quantitative diffusion-weighted MR imaging in the differential diagnosis of breast lesion, *Eur Radiol* 17:2646–2655, 2007.

Marinovich ML, Houssami N, Macaskill P: Meta-analysis of magnetic resonance imaging in detecting residual breast cancer after neoadjuvant therapy, *J Natl Cancer Inst* 105(5):321–333, 2013.

Meeuwis C, Veltman J, van Hall HN, et al.: MR-guided breast biopsy at 3T: diagnostic yield of large core needle biopsy compared with vacuum-assisted biopsy, *Eur Radiol* 22:341–349, 2012.

Meissnitzer M, Dershaw DD, Lee CH, Morris EA: Targeted ultrasound of the breast in women with abnormal MRI findings for whom biopsy has been recommended, *AJR Am J Roentgenol* 193:1025–1029, 2009.

Mercier J, Kwiatkowski F, Abrial C, et al.: The role of tomosynthesis in breast cancer staging in 75 patients, *Diagn Interv Imaging* 96(1):27–35, 2015.

Merckel LG, Verkooijen HM, Peters NH, et al.: The added diagnostic value of dynamic contrast-enhanced MRI at 3.0 T in nonpalpable breast lesions, *PLoS One* 9(4):e94233, 2014.

Millet I, Curros-Doyon F, Molinari N, Bouic-Pages E, Prat X, Alili C, Taourel P: Invasive breast carcinoma: influence of prognosis and patient-related factors on kinetic MR imaging characteristics, *Radiology* 270(1):57–66, 2014.

Monzawa S, Yokokawa M, Sakuma T, et al.: Mucinous carcinoma of the breast: MRI features of pure and mixed forms with histopathologic correlation, *AJR Am J Roentgenol* 192:W125–W131, 2009.

Mori M, Tsunoda H, Takamoto Y: MRI and ultrasound evaluation of invasive lobular carcinoma of the breast after primary systemic therapy, *Breast Cancer* 22:356–365, 2013.

Morris EA, Comstock CE, Lee CH, et al.: ACR BI-RADS® magnetic resonance imaging. *ACR BI-RADS® atlas, breast imaging reporting and data system*, ed 5, Reston, VA, 2013, American College of Radiology.

Morris EA, Liberman L, Ballon DJ, et al.: MRI of occult breast carcinoma in a high-risk population, *AJR Am J Roentgenol* 181:619–626, 2003.

Morris EA, Liberman L, Dershaw DD, et al.: Preoperative MR imaging-guided needle localization of breast lesions, *AJR Am J Roentgenol* 178:1211–1220, 2002.

Morris EA, Schwartz LH, Drotman MB, et al.: Evaluation of pectoralis major muscle in patients with posterior breast tumors on breast MR images: early experience, *Radiology* 214:67–72, 2000.

Morris EA: Illustrated breast MR lexicon, *Semin Roentgenol* 36:238–249, 2001.

Moy L, Elias K, Patel V, et al.: Is breast MRI helpful in the evaluation of inconclusive mammographic findings? *AJR Am J Roentgenol* 193:986–993, 2009.

Moy L, Elias K, Patel V: Is breast MRI helpful in the evaluation of inconclusive mammographic findings? *AJR Am J Roentgenol* 193(4):986–993, 2009.

Muller-Schimpfle M, Ohmenhauser K, Sand J, et al.: Dynamic 3D-MR mammography: is there a benefit of sophisticated evaluation of enhancement curves for clinical routine? *J Magn Reson Imaging* 7:236–240, 1997.

Muttalib M, Ibrahem R, Khashan AS, Hajaj M: Prospective MRI assessment for invasive lobular breast cancer. Correlation with tumour size at histopathology and influence on surgical management, *Clin Radiol* 69(1):23–28, 2014.

Myers KS, Kamel IR, Macura KJ: MRI-guided breast biopsy: outcomes and effect on patient management, *Clin Breast Cancer* 15(2):143–152, 2015.

Nicholson BT, Harvey JA, Cohen MA: Nipple–areolar complex: normal anatomy and benign and malignant processes, *Radiographics* 29:509–523, 2009.

Niell BL, Lee JM, Johansen C, Halpern EF, Rafferty EA: Patient outcomes in canceled MRI-guided breast biopsies, *AJR Am J Roentgenol* 202(1):223–228, 2014.

Nunes LW, Englander SA, Charafeddine R, Schnall MD: Optimal post-contrast timing of breast MR image acquisition for architectural feature analysis, *J Magn Reson Imaging* 16:42–50, 2002.

Nunes LW, Schnall MD, Orel SG: Update of breast MR imaging architectural interpretation model, *Radiology* 219:484–494, 2001.

Obdeijn IM, Brouwers-Kuyper EM, Tilanus-Linthorst MM, et al.: MR imaging-guided sonography followed by Breast J fine-needle aspiration cytology in occult carcinoma of the breast, *AJR Am J Roentgenol* 174:1079–1084, 2000.

Obdeijn IM, Winter-Warnars GA, Mann RM, Hooning MJ, Hunink MG, Tilanus-Linthorst MM: Should we screen BRCA1 mutation carriers only with MRI? A multicenter study, *Breast Cancer Res Treat* 144(3):577–582, 2014.

Offodile RS, Daniel BL, Jeffrey SS, et al.: Magnetic resonance imaging of suspicious breast masses seen on one mammographic view, *Breast J* 10(5):416–422, 2004.

O'Flynn EA, Ledger AE, deSouza NM: Alternative screening for dense breasts: MRI, *AJR Am J Roentgenol* 204(2):W141–W149, 2015.

Ohlinger R, Stomps A, Paepke S, et al.: Ductoscopic detection of intraductal lesions in cases of pathologic nipple discharge in comparison with standard diagnostics: the German multicenter study, *Oncol Res Treat* 37(11):628–632, 2014.

Ojeda-Fournier H, Chloe KA, Mahoney MC: Recognizing and interpreting artifacts and pitfalls in MR imaging of the breast, *Radiographics* 27:147–164, 2007.

O'Neill AC, D'Arcy C, McDermott E, O'Doherty A, Quinn C, McNally S: Magnetic resonance imaging appearances in primary and secondary angiosarcoma of the breast, *J Med Imaging Radiat Oncol* 58:208–212, 2014.

Orel SG, Dougherty CS, Reynolds C, et al.: MR imaging in patients with nipple discharge: initial experience, *Radiology* 216:248–254, 2000.

Orel SG, Rosen M, Mies C, Schnall MD: MR imaging-guided 9-gauge vacuum-assisted core-needle breast biopsy: initial experience, *Radiology* 238:54–61, 2006.

Orel SG, Schnall MD, Newman RW, Powell CM, Torosian MH, Rosato EF: MR imaging-guided localization and biopsy of breast lesions: initial experience, *Radiology* 193:97–102, 1994.

Oxner CR, Vora L, Yim J, et al.: Magnetic resonance imaging-guided breast biopsy in lesions not visualized by mammogram or ultrasound, *Am Surg* 78(10):1087–1090, 2012.

Oztekin PS, Kosar PN: Magnetic resonance imaging of the breast as a problem-solving method: to be or not to be? *Breast J* 20(6):622–631, 2014.

Pallone MJ, Poplack SP, Avutu HB, Paulsen KD, Barth Jr RJ: Supine breast MRI and 3D optical scanning: a novel approach to improve tumor localization for breast conserving surgery, *Ann Surg Oncol* 21(7):2203–2208, 2014.

Parikh J, Selmi M, Charles-Edwards G, et al.: Changes in primary breast cancer heterogeneity may augment midtreatment MR imaging assessment of response to neoadjuvant chemotherapy, *Radiology* 272(1):100–112, 2014.

Partridge SC, DeMartini WB, Kurland BF, et al.: Quantitative diffusion-weighted imaging as an adjunct to conventional breast MRI for improved positive predictive value, *AJR Am J Roentgenol* 193:1716–1722, 2009.

Partridge SC, Gibbs JE, Lu Y, et al.: Accuracy of MR imaging for revealing residual breast cancer in patients who have undergone neoadjuvant chemotherapy, *AJR Am J Roentgenol* 179:1193–1199, 2002.

Partridge SC, McKinnon GC, Henry RG, Hylton NM: Menstrual cycle variation of apparent diffusion coefficients measured in the normal breast using MRI, *J Magn Reson Imaging* 14:433–438, 2001.

Pediconi F, Catalano C, Roselli A, et al.: Contrast-enhanced MR mammography for evaluation of the contralateral breast in patients with diagnosed unilateral breast cancer or high-risk lesions, *Radiology* 243:670–680, 2007.

Pengel KE, Loo CE, Wesseling J, Pijnappel RM, Rutgers EJ, Gilhuijs KG: Avoiding preoperative breast MRI when conventional imaging is sufficient to stage patients eligible for breast conserving therapy, *Eur J Radiol* 83(2):273–278, 2014.

Pereira FP, Martins G, Figueiredo E, et al.: Assessment of breast lesions with diffusion-weighted MRI: comparing the use of different b values, *AJR Am J Roentgenol* 193:1030–1035, 2009.

Perlet C, Heinig A, Prat X, et al.: Multicenter study for the evaluation of a dedicated biopsy device for MR-guided vacuum biopsy of the breast, *Eur Radiol* 12:1463–1470, 2002.

Perlet C, Schneider P, Amaya B, et al.: MR-guided vacuum biopsy of 206 contrast-enhancing breast lesions, *Rofo* 174:88–95, 2002.

Plecha DM, Pham RM, Klein N, et al.: Addition of shear-wave elastography during second-look MR imaging-directed breast US: effect on lesion detection and biopsy targeting, *Radiology* 272(3):657–664, 2014.

Po J, Margolis DJ, Cunningham CH, Herfkens RJ, Ikeda DM, Daniel BL: Water-selective spectral-spatial contrast-enhanced breast MRI for cancer detection in patients with extracapsular and injected free silicone, *Magn Reson Imaging* 24:1363–1367, 2006.

Port ER, Park A, Borgen PI, Morris E, Montgomery LL: Results of MRI screening for breast cancer in high-risk patients with LCIS and atypical hyperplasia, *Ann Surg Oncol* 14:1051–1057, 2007.

Qayyum A, Birdwell RL, Daniel BL, et al.: MR imaging features of infiltrating lobular carcinoma of the breast: histopathologic correlation, *AJR Am J Roentgenol* 178:1227–1232, 2002.

Quinn EM, Coveney AP, Redmond HP: Use of magnetic resonance imaging in detection of breast cancer recurrence: a systematic review, *Ann Surg Oncol* 19:3035–3041, 2012.

Rahbar H, Conlin JL, Parsian S, et al.: Suspicious axillary lymph nodes identified on clinical breast MRI in patients newly diagnosed with breast cancer: can quantitative features improve discrimination of malignant from benign? *Acad Radiol* 22:430–438, 2015.

Rahbar H, Hanna LG, Gatsonis C, et al.: Contralateral prophylactic mastectomy in the American College of Radiology Imaging Network 6667 trial: effect of breast MR imaging assessments and patient characteristics, *Radiology* 273:53–60, 2014.

Rahbar H, DeMartini WB, Lee AY, Partridge SC, Peacock S, Lehman CD: Accuracy of 3T versus 1.5T breast MRI for preoperative assessment of extent of disease in newly diagnosed DCIS, *Eur J Radiol* 84(4):611–616, 2015.

Ralleigh G, Walker AE, Hall-Craggs MA, et al.: MR imaging of the skin and nipple of the breast: differentiation between tumour recurrence and post-treatment change, *Eur Radiol* 11:1651–1658, 2001.

Rieber A, Zeitler H, Rosenthal H, et al.: MRI of breast cancer: influence of chemotherapy on sensitivity, *Br J Radiol* 70:452–458, 1997.

Robertson C, Arcot Ragupathy SK, Boachie C, et al.: The clinical effectiveness and cost-effectiveness of different surveillance mammography regimens after the treatment for primary breast cancer: systematic reviews registry database analyses and economic evaluation, *Health Technol Assess* 15(34):1–322, 2011. v–vi.

Rodenko GN, Harms SE, Pruneda JM, et al.: MR imaging in the management before surgery of lobular carcinoma of the breast: correlation with pathology, *AJR Am J Roentgenol* 167:1415–1419, 1996.

Roebuck JR, Cecil KM, Schnall MD, Lenkinski RE: Human breast lesions: characterization with proton MR spectroscopy, *Radiology* 209:269–227, 1998.

Rubesova E, Grell AS, De Maertelaer V, et al.: Quantitative diffusion imaging in breast cancer: a clinical prospective study, *J Magn Reson Imaging* 24:319–324, 2006.

Santamaria G, Velasco M, Bargallo X, Caparros X, Farrus B, Luis Fernandez P: Radiologic and pathologic findings in breast tumors with high signal intensity on T2-weighted MR images, *Radiographics* 30:533–548, 2010.

Santoro F, Podo F, Sardanelli F: MRI screening of women with hereditary predisposition to breast cancer: diagnostic performance and survival analysis, *Breast Cancer Res Treat* 147:685–687, 2014.

Sardanelli F, Podo F, Santoro F, et al.: Multicenter surveillance of women at high genetic breast cancer risk using mammography, ultrasonography, and contrast-enhanced magnetic resonance imaging (the high breast cancer risk italian 1 study): final results, *Invest Radiol* 46:94–105, 2011.

Sarica O, Uluc F, Tasmali D: Magnetic resonance imaging features of papillary breast lesions, *Eur J Radiol* 83(3):524–530, 2014.

Saslow D, Boetes C, Burke W, et al.: American Cancer Society guidelines for breast screening with MRI as an adjunct to mammography, *CA Cancer J Clin* 57:75–89, 2007.

Schelfout K, Van Goethem M, Kersschot E, et al.: Contrast-enhanced MR imaging of breast lesions and effect on treatment, *Eur J Surg Oncol* 30:501–507, 2004.

Schnall MD, Blume J, Bluemke DA, et al.: MRI detection of distinct incidental cancer in women with primary breast cancer studied in IBMC 6883, *J Surg Oncol* 92:32–38, 2005.

Schnall MD, Rosten S, Englander S, et al.: A combined architectural and kinetic interpretation model for breast MR images, *Acad Radiol* 8:591–597, 2001.

Shah P, Rosen M, Stopfer J, et al.: Prospective study of breast MRI in BRCA1 and BRCA2 mutation carriers: effect of mutation status on cancer incidence, *Breast Cancer Res Treat* 118:539–546, 2009.

Shaylor SD, Heller SL, Melsaether AN, et al.: Short interval follow-up after a benign concordant MR-guided vacuum assisted breast biopsy—is it worthwhile? *Eur Radiol* 24(6):1176–1185, 2014.

Sinha S, Lucas-Quesada FA, Sinha U, et al.: In vivo diffusion-weighted MRI of the breast: potential for lesion characterization, *J Magn Reson Imaging* 15:693–704, 2002.

Slanetz PJ, Edmister WB, Yeh ED, et al.: Occult contralateral breast carcinoma incidentally detected by breast magnetic resonance imaging, *Breast J* 8:145–148, 2002.

Smith H, Chetlen AL, Schetter S, Mack J, Watts M, Zhu JJ: PPV(3) of suspicious breast MRI findings, *Acad Radiol* 21(12):1553–1562, 2014.

Soderstrom CE, Harms SE, Farrell Jr RS, et al.: Detection with MR imaging of residual tumor in the breast soon after surgery, *AJR Am J Roentgenol* 168:485–488, 1997.

Spick C, Baltzer PA: Diagnostic utility of second-look US for breast lesions identified at MR imaging: systematic review and meta-analysis, *Radiology* 273(2):401–409, 2014a.

Spick C, Szolar DH, Baltzer PA, et al.: Rate of malignancy in MRI-detected probably benign (BI-RADS 3) lesions, *AJR Am J Roentgenol* 202(3):684–689, 2014b.

Stehouwer BL, Merckel LG, Verkooijen HM: 3-T breast magnetic resonance imaging in patients with suspicious microcalcifications on mammography, *Eur Radiol* 24(3):603–609, 2014.

Steinbach BG, Hardt NS, Abbitt PL, Lanier L, Caffee HH: Breast implants, common complications, and concurrent breast disease, *Radiographics* 13:95–118, 1993.

Stoutjesdijk MJ, Boetes C, Jager GJ, et al.: Magnetic resonance imaging and mammography in women with a hereditary risk of breast cancer, *J Natl Cancer Inst* 93:1095–1102, 2001.

Sugahara T, Korogi Y, Kochi M, et al.: Usefulness of diffusion-weighted MRI with echo-planar technique in the evaluation of cellularity in gliomas, *J Magn Reson Imaging* 9:53–60, 1999.

Talele AC, Slanetz PJ, Edmister WB, et al.: The lactating breast: MRI findings and literature review, *Breast J* 9:237–240, 2003.

Tan JE, Orel SG, Schnall MD, et al.: Role of magnetic resonance imaging and magnetic resonance imaging-guided surgery in the evaluation of patients with early-stage breast cancer for breast conservation treatment, *Am J Clin Oncol* 22:414–418, 1999.

Tan SL, Rahmat K, Rozalli FI, et al.: Differentiation between benign and malignant breast lesions using quantitative diffusion-weighted sequence on 3 T MRI, *Clin Radiol* 69:63–71, 2014.

Teifke A, Lehr HA, Vomweg TW, et al.: Outcome analysis and rational management of enhancing lesions incidentally detected on contrast-enhanced MRI of the breast, *AJR Am J Roentgenol* 181:655–662, 2003.

Tendulkar RD, Chellman-Jeffers M, Rybicki LA, et al.: Preoperative breast magnetic resonance imaging in early breast cancer: implications for partial breast irradiation, *Cancer* 115:1621–1630, 2009.

Thompson MO, Lipson J, Daniel B, et al.: Why are patients noncompliant with follow-up recommendations after MRI-guided core needle biopsy of suspicious breast lesions? *AJR Am J Roentgenol* 201:1391–1400, 2013.

Tilanus-Linthorst MM, Bartels CC, Obdeijn AI, Oudkerk M: Earlier detection of breast cancer by surveillance of women at familial risk, *Eur J Cancer* 36:514–519, 2000.

Tilanus-Linthorst MM, Obdeijn AI, Bontenbal M, Oudkerk M: MRI in patients with axillary metastases of occult breast carcinoma, *Breast Cancer Res Treat* 44:179–182, 1997.

Trecate G, Tess JD, Vergnaghi D, et al.: Lobular breast cancer: how useful is breast magnetic resonance imaging? *Tumori* 87:232–238, 2001.

Trecate G, Vergnaghi D, Manoukian S, et al.: MRI in the early detection of breast cancer in women with high genetic risk, *Tumori* 92:517–523, 2006.

Trop I, Gilbert G, Ivancevic MK, Beaudoin G: Breast MR imaging at 3T with dual-source radiofrequency transmission offers superior B1 homogeneity: an intraindividual comparison with breast MR imaging at 1.5 T, *Radiology* 267(2):602–608, 2013.

Tsuboi N, Ogawa Y, Inomata T, et al.: Changes in the findings of dynamic MRI by preoperative CAF chemotherapy for patients with breast cancer of stage II and III: pathologic correlation, *Oncol Rep* 6:727–732, 1999.

Tsushima Y, Takahashi-Taketomi A, Endo K: Magnetic resonance (MR) differential diagnosis of breast tumors using apparent diffusion coefficient (ADC) on 1.5-T, *J Magn Reson Imaging* 30:249–255, 2009.

van den Bosch MA, Daniel BL, Pal S, et al.: MRI-guided needle localization of suspicious breast lesions: results of a freehand technique, *Eur Radiol* 16:1811–1817, 2006.

Viehweg P, Heinig A, Lampe D, et al.: Retrospective analysis for evaluation of the value of contrast-enhanced MRI in patients treated with breast conservative therapy, *MAGMA* 7:141–152, 1998.

Viehweg P, Lampe D, Buchmann J, Heywang-Kobrunner SH: In situ and minimally invasive breast cancer: morphologic and kinetic features on contrast-enhanced MR imaging, *MAGMA* 11:129–137, 2000.

Viehweg P, Paprosch I, Strassinopoulou M, Heywang-Kobrunner SH: Contrast-enhanced magnetic resonance imaging of the breast: interpretation guidelines, *Top Magn Reson Imaging* 9:17–43, 1998.

Viehweg P, Rotter K, Laniado M, et al.: MR imaging of the contralateral breast in patients after breast-conserving therapy, *Eur Radiol* 14:402–408, 2004.

Warner E, Plewes DW, Hill KA, et al.: Surveillance of BRCA1 and BRCA2 mutation carriers with magnetic resonance imaging, ultrasound, mammography, and clinical breast examination, *JAMA* 292:1317–1325, 2004.

Warner E, Plewes DB, Shumak RS, et al.: Comparison of breast magnetic resonance imaging, mammography, and ultrasound for surveillance of women at high risk for hereditary breast cancer, *J Clin Oncol* 19:3524–3531, 2001.

Weinfurtner RJ, Patel B, Laronga C, et al.: Magnetic resonance imaging-guided core needle breast biopsies resulting in high-risk histopathologic findings: upstage frequency and lesion characteristics, *Clin Breast Cancer* 15:234–239, 2014.

Wenkel E, Geppert C, Schulz-Wendtland R, et al.: Diffusion weighted imaging in breast MRI: comparison of two different pulse sequences, *Acad Radiol* 14:1077–1083, 2007.

Wiratkapun C, Duke D, Nordmann AS, et al.: Indeterminate or suspicious breast lesions detected initially with MR imaging: value of MRI-directed breast ultrasound, *Acad Radiol* 15:618–625, 2008.

Woodhams R, Matsunaga K, Kan S, et al.: ADC mapping of benign and malignant breast tumors, *Magn Reson Med Sci* 4:35–42, 2005.

Yabuuchi H, Matsuo Y, Okafuji T, et al.: Enhanced mass on contrast-enhanced breast MR imaging: lesion characterization using combination of dynamic contrast-enhanced and diffusion-weighted MR images, *J Magn Reson Imaging* 28:1157–1165, 2008.

Yamaguchi K, Schacht D, Nakazono T, Irie H, Abe H: Diffusion weighted images of metastatic as compared with nonmetastatic axillary lymph nodes in patients with newly diagnosed breast cancer, *J Magn Reson Imaging* 42:771–778, 2014.

Yang Q, Li L, Zhang J, Shao G, et al.: Computer-aided diagnosis of breast DCE-MRI images using bilateral asymmetry of contrast enhancement between two breasts, *J Digit Imaging* 27(1):152–160, 2014.

Yang WT, Hennessy BT, Dryden MJ, Valero V, Hunt KK, Krishnamurthy S: Mammary angiosarcomas: imaging findings in 24 patients, *Radiology* 242:725–734, 2007.

Yeung DK, Cheung HS, Tse GM: Human breast lesions: characterization with contrast-enhanced in vivo proton MR spectroscopy–initial results, *Radiology* 220:40–46, 2001.

Yi A, Cho N, Im SA, et al.: Survival outcomes of breast cancer patients who receive neoadjuvant chemotherapy: association with dynamic contrast-enhanced MR imaging with computer-aided evaluation, *Radiology* 268(3):662–672, 2013.

Yildiz S, Aralasmak A, Kadioglu H, et al.: Radiologic findings of idiopathic granulomatous mastitis, *Med Ultrason* 17:39–44, 2015.

Youk JH, Son EJ, Kim EK: Diagnosis of breast cancer at dynamic MRI in patients with breast augmentation by paraffin or silicone injection, *Clin Radiol* 64:1175–1180, 2009.

Chapter 8

Breast Cancer Treatment-Related Imaging and the Postoperative Breast

Kathleen C. Horst, Kanae K. Miyake, Debra M. Ikeda, and Frederick M. Dirbas

CHAPTER OUTLINE

This chapter provides an overview of clinically driven breast cancer evaluation; the sequence of events after a breast cancer diagnosis; locoregional breast cancer treatment options, including sentinel lymph node (SLN) biopsy; the normal postoperative breast; postradiation therapy change; ipsilateral breast tumor recurrence (IBTR) after lumpectomy; and the appearance of the breast after mastectomy with or without reconstruction.

Suspicious palpable or image-detected breast abnormalities constitute the majority of consultations for breast specialists. The specialist assesses the patient, usually orders a complete imaging workup of suspicious findings, and may ask for fine-needle aspiration (FNA) or percutaneous core biopsy to establish a cancer diagnosis. If percutaneous biopsy results are indeterminate or discordant, or if the patient prefers, a diagnosis may be established by open surgical breast biopsy.

No matter how breast cancer is diagnosed, follow-up treatment depends on the tumor size and stage. Patients usually see a surgeon first, because if the cancer is small surgical management is almost always recommended initially. The two principal surgical options to achieve local control are lumpectomy (almost always followed by breast radiotherapy) and mastectomy. Randomized studies suggest there is equivalent survival with either approach. Lumpectomy (also referred to as *breast-conserving surgery, partial mastectomy,* or *quadrantectomy*) is often offered to patients with small tumors that can be resected with a good cosmetic outcome. In cases where mastectomy is recommended to or preferred by the patient, mastectomy can be performed using various techniques, such as skin-sparing or nipple-areolar-sparing techniques, and can be performed with or without breast reconstruction.

If the cancer is very large, neoadjuvant chemotherapy (NAC; ie, chemotherapy given before excision of the primary tumor) may be recommended before surgery. NAC shrinks the tumor, allows the medical oncologist to determine the chemotherapy's effectiveness in vivo and, if the tumor shrinks to a small enough size, allows the patient to opt for breast-conserving therapy and radiation therapy rather than mastectomy.

At the time of surgery, SLN biopsy (SLNB) commonly accompanies removal of the primary tumor to determine whether axillary lymph nodes harbor metastases. A completion axillary lymph node dissection (ALND; levels I and II) was performed if the sentinel node harbored anything more than isolated tumor cells (*AJCC Staging Manual*); however, the need for ALND is changing after results of the American College of Surgeons Oncology Group Z0011 trial (ACOSOG Z0011) as will be discussed.

Whole-breast, external beam radiotherapy (WB-XRT) usually is performed after lumpectomy to eliminate microscopic residual disease and to suppress tumor recurrence both in the remaining breast parenchyma and in the tissue around the lumpectomy cavity. This typically involves 5 to 7 weeks of whole-breast radiotherapy followed by an electron beam boost dose to the lumpectomy cavity to further eradicate any residual cells near the surgical margins. More recently, studies have demonstrated that in selected patients whole-breast radiotherapy can be delivered safely and effectively in 3 weeks (hypofractionated whole-breast radiotherapy), making the treatment more convenient for the patient. Accelerated partial breast irradiation (APBI) has also emerged as a potential option for selected patients. APBI delivers radiotherapy to the lumpectomy cavity only plus margin and can be safely delivered in one to five treatments. Various APBI techniques include intraoperative radiotherapy (IORT), interstitial brachytherapy, intracavitary brachytherapy, or three-dimensional (3D) conformal external beam radiation. Brachytherapy delivers the radiation dose internally using small radiation-emitting sources inserted into multiple catheters (interstitial brachytherapy) or a balloon catheter (intracavitary brachytherapy) in the biopsy cavity.

It is important for radiologists to understand these steps from workup through cancer diagnosis and treatment because surgery, radiation, and systemic therapy affect imaging of the treated breast. This chapter details each of these steps.

COMBINED CLINICAL AND IMAGING WORKUP OF BREAST ABNORMALITIES

Once the referring physician finds a suspicious breast mass or receives a suspicious mammographic report, the patient undergoes a thorough history and a focused breast examination. Usually a breast cancer specialist (most likely a general surgeon with an interest in breast cancer, a dedicated breast surgeon, or a surgical oncologist) then estimates the patient's risk of having breast cancer, seeks patterns of familial breast cancer, reviews the imaging and pathology, and helps the patient to make an informed decision on immediate intervention or the need to gather more information.

Most patients then undergo a thorough diagnostic imaging workup. Patients with suspicious palpable abnormalities undergo ultrasound, with or without mammography, depending on age, family history, and level of concern over the finding. For example, ultrasound would likely be the sole imaging modality in an 18-year-old woman with a new breast lump and no family history of breast cancer. On the other hand, ultrasound and mammography would likely be used for a 25-year-old woman with a new palpable lesion and an extensive family history of breast cancer in young relatives. The final decision to incorporate mammography into a very young patient's workup is a shared responsibility of the clinician directing the breast workup, the radiologist performing the initial imaging (ultrasound in this case), and the patient. Breast magnetic resonance imaging (MRI) is used sparingly during the initial evaluation of a palpable finding, unless there is an extensive breast or ovarian cancer family history, in which case it serves a dual role as both a diagnostic tool on the affected breast and a screening tool on the contralateral breast.

For patients with nonpalpable findings on screening mammography, workup always includes diagnostic mammography, with or without ultrasound. For suspicious calcifications alone, the radiologist usually obtains magnification mammograms, often not needing ultrasound. An exception might be extensive pleomorphic microcalcifications, in which ultrasound might discover masses suggesting invasive cancer within the calcifications, prompting biopsy. However, if there is an image-detected mass, area of architectural distortion, or palpable mass, the radiologist usually uses both mammography and ultrasound to evaluate the abnormality, estimate its size, and later direct the biopsy. Breast MRI may be valuable in selected cases, as discussed in Chapter 7. Ideally, the radiologist correlates all physical and imaging findings in the report to form a composite picture of all potential abnormalities and their level of suspicion using mammography, ultrasound, and MRI.

Using the combined report, the directing clinician and radiologist plan percutaneous or open biopsy to sample all areas of concern. This sequence varies from patient to patient. This may be as simple as FNA in a young woman with a single area of fibrocystic nodularity and a normal ultrasound or as complex as numerous core biopsies or surgical biopsies in one or both breasts using palpation or image guidance for localization.

Although there are no hard and fast rules about what defines a suspicious palpable abnormality, generally cancers are firm or hard; asymmetric compared with the opposite breast; irregular in shape; and feel as if they are rising up out of the breast tissue, rather than spreading out in the substance of the breast. Physical examination, ultrasound/mammography, and FNA are generally considered the minimum intervention for a suspicious palpable finding and in combination are referred to as the *triple test*. For suspicious palpable findings in which all components of

the triple test are negative, the risk of malignancy is considered approximately 3% or less. Even if all components of the triple test are normal, it is extremely important to inform the patient that there is a low, but measurable, false-negative rate for the triple test and that surgical excision can be performed to completely exclude the possibility of malignancy. This discussion is ideally documented in the medical record. Patients with likely benign palpable findings, unremarkable imaging, and normal percutaneous sampling with FNA (ie, a negative triple test) usually undergo a single follow-up visit 3 to 6 months later with the referring physician for follow-up physical examination and evaluation. Patients who undergo image-guided core biopsy usually undergo repeat imaging at 12 months to assess stability of any residual findings. Progressive findings on repeat palpation or breast imaging at follow-up prompt surgical excision.

For suspicious image-detected nonpalpable lesions, image-guided FNA, percutaneous core biopsy, or wire-localized excisional biopsy is generally considered the minimum intervention. Percutaneous needle core biopsy has become the more common choice. Here, too, it is important to inform the patient of the limitations of percutaneous core biopsy—specifically, that there is a small false-negative rate with needle biopsy. Wire-localized surgical biopsy is usually recommended to exclude malignancy if percutaneous biopsy is indeterminate or discordant with imaging findings or cannot be done. For an anxious patient, wire-localized surgical excision may be a better option initially; the surgeon will usually document this discussion in the medical record. For some patients with lesions close to the chest wall or nipple, wire-localized excisional biopsy may be the safer initial approach.

BREAST CANCER DIAGNOSIS AND TREATMENT

Breast cancer treatment planning usually involves surgery, systemic therapy, and radiation therapy. The goals are removing all the cancer from the breast, optimizing chances for locoregional control, and eradicating occult foci of metastatic disease with systemic treatment (eg, hormone therapy, chemotherapy) as indicated. The team of breast imagers, surgeons, medical oncologists, pathologists, radiation oncologists, and breast reconstruction surgeons plan the sequencing of these events. The pathology report is a key component on which treatment is based. The report details tumor histology; size; estrogen, progesterone, and *her2neu* receptor status; and lymph node involvement. Traditionally, breast tumors are staged using the TNM (tumor, lymph node, metastasis) Classification on Breast Cancer from the American Joint Committee on Cancer (in the 7th edition as of September 2015; Table 8.1). The treatment plan is based on this classification, imaging, physical findings, the patient's wishes, and discussions between the patient and the treating team. A clinical decision algorithm is also available from the National Comprehensive Cancer Network (NCCN) regarding the full spectrum of care.

Locoregional control of breast cancer means eradication of tumor in the breast and treatment to prevent IBTR. If done by surgery first, locoregional control is achieved by either mastectomy or lumpectomy (cancer removal with a margin of normal tissue), and usually is followed by whole-breast or partial breast irradiation. As shown by Protocol B-06 conducted by the National Surgical Adjuvant Breast and Bowel Project (NSABP; Fisher et al., 1985, 1989, 1995), both approaches (lumpectomy with or without breast irradiation and total mastectomy) yield identical disease-free, distant-disease–free and overall survival rates in women with tumors 4 cm or smaller in diameter whether the axillary lymph nodes were positive or negative for metastatic disease. Furthermore, 12 and 20 years of follow-up of subgroups in NSABP B-06 showed that the cumulative incidence of a recurrence of tumor in the ipsilateral breast was significantly higher in the group treated with lumpectomy alone (12 years, 35%; 20 years, 39.2%) compared with the group treated with lumpectomy and breast irradiation

TABLE 8.1 TNM Staging Classification for Breast Cancer

PRIMARY TUMOR (T)[a]

TX	Primary tumor cannot be assessed
T0	No evidence of primary tumor
Tis	Carcinoma in situ
Tis (DCIS)	Ductal carcinoma in situ
Tis (LCIS)	Lobular carcinoma in situ
Tis (Paget)	Paget disease of the nipple *not* associated with invasive carcinoma and/or carcinoma in situ (DCIS and/or LCIS) in the underlying breast parenchyma; carcinomas in the breast parenchyma associated with Paget disease are categorized based on the size and characteristics of the parenchymal disease, although the presence of Paget disease should still be noted
T1	Tumor ≤2 cm in greatest dimension
T1mic	Microinvasion ≤0.1 cm in greatest dimension
T1a	Tumor >0.1 cm but ≤0.5 cm in greatest dimension
T1b	Tumor >0.5 cm but ≤1 cm in greatest dimension
T1c	Tumor >1 cm but ≤2 cm in greatest dimension
T2	Tumor >2 cm but ≤5 cm in greatest dimension
T3	Tumor >5 cm in greatest dimension
T4	Tumor of any size with direct extension to the chest wall and/or skin (ulceration or skin nodules)[b]
T4a	Extension to the chest wall not including only pectoralis muscle adherence/invasion
T4b	Ulceration and/or ipsilateral satellite nodules and/or edema (including peau d'orange) of the skin, which do not meet the criteria for inflammatory carcinoma
T4c	Both T4a and T4b
T4d	Inflammatory carcinoma

REGIONAL LYMPH NODES (N)[a]

NX	Regional lymph nodes cannot be assessed (eg, previously removed)
N0	No regional lymph node metastases
N1	Metastasis to movable ipsilateral level I and II axillary lymph node(s)
N2	Metastases in ipsilateral level I and II axillary lymph nodes that are clinically fixed or matted; or in clinically detected[c] ipsilateral internal mammary nodes in the *absence* of clinically evident axillary lymph node metastases
N2a	Metastases in ipsilateral level I and II axillary lymph nodes fixed to one another (matted) or to other structures
N2b	Metastases only in clinically detected[c] ipsilateral internal mammary nodes and in the *absence* of clinically evident level I and II axillary lymph node metastases
N3	Metastases in ipsilateral infraclavicular (level III axillary) lymph node(s) with or without level I and II axillary lymph node involvement; or in clinically detected[c] ipsilateral internal mammary lymph node(s) with clinically evident level I and II axillary lymph node metastases; or metastases in ipsilateral supraclavicular lymph node(s) with or without axillary or internal mammary lymph node involvement
N3a	Metastases in ipsilateral infraclavicular lymph node(s)
N3b	Metastases in ipsilateral internal mammary lymph node(s) and axillary lymph node(s)
N3c	Metastases in ipsilateral supraclavicular lymph node(s)

PATHOLOGIC (PN)[d]

pNX	Regional lymph nodes cannot be assessed (eg, previously removed, or not removed for pathologic study)
pN0	No regional lymph node metastasis identified histologically
Note: Isolated tumor cell clusters (ITCs) are defined as small clusters of cells not greater than 0.2 mm, or single tumor cells, or a cluster of fewer than 200 cells in a single histologic cross section. ITCs may be detected by routine histology or by immunohistochemical (IHC) methods. Nodes containing only ITCs are excluded from the total positive node count for purposes of N classification but should be included in the total number of nodes evaluated.	
pN0(i−)	No regional lymph node metastases histologically, negative IHC
pN0(i+)	Malignant cells in regional lymph node(s) no greater than 0.2 mm (detected by H&E or IHC including ITC)
pN0(mol−)	No regional lymph node metastases histologically, negative molecular findings (RT-PCR)
pN0(mol+)	Positive molecular findings (RT-PCR), but no regional lymph node metastases detected by histology or IHC
pN1	Micrometastases; or metastases in 1–3 axillary lymph nodes; and/or in internal mammary nodes with metastases detected by sentinel lymph node biopsy (SLNB) but not clinically detected[e]
pN1mi	Micrometastases (>0.2 mm and/or more than 200 cells, but none greater than 2 mm)
pN1a	Metastases in 1–3 axillary lymph nodes, at least one metastasis greater than 2 mm
pN1b	Metastases in internal mammary nodes with micrometastases or macrometastases detected by SLNB biopsy but not clinically detected[e]
pN1c	Metastases in 1–3 axillary lymph nodes and in internal mammary lymph nodes with micrometastases or macrometastases detected by SLNB but not clinically detected
pN2	Metastases in 4–9 axillary lymph nodes; or in clinically detected internal mammary lymph nodes in the absence of axillary lymph node metastases

Continued

TABLE 8.1   TNM Staging Classification for Breast Cancer—cont'd

pN2a	Metastases in 4-9 axillary lymph nodes (at least one tumor deposit greater than 2 mm)
pN2b	Metastases in clinically detected[f] internal mammary lymph nodes in the absence of axillary lymph node metastases
pN3	Metastases in 10 or more axillary lymph nodes; or in infraclavicular (level III axillary) lymph nodes; or in clinically detected[f] ipsilateral internal mammary lymph nodes in the presence of one or more positive level I and II axillary lymph nodes; or in more than three axillary lymph nodes and in internal mammary lymph nodes with micrometastases or macrometastases detected by SLNB but not clinically detected[e]; or in ipsilateral supraclavicular lymph nodes
pN3a	Metastases in 10 or more axillary lymph nodes (at least one tumor deposit greater than 2 mm); or metastases to the infraclavicular (level III axillary lymph) nodes
pN3b	Metastases in clinically detected[f] ipsilateral internal mammary lymph nodes in the presence of one or more positive axillary lymph nodes; or in more than three axillary lymph nodes and in internal mammary lymph nodes with micrometastases or macrometastases detected by SLNB but not clinically detected[e]
pN3c	Metastases in ipsilateral supraclavicular lymph nodes

POSTTREATMENT YPN

Posttreatment yp "N" should be evaluated as for clinical (pretreatment) "N" methods as previously mentioned. The modifier "sn" is used only if a sentinel node evaluation was performed after treatment. If no subscript is attached, it is assumed that the axillary nodal evaluation was by axillary node dissection (AND)

The X classification will be used (ypNX) if no yp posttreatment SN or AND was performed.

N categories are the same as those used for pN.

DISTANT METASTASES (M)

M0	No clinical or radiographic evidence of distant metastases
cM0(i)	No clinical or radiographic evidence of distant metastases, but deposits of molecularly or microscopically detected tumor cells in circulating blood, bone marrow, or other nonregional nodal tissue that are no larger than 0.2 mm in a patient without symptoms or signs of metastases
M1	Distant detectable metastases as determined by classic clinical and radiographic means and/or histologically proven larger than 0.2 mm

ANATOMIC STAGE/PROGNOSTIC GROUP

0	Tis	N0	M0
IA	T1[g]	N0	M0
IB	T0	N1mi	M0
	T1[g]	N1mi	M0
IIA	T0	N1[h]	M0
	T1[g]	N1[h]	M0
	T2	N0	M0
IIB	T2	N1	M0
	T3	N0	M0
IIIA	T0	N2	M0
	T1[g]	N2	M0
	T2	N2	M0
	T3	N1, N2	M0
IIIB	T4	N0, N1, N2	M0
IIIC	Any T	N3	M0
IV	Any T	Any N	M1

[a]The T classification of the primary tumor is the same regardless of whether it is based on clinical or pathologic criteria, or both. Size should be measured to the nearest millimeter. If the tumor size is slightly less than or greater than a cutoff for a given T classification, it is recommended that the size be rounded to the millimeter reading that is closest to the cutoff. For example, a reported size of 1.1 mm is reported as 1 mm, or a size of 2.01 cm is reported as 2 cm. Designation should be made with the subscript "c" or "p" modifier to indicate whether the T classification was determined by clinical (physical examination or radiologic) or pathologic measurements, respectively. Generally, pathologic determination should take precedence over clinical determination of T size.
[b]Invasion of the dermis alone does not qualify as T4.
[c]Clinically detected is defined as detected by imaging studies (excluding lymphoscintigraphy) or by clinical examination and having characteristics highly suspicious for malignancy or a presumed pathologic macrometastasis based on fine-needle aspiration biopsy with cytologic examination. Confirmation of clinically detected metastatic disease by fine-needle aspiration without excision biopsy is designated with an (f) suffix, for example, cN3a(f). Excisional biopsy of a lymph node or biopsy of a sentinel node, in the absence of assignment of a pT, is classified as a clinical N, for example, cN1. Information regarding the confirmation of the nodal status will be designated in site-specific factors as clinical, fine-needle aspiration, core biopsy, or SLNB. Pathologic classification (pN) is used for excision or SLNB only in conjunction with a pathologic T assignment.
[d]Classification is based on axillary lymph node dissection with or without SLNB. Classification based solely on SLNB without subsequent axillary lymph node dissection is designated (sn) for "sentinel node," for example, pN0(sn).
[e]"Not clinically detected" is defined as not detected by imaging studies (excluding lymphoscintigraphy) or not detected by clinical examination.
[f]"Clinically detected" is defined as detected by imaging studies (excluding lymphoscintigraphy) or by clinical examination and having characteristics highly suspicious for malignancy or a presumed pathologic macrometastasis based on fine-needle aspiration biopsy with cytologic examination.
[g]T1 includes T1mi.
[h]T0 and T1 tumors with nodal micrometastases only are excluded from stage IIA and are classified as stage IB.
M0 includes M0(i+). The designation pM0 is not valid; any M0 should be clinical. If a patient presents with M1 before neoadjuvant systemic therapy, the stage is considered stage IV and remains stage IV regardless of response to neoadjuvant therapy. Stage designation may be changed if postsurgical imaging studies reveal the presence of distant metastases, provided that the studies are performed within 4 months of diagnosis in the absence of disease progression and provided the patient has not received neoadjuvant therapy. Postneoadjuvant therapy is designated with the "yc" or "yp" prefix. Of note, no stage group is assigned if there is a complete pathologic response to neoadjuvant therapy, for example, ypT0ypN0cM0.
H&E, hematoxylin and eosin stain; *RT-PCR*, reverse transcriptase polymerase chain reaction.
From American Joint Committee on Cancer (AJCC). Breast. *AJCC cancer staging manual.* New York, 2010, Springer, pp. 347-376.

(12 years, 10%; 20 years, 14.3%), indicating that lumpectomy followed by breast irradiation is appropriate therapy for women with stage I or II breast cancer (Fisher et al., 1995, 2002).

The radiologist helps the team select candidates for breast-conserving surgery or mastectomy by estimating the location and extent of disease with imaging. The critical information is lesion location, size, and extent of disease. This allows the surgeon to form a 3D representation of normal versus malignant tissue, develop a mental image of the tumor within the breast, estimate the amount of additional tissue needed to obtain tumor-free margins, and plan the incision (surgical approach) with the goal of maximizing the probability of tumor removal and maintaining the best cosmetic result. For example, the patient would be recommended for mastectomy if it is not possible to remove an extensive multicentric invasive breast cancer completely with microscopically clear margins. Still, increasingly there is interest in removing multiple lesions from the same breast while preserving the breast. This is being evaluated by an ongoing prospective trial evaluating outcomes in women with multifocal or multicentric disease treated with breast conservation therapy.

Multifocal disease refers to cancers in the same breast quadrant; *multicentric disease* refers to cancers in separate quadrants. As a straightforward example, a 3-mm satellite cancer close to the primary tumor is almost always amenable to surgical resection using breast-conserving techniques with an acceptable cosmetic outcome. In contradistinction, a pair of 3- to 4-cm cancers on opposite sides of the breast is usually treated with mastectomy. There are no hard and fast rules for excising multiple lesions with breast conservation; clinical judgment and experience must be used. For this reason, the surgeon requests information regarding the number and size of cancers, as well as their geographic relationship to each other. If too many foci of invasive cancer or extensive ductal carcinoma in situ (DCIS) is present, the patient is not a candidate for breast-conserving surgery because the surgeon may not be able to excise all the cancer with an acceptable cosmetic result and because of concern over an elevated risk of IBTR.

Patients undergo mastectomy if the entire cancer cannot be excised with a good cosmetic result (as just discussed), if the woman has contraindications to radiotherapy, or if it is her preference. Mastectomy candidates usually are offered immediate or staged ipsilateral breast reconstruction with an autologous tissue flap or a tissue expander, unless there are medical contraindications to reconstruction (eg, multiple comorbidities). Because the contralateral breast may be much larger than the operated cancerous breast after surgery, patients often are offered reduction mammoplasty on the contralateral side for a symmetric postoperative appearance. Characteristic appearances of reduction mammoplasty and breast reconstruction are discussed in Chapter 9.

Breast-conservation patients usually undergo postsurgical whole-breast irradiation to achieve control of residual microscopic disease. Relative contraindications to radiation therapy include pregnancy, previous radiation therapy, and collagen vascular disease such as scleroderma (Box 8.1). Axillary nodal involvement is not a contraindication. Six randomized trials of lumpectomy and radiation therapy showed that the frequency of local recurrence and overall survival (OS) rates are generally comparable to mastectomy. However, IBTRs are reported in 5% of patients at 5 years and in 10% to 15% at 10 years after completion of therapy. Treatment failures (ie, IBTR) usually undergo salvage mastectomy. A trial of women undergoing lumpectomy plus radiation versus mastectomy showed that 9% to 14 % of the lumpectomy plus radiation therapy group had IBTR. With salvage mastectomy, overall and disease-free survival in this group was the same as the mastectomy group at 20 years (Fisher et al., 2002).

Invasive IBTR usually occurs in the lumpectomy site or quadrant within the first 7 years but rarely earlier than 18 months after treatment. IBTR after 7 years will more likely occur in any quadrant, not necessarily at the original site, and is usually considered a new cancer. IBTR near the original lumpectomy site is associated

---

BOX 8.1   Contraindications to Whole-Breast Radiation Therapy

Pregnancy
Previous breast radiation therapy
Multicentric or diffuse disease
Collagen vascular disease (scleroderma)
Poor cosmetic result (relative contraindication)

BOX 8.2   Factors Affecting the Frequency of In-Breast Tumor Recurrence after Radiation Therapy

Invasive ductal cancer with an extensive intraductal component
Residual tumor in the breast
Younger women
Large ductal carcinoma in situ tumors
Lymphatic or vascular invasion
Multicentricity

---

more frequently with systemic relapse than IBTR in other quadrants, which more often reflect a new primary tumor. It is considered more likely in women who have invasive ductal cancer with an extensive intraductal component, residual disease in the breast, extensive DCIS, lymphatic or vascular invasion, or multicentricity, and is more common in younger women (Box 8.2).

Adjuvant systemic therapy is often used after surgery to achieve radical cure. The types of systemic therapy include chemotherapy, endocrine therapy, and anti-HER2 therapy (trastuzumab, etc.). Chemotherapy alone or in these combinations is selected based on the clinician's estimates of the likely risks of breast cancer relapse and death, and the likely benefit of adjuvant therapy. Since 2000, it has been recognized that breast cancer is a heterogeneous collection of genetically distinct disease entities, known as intrinsic subtypes. Genetic features or molecular expression status largely affects the therapeutic response and tumor behavior. Generally, tumors with the expression of hormone receptors (eg, estrogen receptor [ER], progesterone receptor [PgR]) and HER2 receptor can respond well to endocrine therapy and anti-HER2 therapy, respectively. Otherwise, chemotherapy may be required to treat the residual disease. However, the indication for chemotherapy for early breast cancers is complex, because no single biomarker predicts chemotherapy response. Particularly in ER-positive breast cancer, the widespread use of adjuvant chemotherapy has resulted in overtreatment in many patients with chemotherapy, although it has contributed to improved prognosis. Various methods thus are being developed to predict chemotherapy response to stratify breast cancer patients' management, particularly those with ER-positive disease. Adjuvant! Online is an Internet-based tool to provide guidance regarding prognosis and the potential benefit of different chemotherapy protocols by using classic parameters, such as age, histology, lymphatic or vascular invasion, tumor size, nodal stage, ER status, and therapy used (Olivotto, 2005). Gene expression profiling (such as Oncotype DX, MammaPrint, and PAM50) has also been developed, and is becoming useful in managing subsets of early stage breast cancer. These gene signatures are the subject of two large randomized trials, one in the United States (the TAILORx trial for Oncotype DX) and the one in Europe (the MINDACT trial for MammaPrint). Oncotype DX (Genomic Health, Redwood City, CA) is a reverse transcriptase polymerase chain reaction (RT-PCR) assay of 21 selected genes in paraffin-embedded tumor tissue. A validated study showed that Oncotype DX quantifies the likelihood of distant recurrence in patients with node-negative, ER-positive breast cancer treated with tamoxifen alone (Paik, 2004), suggesting Oncotype Dx helps in identifying

TABLE 8.2 Clinicopathologic Surrogate Definition of Intrinsic Subtypes and the Recommended Therapy

Intrinsic Subtype	Clinicopathologic Surrogate Definition	Type of Therapy for Most
Luminal A	Luminal A-like All of ER and PgR positive HER2 negative Ki67 "low" Recurrence rate "low" based on multigene-expression assay (if available)	Endocrine therapy alone
Luminal B	Luminal B-like (HER2 negative) ER positive HER2 negative At least one of Ki67 "high" PgR negative or low Recurrence rate "high" based on multigene-expression assay (if available)	Endocrine therapy + cytotoxics
	Luminal B-like (HER2 positive) ER positive HER2 overexpressed or amplified Any Ki67 Any PgR	Cytotoxics + anti-HER2 + endocrine therapy
Erb-B2 overexpression	HER2 positive (nonluminal) HER2 overexpressed or amplified ER and PgR absent	Cytotoxics + anti-HER2
"Basal-like"	Triple negative (ductal) HER2 negative ER and PgR absent	Cytotoxics

ER, estrogen receptor; *PgR*, progesterone receptor.
From Goldhirsch A, et al: Personalizing the treatment of women with early breast cancer: highlights of the St. Gallen International Expert Consensus on the Primary Therapy of Early Breast Cancer 2013, *Ann Oncol* 24:2206-2223, 2013.

subgroups who will benefit from adding chemotherapy. Mamma-Print (Agendia, Amsterdam, the Netherlands) is a complementary DNA microarray analysis of 70 selected genes in tumor tissue established at the Netherlands Cancer Institute. A prospective clinical study, RASTER, for patients with cT1-3N0M0 breast cancer showed that the MammaPrint is useful in identifying patients who may safely forgo chemotherapy compared with standard clinicopathologic classification (Drukker, 2013). PAM50 (ARUP, Salt Lake City, UT) is a quantitative RT-PCR assay for selected 50 genes that offers intrinsic molecular subtyping and generates a risk of recurrence (ROR) score. Recent studies suggest that the PAM50 ROR score has a significant prognostic value for patients with ER-positive early breast cancer treated with endocrine therapy alone (Nielsen, 2010; Dowsett, 2013; Gnant, 2014).

NCCN guidelines (2015, version 2) propose the indications of systemic adjuvant therapy based on the presence of hormone receptors and HER2 receptor and also use histology and stage of disease. In addition, a gene signature assay (Oncotype Dx) is also recommended to be considered in patients with tumors >0.5 cm, HER2-negative disease, and either N0 or N1mi (micrometastasis) disease. In 2011, the St. Gallen International Breast Cancer Conference determined the clinicopathologic surrogate definition of intrinsic subtypes (updated in 2013) by using immunohistochemical results of Ki67 index in addition to the status of hormone receptors and HER2 receptor (Goldhirsch et al., 2011, 2013; Table 8.2). They recommend systemic treatment according to the subtypes. In this definition, the degrees of Ki67 index and

of PgR expression, and the categories of recurrence risk based on gene signature assays if available, are used to stratify ER-positive HER2-negative early breast cancers into "luminal A-like" in which endocrine therapy alone is recommended for most or "luminal B-like (HER2 negative)" in which endocrine therapy with chemotherapy is recommended for most.

Preoperative NAC, combination chemotherapy given before definitive surgical treatment (lumpectomy or mastectomy), is now a standard option for locally advanced or bulky breast cancers. Locally advanced breast cancer usually includes tumors greater than 5 cm (T3-4); inflammatory breast cancers (T4d); those with spread to other tissues around the breast such as the skin, muscle, or ribs (T4a or b); or those with spread to regional lymph nodes (N2-3), which have no distant metastasis. Thus locally advanced breast cancer mostly belongs to stage III or higher disease. Three distinct benefits of NAC compared with postoperative chemotherapy include enhancing the feasibility of breast-conserving surgery, enabling surgical resection of initially inoperable tumors, and assessing for tumor chemosensitivity. NAC provides tumor shrinkage, decreases tumor burden, and allows some patients to undergo lumpectomy and radiation rather than mastectomy for local control. It also allows some patients with initially inoperable tumors to receive potentially curative surgery. After NAC, surgical resection of the original tumor site establishes the type and extent of residual tumor. This information is important for predicting prognosis. A complete pathologic response (no residual cancer in the original tumor bed by histology) is a good prognostic indicator. Surgical lumpectomy with negative margins also helps to determine whether breast-conserving therapy may be the final surgical step as the patient's best option.

The indication for NAC is now extended to early-stage breast cancer. The NSABP B-18 trial (Fisher et al., 1998; Rastogi et al., 2008) of 1523 women with operable stage I–II breast cancer (T1-3N0M0) showed that NAC with AC (doxorubicin and cyclophosphamide) provided equivalent outcome in disease-free survival (DFS) and OS compared with adjuvant chemotherapy with AC, and that more patients who received NAC than adjuvant chemotherapy underwent breast-conserving surgery. In the neoadjuvant group, the primary tumor response to chemotherapy correlated with outcome, suggesting an advantage of NAC as a predictive factor of outcome. Patients who achieved a pathologic complete response had significantly superior DFS and OS compared with patients who did not. The advantages of NAC found in NSABP B18 have led to greater use of NAC for women with operable breast cancer, especially when they desire a lumpectomy but have large tumors ineligible for conventional conservative surgery at presentation.

EVALUATION OF AXILLARY LYMPH NODES

The treatment of invasive breast cancer historically involved removal of ipsilateral axillary lymph nodes. This was natural, because most women receiving treatment for breast cancer 100 years ago had nodal involvement. With earlier detection of breast cancer, nodal involvement is no longer the norm. In fact, approximately 65% to 70% of women with newly diagnosed invasive breast cancer have normal lymph nodes and therefore will not derive any benefit from ALND.

ALND is a complete en bloc removal of the level I and II lymph nodes (Table 8.3), and is problematic from the standpoint of side effects. It exposes patients to the risk of major complications such as lymphedema, shoulder dysfunction, and sensory changes in and around the axilla. To address this problem, routine level I/level II ALND has evolved to use the SLNB as an initial screen for nodal involvement in patients who are clinically node negative or there are no palpable suspicious axillary lymph nodes on physical examination.

SLNB was initially described for patients with penile cancer, but did not attract much attention until it was broadly adopted

TABLE 8.3   Location of Lymph Nodes Draining the Breast

Level	Location
I	Infralateral to lateral edge of the pectoralis minor muscle
II	Behind the pectoralis minor muscle
III	Between the pectoralis minor and subclavius muscles (Halsted ligament)

BOX 8.3   Sentinel Lymph Node Biopsy Identification Techniques

Radionuclide injection
Blue dye injection
Abnormal palpable lymph node
Combination of the previously mentioned techniques
(Marker or tattoo placed in biopsy-proven positive lymph nodes)
Injection routes: peritumoral, intradermal, subareolar

BOX 8.4   The American Society of Breast Surgeons Indications For Sentinel Lymph Node Biopsy

- T1-2 invasive breast cancer with a clinically negative axilla
- Ductal carcinoma in situ (DCIS) sufficient to require mastectomy, or DCIS with suspected/proved microinvasion
- Patients with clinically negative axillary nodes following neoadjuvant chemotherapy
- Although the evidence is limited, sentinel lymph node (SLN) biopsy may be suitable for selected patients with multicentric cancers, T3 disease, or pregnancy. is not indicated for patients with inflammatory breast cancer.

From The American Society of Breast Surgeons: *Performance and practice guidelines for sentinel lymph node biopsy in breast cancer patients.* https://www.breastsurgeons.org/new_layout/about/statements/PDF_Statements/PerformancePracticeGuidelines_SLN.pdf. Accessed on July 9, 2015.

for use in melanoma patients. In patients with breast cancer, SLNB was first used in 1993, and its proof of concept was established in the 1990s (Giuliano et al., 1994, 1997). SLNB is performed by injecting a tracer material, either a radionuclide, blue dye, or both, into the breast either preoperatively or perioperatively and by looking for evidence of the tracer in one or more sentinel nodes (Box 8.3). SLNB alone does not eliminate, but does significantly decrease, the risk of developing the common complication of lymphedema. The reported sensitivity of SLNB ranges from 88% to 100%, whereas the specificity has been consistently very high, at almost 100% using hematoxylin and eosin (H&E) assessment (Giuliano et al., 1994, 1997; Krag et al., 1998).

NSABP trial B-32 was a randomized controlled phase 3 trial designed to answer the question if SLNB had the same OS, disease-free survival (DFS) and regional control as ALND when the SLN was negative. The trial involved clinically node-negative patients with operable breast cancer stratified by age, tumor size, and surgical treatment (lumpectomy versus mastectomy) who were randomly assigned to ALND versus SLNB. If the SLN was positive, patients went on to completion ALND. Survival results showed no significant difference in OS, DFS, and regional control between SLN-positive patients undergoing ALND versus SLN-negative patients who had no further axillary surgery, suggesting that SLNB without ALND is appropriate when the SLN is negative (Krag et al., 2010).

However, a second central pathology review of paraffin blocks of SLNs that were initially read as negative showed an overall case conversion rate to "positive" of 10.3% of cases (Weaver et al., 2000). Despite the discovery that initially negative SLN cases had occult metastases in up to 10.3% of cases, the entire group of patients with "negative" SLNB with no further treatment had the same OS and DFS as patients undergoing ALND. The occult metastases in the initially negative-SLNB–only group were ≤1 mm in size. This discovery brought into question the significance of tiny metastases and, specifically, if survival was associated with tiny metastases or isolated tumor cells, and if there was need for ALND in the setting of H&E-negative but immunohistochemistry (IHC)-positive SLN. In their follow-up study at 5 years, Weaver et al. (2011) revealed that log-rank tests showed patients with occult metastases had a significant difference in OS ($P = 0.03$), DFS ($P = 0.02$), and distant disease-free interval (DDF; $P = 0.04$) but suggested that the magnitude of the difference in outcome at 5 years was 1.2 percentage points and was small enough to not indicate clinical benefit for ALND.

The ACOSOG Z0010 prospective trial studied the significance and the survival of women with immunohistochemistry (IHC)-detected micrometastases when the SLN was negative by H&E staining. Women had clinical T12N0M0 breast cancer and received breast-conserving therapy and SLN dissection (Giuliano et al., 2011a). If the SLN was negative by H&E staining, the patient had no ALND. OS and DFS were compared between women who were SLN negative by both H&E and IHC staining versus women who were SLN negative by H&E but were positive by IHC. ACOSOG Z0010 revealed that 10.5% of H&E-negative SLNs contained IHC-positive occult metastases. However, the IHC-negative and IHC-positive patients had no difference in OS at a median of 6.3 years. The NSABP B-32 and ACOSOG Z0010 trials suggested that SLNB showing H&E-negative SLNs was acceptable without ALND even when micrometastatic disease was presumed to be present in approximately 10% of patients.

However, the next question to be answered was if women with limited positive SLNs by H&E and no ALND had the same survival as women with positive SLNs undergoing ALND. The ACOSOG Z0011 phase 3 noninferiority trial asked if patients with limited SLN metastatic breast cancer could undergo SLNB and have the same survival as women with limited SLN metastatic breast cancer undergoing ALND (Giuliano et al., 2011b). In this trial, inclusion criteria included women with clinical T1-T2 invasive breast cancer, no palpable adenopathy, and no more than two SLNs containing metastases identified by frozen section, touch preparation, or H&E staining on permanent section after SLNB. All women underwent SLNB and were randomized to SLNB alone or ALND. All patients underwent lumpectomy with postoperative whole-breast radiotherapy. Exclusion criteria were those with three or more involved SLN or planned mastectomy. Of 420 patients randomized to ALND, 106 (27.4%) had additional positive nodes removed beyond the SLN. At a median follow-up of 6.3 years, ALND did not significantly affect OS or DFS in women treated with lumpectomy, systemic therapy, and tangential WB-XRT compared with the use of SLND alone (Giuliano et al., 2011b). Because of ACOSOG Z0011 inclusion criteria, it is important for radiologists to report suspicious-appearing lymph nodes on imaging, particularly if there are three or more suspicious lymph nodes (which would exclude patients for SLND alone).

The American Society of Breast Surgeons (ASBS) suggests that SLNB may be appropriate for T1-T2 invasive breast cancer with a clinically negative axilla, DCIS sufficient to require mastectomy or DCIS with suspected/proved microinvasion, and patients with clinically negative axillary nodes following NAC (Box 8.4). Patients with multicentric cancers, T3 disease, or pregnancy are also indicated as possible candidates for SLNB. ALND has largely been replaced by SLNB for patients with clinical node-negative breast cancer but is still required for a significant proportion of patients (Box 8.5 [ASBS ALND indications]).

The role of the radiologist is to understand the rationale for SLNB and to facilitate its performance. First, tracer is not to be injected into the biopsy cavity or the tumor; tracer injected into a biopsy site cavity is likely to remain in the cavity rather than be transported into the lymphatics. The most common tracers are technetium-99 sulfur colloid and lymphazurin blue dye; some also use methylene blue dye.

Preoperative lymphoscintigraphy is used in some facilities to assist preoperative localization of SLNs in the axilla or in extraaxillary sites (Fig. 8.1). Most commonly these extraaxillary sites are in the supraclavicular, infraclavicular, or internal mammary regions. If tracer does not identify an axillary SLN, the surgeon may choose to harvest an SLN from one of these other sites. Some facilities do not remove an internal mammary SLN or other nonaxillary SLN because of the very low frequency of isolated positive biopsies (usually <3%) and the relatively few cases that would result in meaningful changes in prognosis or therapy. Perhaps not surprisingly, institutions that harvest both axillary and internal mammary SLNs have demonstrated a poorer prognosis when lymph nodes at both sites are involved.

Although there are differences of opinion as to the optimal location of tracer injection, as well as optimal tracer modality, there is general agreement from randomized studies that the technique is sensitive and specific enough to obviate the need for a full ALND in patients whose sentinel nodes test negative for tumor. Generally, the SLN is harvested at the time of surgery and tested with touch preparation or frozen section intraoperatively. If there are tumor cells in more than two SLNs, the surgeon proceeds to a completion level I/level II ALND.

BOX 8.5 The American Society of Breast Surgeons Indications for Axillary Lymph Node Dissection

- The clinically node-positive axilla, confirmed by fine-needle aspiration or core biopsy, in a patient for whom neoadjuvant chemotherapy (NAC) is not planned.
- Occult breast cancer presenting as axillary node metastasis.
- Sentinel lymph node (SLN)-positive patients who fall outside the Z0011 selection criteria (ie, >2 SLN-positive, matted nodes, mastectomy, or breast conservation without whole-breast radiation therapy)
- Inflammatory, clinical stage T4, or high-risk T3 breast cancer.
- Failed SLN mapping.
- Inadequate prior axillary lymph node dissection with residual clinically suspicious nodes
- Sentinel or axillary nodes that remain positive after NAC.
- Axillary recurrence following previous breast cancer treatment.

From The American Society of Breast Surgeons. *Performance and practice guide lines for axillary lymph node dissection in breast cancer patients.* https://www.breastsurgeons.org/new_layout/about/statements/PDF_Statements/PerformancePracticeGuidelines_ALND.pdf. Accessed July 9, 2015.

Nonvisualization of the SLN on lymphoscintigraphy does not preclude SLN identification by the surgeon in the operating room. The SLN may be within thick adipose tissue that can only be identified by the gamma probe in the operating room. The yield for SLN identification in the operating room when it cannot be visualized on lymphoscintigraphy can be increased if blue dye is also used.

Intraoperative evaluation of SLNs occasionally yields false-positive findings. False-negative findings are more common. This can precipitate return of the patient to the operating room weeks after the original SLNB for completion ALND if indicated.

Based on current American Joint Committee on Cancer guidelines, nodal staging is based on the maximal size of the single largest tumor deposit in am SLN (if the SLN is the only involved node) as well as the number of involved lymph nodes. The descriptive category for the smallest extent of disease, isolated tumor cells, means that no single tumor deposit in an axillary node is larger than 0.2 mm. Patients with isolated tumor cells are considered to have normal nodes and are usually not treated with a completion ALND. Proceeding from SLNB alone to the wider axillary node clearance typically requires micrometastatic (>0.2- to 2-mm tumor cell cluster in an SLN) or macrometastatic (>2-mm focus) disease within three or more SLN. In patients with only one or two positive SLNs, ACOSOG Z0011 suggests that no further axillary lymph node surgery may be necessary if they receive adjuvant radiotherapy. In addition, there are new trials evaluating the need for nodal clearance after SLN after NAC. Management of the axilla is performed independent of the decision to pursue lumpectomy or mastectomy.

Not all patients are candidates for SLNB. For example, patients who present with clinically involved axillary nodes may proceed directly to ALND if NAC is not pursued. However, it is important to exercise caution in declaring an axillary lymph node as clinically positive. With the increased frequency of percutaneous core biopsy, more and more patients are presenting to breast cancer specialists with enlarged reactive nodes. A recent study by experienced breast surgeons demonstrated that clinical examination in this setting often overestimates the probability that lymph nodes are involved, which in turn could overestimate the number of patients who proceed directly to ALND. Although SLNB has been widely adopted as a precursor to a full ALND for most patients, many have sought to use imaging studies to determine the need for ALND. Toward this end, investigators have assessed the preoperative appearance of nodes on mammography, ultrasound, MRI, and even positron emission tomography (PET). Among these, only PET with a high standardized uptake value may provide near-definitive proof of nodal involvement preoperatively in the absence of percutaneous sampling. Here, too, one must be careful to distinguish between a reactive node versus an uninvolved node.

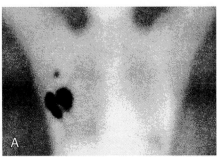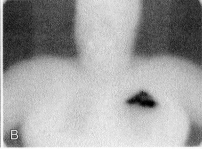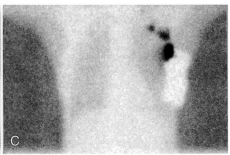

FIG. 8.1 Lymphoscintigraphy for sentinel lymph node (SLN) visualization: three cases. (A) Anterior lymphoscintigram shows activity around the tumor and in the axillary SLN. (B) The lymphoscintigram shows radionuclides injected into the biopsy cavity rather than around it; the radiotracer stayed in the biopsy cavity because it could not be transported to the breast lymphatics. (C) A lymphoscintigram shows activity in the infraclavicular nodes medial to the tumor site. Note the shielding around the injection site and tumor to improve SLN detection.

One preoperative axillary imaging method that has gained a following is axillary lymph node ultrasound with percutaneous FNA of suspicious nodes (Fig. 8.2). Although this test is not a routine part of the initial breast imaging evaluation, there is a new appreciation for preoperative evaluation of ipsilateral axillary lymph nodes in the setting of breast cancer. Axillary ultrasound is particularly helpful when the results of clinical examination of the axilla are suspicious for cancer. Several studies have recently been published using ultrasound-guided FNA or core biopsy to document nodal involvement preoperatively, thus allowing the surgeon to bypass if needed in appropriate clinical settings. This can obviate several known issues with intraoperative assessment of SLNs, such as the time needed to harvest one or more nodes, the intraoperative time needed for pathology to evaluate the node and, most important, the potential for false-negative touch preparation or frozen section at the time of surgery, which may lead to reoperation at a later date. It is possible to mark the biopsied positive lymph nodes by either a metallic marker or by tattoo at the time of biopsy if the nodes are positive to identify them at surgery, as needed.

CLINICAL AND BREAST IMAGING FACTORS IN DETERMINING APPROPRIATE LOCAL THERAPY: LUMPECTOMY OR MASTECTOMY

The therapeutic options for local control of a breast malignancy are lumpectomy (almost always followed by radiotherapy) and mastectomy. Lumpectomy (followed by whole-breast radiotherapy) was introduced approximately 40 years ago and offers equivalent survival to mastectomy. Mastectomy has a slightly lower risk of local recurrence than lumpectomy and obviates the need for radiotherapy in most patients. The use of postmastectomy radiotherapy is controversial in premenopausal women with one to three involved nodes (see the meta-analysis of randomized studies with and without radiotherapy by the Early Breast Cancer Trialists' Collaborative Group [EBCTCG] [Clarke et al. 2005; EBCTCG, 2011]), but it is a common recommendation for women with tumors larger than 5 cm or with four or more involved nodes. The equivalence in OS between lumpectomy with radiotherapy and mastectomy was shown in Protocol B-06 conducted by the NSABP and the Milan I trial conducted in Italy.

The breast imager plays a critical role in aiding the surgeon to make the right therapeutic choice by showing how much cancer is in the breast. There is virtually no disagreement that patients with a unifocal DCIS or invasive cancer may be treated with breast conservation therapy if the entire tumor can be removed with a good cosmetic result and if there are no relative contraindications to radiation therapy (ie, pregnancy, collagen vascular disease, poorly defined or multicentric disease or prior radiotherapy involving the breast).

The controversy regarding the best surgical approach concerns patients with multifocal disease. Some physicians believe that mastectomy is the proper choice for such patients. This preference may be because of results from the original clinical trials comparing lumpectomy with mastectomy, which involved almost exclusively women with unifocal breast cancers. Hence, the safety of breast conservation with respect to local recurrence, distant metastasis, and survival is not as well documented in women with multifocal disease. Still, surgeons are increasingly offering breast conservation to patients with multifocal disease. Thus there is no hard and fast rule regarding how many satellite lesions, or what distance between lesions, constitutes an absolute indication for mastectomy. It is the physician's clinical judgment to avoid predisposing the patient to IBTR; recent data suggest that an IBTR may increase the risk of distant metastasis and death from breast cancer.

Whether the surgeon offers lumpectomy to patients with unifocal disease alone or to patients with multifocal disease, tumor-free margins are a must. For example, offering a woman breast conservation may be reasonable if she has multifocal invasive carcinoma with subcentimeter lesions 3 mm apart and margins that are tumor free by several millimeters. On the other hand, breast conservation may not be offered if a patient has multifocal high-grade DCIS scattered over an area of 5 to 6 cm with only a 1-mm margin; in this example, one would be concerned about additional multifocal disease just beyond the surgical margin.

The definition of *tumor-free margin* has varied among institutions, with some accepting the NSABP model of nontransection and others requiring a 2-mm or greater tumor-free margin. However, a recent consensus guideline from the Society of Surgical Oncology (SSO) and the American Society of Radiation Oncology (ASTRO) has recommended that a negative margin be defined as "no tumor on ink" based on a review of multiple studies. Generally, the margin status must be carefully considered in patients with multifocal disease. Ideally, these patients should have the multiple lesions resected in continuity to gain the best histologic understanding of size, extent, and relationship of lesions to one another, and of the true margins.

Some surgeons offer breast conservation to patients with known multicentric disease, but the less controversial route is with mastectomy as initial treatment. As stated previously, no prospective, randomized study to date has evaluated the safety and effectiveness of breast conservation therapy in the setting of multifocal or multicentric disease. Retrospective studies have been published suggesting that this approach may be safe by demonstrating comparable local recurrence rates in multifocal

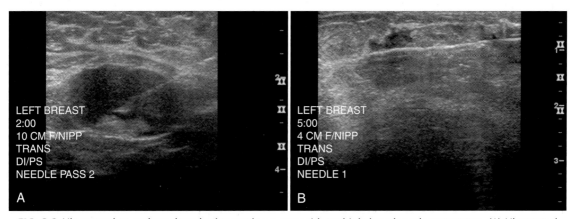

FIG. 8.2 Ultrasound to evaluate lymphadenopathy: a case with multiple lymph node metastases. (A) Ultrasound shows a fine needle aspirating an abnormal lymph node with a very thick cortex that flattened the normal fatty hilum. Aspiration showed breast cancer metastases. (B) Ultrasound shows a core biopsy of a low axillary lymph node that has irregular superficial margins. Biopsy showed cancer metastases.

as well as unifocal disease, whereas others suggest higher IBTR rates. These studies are not powered to draw definitive conclusions but do suggest that further investigation is warranted. There is currently a prospective trial following patients with multifocal or multicentric disease treated with breast conservation therapy to determine the rate of IBTR in this population.

PREOPERATIVE IMAGING

Mammography, ultrasound, and MRI for tumor extent are important tools for selecting appropriate breast conservation therapy candidates and planning surgery (Table 8.4). Mammography is

TABLE 8.4   Breast Imaging Relating to Breast-Conserving Therapy

Timing	Reason	Technique(s)
Preoperative	Ipsilateral tumor extent and contralateral tumor	Bilateral mammography US or MRI as warranted
	Establish diagnosis	Percutaneous biopsy
Perioperative	Tumor excision	Preoperative needle localization (as needed) Specimen radiography
	SLN identification	Radionuclide injection Lymphoscintigraphy (as needed)
Preradiation	Check for residual tumor	Ipsilateral unilateral mammogram US or MRI as needed
Postradiation	Baseline/tumor recurrence	Ipsilateral unilateral mammogram (initial one at 6 months, then every 6–12 months)
	Evaluate ipsilateral and contralateral breast	Bilateral mammogram (12 months)
	Clinical problem	Ipsilateral unilateral mammogram US or MRI as needed

MRI, magnetic resonance imaging; *SLN,* sentinel lymph node; *US,* ultrasound.
Modified from Dershaw DD: The conservatively treated breast. *Diagnosis of diseases of the breast,* Philadelphia, PA, 1997, WB Saunders, p. 553.

the mainstay for determining extent of disease. It identifies diffuse or multicentric disease by finding suspicious breast masses and pleomorphic calcifications (Fig. 8.3). Mammography also can identify benign, extensive, and innumerable bilateral calcifications that could hide early tumor recurrence. Such calcifications are a relative contraindication to breast conservation therapy. Furthermore, mammography finds DCIS that is invisible to MRI. Specifically, approximately 25% of DCIS cases are false-negative on MRI and are discovered only by visualizing pleomorphic calcifications on the mammogram.

On the other hand, MRI has been especially useful in predicting tumor extent before the first surgical procedure (Fig. 8.4). Some investigators have claimed particular effectiveness of MRI in women with invasive lobular carcinoma or showing tumor invasion into the pectoralis muscle or chest wall (Fig. 8.5). With respect to invasive lobular carcinoma, several studies have suggested that MRI may be more effective in detecting the extent of disease than physical examination, mammography, and ultrasound. However, false-negative studies in these series have led to mixed opinions regarding the routine use of MRI in staging invasive lobular carcinoma.

Chest wall tumor invasion on MRI was shown by obliteration of the fat plane between the tumor and the pectoralis muscle, with muscle enhancement, and was proven in five of five cases at surgery (Morris et al., 2000). No muscle involvement was seen at surgery when muscle enhancement was absent in 14 of 14 cases.

MRI also helps exclude candidates for APBI when it finds more than one focus of cancer. Bedrosian et al. (2003) reported a 95% tumor detection rate with MRI and a change in surgical management in 26% (69/267) of patients requiring wider/separate excision or mastectomy, with pathologic verification in 71% (49/69).

Overall, these studies show that MRI may be helpful in surgical planning, but they also indicate that MRI prompts a number of unnecessary biopsies because of a relative lack of specificity. MRI also has false-negative results in invasive lobular carcinoma and DCIS. Other data show that MRI may be associated with treatment delay and an increased mastectomy rate and does not decrease the number of fewer positive margins at surgery. The use of pretreatment MRI before definitive breast cancer surgery remains controversial, particularly if one anticipates whole-breast radiotherapy. The literature on this subject is extensive.

When imaging is complete, additional dialog with the breast imaging team or additional review of imaging studies may be necessary to help the surgeon, medical oncologist, or radiation

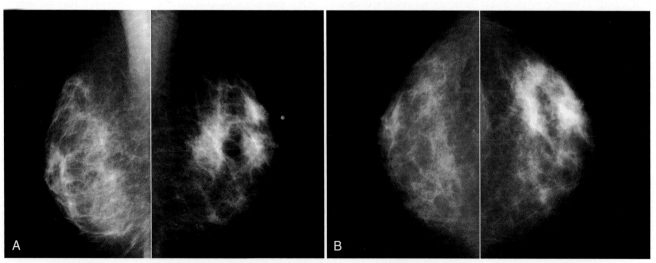

FIG. 8.3 Mammography showing a multicentric left breast cancer. Although this patient felt only one mass in her left breast indicated by the skin marker on the left mediolateral oblique (MLO) mammogram, MLO (A) and craniocaudal (B) mammograms show three spiculated masses over a large region.

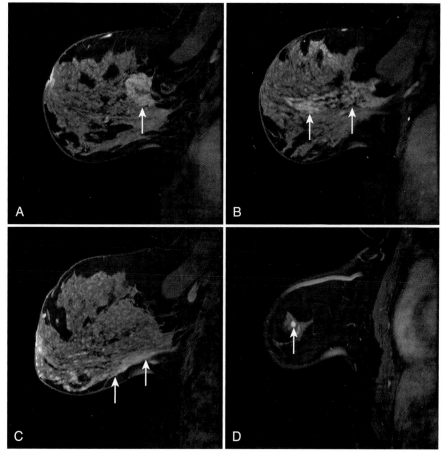

FIG. 8.4 Magnetic resonance imaging (MRI) showing multiple cancers in a woman who felt only a mass in her right breast. (A and B) Postcontrast 3D spectral-spatial excitation magnetization transfer MRI slices of the right breast show a mass near the chest wall (*arrow* in A; invasive ductal cancer) and adjacent segmental clumped enhancement (*arrows* in B) over more than two-thirds of the upper left breast, worrisome for ductal carcinoma in situ (DCIS). (C and D) In the opposite left breast, there is linear enhancement in the lower breast (*arrows* in C) also worrisome for DCIS, and a round, suspicious mass that had fast initial enhancement and late washout on kinetic curves in the extreme medial breast (*arrow* in D). Biopsies of the outer breast showed invasive ductal cancer and DCIS (A and B); core biopsy of the left segmental enhancement showed DCIS (C) and invasive ductal cancer in the inner left breast mass (D). Because of the widespread cancer in both breasts, the patient is not a candidate for breast conservation.

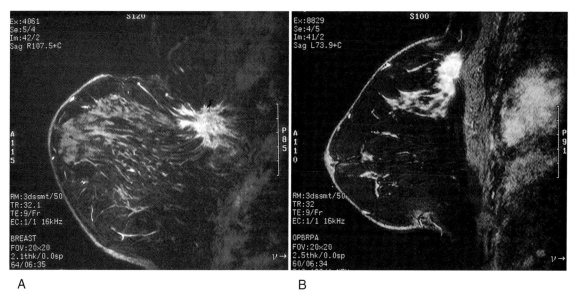

FIG. 8.5 Magnetic resonance imaging (MRI) showing extension into the pectoralis muscle: two cases. (A) Sagittal, contrast-enhanced, 3D spectral-spatial excitation magnetization transfer (3DSSMT) MRI shows a spiculated posterior enhancing mass extending into and enhancing the pectoralis muscle. (B) MRI showing tumor on top of the pectoralis muscle. In contrast to (A), sagittal, contrast-enhanced, 3DSSMT MRI shows an irregular enhancing mass abutting the pectoralis muscle but without enhancing it, suggesting no tumor invasion. Although the surgeon may take some of the pectoralis muscle at surgery to achieve clear margins, the tumor did not extend into the muscle or chest wall at surgery.

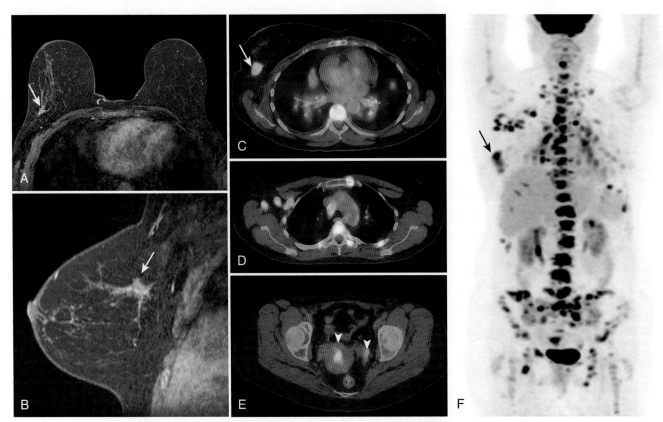

FIG. 8.6 Evaluation of distant metastasis using ^{18}F-FDG positron emission tomography (PET)/computed tomography (CT). A 54-year-old woman with biopsy-proven right invasive breast cancer with ipsilateral axillary nodal metastasis, recently detected with mammography and ultrasonography. (A and B) Axial (A) and sagittal (B) planes of contrast-enhanced fat-suppressed T1-weighted magnetic resonance images show an irregular mass with irregular margins and heterogeneous internal enhancement within the lateral half of the right breast, compatible with biopsy-proven cancer. (C–F) Axial fusion images (C–E) of ^{18}F-FDG PET/CT and a maximum intensity projection PET image show an intense focal uptake in the right breast compatible with the primary cancer (C-F, *arrows*), and diffuse osseous (C–F), pulmonary (C, D, and F), and nodal (D and F) metastatic disease. Hypermetabolic activity involving the endometrial canal and left ovary (E, *arrowheads*) is unlikely to be physiologic given the patient's age, and may represent primary or metastatic disease. ^{18}F-FDG PET/CT depicts systemic metastases, including skeletal and extraskeletal metastases, in a single scan.

oncologist properly counsel the patient regarding appropriate treatment options. This involves a review of the original workup to ensure that all potential abnormalities on physical examination have been evaluated and that the breast imaging workup has been completed (such as up-to-date contralateral mammography as well as additional ultrasound or mammographic imaging for lesions previously considered of secondary concern). The thorough combination of abnormalities identified by palpation or on breast imaging helps ensure that any suspicious foci of tumor are evaluated and incorporated into the treatment plan.

According to NCCN guidelines (2015, version 2), systemic staging using imaging modalities such as chest diagnostic computed tomography (CT), abdominal (±pelvic) CT or MRI, and bone scan (or sodium fluoride PET/CT), is usually recommended for patients with clinically advanced cancer (clinical stage III or IV), and those with clinical stage I and II who have signs or symptoms of distant metastases. ^{18}F-FDG PET/CT is considered as an optional study for those with clinical stage III or IV disease (Fig. 8.6).

NORMAL POSTOPERATIVE IMAGING CHANGES AFTER BREAST BIOPSY OR LUMPECTOMY

To perform a local excision for diagnostic or therapeutic purposes, the surgeon makes a skin incision, removes the mass or wire-localized abnormality, and then closes the subcutaneous tissues and skin. More tissue is excised when removing a cancer to

obtain a margin of normal tissue. Usually, the surgeon allows the surgical cavity to fill in with fluid and granulation tissue.

As a rule, mammograms are not often obtained immediately after diagnostic surgical excisional biopsy. However, in the rare cases when a mammogram is obtained within a few days of surgery, mammography shows a round or oval mass in the postoperative site representing a seroma or hematoma, with or without air. This mass represents the biopsy cavity, filled with fluid that should resolve over time (Fig. 8.7). The adjacent breast tissue shows thickening of trabeculae in subcutaneous fat and increased density caused by local edema or hemorrhage. Skin thickening at the incision is usually present. On MRI the biopsy site is filled with blood or seroma. The fluid in the biopsy cavity is high signal intensity on T2-weighted noncontrast fat-suppressed images (Fig. e8.1).

Over the subsequent weeks, the postoperative site resorbs the air and fluid collection; the collection is replaced by fibrosis and scarring, with residual focal skin thickening and breast edema. On MRI, the immediate postbiopsy cavity is a fluid-filled structure with surrounding normal healing tissue enhancement for up to 18 months after the biopsy. The biopsy cavity shows high signal intensity, architectural distortion, and a scar that can simulate cancer (Fig. 8.8; Box 8.6). The biopsy site usually contains fluid from the seroma, which will be bright on T2-weighted images on MRI. Rim enhancement around the biopsy site is normal even if there is no residual tumor and is caused by healing. In the ipsilateral axilla, reactive lymph nodes may develop that

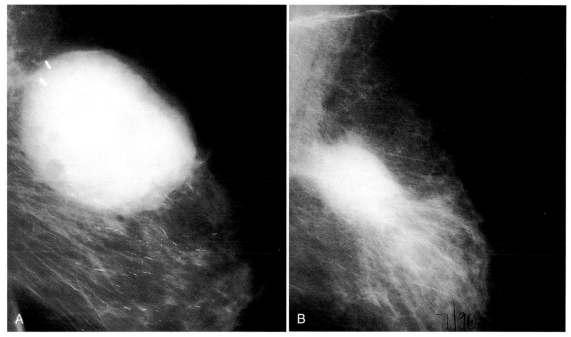

FIG. 8.7 Normal postoperative changes on mammography. (A) Postbiopsy mediolateral oblique (MLO) view shows a large oval mass representing a huge seroma/hematoma after biopsy for cancer, with two adjacent surgical clips. (B) Four years later, the MLO views shows the seroma/hematoma is smaller; the two surgical clips are obscured.

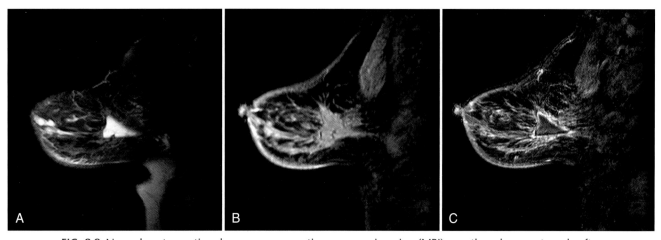

FIG. 8.8 Normal postoperative changes on magnetic resonance imaging (MRI) over the subsequent weeks after surgical excision. (A) In a recently postoperative patient treated for cancer, precontrast sagittal fat-suppressed T2-weighted MRI shows high signal intensity fluid in the biopsy cavity, bright fluid in the retroareolar ducts, and thickened skin with subcutaneous thick fluid-filled trabeculae, compatible with breast edema. (B) Precontrast sagittal 3D spectral-spatial excitation magnetization transfer (3DSSMT) MRI shows the gray fluid-filled postbiopsy scar. (C) Postcontrast sagittal 3DSSMT MRI shows rim enhancement around the dark fluid-filled seroma with the associated skin thickening and breast edema. Note that there are no additional masses in this breast to suggest multifocal cancer.

BOX 8.6   Enhancement on Magnetic Resonance Imaging after Biopsy

Up to 9 months after biopsy and radiation therapy, there is strong enhancement in the biopsy site. From 10 to 18 months after therapy, the enhancement slowly subsides, with no significant enhancement in 94% of cases.

From Heywang-Köbrunner SH, Schlegel A, Beck R, et al: Contrast-enhanced MRI of the breast after limited surgery and radiation therapy, *J Comput Assist Tomogr* 17:891-900, 1993.

---

cannot be distinguished from metastatic disease (Fig. 8.9). MRI after surgery may reveal cancer at the margin edge by showing clumped enhancement or an eccentric residual mass. Although immediate postbiopsy MRI for cancer staging may depict cancer at the biopsy margin, it is more often used to look for cancer elsewhere in the breast away from the biopsy site.

Normal postoperative findings on mammography include architectural distortion, increased density, and parenchymal scarring in at least 50% of patients (Box 8.7). These findings diminish in severity over time (Fig. 8.10). After 3 to 5 years, the findings should be stable on subsequent mammograms. On the

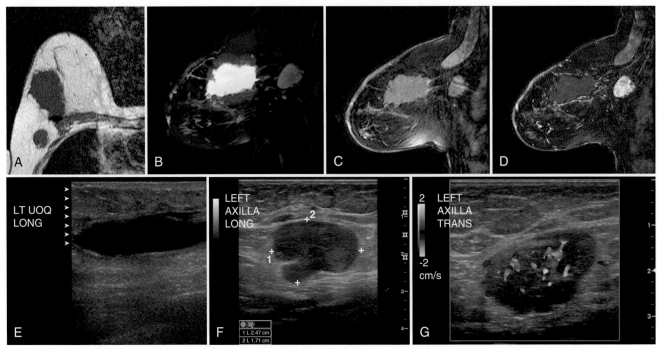

FIG. 8.9 Postbiopsy changes on magnetic resonance imaging (MRI) with abnormal lymphadenopathy. (A) Precontrast axial nonfat-suppressed T1-weighted MRI shows low signal intensity representing fluid in the biopsy cavity soon after surgery. A large lymph node in the left axilla has lost its fatty hilum and is worrisome for metastatic disease. (B) Precontrast fat-suppressed sagittal T2-weighted MRI shows the high signal seroma and the lymph node in the left axilla near the chest wall. Note that the lymph node has abnormal low signal intensity, indicating lymphadenopathy. Normal lymph nodes will usually show a thin high signal intensity cortex with a fatty hilum on T2-weighted images, unlike this case. (C) Precontrast sagittal 3D spectral-spatial excitation magnetization transfer (3DSSMT) MRI shows the seroma and the lymph node in the left axilla. (D) Postcontrast sagittal 3DSSMT MRI shows the nonenhancing seroma and the enhancing abnormal lymph node in the left axilla. (E), Postbiopsy ultrasound shows the fluid-filled biopsy cavity in the left breast corresponding to the fluid cavity seen on MRI. (F) Ultrasound of the abnormal lymph node seen on the MRI shows a thick cortical heterogeneous rim and flattening of the fatty hilum by the abnormal metastatic disease in the lymph node. (G) Doppler ultrasound shows marked vascular flow within the lymph node. The usually thick rim, heterogeneity of the cortex, flattening of the fatty hilum, and increased vascular flow are all abnormal findings worrisome for metastatic disease. Biopsy of the lymph node showed metastatic disease.

---

mammogram, in 50% to 55% of cases, the biopsy cavity resolves so completely that it leaves no scar or distortion in the underlying breast parenchyma, and only comparison with prebiopsy mammograms indicates that breast tissue is missing. In other cases, the scar appears as a chronic architectural distortion or a spiculated mass more evident on one projection than the other.

The remaining 45% to 50% of patients continue to have variable mammographic findings ranging from spiculated masslike scars to slight architectural distortion (Fig. 8.11). In still other, more rare cases, seroma cavities persist, appearing as a round or oval mass as shown in Fig. 8.7.

Postbiopsy scars often have a spiculated masslike appearance that can simulate cancer. Spiculated masses should be viewed with suspicion unless one knows that a biopsy was performed in that location. For this reason, it is important to document the date and location in the breast of previous biopsies on the breast history sheet. Some facilities also place a linear metallic scar marker directly on the skin's biopsy scar before taking the mammogram to show the previous biopsy site. On the mammogram, the linear metallic scar marker on the skin will be near the underlying scar. The skin scar may not be immediately adjacent to the scar inside the breast because the skin is compressed away from the underlying breast parenchyma during the mammogram, but the skin scar is always in close proximity to the postbiopsy scar. If a spiculated mass is seen far from the metallic scar marker, the mass might be cancer rather than a scar. The radiologist reviews the preoperative mammograms to see where the biopsy occurred and correlates the prebiopsy and current mammograms to make this determination (Fig. 8.e8.2).

Fat necrosis is common after a breast biopsy and usually appears as a radiolucent lipid-filled mass. Mammography is pathognomonic for fat necrosis if it shows lipid cysts or typical calcified eggshell-type

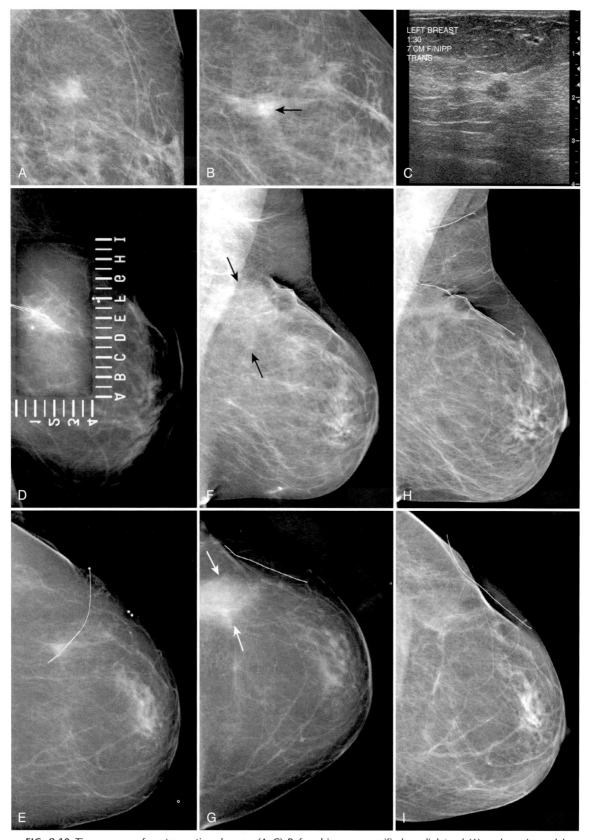

FIG. 8.10 Time course of postoperative change. (A–C) Before biopsy, magnified mediolateral (A) and craniocaudal (CC) (B) mammograms show an ill-defined mass with a few calcifications in the outer left breast. Ultrasound (C) shows an ill-defined hypoechoic mass in the left breast. Core biopsy showed invasive ductal cancer. (D and E) Left mediolateral (D) and CC (E) mammograms show a wire through the mass before excisional biopsy. Pathology showed invasive ductal cancer with negative margins. (F and G) Two years later, postbiopsy mediolateral (F) and CC (G) views show mild architectural distortion, skin deformity, and an ill-defined scar (*arrows*) below a linear metallic scar marker over the skin in which the cancer was removed. Notice skin thickening and architectural distortion in the left axilla from sentinel lymph node dissection. (H and I) Five years later, postbiopsy mediolateral (H) and CC (I) views show only mild architectural distortion and skin deformity, with resolution of most of the skin thickening and scarring shown in F and G.

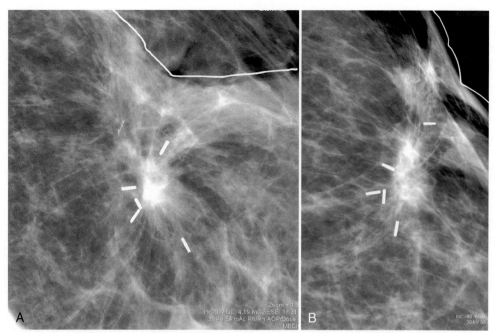

FIG. 8.11 Normal postoperative change on mammography years after surgical excision. Magnification cranio-caudal (A) and mediolateral (B) views show the metallic linear scar marker on the patient's skin with associated skin deformity and skin thickening. Just beneath the marker is the spiculated scar, linear metallic postbiopsy surgical clips outlining the biopsy cavity, and a few faint fat necrosis calcifications, which is typical for a scar.

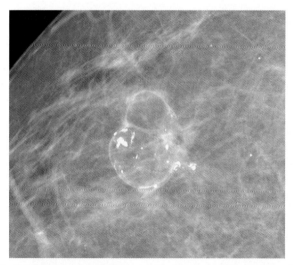

FIG. 8.12 Benign postbiopsy calcifications. A spot compression magnification mammogram shows a calcifying oil cyst in fat necrosis calcifications in a biopsy site. Note the radiolucent center and the calcifications rimming the oil cyst borders.

rims around a radiolucent center (Fig. 8.12). The fat necrosis, lipid cyst, and calcifications usually form in the scar, so these findings should be located near any linear metallic scar markers on the skin. As shown in Chapter 3, calcifications around an oil cyst or fat necrosis can be seen easily with tomosynthesis (see Fig. 3.32).

On ultrasound, the immediate postoperative site shows a seroma or hematoma, breast edema, and focal skin thickening. The fluid collection occasionally contains air. More commonly, the seroma is completely filled with fluid, sometimes containing septa or debris that has varying appearances on ultrasound (Figs. 8.13 and 8.14). Usually the incision can be traced from the biopsy cavity up to the skin and is shown as a linear scar that disturbs the normal breast architecture (Box 8.8).

Later, the fluid in the biopsy cavity resolves and only the fibrotic scar remains. In these cases, ultrasound shows the scar as a hypoechoic spiculated mass that simulates breast cancer, but it should correlate with the postoperative site (Fig. 8.15). Correlating biopsy histories and the physical finding of a scar on the skin distinguishes normal postoperative scarring from cancer. On ultrasound, the spiculated scar often has a "tail" that extends from the scar to the skin, representing the healing biopsy cavity and its adjacent subcutaneous tissue anastomosis (Fig. 8.16).

Postoperative seroma or hematoma is normal and is gradually absorbed. However, if the fluid collection persists or there is a clinical sign of infection, such as fever, erythema, swelling and pain of the skin over the fluid cavity, drainage with subsequent culture of fluid can be performed under the guidance of ultrasound to exclude the possibility of an abscess formation (Fig. 8.17).

WHOLE-BREAST, EXTERNAL BEAM RADIOTHERAPY, AND ACCELERATED PARTIAL BREAST IRRADIATION

An integral part of breast conservation therapy is radiation therapy. Conventional WB-XRT with or without a boost dose to the lumpectomy cavity achieves effective local control of disease within the remaining breast. WB-XRT lowers the frequency of IBTR after breast-conserving therapy. The long-term rates of local recurrence after lumpectomy alone without WB-XRT in the NSABP, Milan, Swedish, and Canadian studies were 39, 23, 24, and 35%, respectively. With the addition of WB-XRT, recurrences were statistically significantly lower at 14, 6, 8, and 11%, respectively. Of note, between 60% to 90% of local recurrences develop near the original primary tumor cavity, so-called *true recurrences,* whereas other recurrences, or *elsewhere failures,* are uncommon. These elsewhere failures occur at the same rate with (0.5%–3.8%) or without (0.5%–3.6%) WB-XRT.

Thus it is important that little or no residual tumor remains after breast surgery and that any residual microscopic tumor foci receive therapeutic doses of radiation. Whole-breast irradiation traditionally is delivered over the course of 5 to 7 weeks,

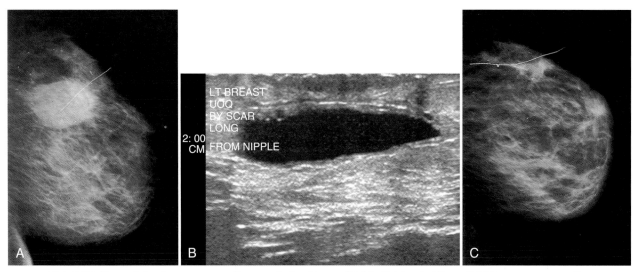

FIG. 8.13 Normal simple seroma on ultrasound after biopsy. (A) Mediolateral oblique (MLO) mammogram after biopsy shows a mass in the biopsy site under the scar marker. (B) Ultrasound under the scar shows a typical fluid collection representing the seroma. The collection was aspirated. (C) An MLO mammogram 2 years later shows the fluid collection has resolved, with only scarring remaining.

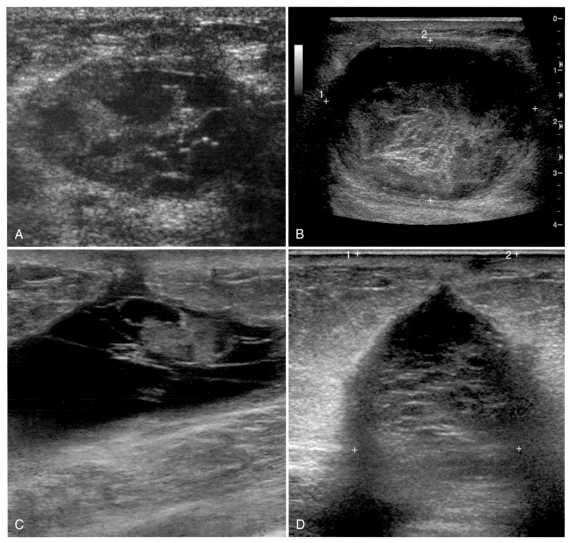

FIG. 8.14 Normal septated seromas in biopsy cavities on ultrasound after surgery: four collections in four different patients. (A) A septated seroma with pockets of fluid and solid components. (B) Another normal seroma with debris and fluid 6 months after biopsy with debris and solid components layering dependently in the inferior aspect of the seroma. (C) Normal 16-week-old seroma with thin septations and a fibrin ball. (D) Normal large seroma cavity with septations and solid components. Notice that the incision from the seroma cavity can be traced to the skin surface in A–C.

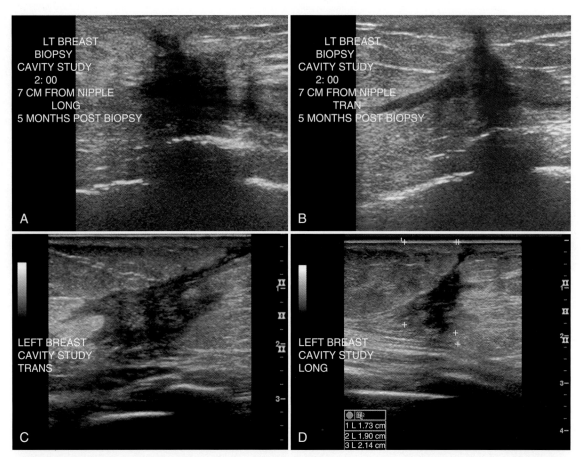

FIG. 8.15 Relatively early-stage of biopsy scars on ultrasound: two cases. (A and B) Five months after biopsy and radiation therapy, longitudinal (A) and transverse (B) scans show a hypoechoic triangular-shaped scar containing fluid, with the incision (filled with fluid) extending to the skin surface. Note the skin thickening and acoustic shadowing of the scar in this case. (C and D) In another patient, 3 months after biopsy and radiation therapy, transverse (C) and longitudinal (D) scans show a typical, spiculated hypoechoic fluid-filled scar and its incision extending from the scar to the skin surface, similar to the biopsy scar in A and B. Note that there is no acoustic shadowing in this case. Note also that the longitudinal study shows distance measurements from the skin surface to the bottom of the cavity and to the chest wall for electron beam boost planning. The radiation oncologist uses these measurements to sterilize the biopsy cavity with an electron beam boost.

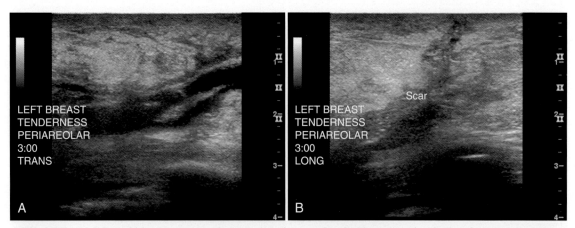

FIG. 8.16 Late-stage of biopsy scars on ultrasound. Eight months after biopsy and radiation therapy, transverse (A) and longitudinal (B) scans show fluid in the scar, but note that the margins are less sharp than those in Fig. 8.15, indicating scar healing and fluid resorption. Note the typical appearance of breast edema on ultrasound in A, shown by the indistinct skin line, gray fat between the skin line and the scar, and dark linear fluid-filled lymphatics in the subcutaneous tissues.

during which the dose is fractionated (ie, given in daily small doses). During WB-XRT the breast skin becomes erythematous and the breast may become edematous, particularly in those patients with larger breasts. The skin may become slightly pitted (*peau d'orange*) because of skin edema, and the breast skin can become tender. A boost dose to the lumpectomy cavity is often added after completion of whole-breast radiotherapy based on a large phase III trial demonstrating reduced recurrence rates with the addition of a boost. After completion of radiotherapy, the breast edema slowly subsides, and the skin becomes less edematous and more normal in appearance as the breast heals.

APBI is a treatment option for selected women with limited early-stage breast cancer after breast-conserving surgery. APBI occurs over a significantly shorter period (*accelerated*) than WB-XRT and targets the tumor bed and defined margin (*partial breast*) rather than the whole breast (Box 8.9).

The shortened time course of radiotherapy increases accessibility of breast conservation treatment and may increase the proportion of women who receive appropriate adjuvant radiotherapy after breast-conserving surgery. In addition, limiting the treatment field to the local tumor bed should, in theory, reduce treatment-related morbidities such as radiation pneumonitis, breast lymphedema, and radiation-induced sarcoma. Because only a part of the breast is irradiated, it is also possible that IBTR after APBI could be treated with repeat breast-conserving surgery and radiation therapy rather than mastectomy. Finally, some investigators suggest that a single fraction of high-dose radiotherapy applied to tumor endothelial cells is more lethal to cancers than fractionated

dosing. Accordingly, single-fraction IORT is potentially the most convenient form of APBI for patients, could provide the most accurate targeting of tissue at risk, and optimally spares normal tissue.

Several different techniques of APBI are used, including interstitial brachytherapy, intracavitary brachytherapy (balloon or multicatheter brachytherapy), IORT, and 3D conformal external beam radiation (3D-CRT). IORT, which delivers radiation directly to the lumpectomy cavity at the time of surgery, is the only APBI technique that allows completion of the surgical and radiation treatment in one hospital visit, saving time for both the patient and the hospital. 3D-CRT is noninvasive and can be performed over 5 to 7 days with twice-daily treatments. All types of APBI use a higher dose per fraction to achieve an effective total dose. Given the higher fractionated dose, posttreatment changes in the breast after APBI may be different from that seen after WB-XRT.

However, the main concern with WB-XRT and APBI is local recurrence and the potential impact of an IBTR on OS. This is particularly true with the use of APBI, in which the entire breast does not receive therapeutic doses of radiation. This means that it is especially important to identify appropriate patients for APBI to prevent failures elsewhere. Several ongoing phase III trials are investigating the role of APBI in selected patients.

BOX 8.8 Postbiopsy Ultrasound Findings

EARLY

Seroma/hematoma
Focal skin thickening
Ability to trace incision from the biopsy cavity to the skin
Fibrin in the seroma (strands, balls)

LATE

Spiculated scar mass (simulates cancer)
±Acoustic shadowing
May see healed incision from the scar to the skin
All ultrasound-detected scars should be correlated to the skin scar and mammographic findings. If there is a mass near the scar but separated by normal tissue, be worried about cancer.

BOX 8.9 Whole-Breast, External Beam Radiotherapy and Accelerated Partial Breast Irradiation

WB-XRT

Treatment encompasses entire breast
Time: 3 to 6 weeks daily therapy
Adds electron beam boost to sterilize the biopsy cavity and a margin of normal tissue
Imaging shows whole-breast edema

ACCELERATED PARTIAL BREAST IRRADIATION

Treatment encompasses biopsy bed and margin only; remainder of breast untreated
Time: varies from 1 to 5 days depending on the technique
Includes:
Interstitial brachytherapy
Intracavitary brachytherapy
Intraoperative radiotherapy
3D conformal external beam radiation
Imaging shows edema in treated site; may have punctate dense calcification in the site

---

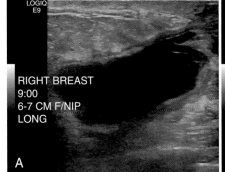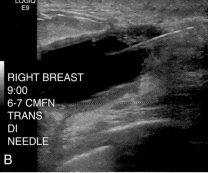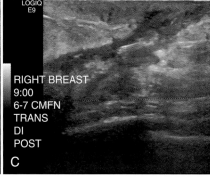

FIG. 8.17 Ultrasound-guided drainage for postoperative abscess. The patient who received lumpectomy for invasive breast cancer 3 months ago developed a painful hot red breast and a fever up to 100°F. (A) Ultrasonography shows a fluid collection with a thick wall at the site of lumpectomy. This could be a postoperative seroma, however, it could be an abscess based on the symptoms. (B and C) Ultrasound-guided fluid drainage was performed. Ultrasound during the drainage (B) shows a needle placed through the cyst wall into the fluid cavity. Ultrasound after the drainage (C) shows that most of the fluid disappeared. A total of 23 cc of fluid was aspirated. The culture was positive for *Staphylococcus lugdunensis*, confirming the diagnosis of an abscess. Patient had antibiotics afterward and her symptoms resolved.

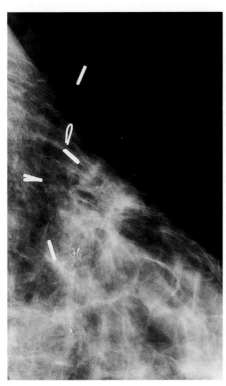

FIG. 8.18 Residual tumor. After biopsy of pleomorphic calcifications showing invasive ductal cancer, the postbiopsy mammogram shows residual calcifications in the biopsy site surrounded by metallic clips in the cavity.

BREAST IMAGING BEFORE REEXCISION LUMPECTOMY OR RADIOTHERAPY

For patients who have undergone an initial cancer excision but have close or involved tumor margins, additional imaging is warranted before reexcision. If, for some reason, ultrasound was not performed for a palpable lesion, ultrasound may visualize previously unanticipated residual disease around the cavity margins or unsuspected satellite lesions. If a specimen radiograph from the original excision had shown microcalcifications at or near the specimen edge and involved margins were seen histologically, repeat mammography (with wire localization) may be helpful in guiding reexcision. Given the difficulty in identifying microscopic residual disease at the time of reoperation, the treatment team should attempt to use any advantage possible to identify residual areas of disease with the intent of targeting them for the surgeon at the time of reexcision.

Patients who have undergone therapeutic excision demonstrating tumor-free margins may still benefit from additional imaging. This is particularly true for women whose lesions presented initially as microcalcifications. Such imaging helps determine the completeness of tumor excision. There is some controversy in the literature as to whether preradiotherapy mammography of the affected breast should become standard to identify possible multifocal disease before committing to radiotherapy. Because the main concern with breast conservation is local recurrence, and because IBTR may affect OS, physicians may order postbiopsy mammograms to determine the completeness of tumor excision if there is any question about residual gross disease or residual microcalcifications (Fig. 8.18). These mammograms are particularly appropriate before the initiation of breast irradiation to make sure there is no residual tumor.

When the biopsy shows unexpected cancer, magnification views of the lumpectomy site and remaining breast before reexcision are especially helpful to show unsuspected, suspicious calcifications

or masses. Calcifications are important because they could be cancer, but they do not always represent tumors. Dershaw et al. (1987) found the positive predictive value of residual microcalcifications representing residual tumor to be 69%, with the likelihood that they represent residual tumor being greatest in cases with DCIS and in those with more than five microcalcifications.

When considering radiation therapy, the number and extent of any calcifications is important, even when they do not indicate tumor. The radiation oncologist must gauge whether they will be able to detect early recurrences on the post–WB-XRT or APBI mammogram. The presence of extensive innumerable calcifications that limit the radiologist's ability to find early cancer is a consideration in patient exclusion from breast conservation.

Pre-ABPI MRI aids patient selection by excluding patients with multifocal or multicentric disease. In one study, Horst et al. (2005) showed that, by using MRI, 9.8% of 51 patients ($n = 5$) had unsuspected disease, including multifocal (3) or multicentric (1) disease, or pectoral fascia involvement (1), precluding enrollment into APBI studies. It is also important to recognize typical MR findings in post-ABPI patients and to distinguish these findings from recurrent or new disease.

NORMAL IMAGING CHANGES AFTER RADIATION THERAPY

Mammography

Recommendations for follow-up mammography after radiation therapy vary by institution. Many facilities obtain a unilateral mammogram 6 to 12 months after the conclusion of radiation therapy, with further follow-up bilateral mammograms at 12-month intervals. Obtaining a mammogram relatively soon after completion of radiation therapy establishes a baseline for future reference (Fig. 8.19).

Normal lumpectomy and WB-XRT alter the normal mammogram. These include the usual postbiopsy changes in the surgical site plus diffuse skin thickening and breast edema from WB-XRT (Box 8.10; Fig. e8.3). Unlike normal focal postoperative edema, breast edema from WB-XRT encompasses the entire breast and not just the region around the postoperative site. On physical examination, the breast commonly shows *peau d'orange,* a large swollen areola or nipple, occasional brownish or red skin, and occasional breast tenderness and swelling. Skin thickening in the immediate postradiation therapy period is caused by breast edema from small-vessel damage; later, it is caused by fibrotic change. Findings of breast edema are most obvious compared with the contralateral side or older mammograms.

On the mammogram, the indications of breast edema are skin and stromal thickening, diffuse increased breast density, and trabecular thickening in subcutaneous fat. The usual changes of the postbiopsy scar are superimposed on the findings of whole-breast edema. The biopsy cavity, seen initially as a fluid-filled mass, may be partially obscured by surrounding breast edema from radiation therapy. These changes usually decrease somewhat over a period of 2.5 to 3 years or may remain stable. With resolution of the surrounding breast edema, the biopsy cavity may become more apparent but should not grow in size.

Progression of breast edema is abnormal and should be investigated. Etiologies of unilateral breast edema other than radiation therapy are inflammatory breast cancer, mastitis, trauma, and obstructed breast lymphatic or venous drainage.

After completion of whole-breast irradiation, many facilities use a lumpectomy cavity boost to sterilize the operative site. Some facilities have the surgeon line the cavity with radiopaque markers to guide the cavity boost and use x-ray or CT imaging for guidance (Fig. 8.20). Other facilities use breast ultrasound to delineate and mark the skin over the breast biopsy cavity for the boost treatment.

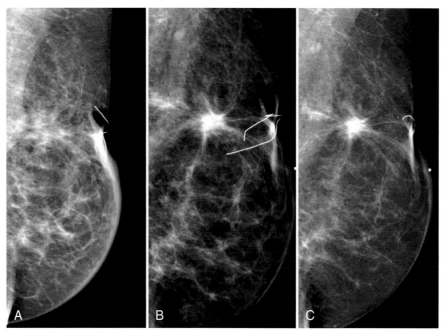

FIG. 8.19 Normal postbiopsy/radiation therapy changes over time. (A) Mediolateral oblique (MLO) mammogram immediately after biopsy and radiation therapy for cancer shows architectural distortion in the biopsy site and overlying skin retraction; metallic markers are seen on the scar. Edema is present, as shown by skin thickening, especially in the lower breast on the MLO view. (B) MLO mammogram 1 year later shows diminishing breast edema and retraction of the biopsy scar, which is more apparent than the year before. It looks like a spiculated mass or possibly cancer. Note that its proximity to the metallic linear skin scar markers shows that it clearly corresponds to the biopsy site. (C) MLO mammogram 3 years later shows resolution of breast edema, with some residual skin thickening. Further retraction of the skin over the biopsy scar has occurred, and the scar still looks like a spiculated mass, simulating cancer, but is unchanged, indicating its benign etiology.

BOX 8.10   Mammographic Findings after Breast Conservation and Radiation Therapy

Whole-breast edema
Postbiopsy scar
Skin retraction/deformity (variable)
Axillary node dissection distortion (if performed)
Metallic clips outlining the biopsy cavity (variable)
The findings are worst at 6 months, diminish, and then stabilize at 2 to 3 years.

In about 25% of women, calcifications develop in the treated breast at the biopsy site; these calcifications can be extreme if the radiation therapy was done many years ago with higher orthovoltage radiation compared with current therapy (Fig. 8.21). Although most of these calcifications will be caused by benign dystrophic calcification, fat necrosis, or calcifying suture material, magnification views of calcifications in the biopsy site are required to distinguish them from the pleomorphic calcifications of cancer recurrence. Calcifications from fat necrosis or calcifying oil cysts have a typical dystrophic appearance, with the latter forming around a radiolucent center (Fig. 8.22). The dystrophic calcifications in fat necrosis can simulate malignancy, but tomosynthesis may show the calcifications forming around fat. Magnification orthogonal projections may show the beginnings of the typical curvilinear shape of fat necrosis. Careful inspection of the previous mammogram may also help by showing that the calcifications are forming around a radiolucent center of fat. When there are no distinguishing features to diagnose dystrophic or fat necrosis calcifications, these calcifications cannot be distinguished from cancer and prompt biopsy (Fig. 8.23).

Biopsy should be performed on suspicious pleomorphic calcifications. Some suspicious calcifications represent incompletely resected tumor, especially in the absence of postbiopsy, preradiotherapy mammograms or if the specimen radiograph suggests that the calcifications were incompletely excised. Comparison with the original prebiopsy mammograms is important to determine whether the original microcalcifications were not totally excised and should undergo reexcision.

Nonspecific microcalcifications forming in or near the biopsy site are a problem. Such calcifications may be benign or malignant. Calcifications that diminish or disappear represent either resolving benign calcifications or represent residual tumor that has responded to therapy. Disappearing calcifications are especially worrisome if they are replaced by a suspicious mass, which should be biopsied. Unchanging nonspecific calcifications should be monitored because they may represent either benign findings (monitor) or incompletely resected tumor (will increase, prompting biopsy).

Increasing microcalcifications are suggestive of breast cancer recurrence and should prompt biopsy unless they are specific for dystrophic calcifications or fat necrosis.

When using APBI in lieu of standard WB-XRT, the higher doses per fraction used with APBI have led to a variety of findings in several phase I/phase II studies. Some groups have reported a higher incidence of posttreatment calcifications, leading to fairly high rates of early postlumpectomy biopsy. It has not been clear from these studies whether a lower threshold for biopsy was set because of the experimental nature of APBI. Other studies have suggested that the incidence of calcifications, attributed to asymptomatic fat necrosis, increases with time after APBI. There has been no systematic evaluation of mammographic findings after APBI either with prior phase I or phase II studies, or from the limited reports from phase III studies published to date. It is fairly clear, however, that APBI will likely become a standard treatment option for at least some women with

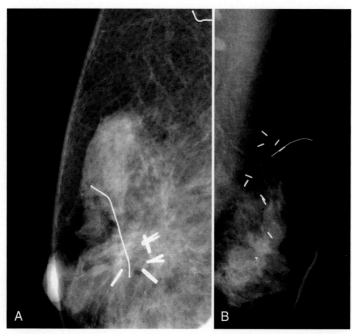

FIG. 8.20 Markers in the biopsy site for electron beam boost: two cases. (A) Mediolateral oblique (MLO) cropped mammogram shows postbiopsy change under a linear scar marker in the upper outer portion of the right breast, with metallic surgical clips lining the biopsy site. The markers are used as a guide for radiation therapy ports. There is another scar marker in the axilla incidentally marking the site. (B) In another patient, left MLO mammogram shows postbiopsy change in the upper left breast, with metallic surgical clips lining a large biopsy cavity and a linear metallic skin marker showing the skin scar.

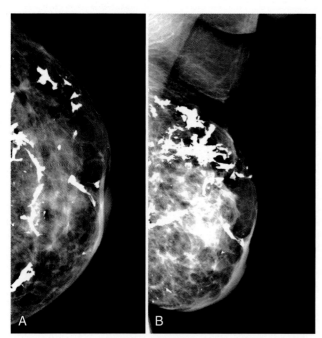

FIG. 8.21 Dense dystrophic calcifications after radiation therapy. Craniocaudal (A) and mediolateral oblique (B) views after an older type of whole-breast radiation therapy that used a higher orthovoltage radiation compared with current methods shows a small left breast, skin thickening, and large, coarse, and bizarre dystrophic calcifications. Breast shrinkage and these types of calcifications are not usually seen with whole-breast radiation therapy today.

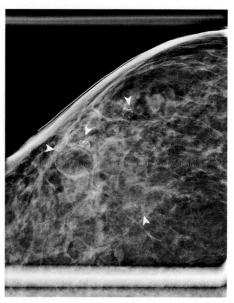

FIG. 8.22 Calcified oil cysts after radiation therapy and lumpectomy. Magnification of right craniocaudal mammogram obtained 3 years after lumpectomy and whole-breast radiation therapy for invasive breast cancer shows rim, eggshell-type, or curvilinear calcifications and round fat density (*arrowheads*), representing oil cysts, associated with architectural distortion and skin thickening caused by whole-breast radiation therapy. Note the linear metallic skin scar marker on the incision site.

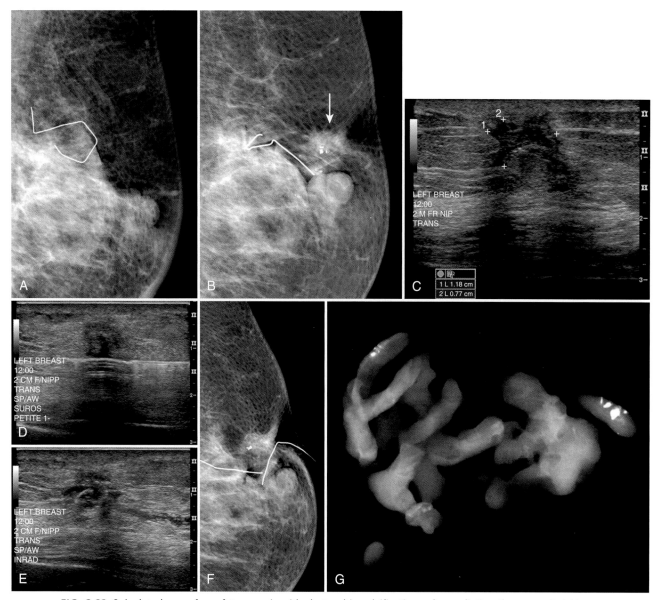

FIG. 8.23 Spiculated mass from fat necrosis with dystrophic calcifications after radiation therapy, mimicking a recurrent cancer. (A) Cropped mammogram shows scarring in the upper left breast and skin thickening from radiation therapy after cancer biopsy, with a metallic skin scar marker over the biopsy site. (B) Two years later, a new spiculated mass containing dystrophic calcifications (*arrow*) is noted near the scar and is worrisome for cancer. (C) Ultrasound shows the spiculated mass and calcifications corresponding to the mammographic finding. (D) Ultrasound shows a core biopsy needle through the mass and calcifications. (E), Postbiopsy ultrasound shows the residual mass, a marker, and surrounding hematoma. (F) Postbiopsy mammogram shows removal of the calcifications, a hematoma, and the marker. Note the linear scar markers and skin deformity from the prior biopsy. (G) Specimen radiograph shows the calcifications within the core biopsy samples. Histology showed fat necrosis and scar. This demonstrates how fat necrosis can simulate recurrent cancer when it forms a spiculated mass and calcifications.

early-stage breast cancer pursuing breast conservation. Because radiologists may see the findings of a large seroma cavity extending from the skin surface to the chest wall (Fig. 8.24) or increased calcifications in and around the lumpectomy cavity resulting from fat necrosis from ABPI, it will be important to contrast normal post-APBI changes to normal postbiopsy changes when the scar is small (Fig. 8.25). An example is the typical very dense, almost metallic pattern of calcifications caused by APBI or IORT (Fig. 8.26; Fig. e8.4). Recognition of post-APBI findings will minimize both false-positive, as well as false-negative, interpretations of post-APBI mammograms as this new paradigm emerges.

Magnetic Resonance Imaging

On MRI, the breast biopsy scar enhances for up to 18 months with rapid uptake and washout kinetics and is a common cause for false-positive readings. On MRI, normal postbiopsy fat necrosis produces a spiculated mass that enhances rapidly and washes out on the kinetic curve. This common false-positive MRI finding can result in biopsy unless the radiologist investigates the patient's history and correlates the MRI to other imaging (Fig. 8.27).

Recurrent invasive cancers usually appear as a mass in or near the biopsy site in the first few years. Cancers recurring as DCIS

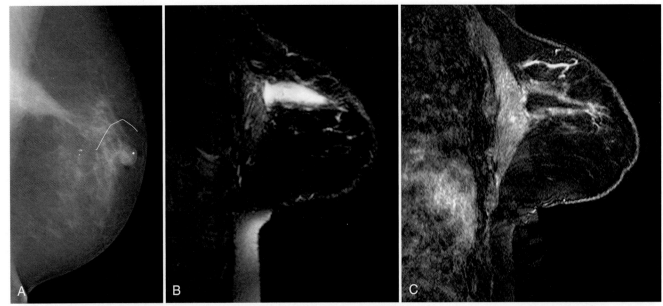

FIG. 8.24 Mammography and magnetic resonance imaging (MRI) after accelerated partial breast irradiation (APBI). (A) Mediolateral oblique mammogram shows postbiopsy change in a cylindrical scar extending from the skin surface (marked by a metallic linear scar marker) to the chest wall of the left breast after intraoperative radiation therapy. Note that after ABPI there is very little breast edema, skin thickening, or skin deformity, unlike with whole-breast irradiation changes shown in Figs. 8.19 and 8.23, in which almost the entire breast shows breast edema and generalized skin thickening. (B) Sagittal fat-suppressed T2-weighted MRI shows the fluid-filled biopsy site extending from the skin to the chest wall, corresponding to the scar seen on the mammogram. (C) Sagittal postcontrast 3D magnetization transfer MRIs show the fluid-filled biopsy site extending from the skin to the chest wall, with enhancement on the periphery of the biopsy cavity. Note that edema is limited to the operative site, unlike with whole-breast irradiation.

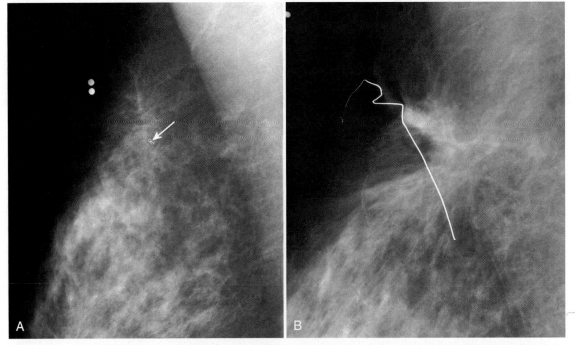

FIG. 8.25 Normal scarring at a biopsy site. (A) Prebiopsy cropped mediolateral oblique (MLO) view shows a postbiopsy marker (*arrow*) in which cancer was biopsied by stereotaxis; two BBs show the previous needle entry site. (B) Postbiopsy cropped MLO view shows limited architectural distortion and skin deformity at the biopsy scar after definitive cancer surgery. Cancer recurrences display pleomorphic calcifications, increasing density, or mass-like change in the scar, which are not present here. Contrast B to the residual calcifications in malignancy in Fig. 8.32.

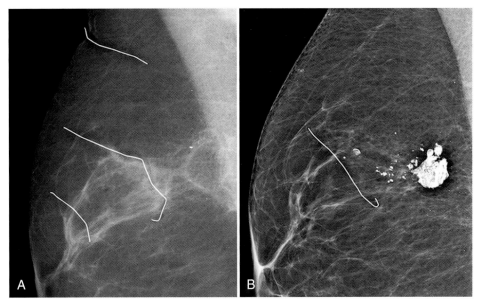

FIG. 8.26 Typical dense benign calcifications after intraoperative radiotherapy (IORT). (A) Mediolateral oblique (MLO) mammogram 2 years after IORT shows architectural distortion with microcalcifications at the site of IORT, which was performed at the time of lumpectomy for invasive ductal cancer with ductal carcinoma in situ. (B) MLO mammogram 9 years after IORT shows dense, sharply demarcated metal-like calcifications developing at the site of IORT. Note linear scar markers.

are difficult to identify on MRI, because DCIS may not produce the characteristic rapid initial and late-phase plateau or washout kinetic curve of invasive cancer and are identified only by their linear or segmental morphology. Moreover, chemotherapy changes the enhancement pattern of the breast by diminishing enhancement of normal breast parenchyma and tumor alike.

Chemotherapy response shows decreased breast cancer size and often changes suspicious kinetic curves to benign linetic patterns (slow early and persistent late kinetics), even when invasive breast cancer is still present. The change in the kinetic curve pattern is thought to be caused by loss of abnormal tumor vascularity. Thus enhancement at the site of prior cancer should be considered residual tumor even if the kinetic curves are benign.

APBI using either IORT or 3D-CRT results in characteristic posttreatment MRI changes, which extend from the skin to the chest wall. Typically, there is only localized skin thickening in the APBI area and an absence of the generalized skin thickening seen with WB-XRT. In addition, signal voids are common in the postoperative breast after APBI. These signal voids may persist up to 25 months after treatment. Some signal voids may resolve between 6 and 33 months after treatment, whereas others persist. The reason for persistent signal voids in the breast lumpectomy cavities not containing metal at 25 months is uncertain but is related to altered paramagnetic properties of the treated biopsy site or methemoglobin. Radiologists should be aware of the characteristic MRI appearance of the APBI field to avoid false-positive diagnoses.

TREATMENT FAILURE OR IPSILATERAL BREAST TUMOR RECURRENCE (IBTR)

The incidence of treatment failure is approximately 1% per year. Women who are at greatest risk for failure include those younger than age 35 (and especially those younger than age 30); those treated for invasive cancer with an extensive intraductal component or infiltrating ductal carcinoma with a large intraductal component; those with intraductal carcinoma of the comedo type; those with intraductal cancer measuring 2.5 cm or greater in diameter; those with multicentric lesions, as suggested in the studies discussed in this chapter, and those treated for more than one synchronous cancer in the same breast; and

those with angiolymphatic invasion. Gross residual tumor also has a poor prognosis, but microscopic residual disease may not infer a greater risk of IBTR. Despite the slightly higher tendency for recurrence in these groups, no risk factor is an absolute contraindication to breast conservation; data on lesions with these features in randomized studies more often than not suggest a trend for increased recurrence rather than a statistically significant association.

For women who choose lumpectomy, IBTR rates are approximately 5% at 5 years and between 10% and 15% at 10 years after therapy. Invasive IBTR is most common between 18 months and 7 years after treatment; during this period IBTR is more common in or around the lumpectomy cavity. IBTR after 7 years more frequently is a random event in any quadrant of the affected breast, not necessarily at the original site, and is usually unrelated to the original lesion in the breast.

Late ipsilateral breast treatment failures consisting of DCIS or invasive tumors smaller than 2 cm may have a better prognosis than larger recurrences; thus, some feel it is important to diagnose recurrences near the original tumor or new cancers elsewhere in the breast as early as possible. However, there is no clinical trial evidence supporting this belief. Treatment failures after lumpectomy and WB-XRT are usually treated by salvage mastectomy.

Treatment failures detected on mammography manifest as new pleomorphic calcifications or masses developing in the biopsy site. At times, a breast cancer recurrence is hard to distinguish from the normal postbiopsy scar, which mimics cancer. However, unlike cancer recurrences, the normal postbiopsy scar becomes smaller and less apparent over time on the mammogram, with stabilization at 2 to 3 years. Central fat necrosis may produce a radiolucent center in the biopsy cavity. Thus it is not normal if the scar grows in size or becomes denser or more masslike. The radiologist suspects recurrent carcinoma and prompts biopsy if the scar develops new pleomorphic calcifications or becomes more dense, if the scar edge becomes rounder, or if the scar grows (Figs. 8.28 and 8.29).

Breast cancer in the irradiated breast may arise at the site of the original tumor or elsewhere in the breast (Fig. 8.30). Recurrences at the original tumor site are usually caused by failure to

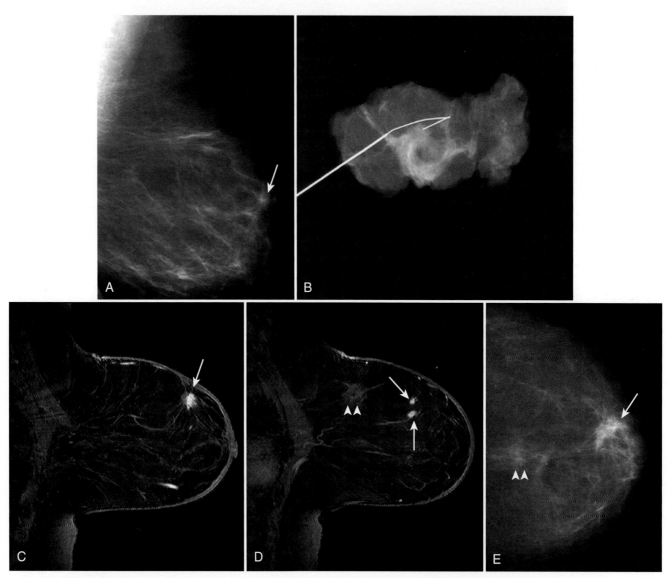

FIG. 8.27 Fat necrosis at a biopsy site on magnetic resonance imaging (MRI), mimicking cancer. (A) Prebiopsy mediolateral oblique view shows a spiculated mass (*arrow*) in the upper breast, which later was biopsied and showed cancer. (B) The specimen radiograph shows the cancer (invasive ductal cancer) and localizing wire. (C) Six months later, a postcontrast sagittal 3D spectral-spatial excitation magnetization transfer (3DSSMT) MRI shows an enhancing spiculated mass (*arrow*) in the upper breast and skin thickening. (D) On another slice, the postcontrast sagittal 3DSSMT MRI shows two enhancing masses representing fat necrosis (*arrows*), and a posterior nonenhancing low-intensity architectural distortion representing an old biopsy scar (*arrowheads*). Note that the breast biopsy scar enhances for up to 18 months, whereas scarring older than 18 months does not enhance. (E), Craniocaudal mammogram after the MRI shows the old architectural distortion in the central breast (*arrowheads*) and postbiopsy scarring closer to the nipple (*arrow*), corresponding to the spiculated enhancing mass on MRI, which represented normal fat necrosis. Note how fat necrosis can simulate cancer on MRI.

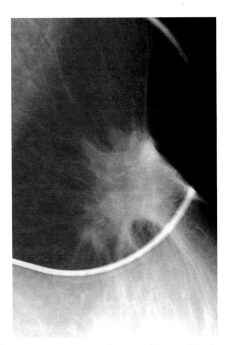

FIG. 8.28 Breast cancer occurring at a biopsy site. A postbiopsy spot compression mediolateral oblique mammogram shows architectural distortion, skin retraction, and deformity at a biopsy scar. Unlike normal biopsy scars, which have a little density in their central part, this spot view shows a moderately masslike area in the scar, which was invasive ductal cancer. Contrast this tumor with the normal postbiopsy scar in Fig. 8.25B.

eradicate the original cancer and represent true treatment failures; they occur sooner than a tumor developing elsewhere in the breast. Tumors developing outside the treated area occur at the same rate as tumors forming in the contralateral breast.

Recurrent disease is diagnosed by mammography or physical examination. About half of the recurrences are detected by mammography and half by physical examination. Those that are mammographically detected usually contain pleomorphic microcalcifications or masses (Box 8.11). Palpable recurrences usually manifest as masses, are more frequently invasive cancer, and may be displayed on the mammogram as developing asymmetries or masses. On ultrasound, an IBTR shows as a mass separate from or in continuity with the biopsy scar (Fig. 8.31) if it occurs near the original biopsy site.

On mammography, breast cancer recurrences contain pleomorphic calcifications (Fig. 8.32) or are shown as masses with or without calcifications. This is why radiologists investigate any new mass, because even benign-appearing new solid masses may represent a new cancer (Figs. 8.33 and 8.34; Fig. e8.5)

There are no absolute guidelines for management of an IBTR after lumpectomy and radiotherapy. Traditionally, because of concern of increased fibrosis and breast shrinkage with repeat radiotherapy, most IBTRs are treated with completion mastectomy with or without reconstruction. Some patients and physicians will attempt repeat lumpectomy without additional radiotherapy, but little long-term data on the safety and effectiveness of this approach are available. Recently investigators have treated patients with IBTR using repeat lumpectomy and APBI. Here as well, isolated case reports alone exist and little long-term data on safety or effectiveness are available. Thus, generally, recurrent tumor is usually treated with salvage mastectomy.

MASTECTOMY

Mastectomy is used when it is not possible to excise the entire breast tumor with a good cosmetic result, if there is a

contraindication to radiotherapy, or if it is the patient's preference to have a mastectomy. Although there is no strict size cutoff when choosing lumpectomy or mastectomy, lesions larger than 5 cm or patients with multifocal disease are usually approached with mastectomy.

There are exceptions to this paradigm. For a patient with newly diagnosed breast cancer, if the workup reveals an invasive tumor larger than 5 cm, NAC may be offered before surgery because it might decrease tumor size and facilitate breast conservation.

Also, the demonstration of multifocal disease is now considered a relative contraindication to breast conservation rather than an absolute contraindication.

Various types of mastectomies are performed. With a traditional mastectomy, the nipple–areolar complex is removed with an ellipse of skin and underlying breast tissue. A skin-sparing mastectomy suggests that some of the breast skin that would normally have been removed is allowed to remain. The postoperative appearance of a skin-sparing mastectomy is variable in terms of the amount of skin remaining. In some patients, the skin left behind may simply be in one quadrant; at its extreme, a total skin-sparing mastectomy removes the nipple–areolar complex but leaves all the remaining breast skin intact.

In the case of a subcutaneous mastectomy, the breast tissue is removed as with a simple (total) mastectomy, except that the nipple–areolar complex is preserved. This is occasionally requested by patients who are having mastectomy for prophylactic reasons and do not want to lose the nipple–areolar complex.

More recently areolar- and nipple-sparing mastectomies have been offered to patients with invasive breast cancer; hence, the slightly differing nomenclature in contrast to subcutaneous mastectomy. There is more oncologic soundness in areolar-sparing mastectomy, because breast ductal tissue does not involve the skin of the areola and therefore can be removed with the underlying breast as part of the mastectomy. In nipple-sparing mastectomy, by definition, some ductal tissue may remain within the nipple itself, as well as in the underlying bud of tissue, which ensures adequate vascularity to the nipple. Although the risk of direct nipple involvement varies among patient subgroups, it is important to point out that no randomized trials have demonstrated the safety of nipple-sparing mastectomy compared with a traditional simple mastectomy. Typically, radiotherapy is not routinely performed after a nipple-sparing mastectomy unless there are pathologic indications such as multiple involved nodes or a large tumor.

After mastectomy, breast reconstruction options include an implant, a latissimus dorsi flap with an implant when significant breast skin has been lost, or a transverse rectus abdominis myocutaneous (TRAM) flap or one of its derivative procedures, such as a deep inferior epigastric perforator (DIEP) flap. Images of reconstructed breasts are shown in Chapter 9. In the case of skin-sparing subcutaneous mastectomy, the surgeon removes the breast tissue as for a simple (total) mastectomy but preserves the nipple–areolar complex and inserts a tissue expander. Unless there is a medical contraindication to breast reconstruction, patients who choose mastectomy are always offered breast reconstruction with a tissue expander/implant or autologous tissue flap. Imaging of the reconstructed breast is typically not performed after expander or implant placement or after autologous tissue reconstruction.

Sometimes, reduction mammoplasty may be required on the contralateral, unaffected breast to achieve symmetry with the treated breast. The appearances of breasts reconstructed with autologous tissue and contralateral normal breasts that have undergone reduction mammoplasty are characteristic and should not be mistaken for cancer. These are shown in Chapter 9.

Breast cancer recurrences in the unreconstructed mastectomy site are usually detected by physical examination. Because of the low yield of breast cancer detection from the small amount of

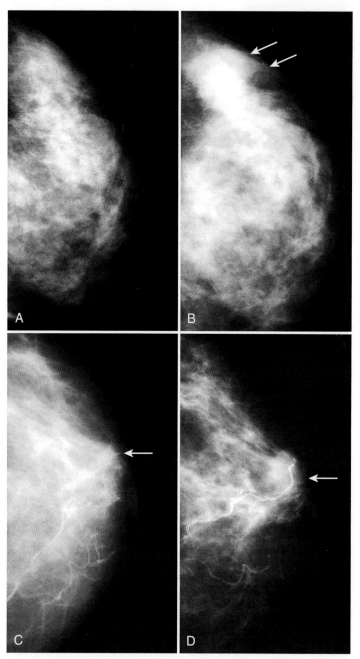

FIG. 8.29 Breast cancer recurring at a biopsy site, manifested as developing asymmetry/mass: two cases. (A and B) Postbiopsy craniocaudal (CC) mammogram (A) shows architectural distortion in the outer portion of the breast after biopsy and radiation therapy for cancer. Five years later (B), a developing asymmetry (*arrows*) has grown in the outer part of the breast. Biopsy showed recurrent cancer. (C and D) In another patient, postbiopsy CC view (C) shows minimal architectural distortion near the nipple after biopsy and radiation therapy for cancer (*arrow*). The next year a developing mass (D, *arrow*) was noted in the biopsy site. Biopsy showed recurrent cancer.

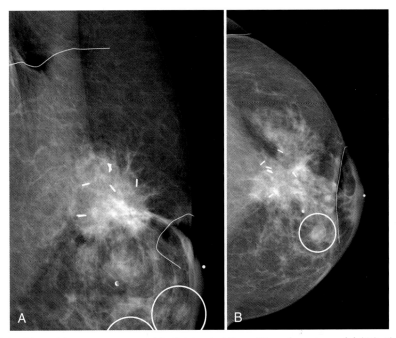

FIG. 8.30 Ipsilateral breast tumor recurrence. Mediolateral oblique (A) and craniocaudal (CC; B) mammograms 2 years after radiation therapy show postbiopsy scarring and surgical clips in the retroareolar region, with skin thickening. There is a new round mass in the medial left breast best seen and circled on the CC view (B), and seen and circled in the MLO view (A), separated from the old biopsy site by normal tissue. Additional views confirmed that a mass was present, and biopsy showed a new invasive ductal cancer in a site other than the original biopsy site.

BOX 8.11 Benign and Suspicious Mammographic Findings Developing in the Biopsy Site after Breast Conservation and Radiation Therapy

Pleomorphic calcifications (cancer recurrence or residual)
Nonspecific calcifications (benign or malignant)
Dystrophic calcifications (benign)
Suture calcifications (benign)
Oil cyst (benign)
Developing density or mass (suspicious)

---

breast tissue remaining, surveillance mammography of the mastectomy site is usually not performed.

BREAST IMAGING FOR ASSESSING RESPONSE TO NEOADJUVANT CHEMOTHERAPY

In the setting of NAC, breast imaging is important for monitoring tumor response and for identifying residual disease after chemotherapy. Currently, the tumor response is determined based on changes of the tumor size (Response Evaluation Criteria in Solid Tumors response [RECIST] criteria or World Health Organization [WHO] criteria). After completion of chemotherapy, breast imaging compares residual tumor size with prechemotherapy measurements so that chemotherapy response may be characterized as complete or partial response, no response, or tumor progression. For surgical planning, breast imaging identifies and localizes residual tumor for surgical treatment planning (breast conservative surgery or mastectomy), even in patients who have had a complete clinical response. The goal of imaging is to provide information to achieve resection of all residual, or, in the setting of complete response, to guide the surgery to the prechemotherapy tumor location to confirm complete histopathology response with excision. Thus identification of tumors and

evaluation of residual tumor size and extent are essential components in tumor response assessment using breast imaging.

Physical examination, mammography, and ultrasound are classic ways to assess tumor size; however, they have been known to be only moderately useful in predicting residual tumor size with a moderate correlation to the pathologic tumor size (correlation coefficient 0.41–0.42), with a limited accuracy of 66% to 75% (Chagpar et al., 2006).

MRI is another imaging tool that is potentially useful in response assessment in patients with NAC. Thus far, studies evaluating the accuracy of MRI in predicting postchemotherapy tumor size, however, have shown inconsistent results. Correlation between tumor size on post-NAC MRI and pathologic tumor size has varied from high (correlation coefficient 0.89; Partridge et al., 2002) to low (correlation coefficient 0.49; Wright et al., 2010). Straver et al. (2010) reported that MRI incorrectly indicated the post-NAC surgical treatment in 17% (36/208) of patients, including 13% (27/208) with underestimation of disease extent on MRI leading to incorrect indication of breast conservative therapy and 4% (9/208) with overestimation of disease extent on MRI leading to correct indication of breast mastectomy, when a correct indication of breast conservative therapy was defined as a preoperatively feasible breast conservative therapy combined with tumor size <30 mm at pathology (Straver et al. 2010). Among patients who were diagnosed as complete remission (CR) on post-NAC MRI, 56% to 75% had residual disease at pathologic examination (Chen et al., 2008; Straver et al., 2010). Pitfalls in interpreting post-NAC MRI include alternation of tumor vascularity on MRI because alternated angiogenic abnormal tumor vascularity may change dynamic enhancement of tumors to resemble benign disease. Thus any residual enhancement at the site of a previously known tumor is suspicious (Fig. 8.35), even if its kinetics is benign appearing. Because of the poor specificity of MRI findings after chemotherapy, pretreatment MRI is essential as a baseline for comparison.

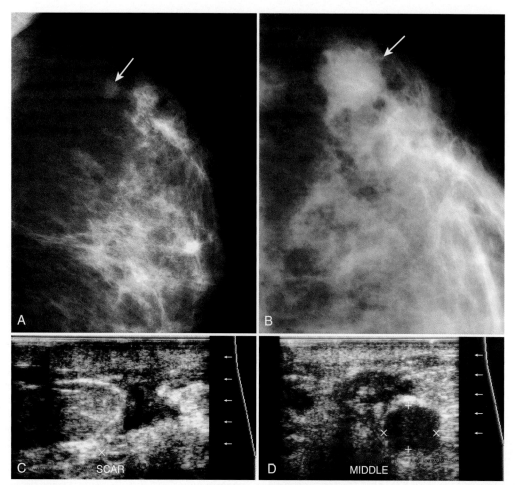

FIG. 8.31 Treatment failure. (A and B) Mediolateral oblique views 1 year (A) and 1.5 years (B) after radiation therapy show a palpable round ill-defined mass (*arrows*) in the biopsy site in the upper part of the breast. (C and D) Ultrasound at 1.5 years shows a fluid-filled scar (C) at the biopsy site. Separate from the biopsy site is a round hypoechoic solid mass marked by calipers (D). Note that because the round mass is separate from the fluid collection, it cannot represent a part of the biopsy scar and must be considered suspicious. Biopsy showed an invasive ductal cancer.

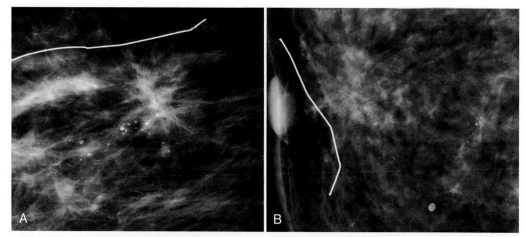

FIG. 8.32 Treatment failure: two cases with calcifications. (A) Magnified cropped mammogram shows a linear metallic scar marker overlying a spiculated but stable postlumpectomy scar. However, there are new pleomorphic calcifications in and near the scar, representing ductal carcinoma in situ in the biopsy site. (B) In another patient, a stable spiculated scar is seen under the linear metallic marker in the periareolar region. Note the pleomorphic calcifications in and extending posteriorly to the scar, representing recurrent cancer.

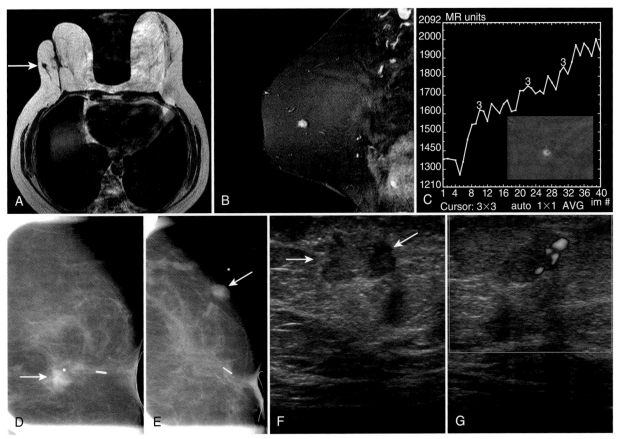

FIG. 8.33 Atypical ipsilateral breast tumor recurrence on magnetic resonance imaging (MRI), mammography, and ultrasound. (A) Axial nonfat-suppressed T1-weighted localizer shows architectural distortion in skin from the prior biopsy for cancer and a small round, low signal intensity mass (*arrow*) in the outer right breast. (B) Sagittal postcontrast 3D spectral-spatial excitation magnetization transfer (3DSSMT) shows an enhancing round mass against a fatty background. (C) Kinetic curve for a region of interest over the outer round mass shows a benign kinetic curve characterized by a slow initial rise and persistent late phase. However, because the mass was not present previously, it was considered suspicious. (D and E) Magnified mediolateral (D) and craniocaudal (E) mammograms show architectural distortion and a marker in the retroareolar region after biopsy and radiation therapy for cancer. In the outer left breast, lateral to the scar, there is a palpable oval mass (*arrows*), marked by a BB and corresponding to the mass seen on MRI in B. (F and G) Ultrasound over the mass shows a solid mass with microlobulated margins (F, *arrows*), that shows marked vascularity on color Doppler ultrasound (G). Biopsy showed invasive ductal cancer and the patient underwent mastectomy.

Early response assessment with interim MRI examinations obtained during the midtreatment, usually after the first one or two cycles, is also another potential role of MRI. Accurate early response assessment can contribute to a timely adjustment of treatment protocol if necessary, avoiding unnecessary toxicity of ineffective treatments. Several studies have been performed to investigate the accuracy of interim MRI using various parameters, including changes in unidimensional or bidimensional tumor size, 3D volume, quantitative dynamic contrast measurements (volume transfer constant, exchange rate constant, early contrast uptake), heterogeneity (tumor entropy and uniformity), descriptive patterns of tumor reduction, and quantitative ^{1}H MR spectroscopy. However, because of unpowered studies with heterogeneous techniques, the evidence of MRI in the early prediction of therapeutic response is still insufficient (Prevos, 2012). Because of this and other studies, interim MRI examinations are often not reimbursed in the United States. More studies with sufficient statistical power are warranted to determine the value of breast MRI in response evaluation in patients with NAC.

On occasion, NAC may produce a complete clinical response and the tumor is undetectable by both physical examination and imaging after NAC, making identification of the original tumor difficult to identify for surgeons to excise to confirm a complete histopathological response. To avoid this problem, radiologists place a small metallic marker in the tumor under imaging guidance before the patient undergoes chemotherapy (see Fig. 8.35). Then, if all traces of the tumor fade with chemotherapy, the marker shows the original tumor location as a target for subsequent preoperative needle localization to excise the now-invisible tumor bed. Recent NCCN guidelines encourage the use of percutaneously placed markers into the breast before NAC.

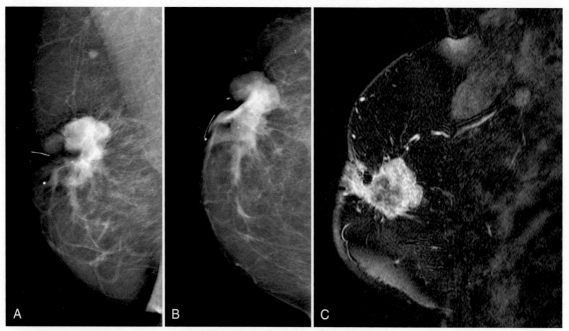

FIG. 8.34 Ipsilateral breast tumor recurrence on mammography and magnetic resonance imaging (MRI). (A and B) Mediolateral (A) and craniocaudal (B) mammograms show a dense, lobulated, suspicious mass invading and puckering the skin, growing in the biopsy site shown by the linear metallic skin scar marker. The cancer had been resected years ago, and the mass was worrisome for cancer recurrence. (C) Sagittal T1-weighted postcontrast 3D spectral-spatial excitation magnetization transfer MRI shows an enhancing irregular mass with central necrosis that extends to and infiltrates the skin, in the outer right breast. A round signal void is seen in the anterior aspect of the mass from a recent fine-needle biopsy resulting in air or methemoglobin.

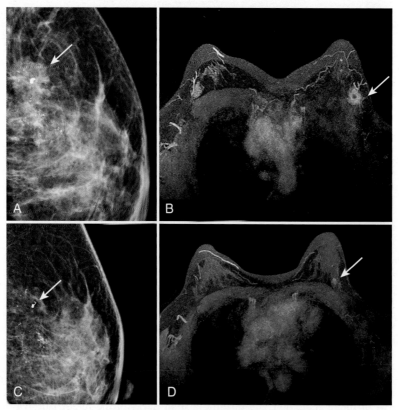

FIG. 8.35 Residual cancer after neoadjuvant chemotherapy (NAC). (A) Before NAC, photographically magnified mediolateral oblique mammogram shows a spiculated 14-mm mass (*arrow*) and fine pleomorphic microcalcifications in the left upper breast, representing breast cancer (an invasive breast cancer with ductal carcinoma in situ) shown by ultrasound-guided biopsy with a coil-shaped marker. (B) Partial maximum intensity projection (MIP) image from contrast-enhanced water-specific T1-weighted magnetic resonance imaging (MRI), obtained before NAC, shows the enhancing irregular cancer with a signal void caused by the marker (*arrow*) with rapid washin and washout kinetics in the left upper outer quadrant. (C) This patient received NAC before surgery. On post-NAC magnified lateromedial mammography, there is architectural distortion and microcalcifications; but no residual mass around the marker (*arrow*) caused by tumor response. (D) MRI (partial MIP image from contrast-enhanced imaging) after NAC shows resolution of abnormal tumor enhancement (partial response), but there is still abnormal enhancement (*arrow*) inferior to the biopsy marker, which is worrisome for residual disease. After x-ray–guided bracket wire localization for the biopsy marker, minimal foci of residual invasive and in situ ductal carcinoma was identified.

Key Elements

Immediate postsurgical breast changes on mammography include increased density (local edema), oval or round masses (seroma/hematoma) with or without air, and skin thickening.

The fluid in the surgical site resolves over the next few weeks and months in most cases.

Postsurgical changes diminish in severity over time and are stable at 3 to 5 years.

From 50% to 55% of patients undergoing surgical breast biopsy for benign disease have no mammographic findings at 3 years.

The remaining 45% to 50% of patients show architectural distortion, parenchymal changes (scarring) that may be spiculated, or increased density that can simulate breast cancer.

To determine whether a spiculated density on the mammogram is a postbiopsy scar or cancer, it is important to correlate the postsurgical site with the location of the spiculated finding.

Fat necrosis occurring in a biopsy site is visualized as radiolucent lipid-filled masses, with occasional curvilinear calcifications forming around the lucent center.

On ultrasound, the immediate postsurgical site appears as a fluid-filled mass representing the seroma; it occasionally displays septa, debris, or fluid tracking up to the skin incision.

If only the fibrotic scar remains, ultrasound reveals a hypoechoic spiculated mass that simulates breast cancer, but it should correlate with the postoperative site.

On MRI, the immediate postbiopsy cavity is a fluid-filled structure with surrounding tissue enhancement.

Postbiopsy scarring enhancement persists for up to 18 months and should then subside.

Breast tumors are staged by the TNM (tumor, lymph node, metastasis) classification of breast cancer from the American Joint Committee on Cancer.

Local control of breast cancer requires surgical eradication of tumor by mastectomy or lumpectomy, followed by radiotherapy.

The breast imager aids the surgeon in selecting candidates for breast-conserving surgery by determining the extent of tumor.

Relative contraindications to radiation therapy include previous radiation therapy, pregnancy, collagen vascular disease, and multicentric or diffuse disease.

Ipsilateral breast tumor recurrences are reported in 5% of women at 5 years and in 10% to approximately 15% at 10 years after completion of therapy.

Treatment failures after breast conservation are managed by salvage mastectomy.

The sentinel lymph node (SLN) biopsy technique identifies the lymph node most likely to harbor metastasis. Radionuclide tracers or blue dye is injected into the breast and later carried into the breast lymphatics draining the tumor or biopsy cavity.

A "hot" node, a blue node, or an abnormal palpable node identified at surgery is an SLN.

The SLN may be examined by hematoxylin and eosin staining, as well as by immunohistochemistry staining for low molecular weight cytokeratins.

The SLN may be identified at surgery even with nonvisualization of an SLN at lymphoscintigraphy.

Magnetic resonance imaging (MRI) has been used for predicting the extent of tumor before the initial breast cancer surgical procedure, with some false-negative results in women with invasive lobular carcinoma and ductal carcinoma in situ (DCIS).

If preoperative needle localization has been performed, specimen radiography or specimen sonography is used to determine whether the suspicious finding has been adequately removed.

As needed, postbiopsy mammograms determine the completeness of tumor excision, are particularly appropriate before the initiation of breast irradiation, and should be performed if residual tumor is suspected.

Most facilities obtain a unilateral mammogram 6 months after the conclusion of radiation therapy, with further follow-up bilateral mammograms at 12-month intervals.

Breast edema from whole-breast radiation therapy encompasses the entire breast and manifests as diffuse increased parenchymal density, skin thickening, and trabecular thickening in subcutaneous fat.

Postsurgical and postradiation therapy changes usually decrease somewhat over a period of 2.5 to 3 years or may remain stable.

Calcifications in the biopsy site in an irradiated breast represent fat necrosis, dystrophic calcifications, calcifying suture material, or breast cancer recurrence.

Chemotherapy changes the MRI enhancement pattern of the breast by diminishing enhancement of normal breast parenchyma and tumor alike.

On MRI, suspicious postchemotherapy kinetic late-phase plateau or washout curve patterns can change to a benign persistent late-phase pattern despite the presence of viable breast cancer.

Recurrent cancer on mammography shown by pleomorphic microcalcifications frequently represents DCIS.

Palpable recurrences are usually seen as mammographic masses and are more frequently invasive cancers.

Breast reconstruction includes an implant, a latissimus dorsi flap, or a transverse rectus abdominis myocutaneous flap.

Breast cancer recurrence in an unreconstructed mastectomy site is usually detected by physical examination.

SUGGESTED READINGS

Abe H, Schmidt RA, Kulkarni K, et al.: Axillary lymph nodes suspicious for breast cancer metastasis: sampling with US-guided 14-gauge core-needle biopsy—clinical experience in 100 patients, *Radiology* 250:41–49, 2009.

Alazraki NP, Styblo T, Grant SF, et al.: Sentinel node staging of early breast cancer using lymphoscintigraphy and the intraoperative gamma-detecting probe, *Semin Nucl Med* 30:56–64, 2000.

Al-Hallaq HA, Mell LK, Bradley JA, et al.: Magnetic resonance imaging identifies multifocal and multicentric disease in breast cancer patients who are eligible for partial breast irradiation, *Cancer* 113:2408–2414, 2008.

American Joint Committee on Cancer (AJCC). Breast: *AJCC cancer staging manual*, New York, 2010, Springer, pp 347–376.

The American Society of Breast Surgeons: Performance and practice guidelines for axillary lymph node dissection in breast cancer patients. https://www.breastsurgeons.org/new_layout/about/statements/PDF_Statements/PerformancePracticeGuidelines_ALND.pdf Accessed July 9, 2015.

The American Society of Breast Surgeons: Performance and practice guidelines for sentinel lymph node biopsy in breast cancer patients. https://www.breastsurgeons.org/new_layout/about/statements/PDF_Statements/PerformancePracticeGuidelines_SLN.pdf Accessed on July 9, 2015.

Bauer TW, Spitz FR, Callans LS, et al.: Subareolar and peritumoral injection identify similar sentinel nodes for breast cancer, *Ann Surg Oncol* 9:169–176, 2002.

Bedrosian I, Mick R, Orel SG, et al.: Changes in the surgical management of patients with breast carcinoma based on preoperative magnetic resonance imaging, *Cancer* 98:468–473, 2003.

Bedrosian I, Reynolds C, Mick R, et al.: Accuracy of sentinel lymph node biopsy in patients with large primary breast tumors, *Cancer* 88:2540–2545, 2000.

Bevilacqua JL, Gucciardo G, Cody HS, et al.: A selection algorithm for internal mammary sentinel lymph node biopsy in breast cancer, *Eur J Surg Oncol* 28:603–614, 2002.

Birdwell RL, Smith KL, Betts BJ, et al.: Breast cancer: variables affecting sentinel lymph node visualization at preoperative lymphoscintigraphy, *Radiology* 220:47–53, 2001.

Bleicher RJ, Ciocca RM, Egleston BL, et al.: Association of routine pretreatment magnetic resonance imaging with time to surgery, mastectomy rate, and margin status, *J Am Coll Surg* 209:180–187, 2009.

Bleicher RJ, Morrow M: MRI and breast cancer: role in detection, diagnosis, and staging, *Oncology (Williston Park)* 21:1521–1533, 2007.

Boughey JC, Middleton LP, Harker L, et al.: Utility of ultrasound and fine-needle aspiration biopsy of the axilla in the assessment of invasive lobular carcinoma of the breast, *Am J Surg* 194:450–455, 2007.

Brennan ME, Houssami N, Lord S, et al.: Magnetic resonance imaging screening of the contralateral breast in women with newly diagnosed breast cancer: systematic review and meta-analysis of incremental cancer detection and impact on surgical management, *J Clin Oncol* 27:5640-5649, 2009.

Brenner RJ, Pfaff JM: Mammographic features after conservation therapy for malignant breast disease: findings standardized by regression analysis, *AJR Am J Roentgenol* 167:171-178, 1996a.

Brenner RJ, Pfaff JM: Mammographic changes after excisional breast biopsy for benign disease, *AJR Am J Roentgenol* 167:1047-1052, 1996b.

Budrukkar A: Accelerated partial breast irradiation: an advanced form of hypofractionation, *J Cancer Res Ther* 4:46-47, 2008.

Chagpar AB, Middleton LP, Sahin AA, et al.: Accuracy of physical examination, ultrasonography, and mammography in predicting residual pathologic tumor size in patients treated with neoadjuvant chemotherapy, *Ann Surg* 243:257-264, 2006.

Chen JH, Feig B, Agrawal G, et al.: MRI evaluation of pathologically complete response and residual tumors in breast cancer after neoadjuvant chemotherapy, *Cancer* 112:17-26, 2008.

Chen PY, Vicini FA, Benitez P, et al.: Long-term cosmetic results and toxicity after accelerated partial-breast irradiation: a method of radiation delivery by interstitial brachytherapy for the treatment of early-stage breast carcinoma, *Cancer* 106:991-999, 2006.

Choi YJ, Ko EY, Han BK, et al.: High-resolution ultrasonographic features of axillary lymph node metastasis in patients with breast cancer, *Breast* 18:119-122, 2009.

Choy N, Lipson J, Porter C, et al.: Initial results with preoperative tattooing of biopsied axillary lymph nodes and correlation to sentinel lymph nodes in breast cancer patients, *Ann Surg Oncol* 22:377-382, 2015.

Clarke M, Collins R, Darby S, et al.: Effects of radiotherapy and of differences in the extent of surgery for early breast cancer on local recurrence and 15-year survival: an overview of the randomised trials, *Lancet* 366(9503):2087-2106, 2005.

Cody 3rd HS, Fey J, Akhurst T, et al.: Complementarity of blue dye and isotope in sentinel node localization for breast cancer: univariate and multivariate analysis of 966 procedures, *Ann Surg Oncol* 8:13-19, 2001.

Cody 3rd HS, Urban JA: Internal mammary node status: a major prognosticator in axillary node-negative breast cancer, *Ann Surg Oncol* 2:32-37, 1995.

Cote RJ, Peterson HF, Chaiwun B, et al.: For the International Breast Cancer Study Group: role of immunohistochemical detection of lymph-node metastases in management of breast cancer, *Lancet* 354:896-900, 1999.

Cox BW, Horst KC, Thornton S, Dirbas FM: Impact of increasing margin around the lumpectomy cavity to define the planning target volume for 3D conformal external beam accelerated partial breast irradiation, *Med Dosim* 32:254-262, 2007.

Crivellaro M, Senna G, Dama A, et al.: Anaphylaxis due to patent blue dye during lymphography, with negative skin prick test, *J Investig Allergol Clin Immunol* 13:71-72, 2003.

Damle S, Teal CB: Can axillary lymph node dissection be safely omitted for early-stage breast cancer patients with sentinel lymph node micrometastasis? *Ann Surg Oncol* 16(12):3215-3216, 2009.

Dang CM, Zaghiyan K, Karlan SR, Phillips EH: Increased use of MRI for breast cancer surveillance and staging is not associated with increased rate of mastectomy, *Am Surg* 75:937-940, 2009.

Denison CM, Ward VL, Lester SC, et al.: Epidermal inclusion cysts of the breast: three lesions with calcifications, *Radiology* 204:493-496, 1997.

Dershaw DD: *The conservatively treated breast. Diagnosis of diseases of the breast*, Philadelphia, PA, 1997, WB Saunders, p 553.

Dershaw DD, Shank B, Reisinger S: Mammographic findings after breast cancer treatment with local excision and definitive irradiation, *Radiology* 164:455-461, 1987.

Dirbas FM: Accelerated partial breast irradiation: where do we stand? *J Natl Compr Canc Netw* 7:215-225, 2009.

Dirbas FM, Jeffrey SS, Goffinet DR: The evolution of accelerated, partial breast irradiation as a potential treatment option for women with newly diagnosed breast cancer considering breast conservation, *Cancer Biother Radiopharm* 19:673-705, 2004.

D'Orsi CJ, Sickles EA, Mendelson EB, Morris EA, et al.: *ACR BI-RADS® atlas, breast imaging and reporting and data system*, Reston, VA, 2013, American College of Radiology.

Dowlatshahi K, Fan M, Anderson JM, Bloom KJ: Occult metastases in sentinel nodes of 200 patients with operable breast cancer, *Ann Surg Oncol* 8:675-681, 2001.

Dowlatshahi K, Fan M, Snider HC, Habib FA: Lymph node micrometastases from breast carcinoma: reviewing the dilemma, *Cancer* 80:1188-1197, 1997.

Dowsett M, Sestak I, Lopez-Knowles E, et al.: Comparison of PAM50 risk of recurrence score with oncotype DX and IHC4 for predicting risk of distant recurrence after endocrine therapy, *J Clin Oncol* 31:2783-2790, 2013.

Drukker CA, Bueno-de-Mesquita JM, Retel VP, et al.: A prospective evaluation of a breast cancer prognosis signature in the observational RASTER study, *Int J Cancer* 133:929-936, 2013.

Dupont EL, Kuhn MA, McCann C, et al.: The role of sentinel lymph node biopsy in women undergoing prophylactic mastectomy, *Am J Surg* 180:274-277, 2000.

Early Breast Cancer Trialists' Collaborative Group (EBCTCG): Effect of radiotherapy after mastectomy and axillary surgery on 10-year recurrence and 10-year breast cancer mortality: meta-analysis of individual patient data for 8135 women in 22 randomized trials, *Lancet* 383:2127-2135, 2014.

Evans SB, Kaufman SA, Price LL, et al.: Persistent seroma after intraoperative placement of MammoSite for accelerated partial breast irradiation: incidence, pathologic anatomy, and contributing factors, *Int J Radiat Oncol Biol Phys* 65:333-339, 2006.

Fischer U, Kopka L, Grabbe E: Breast carcinoma: effect of preoperative contrast-enhanced MR imaging on the therapeutic approach, *Radiology* 213:881-888, 1999.

Fisher B, Anderson S, Bryant J, et al.: Twenty-year follow-up of a randomized trial comparing total mastectomy, lumpectomy, and lumpectomy plus irradiation for the treatment of invasive breast cancer, *N Engl J Med* 347:1233-1241, 2002.

Fisher B, Anderson S, Redmond CK, Wolmark N, Wickerham DL, Cronin WM: Reanalysis and results after 12 years of follow-up in a randomized clinical trial comparing total mastectomy with lumpectomy with or without irradiation in the treatment of breast cancer, *N Engl J Med* 333:1456-1461, 1995.

Fisher B, Bauer M, Margolese R, et al.: Five-year results of a randomized clinical trial comparing total mastectomy and segmental mastectomy with or without radiation in the treatment of breast cancer, *N Engl J Med* 312:665-673, 1985.

Fisher B, Dignam J, Wolmark N, et al.: Lumpectomy and radiation therapy for the treatment of intraductal breast cancer: findings from National Surgical Adjuvant Breast and Bowel Project B-17, *J Clin Oncol* 16:441-452, 1998.

Fisher B, Redmond C, Poisson R, et al.: Eight-year results of a randomized clinical trial comparing total mastectomy and lumpectomy with or without irradiation in the treatment of breast cancer, *N Engl J Med* 320:822-828, 1989.

Freedman GM, Fowble BL, Nicolaou N, et al.: Should internal mammary lymph nodes in breast cancer be a target for the radiation oncologist? *Int J Radiat Oncol Biol Phys* 46:805-814, 2000.

Garcia-Barros M, Paris F, Cordon-Cardo C, et al.: Tumor response to radiotherapy regulated by endothelial cell apoptosis, *Science* 300:1155-1159, 2003.

Giuliano AE, Hawes D, Ballman KV, et al.: Association of occult metastases in sentinel lymph nodes and bone marrow with survival among women with early stage invasive breast cancer, *JAMA* 306:385-393, 2011a.

Giuliano AE, Hung KK, Ballman KV, et al.: Axillary dissection vs no axillary dissection in women with invasive breast cancer and sentinel node metastasis: a randomized clinical trial, *JAMA* 305:569-575, 2011b.

Guiliano AE, Jones RC, Brennan M Statman R: Sentinel lymphadenectomy in breast cancer, *J Clin Oncol* 15(6):2345-2350, 1997.

Giuliano AE, Kirgan DM, Guenther JM, Morton DL: Lymphatic mapping and sentinel lymphadenectomy for breast cancer, *Ann Surg* 220:391-398, 1994. discussion 398-401.

Gnant M, Filipits M, Greil R, et al.: Predicting distant recurrence in receptor-positive breast cancer patients with limited clinicopathological risk: using the PAM50 Risk of Recurrence score in 1478 postmenopausal patients of the ABCSG-8 trial treated with adjuvant endocrine therapy alone, *Ann Oncol* 25:339-345, 2014.

Godinez J, Gombos EC, Chikarmane SA, et al.: Breast MRI in the evaluation of eligibility for accelerated partial breast irradiation, *AJR Am J Roentgenol* 191:272-277, 2008.

Goldhirsch A, Winer EP, Coates AS, et al.: Personalizing the treatment of women with early breast cancer: highlights of the St. Gallen International Expert Consensus on the Primary Therapy of Early Breast Cancer 2013, *Ann Oncol* 24:2206-2223, 2013.

Goldhirsch A, Wood WC, Coates AS, et al.: Strategies for subtypes—dealing with the diversity of breast cancer: highlights of the St. Gallen International Expert Consensus on the Primary Therapy of Early Breast Cancer 2011, *Ann Oncol* 22:1736-1747, 2011.

Golshan M, Martin WJ, Dowlatshahi K: Sentinel lymph node biopsy lowers the rate of lymphedema when compared with standard axillary lymph node dissection, *Am Surg* 69:209-212, 2003.

Gorechlad JW, McCabe EB, Higgins JH, et al.: Screening for recurrences in patients treated with breast-conserving surgery: is there a role for MRI? *Ann Surg Oncol* 15:1703-1709, 2008.

Goyal S, Khan AJ, Vicini F, et al.: Factors associated with optimal cosmetic results at 36 months in patients treated with accelerated partial breast irradiation (APBI) on the American Society of Breast Surgeons (ASBrS) MammoSite Breast Brachytherapy Registry Trial, *Ann Surg Oncol* 16:2450-2458, 2009.

Heywang SH, Hilbertz T, Beck R, et al.: Gd-DTPA enhanced MR imaging of the breast in patients with postoperative scarring and silicone implants, *J Comput Assist Tomogr* 14:348-356, 1990.

Heywang-Köbrunner SH, Schlegel A, Beck R, et al.: Contrast-enhanced MRI of the breast after limited surgery and radiation therapy, *J Comput Assist Tomogr* 17:891-900, 1993.

Hill AD, Tran KN, Akhurst T, et al.: Lessons learned from 500 cases of lymphatic mapping for breast cancer, *Ann Surg* 229:528-535, 1999.

Holwitt DM, Swatske ME, Gillanders WE, et al.: Scientific Presentation Award: the combination of axillary ultrasound and ultrasound-guided biopsy is an accurate predictor of axillary stage in clinically node-negative breast cancer patients, *Am J Surg* 196:477-482, 2008.

Horst KC, Ikeda DM, Birdwell RL, et al.: Breast magnetic resonance imaging alters patient selection for accelerated, partial breast irradiation. Proceedings of the American Society for Therapeutic Radiology and Oncology 47th annual meeting, *Int J Radiat Oncol Biol Phys* 63(Suppl 1):S4-S5, 2005.

Houssami N, Hayes DF: Review of preoperative magnetic resonance imaging (MRI) in breast cancer: should MRI be performed on all women with newly diagnosed, early stage breast cancer? *CA Cancer J Clin* 59:290-302, 2009.

Huvos AG, Hutter RV, Berg JW: Significance of axillary macrometastases and micrometastases in mammary cancer, *Ann Surg* 173:44-46, 1971.

Jannink I, Fan M, Nagy S, et al.: Serial sectioning of sentinel nodes in patients with breast cancer: a pilot study, *Ann Surg Oncol* 5:310-314, 1998.

Jothy Basu KS, Bahl A, Subramani V, et al.: Normal tissue complication probability of fibrosis in radiotherapy of breast cancer: accelerated partial breast irradiation vs conventional external-beam radiotherapy, *J Cancer Res Ther* 4:126-130, 2008.

Jozsef G, Luxton G, Formenti SC: Application of radiosurgery principles to a target in the breast: a dosimetric study, *Med Phys* 27:1005-1110, 2000.

Karamlou T, Johnson NM, Chan B, et al.: Accuracy of intraoperative touch imprint cytologic analysis of sentinel lymph nodes in breast cancer, *Am J Surg* 185:425–428, 2003.

Keshtgar MR, Ell PJ: Clinical role of sentinel lymph node biopsy in breast cancer, *Lancet Oncol* 3:105–110, 2002.

Kiluk JV, Ly QP, Meade T, et al: Axillary recurrence rate following negative sentinel node biopsy for invasive breast cancer: long-term follow-up, *Ann Surg Oncol* 18(Suppl 3):S339–S342.

Krag D, Weaver D, Ashikaga T, et al.: The sentinel node in breast cancer—a multicenter validation study, *N Engl J Med* 339:941–946, 1998.

Krag DN, Anderson SJ, Julian TB, et al.: Sentinel-lymph-node resection compared with conventional axillary-lymph-node dissection in clinically node-negative patients with breast cancer: overall survival findings from the NSABP B-32 randomised phase 3 trial, *Lancet Oncol* 11:927–933, 2010.

Kuzmiak CM, Zeng D, Cole E, Pisano ED: Mammographic findings of partial breast irradiation, *Acad Radiol* 16(7):819–825, 2009.

Lacour J, Le M, Caceres E, et al.: Radical mastectomy versus radical mastectomy plus internal mammary dissection. Ten year results of an international cooperative trial in breast cancer, *Cancer* 51:1941–1943, 1983.

Lagios MD: Clinical significance of immunohistochemically detectable epithelial cells in sentinel lymph node and bone marrow in breast cancer, *J Surg Oncol* 83:1–4, 2003.

Langer I, Guller U, Viehl CT, et al.: Axillary lymph node dissection for sentinel lymph node micrometastases may be safely omitted in early-stage breast cancer patients: long-term outcomes of a prospective study, *Ann Surg Oncol* 16(12):3366–3374, 2009.

Lehman CD, DeMartini W, Anderson BO, Edge SB: Indications for breast MRI in the patient with newly diagnosed breast cancer, *J Natl Compr Canc Netw* 7:193–201, 2009.

Liberman L: Lymphoscintigraphy for lymphatic mapping in breast carcinoma, *Radiology* 228:313–315, 2003.

Liberman L, Van Zee KJ, Dershaw DD, et al.: Mammographic features of local recurrence in women who have undergone breast-conserving therapy for ductal carcinoma in situ, *AJR Am J Roentgenol* 168:489–493, 1997.

Lu WL, Jansen L, Post WJ, et al.: Impact on survival of early detection of isolated breast recurrences after the primary treatment for breast cancer: a meta-analysis, *Breast Cancer Res Treat* 114:403–412, 2009.

Mamounas EP: Sentinel lymph node biopsy after neoadjuvant systemic therapy, *Surg Clin North Am* 83:931–942, 2003.

Mariani L, Salvadori B, Marubini E, et al.: Ten year results of a randomised trial comparing two conservative treatment strategies for small size breast cancer, *Eur J Cancer* 34:1156–1162, 1998.

Martin RC, Derossis AM, Fey J, et al.: Intradermal isotope injection is superior to intramammary in sentinel node biopsy for breast cancer, *Surgery* 130:432–438, 2001.

McCarter MD, Yeung H, Fey J, et al.: The breast cancer patient with multiple sentinel nodes: when to stop? *J Am Coll Surg* 192:692–697, 2001a.

McCarter MD, Yeung H, Yeh S, et al.: Localization of the sentinel node in breast cancer: identical results with same-day and day-before isotope injection, *Ann Surg Oncol* 8:682–686, 2001b.

McMasters KM, Chao C, Wong SL, et al.: Sentinel lymph node biopsy in patients with ductal carcinoma in situ: a proposal, *Cancer* 95:15–20, 2002.

McMasters KM, Tuttle TM, Carlson DJ, et al.: Sentinel lymph node biopsy for breast cancer: a suitable alternative to routine axillary dissection in multi-institutional practice when optimal technique is used, *J Clin Oncol* 18:2560–2566, 2000.

McMasters KM, Wong SL, Martin 2nd RC, et al.: Dermal injection of radioactive colloid is superior to peritumoral injection for breast cancer sentinel lymph node biopsy: results of a multi-institutional study, *Ann Surg* 233:676–687, 2001.

Mendelson EB: Evaluation of the postoperative breast, *Radiol Clin North Am* 30:107–138, 1992.

Montague ED: Conservation surgery and radiation therapy in the treatment of operable breast cancer, *Cancer* 53(Suppl):700–704, 1984.

Montague ED, Fletcher GH: Local regional effectiveness of surgery and radiation therapy in the treatment of breast cancer, *Cancer* 55(Suppl):2266–2272, 1985.

Morris EA, Schwartz LH, Drotman MB, et al.: Evaluation of pectoralis major muscle in patients with posterior breast tumors on breast MR images: early experience, *Radiology* 214:67–72, 2000.

Morrow M: Should routine breast cancer staging include MRI? *Nat Clin Pract Oncol* 6:72–73, 2009.

Mortellaro VE, Marshall J, Singer L, et al.: Magnetic resonance imaging for axillary staging in patients with breast cancer, *J Magn Reson Imaging* 30:309–312, 2009.

Mumtaz H, Hall-Craggs MA, Davidson T, et al.: Staging of symptomatic primary breast cancer with MR imaging, *AJR Am J Roentgenol* 169:417–424, 1997.

Nathanson SD, Wachna DL, Gilman D, et al.: Pathways of lymphatic drainage from the breast, *Ann Surg Oncol* 8:837–843, 2001.

National Comprehensive Cancer Network (NCCN): *NCCN clinical practice guidelines in oncology. breast cancer, version 2*, 2015.

National Comprehensive Cancer Network (NCCN): *NCCN guidelines breast cancer screening and diagnosis, version 1*, 2014.

Nelson JC, Beitsch PD, Vicini FA, et al.: Four-year clinical update from the American Society of Breast Surgeons MammoSite brachytherapy trial, *Am J Surg* 198(1):83–91, 2009.

Nielsen TO, Parker JS, Leung S, et al.: A comparison of PAM50 intrinsic subtyping with immunohistochemistry and clinical prognostic factors in tamoxifen-treated estrogen receptor-positive breast cancer, *Clin Cancer Res* 16:5222–5232, 2010.

Offersen BV, Overgaard M, Kroman N, Overgaard J: Accelerated partial breast irradiation as part of breast conserving therapy of early breast carcinoma: a systematic review, *Radiother Oncol* 90:1–13, 2009.

Olivotto IA, Bajdik CD, Ravdin PM, et al.: Population-based validation of the prognostic model ADJUVANT! for early breast cancer, *J Clin Oncol* 23:2716–2725, 2005.

Ollila DW, Klauber-DeMore N, Tesche LJ, et al.: Feasibility of breast preserving therapy with single fraction in situ radiotherapy delivered intraoperatively, *Ann Surg Oncol* 14:660–669, 2007.

Orel SG, Schnall MD, Powell CM, et al.: Staging of suspected breast cancer: effect of MR imaging and MR-guided biopsy, *Radiology* 196:115–122, 1995.

Orel SG, Troupin RH, Patterson EA, Fowble BL: Breast cancer recurrence after lumpectomy and irradiation: role of mammography in detection, *Radiology* 183:201–206, 1992.

Paik S, Shak S, Tang G, et al.: A multigene assay to predict recurrence of tamoxifen-treated, node-negative breast cancer, *N Engl J Med* 351:2817–2826, 2004.

Partridge SC, Gibbs JE, Lu Y, Esserman LJ, Sudilovsky D, Hylton NM: Accuracy of MR imaging for revealing residual breast cancer in patients who have undergone neoadjuvant chemotherapy, *AJR Am J Roentgenol* 179:1193–1199, 2002.

Pendas S, Dauway E, Giuliano R, et al.: Sentinel node biopsy in ductal carcinoma in situ patients, *Ann Surg Oncol* 7:15–20, 2000.

Pernas S, Gil M, Benitez A, et al.: Avoiding axillary treatment in sentinel lymph node micrometastases of breast cancer: a prospective analysis of axillary or distant recurrence, *Ann Surg Oncol* 17:772–777, 2010.

Perou CM, Sorlie T, Eisen MB, et al.: Molecular portraits of human breast tumours, *Nature* 406:747–752, 2000.

Philpotts LE, Lee CH, Haffty BG, et al.: Mammographic findings of recurrent breast cancer after lumpectomy and radiation therapy: comparison with the primary tumor, *Radiology* 201:767–771, 1996.

Polgar C, Strnad V, Major T: Brachytherapy for partial breast irradiation: the European experience, *Semin Radiat Oncol* 15:116–122, 2005.

Prevos R, Smidt ML, Tjan-Heijnen VC, et al.: Pre-treatment differences and early response monitoring of neoadjuvant chemotherapy in breast cancer patients using magnetic resonance imaging: a systematic review, *Eur Radiol* 22:2607–2616, 2012.

Rao R, Lilley L, Andrews V, et al.: Axillary staging by percutaneous biopsy: sensitivity of fine-needle aspiration versus core needle biopsy, *Ann Surg Oncol* 16:1170–1175, 2009.

Rastogi P, Anderson SJ, Bear HD, et al.: Preoperative chemotherapy: updates of National Surgical Adjuvant Breast and Bowel Project Protocols B-18 and B-27, *J Clin Oncol* 26:778–785, 2008.

Sandrucci S, Mussa A: Sentinel lymph node biopsy and axillary staging of T1-T2 N0 breast cancer: a multicenter study, *Semin Radiat Oncol* 15:278–283, 1998.

Schwartz GF, Giuliano AE, Veronesi U: Proceedings of the consensus conference of the role of sentinel lymph node biopsy in carcinoma of the breast, 19–April 22, 2001, Philadelphia, *Breast J* 8:124–138, 2002.

Shen P, Glass EC, DiFronzo LA, Giuliano AE: Dermal versus intraparenchymal lymphoscintigraphy of the breast, *Ann Surg Oncol* 8:241–248, 2001.

Sickles EA, D'Orsi CJ, Bassett LW, ACR BI-RADS®—mammography, et al.: *ACR BI-RADS® atlas, breast imaging reporting and data system*, Reston, VA, 2013, American College of Radiology.

Sickles EA, Herzog KA: Mammography of the postsurgical breast, *AJR Am J Roentgenol* 136:585–588, 1981.

Singletary SE, Greene FL: Revision of breast cancer staging: the 6th edition of the TNM Classification, *Semin Surg Oncol* 21:53–59, 2003.

Smith BD, Arthur DW, Buchholz TA, et al.: Accelerated partial breast irradiation consensus statement from the American Society for Radiation Oncology (ASTRO), *Int J Radiat Oncol Biol Phys* 74:987–1001, 2009.

Steinhoff MM: Axillary node micrometastases: detection and biologic significance, *Breast J* 5:325–329, 1999.

Straver ME, Loo CE, Rutgers EJ, et al.: MRI-model to guide the surgical treatment in breast cancer patients after neoadjuvant chemotherapy, *Ann Surg* 251:701–707, 2010.

Tendulkar RD, Chellman-Jeffers M, Rybicki LA, et al.: Preoperative breast magnetic resonance imaging in early breast cancer: implications for partial breast irradiation, *Cancer* 115:1621–1630, 2009.

Tuli R, Christodouleas J, Roberts L, et al.: Prognostic indicators following ipsilateral tumor recurrence in patients treated with breast-conserving therapy, *Am J Surg* 198:557–561, 2009.

Turner RR, Ollila DW, Krasne DL, Giuliano AE: Histopathologic validation of the sentinel lymph node hypothesis for breast carcinoma, *Ann Surg* 226:271–278, 1997.

Veronesi U, Luini A, Del Vecchio M, et al.: Radiotherapy after breast-preserving surgery in women with localized cancer of the breast, *N Engl J Med* 328:1587–1591, 1993.

Veronesi U, Orecchia R, Luini A, et al.: Full-dose intraoperative radiotherapy with electrons during breast-conserving surgery: experience with 590 cases, *Ann Surg* 242:101–106, 2005.

Veronesi U, Paganelli G, Viale G, et al.: Sentinel lymph node biopsy and axillary dissection in breast cancer: results in a large series, *J Natl Cancer Inst* 91:368–373, 1999.

Veronesi U, Paganelli G, Viale G, et al.: A randomized comparison of sentinel-node biopsy with routine axillary dissection in breast cancer, *N Engl J Med* 349:546–553, 2003.

Veronesi U, Zurrida S, Mazzaro G, Viale G: Extensive frozen section examination of axillary sentinel nodes to determine selective axillary dissection, *World J Surg* 25:806–808, 2001.

Vicini FA, Kestin L, Huang R, Martinez A: Does local recurrence affect the rate of distant metastases and survival in patients with early-stage breast carcinoma treated with breast-conserving therapy? *Cancer* 97:910–919, 2003a.

Vicini FA, Remouchamps V, Wallace M, et al.: Ongoing clinical experience utilizing 3D conformal external beam radiotherapy to deliver partial-breast irradiation in patients with early-stage breast cancer treated with breast-conserving therapy, *Int J Radiat Oncol Biol Phys* 57:1247–1253, 2003b.

Wazer DE, Kaufman S, Cuttino L, et al.: Accelerated partial breast irradiation: an analysis of variables associated with late toxicity and long-term cosmetic outcome after high-dose-rate interstitial brachytherapy, *Int J Radiat Oncol Biol Phys* 64:489–495, 2006.

Weaver DL, Ashikaga T, Krag DN, et al.: Effect of occult metastases on survival in node-negative breast cancer, *N Eng J Med* 364:412–421, 2011.

Weaver DL, Krag DN, Ashikaga T, Harlow SP, O'Connell M: Pathologic analysis of sentinel and nonsentinel lymph nodes in breast carcinoma: a multicenter study, *Cancer* 88:1099–1107, 2000.

Wright FC, Zubovits J, Gardner S, et al.: Optimal assessment of residual disease after neo-adjuvant therapy for locally advanced and inflammatory breast cancer—clinical examination, mammography, or magnetic resonance imaging? *J Surg Oncol* 101:604–610, 2010.

Yarbro JW, Page DL, Fielding LP, et al.: American Joint Committee on Cancer prognostic factors consensus conference, *Cancer* 86:2436–2446, 1999.

Zafrani B, Fourquet A, Vilcoq JR, et al.: Conservative management of intraductal breast carcinoma with tumorectomy and radiation therapy, *Cancer* 57:1299–1301, 1986.

Chapter 9
Breast Implants and the Reconstructed Breast

Kanae K. Miyake, Debra M. Ikeda, Dung H. Nguyen, and Bruce L. Daniel

CHAPTER OUTLINE

Breast reconstruction is commonly performed for breast augmentation, for breast reduction, or for reconstruction after breast cancer surgery. Current breast reconstruction techniques are diverse and may involve the use of an implant, autologous tissue, or a combination of the two. Radiologists should be familiar with the normal postoperative imaging appearances of breast implants and reconstructed breasts; be able to diagnose complications related to breast reconstruction, such as implant rupture; and be able to distinguish normal postoperative and reconstruction findings from postsurgical/implant complications or breast cancer recurrences. This chapter reviews the basics of breast implant placement for augmentation, autologous tissue reconstruction techniques, and reduction mammoplasty as well as reviews mammographic, ultrasound, and magnetic resonance imaging (MRI) techniques of implants and reconstructed breasts, showing normal and ruptured breast implants, the normal postoperative or reconstructed breast, and complications related to breast reconstruction.

BREAST IMPLANTS

History in the United States

Silicone breast implants were introduced in 1964 by Cronin and Gerow (Derby, 2015). An estimated 2 million women in the United States have silicone breast implants, with approximately 80% placed for breast augmentation and the remainder for breast reconstruction after mastectomy. On April 16, 1992, the U.S. Food and Drug Administration (FDA) restricted the use of silicone implants to women undergoing breast reconstruction for mastectomy because of concern about implant rupture and a possible association with connective tissue disease.

Addressing these concerns, an article by Tugwell et al. (2001) reported a U.S. District Court order establishing a national science panel to assess whether existing scientific studies showed an association between silicone breast implants and connective tissue disease. They concluded that no scientific evidence of such a relationship exists, and there is no evidence of a relationship between silicone breast implants and breast cancer. At that time, silicone gel breast implants were used for breast reconstruction after mastectomy in the United States. Saline-filled implants were used for cosmetic breast augmentation.

In 2007, a review article by McLaughlin et al. restated that there was no "causal association between breast implants and breast or any other type of cancer, definite or atypical connective tissue disease, adverse offspring effects, or neurologic disease." A subsequent study by Lipworth et al. in 2011 showed no association with silicone breast implants and connective tissue disease. A separate meta-analysis of 17 studies representing 7 cohorts in 2015 showed no association between breast implants and risk of breast cancer (Noels, 2015). There is, however, a rare but reported primary breast anaplastic large cell lymphoma (ALCL) seen in patients with implants. This rare lymphoma is a disease of the fibrous capsule surrounding the implant and not of the breast tissue around the implant.

The FDA reapproved and lifted the moratorium on silicone breast implants for both augmentation and reconstruction after extensive study and analysis in 2006. In a document issued by the FDA (http://www.fda.gov/medicaldevices/deviceregulationandgui dance/guidancedocuments/ucm071228.htm), breast implant types, testing, and recommending the development of Core Study Clinical Data Groups to review patient cohorts of different breast implant types from manufacturers were described. The FDA recommended studying cohorts of patients separated into indications for primary augmentation, primary reconstruction, revision augmentation, and revision reconstruction at entry to review data of 10 years or more of prospective follow-up (this could include data with premarket and postmarket approval follow-up). On the FDA website (accessed February 2015), routine MRI evaluations in all patients at 1, 2, 4, 6, 8, and 10 years were recommended to monitor patients for silent rupture for the Core Studies for silicone breast implants. Many of the studies on breast implant complications and rupture now arise from FDA-recommended Core Study data.

Implant Types

There are several types of implants available in United States, in terms of material type, shape, surface texturing, and the number of chambers (Table 9.1; Box 9.1). The most common breast implants are single-lumen silicone implants. Silicone implants are composed of a silicone elastomer shell filled with silicone made from a synthetic polymer of cross-linked chains of dimethyl siloxane, which makes the implant soft and movable. The inner silicone can be a gel, a liquid, or a solid form (Fig. 9.1). The outer envelope can be textured (polyurethane coated) or smooth (uncoated; Fig. 9.2). Textured silicone implants are now comprised of first-generation through fifth-generation types (Table 9.2). The newer generations of silicone implants are more stable and have had a very small rupture rate.

Saline implants are composed of an outer silicone shell and an inner envelope filled with saline. Double- or triple-lumen implants have two or more envelopes inside one another, and each can contain saline or silicone gel. A common double-lumen implant is the saline outer, silicone inner implant. More recent common double-lumen implants have silicone outer and saline inner components.

Less common implants include those filled with a polyvinyl alcohol sponge or a lipid substance (Trilucent implant), the latter of which may show a serous/lipid level on MRI if ruptured. Stacked implants are two single-lumen implants placed one on top of the other in the breast for aesthetic purposes. An implant type that is no longer used was covered with a finely textured meshlike surface over the outer envelope that was composed of a polyurethane-coated material to prevent fibrous capsular formation. This implant was banned because of the release of 2,4-toluenediamine, a by-product suspected to cause cancer in laboratory animals.

TABLE 9.1 Variation of Implants

Category	Types
Fill	Saline, silicone, miscellaneous (polyvinyl alcohol sponge, lipid, etc.)
Shape	Round, anatomic
Surface	Smooth, texture
Chamber	Single-lumen, multilumen

BOX 9.1 Examples of Implant Types

Single-lumen silicone
Single-lumen saline
Double-lumen: saline outer, silicone inner
Single-lumen silicone, outer polyurethane mesh coating
Single-lumen, lipid-filled
Complex or custom implants
Stacked implants
Direct silicone or paraffin injections

All implants are placed behind the breast tissue, and some implants are placed behind the pectoralis muscle (Fig. 9.3).

MAMMOGRAPHY AND IMPLANTS

Mammographic Limited-Compression Views and Implant-Displaced Views

An implant is not as compressible as breast tissue and can be ruptured if compressed too hard during either mammography (in breast imaging) or during closed capsulotomy (by the surgeon's fingers). Because limited mammographic compression decreases visualization of cancers, the Mammography Quality Standards Act recommends two specific views of each implanted breast (Box 9.2): one to look at the implant and one to look at the breast tissues for cancer. These two views include one limited-compression view that includes the implant and the tissue around it but does not use much compression (to not rupture the implant), and two implant-displaced views in which the technologist carefully strongly compresses only the breast tissue in front of the implant by carefully displacing the implant out of the field of view (Figs. 9.4 and 9.5). The limited-compression mammogram in which the implant

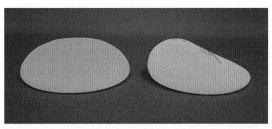

FIG. 9.1 Shapes of implants: round versus anatomic. Lateral view of silicone implants. The left implant is round shaped, and the right implant is anatomic shaped. Anatomic-shaped implants provide a more natural shape that resembles a breast.

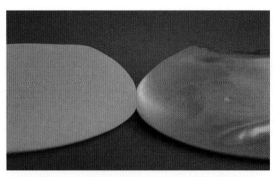

FIG. 9.2 Surfaces of implants: texture versus smooth. Lateral view of silicone implants. Polyurethane-coated outer envelope makes a textured gray-white surface (*left*), and the uncoated envelope is smooth (*right*).

TABLE 9.2 Generational Differences of Textured Silicone Implants

Generation	Years	Shell Thickness (mm)	Gel	Internal Barrier Lining	Shaped
First	1963–1972	0.75	Thick	No	No
Second	1972–1980	0.13	Thin	No	No
Third	1981 onward	0.28–0.30	Thick	Yes	No
Fourth	1993 onward	0.5	More cohesive, form stable	Yes	No
Fifth	1993 onward	0.075–0.75	Highly cohesive, form stable	Yes	Yes

From Derby BM, Codner MA: Textured silicone breast implant use in primary augmentation: core data update and review, *Plast Reconstr Surg* 135:113–124, 2015.

is surrounded by noncompressed breast tissue looks at both the breast tissue and the implant integrity. The second view, the strongly compressed tissue implant-displaced view, looks specifically at the breast tissue for cancer. However, even with the implant-displaced views, the radiologist sees only about 80% of the breast tissue because some breast tissue will always be hidden by the implant.

Normal Implants on Mammography

A normal silicone implant is quite dense and completely opaque and obscures and displaces much of the surrounding breast tissue. On mammography the silicone implant appears as a smooth, white oval opacity near the chest wall (Fig. 9.4A). Unlike opaque silicone implants, saline implants contain radiolucent saline surrounded by a dense silicone outer envelope (Fig. 9.5A). Wrinkles on saline implants are easily detected, unlike on opaque silicone implants, which are completely white (Fig. 9.5A). Wrinkles are normal findings that are accentuated by mammography because the implant envelope is easily folded when compressed (Fig. 9.6). Another common type of implant is the saline outer, silicone inner double-lumen implant, which appears as an opaque opacity (inner silicone implant) surrounded by lucent opacity (outer saline lumen implant; Fig. 9.7).

Breast implants are always placed behind the breast tissue for augmentation. If the implant is behind the glandular tissue and on top of the pectoralis muscle, it is in the subglandular position. If the implant is behind the glandular tissue and behind the pectoralis muscle, it is in the subpectoral position (see Fig. 9.3). When an implant is in the subglandular position, the shadow of the pectoralis muscle is underneath the implant on the mediolateral oblique view (Fig. 9.8A). In contrast, the pectoralis muscle curves over the implant for implants placed in the subpectoral position (Fig. 9.8B).

The body generally forms a fibrous capsule around the implant, no matter what type of implant. The fibrous capsule is usually soft, nonpalpable, and undetectable to physical examination, but with time, the capsule may harden or calcify. On mammography, the fibrous capsule surrounding implants is not usually visible unless it calcifies. A calcified fibrous capsule contains dystrophic sheetlike calcifications and appears white, thin, and bumpy next to the implant on the nonimplant-displaced views (Fig. 9.9). Another specific type of capsular calcification that can be mistaken for cancer and will sometimes prompt biopsy is from calcifying polyurethane-covered implants. These implants are covered with a spongelike material, and when they calcify they produce a typical fine mesh-like calcification (Fig. 9.10). Implant-displaced views displace the capsular calcifications away from the implant. These views, with or without spot magnification, help analyze calcifications if the concern is that the calcifications are in the breast parenchyma rather than in the implant capsule.

Mammographic Findings after Implant Removal

As many as 20% of women who receive breast implants for augmentation have their implants removed (with or without replacement) within 8 to 10 years for some reason, such as implant rupture, cosmetic issue, or other complications. When surgeons remove the implants, they often leave the fibrous capsules in the breasts, which may be seen on subsequent imaging studies. Typically, the postremoval implant cavity is on the chest wall. The post removal mammogram may or may not show the implant cavity at all. The cavity may resolve completely, or may scar and cause architectural distortion, or may fill with fluid and look like a mass (Fig. 9.11). If the fibrous capsule had calcified and is retained in the breast, the mammogram may show dystrophic calcifications that reside in the fibrous capsule. These calcifications typically appear in a sheetlike curvilinear pattern at the chest wall (Fig. 9.12), but occasionally can show a nonspecific pattern, which can be hard to distinguish from cancer and can prompt biopsy (Fig. 9.13). If the retained implant envelope has calcifying polyurethane, the resulting meshlike calcification can mimic ductal carcinoma in situ (DCIS; Fig. 9.14). In women with a history of the removal of an extracapsular ruptured implant, some extravasated silicone may be left in the breast, because it is difficult to remove all the silicone gel without removing much of the breast.

Screening for Breast Cancer in Women with Implants

When evaluating breast tissue for cancer in women with implants, it is important to inspect both the implant-displaced views and the breast tissue adjacent to the implant on the nonimplant-displaced limited-compression standard views. Breast tissue and breast cancers are basically visualized better with the implant-displaced views compared with the limited-compression views that include the implant (Fig. 9.15). The implant-displaced technique does optimize the amount of breast tissue displayed on the mammogram, but even with the implant-displaced views, only about 80% of the breast tissue can be seen. The standard views with limited compression may display a mass near the implant or the fibrous capsule not evident on implant-displaced views, because masses on the fibrous capsule can be pushed away from the field of view with the implant-displaced views (Fig. e9.1). Spot compression, other fine-detail views, or tomosynthesis may be useful for evaluating masses or suspicious calcifications in women with implants (Fig. 9.16). Needle localization, ultrasound-guided core biopsy, and stereotactic core biopsy all can be performed in

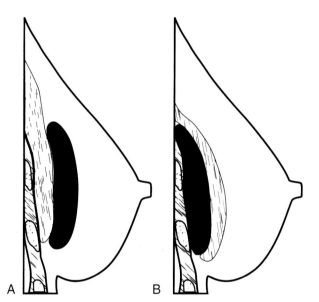

FIG. 9.3 Schematic of implant placement: subglandular versus subpectoral. (A) Subglandular implant placement in which the implant is placed on top of the pectoralis muscle. (B) Subpectoral implant placement in which the implant is placed underneath the pectoralis muscle, which curves over the implant.

BOX 9.2   Mammography of Implants

Four views of each breast:
    CC and ML or MLO with the implant
    CC and ML or MLO implant-displaced views
Magnification, spot, and other fine-detail views can be performed
    in the implanted breast
5% of screenings show asymptomatic rupture

CC, craniocaudal; *ML,* mediolateral; *MLO,* mediolateral oblique.

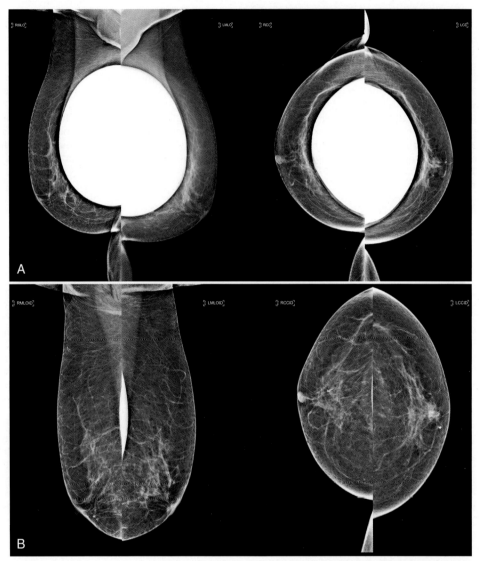

FIG. 9.4 Standard and implant-displaced mammograms of breasts with normal silicone implants. (A) Standard mediolateral oblique (MLO; *left*) craniocaudal (CC; *right*) mammograms obtained under limited compression show subpectoral silicone implants. Silicone implants are depicted as completely opaque white oval structures near the chest wall. Note the pectoralis muscle curving over the implant on the MLO view in A. The technologist uses very little compression to avoid rupturing the implant, but it is hard to find breast cancer in uncompressed breast tissue. (B) Implant-displaced MLO (*left*) and CC (*right*) mammograms show well-compressed breast tissue anterior to the implant. Note that the breast tissue is spread apart on the implant-displaced views, making it easier to find early cancer. However, even with the best implant-displaced views, the radiologist can see at most only 80% of the breast tissue, because the implant obscures the rest of the tissue.

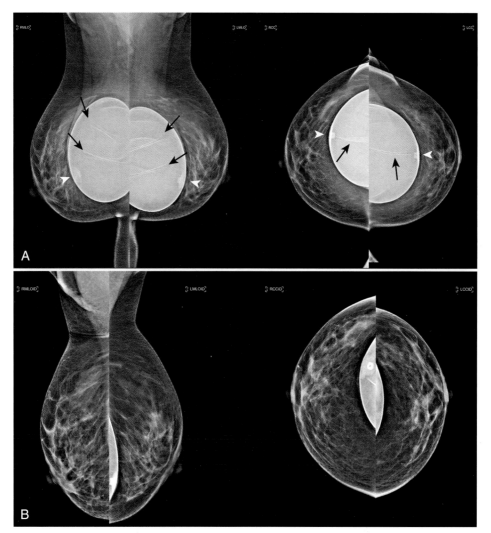

FIG. 9.5 Standard and implant-displaced mammograms of breasts with normal saline implants. (A) Standard mediolateral oblique (MLO; *left*) and craniocaudal (CC; *right*) mammograms obtained under limited compression show subpectoral saline implants. The lucent saline implants are surrounded by an envelope made out of stretchy silicone. Note the implant envelope wrinkles (*arrows*) and the injection ports in which the surgeon adds saline to increase or decrease the implant size at the time of surgery (*arrowheads*). (B) Implant-displaced MLO (*left*) and CC (right) mammograms show well-compressed breast tissue anterior to the implant. In this case the technologist included a tiny bit of the anterior aspect of the implant but did not rupture it on the mammogram.

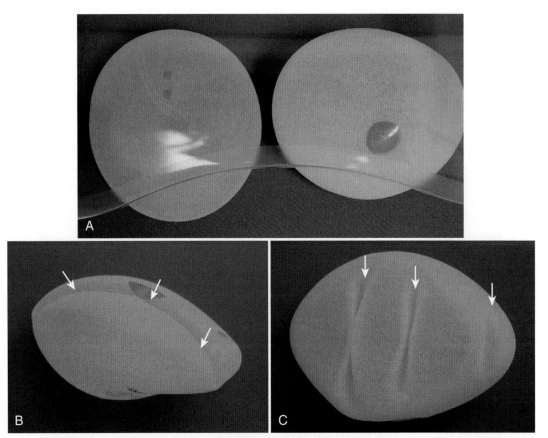

FIG. 9.6 Wrinkles in compressed implants. (A) Silicone implant (*left*) and a saline implant (*right*) are compressed from the top by a clear plastic board. Implants have no wrinkles. (B and C) The same silicone implant (B) and the same saline implant (C) as those used in A are compressed from the sides and now show wrinkles (*arrows*) in the implant envelope. This experiment indicates mammography can generate and enhance temporal implant envelope wrinkles, because implants are deformable and are compressed from the sides at the time of mammography.

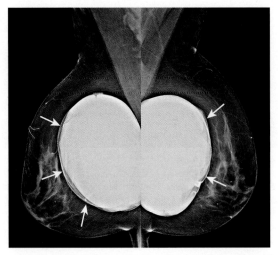

FIG. 9.7 Saline outer, silicone inner double-lumen subglandular implants. Bilateral mediolateral oblique mammograms show the outer envelope containing lucent saline in the outer lumen (*arrows*) surrounding the inner silicone lumen shown as the oval opaque opacity.

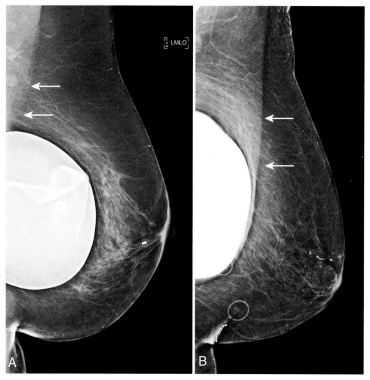

FIG. 9.8 Implant positions on mammography: subglandular versus subpectoral placement. (A) Mediolateral oblique (MLO) mammogram shows a subglandular saline implant. The pectoralis muscle (*arrows*) lies underneath the implant, which has a wrinkle and injection port visible. (B) In another patient, an MLO mammogram shows a subpectoral silicone implant. The pectoralis muscle (*arrows*) curves over the implant. In the lower breast there is a circle marker around a normal skin mole. (See the schematic in Fig. 9.3.)

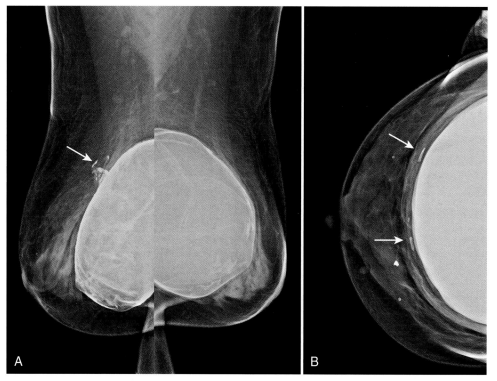

FIG. 9.9 Examples with calcifications in the implant fibrous capsule. (A) Bilateral mediolateral oblique mammograms show a thin rim of dystrophic calcifications that outline the bilateral saline implants and a nodular dystrophic calcification (*arrow*) around the right implant. They represent calcifications in the fibrous capsules that develop around breast implants. (B) In another patient, a craniocaudal mammogram shows thin, dense linear calcifications in the fibrous capsule surrounding a silicone implant.

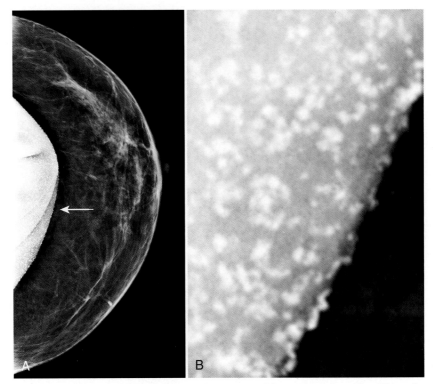

FIG. 9.10 Calcifications of the implant envelope. Left craniocaudal mammogram (A) and its photographically magnified view (B) show multiple tiny calcifications formed on the polyurethane-coated outer envelope of an intact subglandular saline implant (*arrow*).

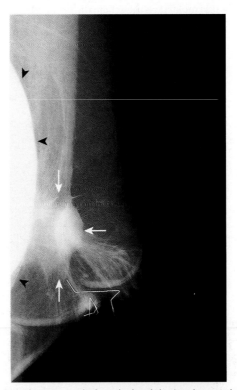

FIG. 9.11 Removed-implant cavity. After removal of a subglandular implant and placement of a new subpectoral implant (*arrowheads*), this patient has a characteristic "removed-implant cavity" (*arrows*) in the breast tissue. The removed subglandular implant cavity on top of the pectoralis muscle has now filled with fluid producing a small, smooth oval mass in the prior implant site. Note the metallic linear scar markers showing the scars in the lower part of the breast, with skin distortion and deformity from surgery.

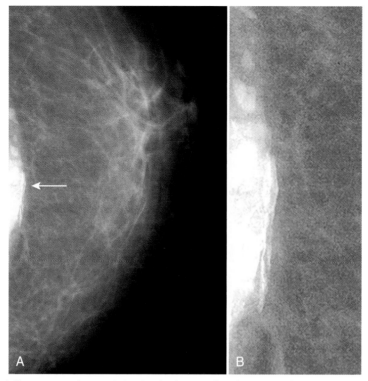

FIG. 9.12 Calcified fibrous capsule remaining in the breast after the removal of an implant. This patient's implants were removed but the fibrous capsule that formed around the implant was left in the breast near the chest wall after surgery (*arrow*). Left craniocaudal mammogram (A) and its photographically magnified view (B) show the typical sheetlike dystrophic calcification forming in the fibrous capsule that originally surrounded the implant.

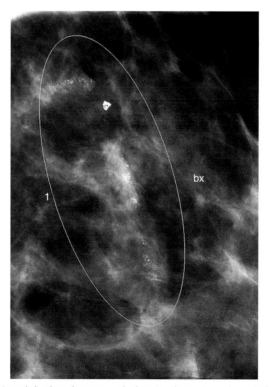

FIG. 9.13 Capsular calcifications left after the removal of an implant. Capsular calcifications in a line mimic ductal carcinoma in situ. Biopsy showed dystrophic calcifications in the retained fibrous capsule after the implant removal.

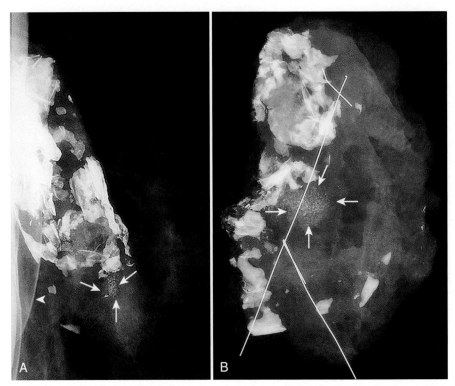

FIG. 9.14 Calcifying mesh of the polyurethane-coated outer envelope left after the implant removal. (A) Implant-displaced mediolateral oblique mammogram shows the second subpectoral saline implant (*arrowhead*) and dystrophic sheetlike calcifications from retained fibrous capsule of the previously removed first subglandular polyurethane-covered implant. Notice grouped microcalcifications (*arrows*), mimicking ductal carcinoma in situ, located near the dystrophic calcifications. (B) Specimen radiography shows a preoperative localization wire tip near the tiny meshlike microcalcifications (*arrows*) near the dystrophic implant capsule that were removed by surgery. These microcalcifications represented the calcifying mesh of the outer polyurethane coating.

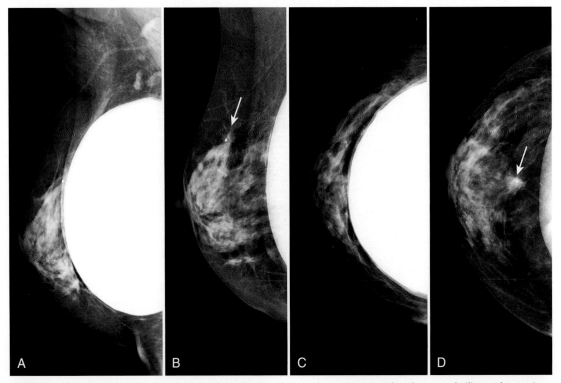

FIG. 9.15 Breast cancer visualized on implant-displaced views in a patient with subpectoral silicone breast implants. Mediolateral oblique mammograms of limited-compression view (A) and implant-displaced view (B) and craniocaudal mammograms of limited-compression view (C) and implant-displaced view (D) show invasive breast cancer in the upper middle right breast (*arrows*), which is visualized only on implant-displaced views (B and D). Note the biopsy marker within the tumor.

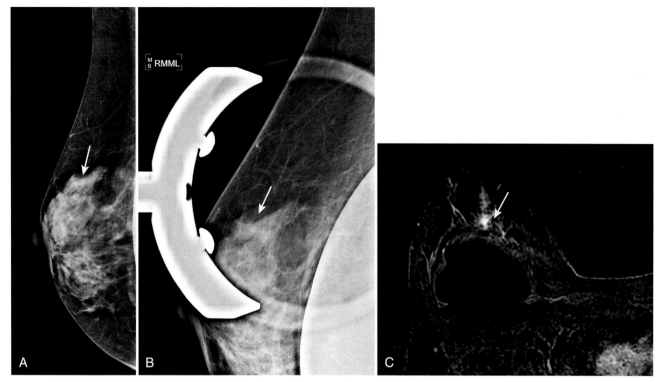

FIG. 9.16 Spot view for suspicious density in a patient with an implant. Implant-displaced mediolateral oblique mammogram (A) shows a suspicious density (*arrow*) with architectural distortion in the right upper breast. Spot compression magnification (B) was successfully applied in the lateral view showing a suspicious lesion (*arrow*), visualized more clearly than A. Fat-suppressed contrast-enhanced T1-weighted magnetic resonance image (C) shows an enhancing mass (*arrow*) at the corresponding location. Final diagnosis was invasive ductal cancer.

women with implants as well. The radiologist just has to obtain informed consent, which includes implant rupture as a possible complication for percutaneous biopsies.

Both physical examination and breast ultrasound as an adjunct to mammography are also helpful in evaluating mammographically detected breast masses or palpable findings, because mammography is limited with implants in place. Ultrasound can be especially helpful in determining whether a true mass exists, because it can evaluate the entire breadth of the breast tissue down to the implant (Fig. 9.17). Ultrasound is also helpful to distinguish breast masses from the snowstorm appearance of silicone granulomas caused by ruptured implants.

IMPLANT COMPLICATIONS

Complications associated with silicone gel-filled breast implants include contracture of the fibrous capsule, calcification of the fibrous capsule, implant rippling, seroma, malposition, hematoma, infection, breast pain, implant rupture, and silicone gel "bleed" (Box 9.3). Breast implant-associated ALCL is a recently described rare clinicopathologic entity that could be associated with implants.

Capsular Contraction

Implants can undergo capsular contraction, becoming hard and resistant, leading to a round, hard implant appearance and feel. It is the most common implant complication, with a reported incidence of more than 70% in some older series and only about a 20% incidence in more recent series. The hardened capsule may be due in part to *Staphylococcus epidermidis* from the breast ducts causing a subclinical implant infection, among other causes (Derby, 2015). The classic Baker Classification is used clinically to describe increasing levels of capsular formation, contracture,

and hardening of breast implants on physical inspection and examination (Table 9.3). The highest incidence of capsular contracture occurs if a breast implant is in a subglandular location and the lowest incidence of capsular contracture is associated with use of a textured implant in a submuscular location (Wazir et al., 2015). Open surgical capsulotomy, in which the hardened implant capsule is removed, was used to solve the problem of capsular contracture. Alternatively, surgeons would squeeze the implant to break the hardened fibrous capsule to allow the implant to become soft and pliable again. This is called a *closed capsulotomy* and, unfortunately, could result in implant rupture.

Different types of fillers for implants were examined in trials, resulting in varying rates of fibrous capsule contracture. Munker et al. (2001) reported on Trilucent implants in 27 patients who elected to exchange their implants for a fourth-generation cohesive silicone implant. Of these 27 patients, 14 had a change in the volume of their implants but not all were aware of the change, and capsular contracture was not present (Baker grade II; see Table 9.3); 55% of the implants had thickening or color changes caused by peroxidation of the triglyceride contents, and the implant capsule was adherent to breast tissues—in particular, the pectoralis muscle—which led to prolonged operative times. Rizkalla et al. (2001) reported similar results, with a reoperation rate of 20% (10/50) and an implant deflation rate of 10% (5/50). The Medical Devices Agency in the United Kingdom (which merged with the Medicines Control Agency in April 2003 to form the Medicines and Healthcare Products Regulatory Agency) withdrew the Trilucent implant from the market in March 1999, with a subsequent recommendation in June 2000 that the implants be removed from patients.

A new type of alloplastic material for implants that contains carboxymethylcellulose, called Hydrogel, was introduced into the European market. Of 12 patients with 20 implants placed

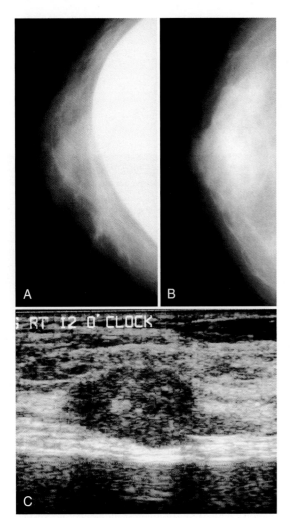

FIG. 9.17 The usefulness of ultrasonography to find a mass in a woman with implants. Limited-compression standard mammogram (A) shows that the dense silicone implant near the chest wall obscures most of the breast tissue in this patient with a palpable mass at the 12 o'clock position of the right breast. On implant-displaced mammogram (B), even when the implant is displaced, not all the breast tissue can be seen and the palpable mass is displaced with the implant out of the field of view. At the 12 o'clock position of the right breast, ultrasound (C) shows a suspicious irregular mass containing calcification on the fibrous capsule of the implant, which is not seen on the mammogram because it was pushed away from the field of view on the implant-displaced compressed images. Biopsy revealed invasive ductal cancer.

BOX 9.3   Untoward Effects of Breast Implants

Contraction of the fibrous capsule
Calcification of the fibrous capsule
Seroma around the implant
Hematoma
Rupture
Silicone gel "bleed"
Infection
Implant displacement, malposition, or extrusion
Breast pain
Breast feeding difficulties
Breast implant-associated anaplastic large cell lymphoma

TABLE 9.3   Baker Classification for Capsular Contraction

Grade	Breast Firmness	Implant	Implant Visibility
I	Soft	Nonpalpable	Nonvisible
II	Minimal	Palpable	Nonvisible
III	Moderate	Easily palpable	Distortion visible
IV	Severe	Hard, tender, cold	Distortion may be marked

From Baker JL Jr: Augmentation mammaplasty. In Owsley JQ Jr, Peterson RA, editors: *Symposium on aesthetic surgery of the breast*, St. Louis, 1978, CV Mosby.

between 1996 and 1997, as reported by Cicchetti et al. (2002), none showed immediate complications and had Baker grade I or II capsular contracture at 3.5 years of follow-up.

Implant Rupture

Silicone breast implant ruptures were attributed or associated with subpectoral location and older implant age, especially implants manufactured in the late 1970s and early 1980s (ie, second-generation implants). The older generation implant models (first, second, or third generation) have not been manufactured for many decades; many of the initial implant rupture reports from the 1990s were of these older implants. Newer generation silicone implants (fourth and fifth generation) have very small rupture rates in primary breast augmentation patients (Bengston, 2012) with 2.0% to 3.8% 6-year rupture rates for fifth-generation implants (Wazir, 2015). However, the actual rupture rate calculations can be complex, because a study of a single manufacturer's breast implant Core Study showed a 9.0% to 12.2% single time point rupture rate (Handel, 2013). A great controversy arose in 2012 when the Poly Implant Prothèse (PIP) silicone implant, marketed in Europe, was found to contain nonmedical industrial grade silicone and had a high reported rupture rate of 16.6% at 5 to 6 years and 24% to 30% at 10 years (Wazir, 2015). The overall average calculated rupture rate of 14.4% for PIP implants (Wazir, 2015) is high compared with a 7.7% 10-year Natrelle implant rupture rate (Spear, 2014, Core Clinical Study Group). Most of the PIP implants were placed in Europe and not in the United States. Closed capsulotomy, or manual breaking of the fibrous capsule, is also associated with implant rupture, as previously mentioned.

When silicone breast implants rupture, silicone gel, which consists of thick and sticky synthetic polymers, does not get absorbed and stays within the breast tissue. In contradistinction, when a saline implant ruptures, the saline diffuses into the breast tissue and the envelope shrinks back against the chest wall. Because saline is a mixture of salt and water, the saline is absorbed into the body with no major complications. The deflation of the saline breast implant is usually noticeable to the patient because her breast becomes noticeably smaller.

On the other hand, when a silicone gel breast implant envelope ruptures, the implant may retain much of its shape and volume if the fibrous capsule is intact and continues to contain the free silicone. Thus silicone implant rupture can be silent clinically, symptomatic, and without noticeable reduction in breast size. Silicone implant integrity is classified as intact, intact with gel bleed, intracapsular rupture, or extracapsular rupture (Table 9.4; Fig. 9.18). *Extracapsular rupture* is defined as implant rupture with silicone gel extruded outside a broken fibrous capsule. *Intracapsular rupture* is defined as rupture of the implant envelope, and the surrounding fibrous capsule is intact. Silicone gel extrudes though a broken implant envelope, but is still contained within an intact fibrous capsule surrounding the implant. *Gel bleed* is defined as silicone gel leakage through an intact implant envelope, although the existence of gel bleed versus small, undetected ruptures remains controversial.

TABLE 9.4   Implant Rupture Types for Silicon implant

Rupture Types	Silicone Location	Envelope Status
Intracapsular rupture	Fibrous capsule contains silicone gel	Envelope ruptured
Extracapsular rupture	Silicone gel outside fibrous capsule	Envelope ruptured
Gel bleed (controversial)	Silicone outside envelope	Envelope intact

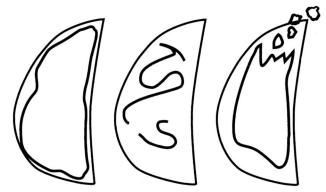

FIG. 9.18 Schematic of implant rupture. On the left, a fibrous capsule forms around an intact implant. In the middle, the implant shell may rupture, but the silicone is contained in the fibrous capsule (intracapsular rupture). On the right, the implant capsule and the fibrous capsule are ruptured, with silicone outside the fibrous capsule (extracapsular rupture).

A clinical diagnosis of silicone implant rupture is often difficult to make. Feng and Amini (1991) reported significant risk factors for silicone implant rupture as older implants age (this was a report of first-, second-, or third-generation implant series): retroglandular location, capsular contracture, local symptoms, implant type (they describe that double-lumen and polyurethane-covered implants rupture less frequently than smooth gel implants), and manufacturer. The clinical history, signs, and symptoms are frequently nonspecific for implant rupture. Rosculet (1992) reported that of 19 symptomatic patients with ruptured implants, women complained of palpable axillary, breast, or chest wall masses; pain; or changes in the size, shape, or texture of the breast. In one surgical series, 3 of the 32 patients reviewed were asymptomatic. Because physical examination misses approximately 50% of ruptures, clinicians turned to imaging to help diagnose ruptured implants when the clinical findings were questionable.

Thus imaging assessment plays a main role in the detection of implant ruptures, particularly ruptured silicone implants. Details will be discussed later (see section: Imaging Evaluation of Implant Rupture).

Breast Implant-Associated Anaplastic Large Cell Lymphoma

Primary breast ALCL is an extremely rare lymphoma reported in patients with implants. It is a disease of the fibrous capsule surrounding the implant and not of the breast tissue around the implant. In the few clinical reports in the literature, the patient's clinical presentation is usually an effusion around the implant, and rarely there is a solid mass present. Miranda et al. (2014) reported on 60 patients with ALCL of whom 42 (70%) presented with an effusion versus 18 (30%) who presented with a mass, with a wide 1- to 32-year time interval between surgery and lymphoma diagnosis (reported median time interval 9 years and mean of 10.9

years). Miranda et al. (2014) and Adrada et al. (2014) both showed that patients who presented with a mass had a worse prognosis than patients who presented with an effusion. Also, Adrada et al. (2014) reported imaging study performance in the detection of an effusion or a mass related to ALCL in 44 patients. The sensitivity for detecting an effusion was 84, 55, 82, and 38% and for detecting a mass was 46, 50, 50, and 64%, by ultrasound, computed tomography, MRI, and positron emission tomography, respectively. The sensitivity of mammography in the detection of an abnormality without distinction of effusion or mass was 73%, and specificity 50%. Ultrasound and MRI seem most sensitive for detecting effusions around breast implants. Adrada et al. (2014) went on to state that nonspecific effusions around implants are common in the postoperative period and that delayed seromas beyond 1 year after implant placement are much less common (estimated at less than 1%). They suggested that if there is a delayed effusion or concern for ALCL with delayed seroma, cytology can be considered. Of the 44 patients in their series, 21 (48%) patients had an effusion only, 12 (27%) had both an effusion and a mass, and eight (18%) had a mass only. Cytology was done in 24 patients with effusions (with or without a mass) and was positive in 19 (78%).

Currently, available data are limited in terms of the imaging features and the diagnostic strategy of implant-associated ALCL. Awareness of this disease and better understanding of the spectrum of imaging findings may improve the detection and the proper management of implant-associated ALCL in the future.

IMAGING EVALUATION OF IMPLANT RUPTURE

Mammography

A retrospective review of screening mammograms in 350 asymptomatic women with breast implants, including first-, second-, or third-generation implants, showed an incidence of asymptomatic silicone implant rupture of 5% (Destouet, 1992). Table 9.5 summarizes the imaging findings of ruptures of silicone implants, including intracapsular rupture, extracapsular rupture, and gel bleed.

A blob of silicon outside of the implant and beyond the fibrous capsule is a typical and specific finding of silicone implant rupture on mammogram, and is seen only when a woman develops an extracapsular rupture (Fig. 9.19). However, some women with extracapsular rupture may show only contour abnormality of the ruptured implant because the extruded silicone does not separate far enough from the bulk of the implant to be seen as a separate blob (Figs. 9.20 and 9.21). Thus extracapsular rupture may have no apparent abnormality on mammograms, and the diagnosis must be made by either ultrasound or MRI.

Silicone within axillary lymph nodes is a rare finding, but is highly suggestive of an extracapsular rupture (Fig. 9.22). This finding is observed when the silicone extravasates outside the fibrous capsule, enters the lymphatics, and is trapped in the lymph nodes.

Intracapsular rupture of a silicone implant is almost impossible to detect on mammography, because the silicone gel is still contained within an intact fibrous capsule. An implant with intracapsular rupture is often depicted as a normal-looking implant on mammography. Sometimes, a bulging contour suggests, but is not definitive of, intracapsular rupture, because a lobulated contour also can be seen in capsular contracture or herniation of an intact implant envelope through a break in the surrounding fibrous capsule (Table 9.6). When mammographic findings are equivocal, radiologists use ultrasound and MRI to make the diagnosis of a rupture.

After removal of an extracapsular ruptured implant, inevitably some extravasated silicone is left in the breast. This happens because it is sometimes impossible to remove all the silicone gel without removing much of the breast tissue, and the gel stays within the breast tissue without absorption (Fig. 9.23). If

TABLE 9.5   Imaging Findings with Rupture of Silicone Implant

Imaging Modality	Intracapsular	Extracapsular	Gel Bleed
Mammography	Not present	Silicone globs in breast tissue Silicone in lymph nodes Silicone in ducts Implant contour deformity (occasionally seen)	Occasionally seen
Ultrasound	Stepladder sign	Snowstorm or echodense noise Hypoechoic mass	Snowstorm or echodense noise
Magnetic resonance imaging	Linguine sign Teardrop/keyhole sign Subcapsular lines Water droplets (occasionally seen)	Silicone outside the envelope Signs of intracapsular rupture	Teardrop/keyhole sign Subcapsular lines

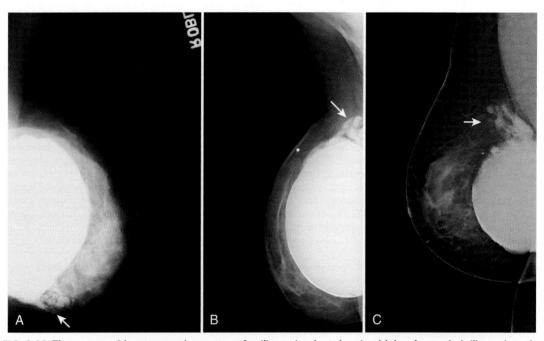

FIG. 9.19 Three cases with extracapsular rupture of a silicone implant showing blobs of extruded silicone into the breast tissue. (A) Mediolateral oblique (MLO) mammogram shows blobs of silicone (*arrow*) extruded into tissue inferior to the implant on an analog mammogram. (B) This patient felt a mass in her upper right breast, marked by a BB, corresponding to extruded silicone (*arrow*) above the implant on MLO view. (C) Right MLO view shows extruded silicone (*arrow*) above the implant. Incidentally, note capsular calcification in this patient.

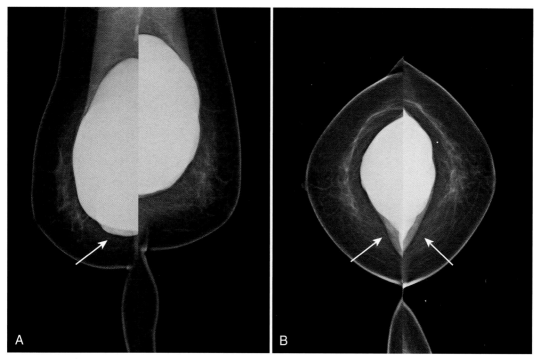

FIG. 9.20 Extracapsular rupture of silicone implant: abnormal contour. Mediolateral oblique (MLO; A) and craniocaudal (CC; B) mammograms show only contour abnormality of both implants, with the suggestion of extrusion of silicone in the lower right breast on the MLO view (A; *arrow*) and in the medial aspect of both CC mammograms (B; *arrows*). Bilateral extracapsular ruptures were confirmed by surgery. It is not easy to differentiate extracapsular rupture from normal implant or intracapsular rupture.

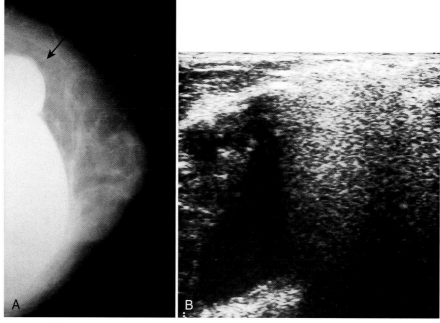

FIG. 9.21 Extracapsular rupture of silicone implant: abnormal contour. A craniocaudal mammogram (A) shows an unusual bulge (*arrow*) of the implant's outer contour that represents either rupture or a herniation of the implant through a tear in the fibrous capsule; surgery showed extracapsular rupture. Ultrasound (B) shows echodense noise or snowstorm sign over the bulge in A, confirming a rupture.

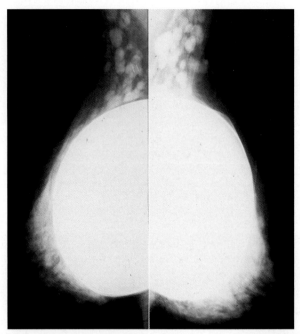

FIG. 9.22 Extracapsular rupture of silicone implant: silicone in axillary lymph nodes. Mediolateral oblique mammograms show retained silicone in bilateral axillary lymph nodes. The patient has a history of removal of ruptured silicone implants and replacement with new implants.

TABLE 9.6   False-Positive Imaging Findings for Rupture

Imaging Modality	Sign	Differential Diagnosis
Mammography	Implant contour deformity	Contained rupture Capsular contracture Herniation through a capsule tear
	Intraparenchymal silicone	Previous leak with the ruptured implant removed
Ultrasound	Stepladder sign	Intracapsular rupture Intact multilumen implant
Magnetic resonance imaging	Linguine sign Water droplets (occasionally seen)	Intracapsular rupture Intact multilumen implant

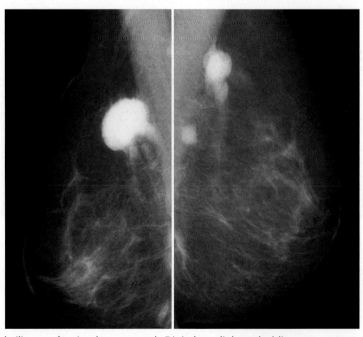

FIG. 9.23 Retained silicone after implant removal. Digital mediolateral oblique mammograms show retained silicone in the upper breasts after removal of ruptured bilateral silicone implants. Complete removal of all the extravasated silicone is sometimes difficult without removing some breast tissue.

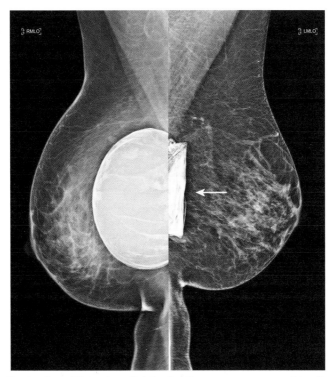

FIG. 9.24 Ruptured saline implant. Bilateral mediolateral oblique mammograms show that the saline implant in the left breast ruptured. Note the collapsed saline envelope at the chest wall (*arrow*).

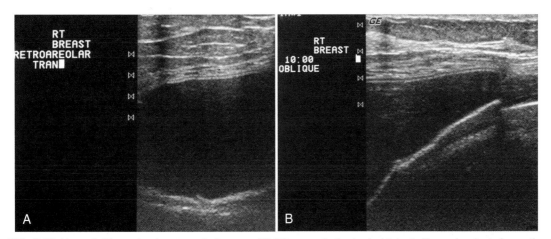

FIG. 9.25 Normal silicone implant: anechoic mass. (A) Ultrasound of a typical intact silicone implant shows the breast tissue in the near field and the oval hypoechoic implant near the chest wall. Note that the appearance of a normal silicone implant is almost anechoic and simulates a very, very large cyst. (B) Ultrasound of an intact silicone implant shows a typical normal edge artifact causing shadowing where the edge of the implant meets breast tissue.

a new silicone implant is placed later, the residual silicone from the old ruptured implant makes it impossible to tell on subsequent mammography if the new implant has ruptured.

Saline implants provide different imaging finding from those of silicone implants after rupture. Because the saline is absorbed into the body, mammography usually shows only a collapsed envelope at the chest wall when a saline breast implant ruptures (Fig. 9.24).

Ultrasound

Ultrasound is an adjunct to mammography in the diagnosis of ruptured breast implants. Ultrasound signs of rupture have varying sensitivities of 25% to 65% and specificities of 57% to 98%.

Ultrasound is less expensive than MRI and is more cost-effective than MRI in diagnosing ruptures.

On ultrasound, the normal single-lumen implant, either silicone or saline, appears as an anechoic mass with a smooth echogenic edge (Fig. 9.25), with or without *reverberation artifacts* and *radial folds.* Reverberation artifacts are multiple bands of noise caused by repeat reflections of the beam between the skin surface and the anterior wall of the implant. Reverberation artifacts are characteristically seen in the near field, parallel the anterior wall of implant, and have the same width as the breast tissue anterior to the implant (Fig. 9.26). Reverberation artifacts are easily distinguished from echodense noise observed in ruptures. The radial folds are infoldings of the intact envelope that look like white lines extending to the periphery of the envelope (see Fig. 9.26).

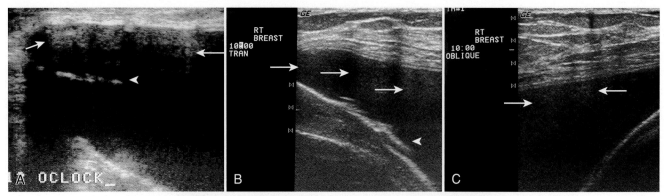

FIG. 9.26 Intact silicone implants: examples of reverberation artifacts and radial folds. (A) Ultrasound shows a normal anechoic implant with normal reverberation artifacts (*arrows*) in the near field of the implant that are as thick as the breast tissue above it; the bright line within the implant represents a normal radial fold (*arrowhead*) that extends to the periphery of the implant when scanned from multiple angles. (B) Reverberation artifact (*arrows*) is shown as gray speckles in the near field of a normal silicone implant with normal radial folds (*arrowhead*) on its inferior aspect. (C) Reverberation artifact (*arrows*) is seen in the near field of a normal silicone implant. Note that rupture produces a bright shadow that obscures all features of structures deep to the extruded silicone, whereas reverberation artifact occurs only in the near field and does not obscure deeper structures.

Extracapsular rupture of a silicone implant has the classic snowstorm sign or echodense noise, which is a characteristic echogenic finding caused by the slow velocity of sound in silicone with respect to the surrounding breast parenchyma (Fig. 9.27). Snowstorm, or echodense noise, looks like air in the bowel, has an intense echogenic appearance, and obscures all findings beneath it. It can be distinguished from edge artifact by scanning at different angles, because extruded silicone produces the echogenic snowstorm appearance when scanned from all angles, whereas edge artifact changes or disappears.

Another sign of extracapsular rupture is a hypoechoic mass corresponding to large globules of silicone extruded away from the implant (Fig. 9.28). In this situation, so much silicone is extruded that the silicone glob appears as a hypoechoic mass, similar to the intact implant. To ensure the correct diagnosis, the sonographer places a skin marker on the hypoechoic mass and repeats the mammogram to correlate the silicone on the radiograph with the ultrasound finding. Direct silicone or paraffin injections have an appearance similar to extracapsular rupture and are characterized by echodense noise. Usually there is so much artifact from the snowstorm with silicone/paraffin injections that the ultrasound is nondiagnostic.

Gel bleed is defined as silicone gel outside an intact implant envelope. Ultrasound shows gel bleed as snowstorm or echodense noise. By definition, gel bleed indicates extracapsular silicone surrounding an intact implant, but this definition is controversial because some investigators believe that there will always be a tiny rupture accompanying gel bleed. Given that ultrasound examinations demonstrating echodense noise can be caused by severe gel bleed, it is controversial whether the scan should be classified as a true-positive or false-positive examination. Patients with gel bleed usually have their implants removed because silicone is outside the implant and is in direct contact with breast tissue.

Intracapsular rupture means that the envelope is ruptured but the silicone is still inside an intact fibrous capsule. This means that there will be no snowstorm, unless silicone has leaked into the surrounding tissue (making it an extracapsular rupture). Intracapsular rupture produces a stepladder sign, which represents the collapsing ruptured implant shell within the intact fibrous capsule (Figs. 9.29 and 9.30). The stepladder sign is characterized by multiple thin echogenic lines within the implant that do not extend to the periphery of the implant and look like the steps of a stepladder. The thin lines represent echoes of the collapsing implant wall folding in on itself. The stepladder sign is seen with both intracapsular and extracapsular rupture.

Normal radial folds can simulate the stepladder sign. However, radial folds always extend to the implant periphery, whereas stepladder lines do not. False-positive stepladder signs are also caused by intact multilumen implants producing multiple linear echoes in the implant, similar to an intracapsular rupture (Fig. 9.31).

Diffuse linear echoes, debris, or diffuse low-level echoes within the implant may also indicate intracapsular rupture, but they are less definitive. In a small percentage of studies, the ultrasound is false-negative for rupture. In one series, Rietjens et al. (2014) showed that ultrasound had a negative predictive value (NPV) of 85%, and suggested that if the ultrasound is negative, MRI might be avoided, even though MRI generally has a higher overall accuracy, because of the high NPV of ultrasound.

Magnetic Resonance Imaging

When possible, silicone implant rupture should be evaluated by MRI, because it is most often silent and because MRI has a higher sensitivity in detecting rupture than other imaging methods. As noted in product information sheets of commercially available implants in the United States, routine MRI surveillance for silicone gel implants has been recommended at first 3 years postoperatively, then every 2 years, by the FDA for detecting silent rupture or leaks.

MRI distinguishes silicone gel from fat, water, glandular tissue, and any other tissues in the breast based on their unique MR relaxation properties using specific pulse sequences. At 1.5 t, silicone gel has a 100-Hz chemical shift from the aliphatic proton resonance of lipid and a 320-Hz chemical shift from the proton resonance of water, which makes it possible to separate silicone from water and fat. Various MRI techniques have been developed to acquire silicone-specific images that are mainly classified into the following two types: (1) T2-weighted fast spin-echo (FSE) technique with short tau inversion recovery (STIR) and with water-saturation (so-called "water-sat STIR") and (2) T2-weighted FSE technique with STIR (T2-STIR) and with phase-based separation of water and silicone. The first technique, water-sat STIR, uses a short T1 inversion recovery pulse sequence to suppress the fat component of the signal and a chemical shift presaturation pulse to eliminate the water component of the signal. This is a commercially available technique (Table 9.7). However, water-saturation used in this sequence is shim dependent, and thus may be associated with inhomogeneous water suppression. The second technique, T2-weighted FSE technique with STIR and with phase-based separation of water and silicone, also uses a short T1 inversion recovery pulse sequence to suppress the fat component of the signal, but it

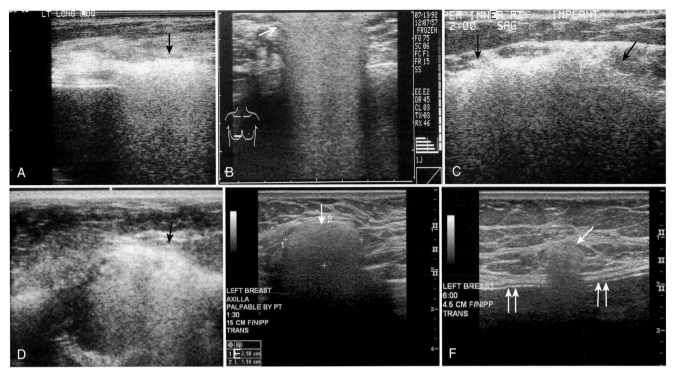

FIG. 9.27 Extracapsular rupture of silicone implants: examples of snowstorm sign. (A) Ultrasound shows echodense noise or snowstorm artifact (*arrow*), representing extracapsular silicone. Compare with normal implants and normal reverberation artifact in Fig. 9.26. Note that rupture produces a bright shadow that obscures all features of structures deep to the extruded silicone, whereas reverberation artifact occurs only in the near field and does not obscure deeper structures. (B) Ultrasound of extracapsular silicone shows the bright gray echodense noise or snowstorm artifact (*arrow*) that obscures the implant below. (C) In another patient with a large extracapsular rupture, the snowstorm (*arrows*) fills the image and obscures all adjacent structures, including the breast tissue and implant below. (D) The snowstorm appearance (*arrow*) on the right side almost obscures the implant below. (E) This silicone granuloma was palpable, forming a round mass that had the snowstorm appearance (*arrow*). (F) Another silicone granuloma (*arrow*) above the normal intact implant (*double arrows*).

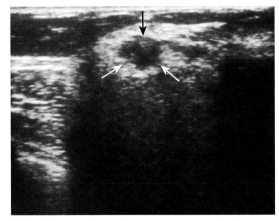

FIG. 9.28 Extracapsular rupture of silicone implant: hypoechoic mass. An extracapsular rupture in a patient who had a glob of silicone is producing a hypoechoic mass (*arrows*) in the breast tissue above the implant, but surrounded by echodense noise. The extruded glob of silicone was confirmed by placing a marker over the finding and obtaining a mammogram, which showed silicone. Note that the larger silicone glob produces a mass similar to the intact implant in the lower right corner of the image.

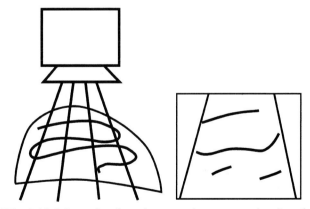

FIG. 9.29 Schematic of an intracapsular rupture showing the "stepladder sign." The transducer shows the collapsing implant envelope, which is producing multiple lines, or a stepladder sign, on ultrasound. This sign can be seen in an extracapsular rupture too, as long as there is a snowstorm or echodense noise sign accompanying the stepladder.

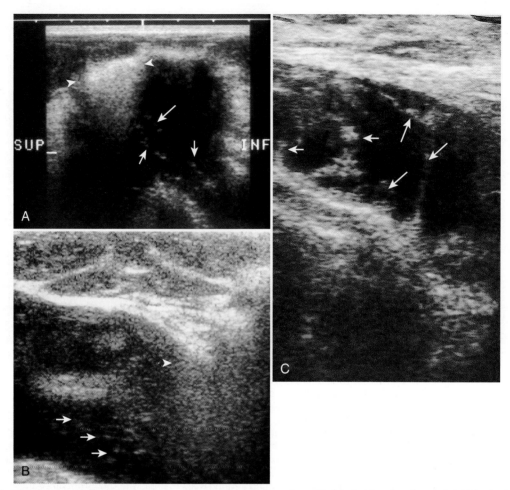

FIG. 9.30 Ruptured silicone implants: examples of stepladder sign. (A) Stepladder sign (*arrows*) within the inferior breast is shown as thin white lines within the implant on the right side of the image. There is a snowstorm sign on the left side of the image, representing extracapsular silicone (*arrowheads*). (B) Stepladder sign (*arrows*) and multiple tiny linear echoes in the implant in a patient with an extracapsular rupture and a snowstorm artifact on the right (*arrowhead*). (C) Stepladder sign (*arrows*) in intracapsular rupture consists of multiple thick and thin linear echoes in the implant that do not always extend to the periphery.

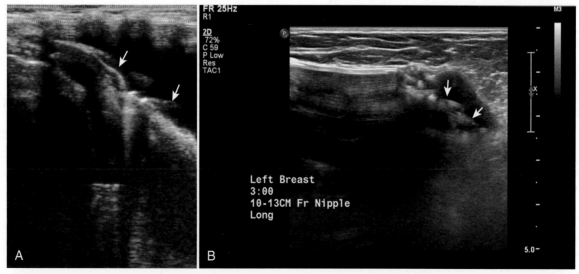

FIG. 9.31 Intact implants: examples of false-positive stepladder sign in multilumen implants. (A) Multilumen saline implant. (B) Saline outer, silicone inner double-lumen implant. Multiple lines (*arrows*) representing the multiple envelopes in intact multilumen implants mimic stepladder sign and could lead to a false-positive diagnosis of intracapsular rupture. It is critical to know the implant type before diagnosing implant rupture.

uses a phase-based approach to separate the silicone component of the signal from the water component. The phase-based methods are robust techniques to separate the silicone signal component and the water signal component and can generate several types of images, including silicone-specific images, water-specific images, and combined water and silicone images, from a single scan acquisition. There have been various phase-based methods developed, such as 2-point Dixon, FLEX, MEDAL, 3-point DIXON, and IDEAL. A disadvantage of phase-based approach is that images are artifacts from motion, aliasing, and metal clips.

An MRI protocol to evaluate silicone breast implants consists of T1-weighted imaging, T2-weighted (FSE) imaging, silicone-specific imaging, and optionally water-specific imaging (Box 9.4). Intravenous contrast (IV), which is essential for the

diagnosis of breast cancers, is unnecessary for the detection of implant rupture. However, IV contrast may be useful when evaluating for other implant-related conditions such as the rare implant-associated ALCL, implant-associated infections, and in patients with known or suspected breast cancer in a patient with implants. Table 9.8 summarizes the property of signal intensities of fat, water, and silicone gel on various MRI sequences, including silicone-specific images. Both silicone gel and water are high signals on T2-weighted images and combined silicone and water images, but signal suppression of either the silicone component or water component makes it possible to distinguish these components. The silicone gel filling an implant has a high intensity on silicone-specific images and a low signal intensity on water-specific images (Fig. 9.32). In contrast, MRI of a normal saline implant shows the intact implant envelope filled with water, which is a high signal on water-specific images but dark on silicone-specific images (Fig. 9.33).

Patients are scanned prone in a dedicated breast coil to diminish breathing artifacts from chest wall movement. The implant is usually scanned in the axial and sagittal/oblique planes to look at all implant contours and to see radial folds versus ruptured envelopes. Newer three-dimensional (3D) T2W1 techniques (CUBE, SPACE, etc.) are being developed that will allow reformatted images in any place from a single scan acquisition. MRI images of a normal single-lumen silicone implant show high signal from the silicone gel with a smooth oval implant border on silicone-specific images. Minor implant bulges or herniations and short and long radial folds are noted as incidental normal findings. Radial folds are dark lines that extend to the periphery of the implant and represent folds in the implant envelope (Figs. 9.34 and 9.35; Video 9.1). Reactive fluid around the implant and water droplets in a radial fold but topologically outside the envelope are classified as nonspecific findings but are noted in the report (Box 9.5), particularly if the findings are marked or implant infection is suspected.

Intracapsular rupture is characterized by the keyhole or teardrop sign, the subcapsular line, and the linguine sign (Fig. 9.36). The keyhole or inverted teardrop sign represents silicone outside the implant envelope within a short radial fold outside the implant envelope (Fig. 9.37; see the left breast in Video 9.2). A tip to differentiate between a normal radial fold and a keyhole sign is the signal intensity within the fold on silicone-specific images. On these images, a normal radial fold is totally black inside, whereas a teardrop sign is white inside because of the leaked silicone that intersperses between the implant envelope and the fibrous capsule (Figs. 9.34B and 9.36A). Note that the inside of a fold is topologically outside of the envelope. A subcapsular line is a dark

TABLE 9.7 Advantages and Disadvantages of Silicone-Specific Imaging Techniques

	Techniques	Advantages	Disadvantages
A	Water-sat T2-STIR	Commercially available	Shim dependent
B	T2-STIR with phase-based separation of water and silicone	Robust separation of water and silicone independent of shim Gives both water only and silicone only images, and combined water and silicone images from a single sequence	Artifacts from motion, aliasing, and clips

STIR; short tau inversion recovery.

BOX 9.4 Magnetic Resonance Imaging Techniques for Implants

T1-weighted imaging
T2-weighted fast spin-echo (optional; fat-suppression with short tau inversion recovery [STIR])
Silicone-specific T2-weighted imaging (water-sat T2-STIR or T2-STIR with phase-based[a] separation of water and silicone)
Optional; water-specific T2-weighted imaging (silicone-sat T2-STIR or T2-STIR with phase-based[a] separation of water and silicone)

[a]Phase-based technique includes 2-point Dixon, FLEX, MEDAL, 3-point Dixon, and IDEAL.

TABLE 9.8 Signal Intensity of Fat, Water, and Silicone on Magnetic Resonance Imaging Sequences

Basis	Suppression of Fat Signal	Suppression of Water or Silicone Signal	MRI Sequences	Signal Intensity on MRI		
				Fat	Water	Silicone Gel
T2	NA	NA	T2 FSE	High	High	High
	Inversion recovery		T2 FSE + STIR	Dark	High	High
		Saturation pulse	T2 FSE + STIR + Water-sat[a]	Dark	Dark	High[c]
			T2 FSE + STIR + silicone-sat	Dark	High	Dark
		PBS[b]	T2 FSE + STIR + PBS; water only	Dark	High	Dark
			T2 FSE + STIR + PBS; silicone only	Dark	Dark	High[c]
			T2 FSE + STIR + PBS; combined	Dark	High	High
T1	NA	NA	T1	High	Very low	Low

[a]Water-sat T2-STIR.
[b]T2-STIR with PBS of water and silicone.
[c]Silicone-specific image.
FSE, fast spin-echo; *MRI,* magnetic resonance imaging; *NA,* not applied; *PBS,* phase-based separation; *sat,* saturation; *STIR,* short tau inversion recovery.

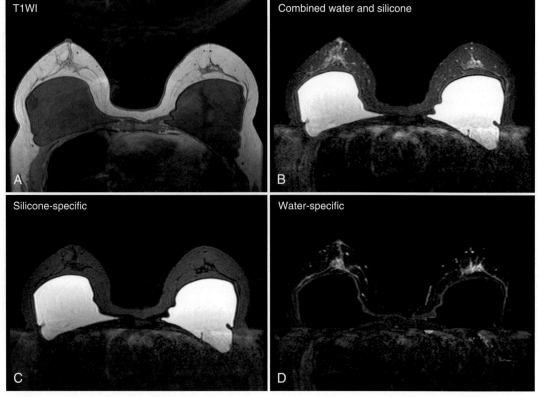

FIG. 9.32 Bilateral normal silicone implant on magnetic resonance image. (A) T1-weighted image. (B) Combined water and silicone image. (C) Silicone-specific image. (D) Water-specific image. Silicone gel appears in low intensity on T1-weighted image (A), high intensity on combined image (B), high intensity on silicone-specific image (C), and low intensity on water-specific image (D). High intensity on silicone-specific image (C) allows the selective identification of silicone.

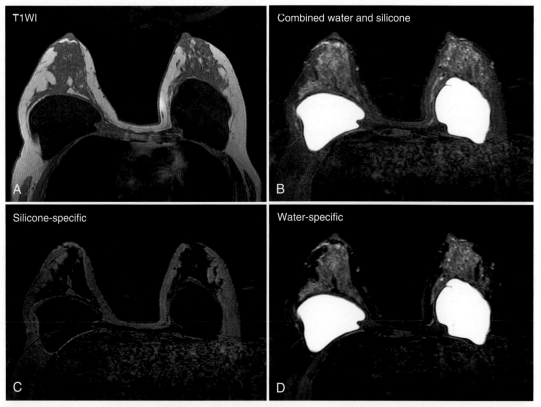

FIG. 9.33 Bilateral normal saline implants on magnetic resonance image (MRI). (A) T1-weighted image. (B) Combined water and silicone image. (C) Silicone-specific image. (D) Water-specific image. Water or saline appears in very low intensity on T1-weighted image (A), high intensity on combined image (B), low intensity on silicone-specific image (C), and high intensity on water-specific image (D). High intensity on water-specific image (D) is characteristic for saline implants. Note that the silicone-specific image (C) shows low intensity within the saline implants, contrasting with high intensity observed in silicone implants (Fig. 9.32C). Generally, MRI studies including silicone-specific imaging are not performed for the evaluation of saline implants, but in this case, they were performed because the patient had residual silicone droplets from a prior silicone implant rupture (images not shown).

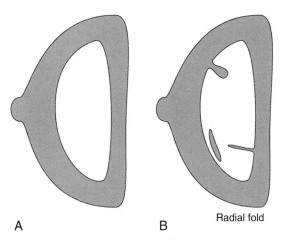

A   B   Radial fold

FIG. 9.34 Schematic of normal silicone implant. (A) No wrinkles. (B) Radial folds. An intact implant can fold on itself and produce dark lines called radial folds that extend to the periphery of the implant and are totally black inside on silicone-specific images.

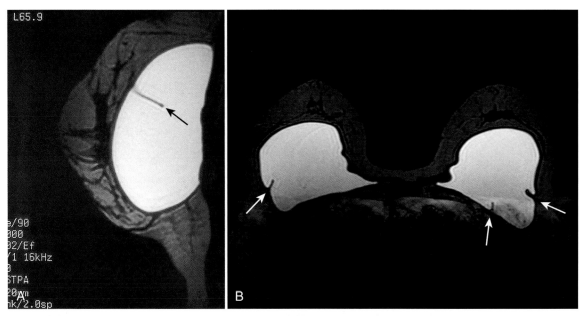

FIG. 9.35 Intact silicone implants: examples of radial fold. (A) Sagittal silicone-specific magnetic resonance image (MRI) shows a single radial fold (*arrow*). (B) Axial silicone-specific image shows multiple radial folds (*arrows*). Video 9.1 shows radial folds depicted as dark lines that extend to the periphery of the implant.

BOX 9.5 Nonspecific Findings on Magnetic Resonance Imaging

Water droplets
Reactive fluid around the implant
Bulges in contour
Radial folds (normal finding)

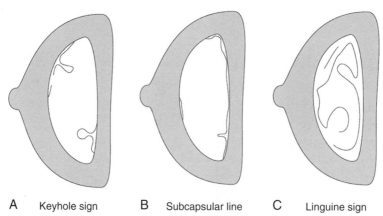

FIG. 9.36 Schematic of intracapsular rupture of silicone implant: keyhole sign, subcapsular line, and linguine sign. (A) Keyhole (or teardrop) sign. Silicone that intersperses between the collapsing envelope and the fibrous capsule produces a high-intensity center inside the fold on silicone-specific images called a keyhole or inverted teardrop. Compare the keyhole sign with a normal radial fold illustrated in Fig. 9.34B. (B) Subcapsular line. When the implant shell breaks, the shell pulls away from the fibrous capsule and produces the subcapsular line. The space between the subcapsular line and the capsule is a high signal on silicone-specific images. (C) Linguine sign. Later, when the entire shell collapses into the fibrous capsule, the linguine sign is produced, which looks like a loose thread.

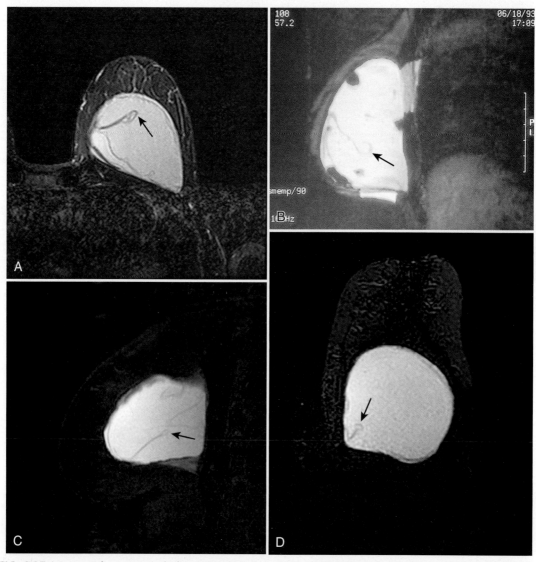

FIG. 9.37 Intracapsular rupture of silicone implants: examples of keyhole sign (teardrop sign). (A) Axial combined water and silicone magnetic resonance image (MRI) shows a keyhole sign (*arrow*) and subcapsular lines. (B) Sagittal silicone-specific MRI shows a keyhole sign (*arrow*), subcapsular lines, a linguine sign, and nonspecific water droplets. (C) Sagittal silicone-specific MRI shows a keyhole sign (*arrow*), subcapsular lines, and a linguine sign. (D) Axial silicone-specific MRI of left breast shows a keyhole sign (*arrow*) and a subcapsular line (see Video 9.2).

line that parallels the implant shell and cannot be traced to the periphery of the implant, representing incomplete shell collapse (Fig. 9.38). Silicone between the subcapsular line and the implant capsule is high on silicone-specific images and indicates intracapsular rupture. The linguine sign is the curvy noodle-shaped dark lines inside the implant that do not extend to the periphery, representing the collapsing ruptured implant shell within an intact fibrous capsule that contains the silicone gel (Fig. 9.39).

Silicone outside the fibrous capsule, within the breast parenchyma or axilla, represents extracapsular rupture (Fig. 9.40; see right breast in Video 9.2). Signs of intracapsular rupture will nearly always be present with the finding of extracapsular rupture. Severe gel bleed is diagnosed if a thin coating of silicone is identified around the periphery of the implant but the implant is intact.

Pitfalls in imaging interpretation that can result in misinterpreting intact implants as ruptured implants include the uncommon types of implant with multilumen structures or rare implant materials, poor positioning of breast at the time of MRI study, and a "redo" from a prior rupture (Box 9.6). Knowing the surgical history and implant type before imaging is crucial for accurate interpretation to prevent overdiagnosis of ruptures in cases with complex multilumen implants or stacked implants (Fig. 9.41). Proper positioning is necessary to obtain appropriate MR images, because wrong positioning produces artificial bulges by squeezing a part of implant between the coil and the chest wall (Fig. 9.42). Knowing a history of previous ruptures and subsequent implant replacement is also important. Implant replacement after rupture (a redo) may not completely remove all silicone material extruded from the rupture. This makes a confusing appearance of residual silicone droplets next to the new intact implant and can result in misinterpretation as extracapsular rupture of the new implant (Fig. 9.43).

In an early series of 143 patients with 281 silicone implants (Gorczyca, 1994), MRI showed a sensitivity of 76% and a specificity of 97% for implant rupture. This series used a T2-weighted FSE technique, a T2-weighted FSE technique with water suppression,

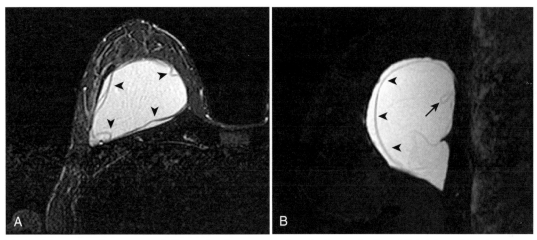

FIG. 9.38 Intracapsular rupture of silicone implants: examples of subcapsular line. (A) Axial combined water and silicone magnetic resonance image (MRI) shows subcapsular lines (*arrowheads*). (B) Sagittal silicone-specific MRI shows subcapsular lines (*arrowheads*) and a keyhole sign (*arrow*).

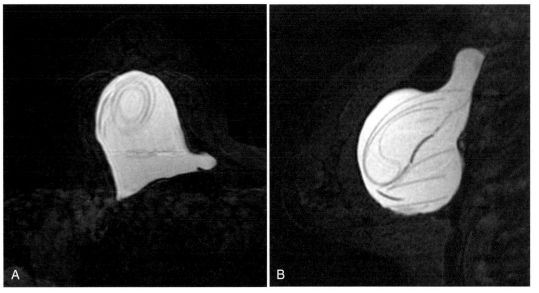

FIG. 9.39 Intracapsular rupture of silicone implants: examples of linguine sign. (A) Axial silicone-specific magnetic resonance image (MRI) shows a linguine sign. (B) Sagittal silicone-specific MRI shows a linguine sign.

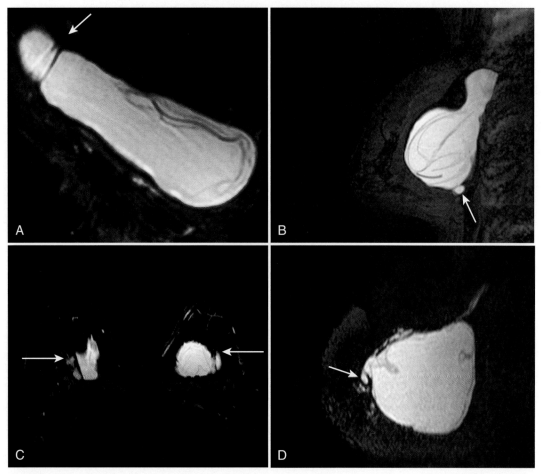

FIG. 9.40 Extracapsular rupture of silicone implants: examples of bulges of silicone. (A) Axial silicone-specific magnetic resonance image (MRI) shows extravasated silicone (*arrow*), seen as a bulge in the axillary portion of the implant. The linguine sign is seen within the implant. Silicone outside the fibrous capsule is a definitive sign of extracapsular rupture. (B) Sagittal silicone-specific MRI shows extravasated silicone (*arrow*), which is seen as a bulge in the lower posterior portion of the implant. The linguine sign is also seen within the implant. (C) Axial silicone-specific MRI shows extravasated silicone (*arrows*) in the outer portions of bilateral implants. (D) Sagittal silicone-specific MRI of the right breast reconstructed from 3D CUBE images shows bulges (*arrow*) and droplets of silicone with the high signal intensity in the anterior portion of the implant. Keyhole signs are also observed within the implant (see axial images of this case in Video 9.2).

BOX 9.6   Causes of False-Positive Magnetic Resonance Imaging Diagnoses of Implant Rupture

Implants with multilumen structures or rare implant materials
Poor positioning at the time of magnetic resonance imaging study
Implant replacement after rupture (a "redo")

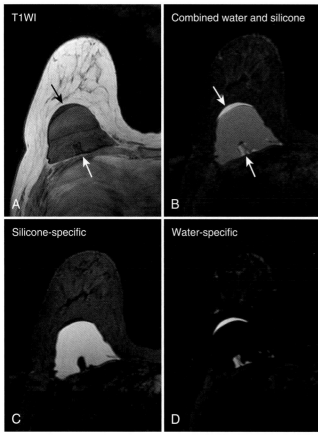

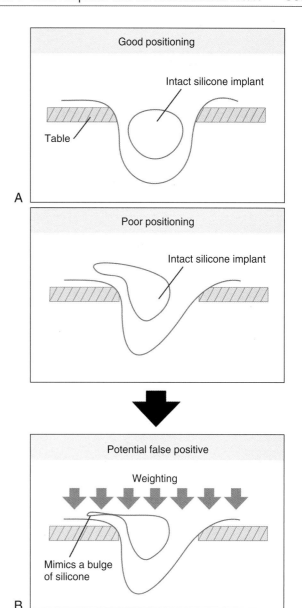

FIG. 9.41 Saline outer, silicone inner double-lumen implant producing a confusing appearance. (A) T1-weighted image. (B) Combined water and silicone image. (C) Silicone-specific image. (D) Water-specific image. Under the implant capsule there are very low intensity spaces on T1-weighted image (A) and high intensity on combined image (B) that could be mistaken as a subcapsular line and a keyhole sign of intracapsular rupture. However, these spaces appear in low signal on silicone-specific image (C) and high signal on water-specific image (D), allowing the identification of water, not silicone, within the spaces. This implant was a normal saline outer, silicone inner, double-lumen implant without intracapsular rupture. Careful image interpretation and knowing the type of implants may avoid the misdiagnosis. Note signal dropout is seen along the places in which silicone meets saline, which is caused by the chemical shift on combined water and silicone images (B).

FIG. 9.42 Poor positioning can cause false-positive magnetic resonance (MR) imaging diagnosis of silicone implant rupture. (A) Schematic of good positioning. (B) Schematic of poor positioning. When a breast is wrongly positioned in the coil, a part of implant may be captured between the coil and the chest wall. The squeezed implant may mimic bulges of implant and may lead to the misdiagnosis as extracapsular rupture. Proper positioning is essential to evaluate MR images correctly.

and a T1-weighted spin-echo technique with fat suppression. In a 2001 meta-analysis of studies published between 1992 and 1998 performed with varying MRI procedures and technologies (Cher, 2001), the summary MRI sensitivity for rupture was 78% (95% confidence interval [CI] 71%–83%) and summary specificity was 91% (95% CI 86–94%), with an odds ratio for overall test accuracy of 40.1 (range 18.8–85.4), using receiver operating characteristics meta-analysis methodology.

More recent studies using improved silicone-specific MR images found higher sensitivity. In a series of 30 patients with 59 implants (Ikeda, 1999), MRI had a sensitivity of 100%, a specificity of 63%, a positive predictive value (PPV) of 71%, an NPV of 100%, and an accuracy of 81% in the detection of rupture/bleed. The linguine sign was the most sensitive (93%) and specific (65%) finding for rupture. The nonspecific sign of water droplets within the implant had a sensitivity of 92% and a low specificity of 44%. Linear extension of silicone along the

chest wall and the presence of reactive fluid were not sensitive or specific for rupture and can be caused by poor positioning. Nonspecific signs such as contour deformity (77%, 10/13), water droplets (54%, 7/13), and reactive fluid (23%, 3/13) were common. In this series, MRI was shown to be more sensitive and accurate than mammography and ultrasound in detecting breast implant rupture or bleed. Another study of 107 women with 214 PIP silicone implants recalled from the European market (Maijers, 2013) showed a sensitivity of 93%, a specificity of 93%, a PPV of 77%, and an NPV of 98% in detecting implant rupture/leakage. In summary, MRI is a highly accurate diagnostic tool in identifying implant rupture along with sophisticated silicone imaging techniques.

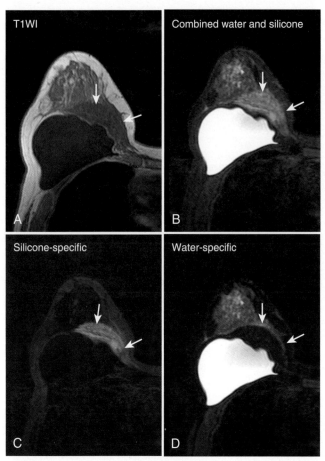

FIG. 9.43 Residual silicone from a prior extracapsular rupture producing a confusing appearance. (A) T1-weighted image. (B) Combined water and silicone image. (C) Silicone-specific image. (D) Water-specific image. Anterior to a saline implant, there is a mass that is low intensity on T1-weighted image (A), high intensity on combined image (B), high intensity on silicone-specific image (C), and low intensity on water-specific image (D), representing silicone (*arrows*) within the breast tissue. This patient has a history of extracapsular rupture of a silicone implant and implant replacement (a "redo") with a saline implant and has residual silicone from the prior rupture within the breast tissue. Residual silicone could be mistaken as a tumor if the silicone-specific study and contrast-enhanced study are not performed, and as a bulge from a replaced intact implant if a silicone implant is used for the replacement. Knowing the patient's history is important to avoid the misdiagnosis.

DIRECT SILICONE/PARAFFIN INJECTION

Silicone within the breast and extensive fat necrosis type calcifications are seen in women with a history of direct silicone injections. Direct silicone or paraffin injections were used overseas for breast augmentation; free silicone, paraffin, or other materials were injected directly into the breast tissue. Direct silicone injection was performed in the United States in the 1950s and 1960s, but the FDA prohibited it in the 1970s because of reported adverse effects, including formation of granulomatous masses, fibrosis, lymphadenopathy, and infection. Granulomatous masses are generated because the silicone globules are foreign bodies, are often associated with calcification, and may sometimes form hard masses that the patients can feel on palpation. On mammography, silicone globules appear as multiple radiopaque masses with or without a round rim (former eggshell-type) calcifications that obscure the underlying breast tissue (Fig. 9.44;

Video 9.3). Ultrasound of silicone granulomas shows the snowstorm sign, also known as echodense noise, which obscures all findings beneath it. The nodular silicone mastopathy may mimic breast cancers. However, because these silicone or injection granulomas may become quite hard and obscure the underlying breast tissue, the assessment for breast cancer with physical examination, mammographic examination, and ultrasound can be quite challenging. MRI may be required for the further assessment (Fig. 9.45; Video 9.4).

BREAST RECONSTRUCTION

After mastectomy, the breast may be reconstructed with a tissue expander followed by an implant, autologous tissue, or a combination of the two. Implant reconstruction usually requires placement of a tissue expander at the time of mastectomy and subsequent expansion of the skin (Figs. 9.46 and 9.47). At a subsequent surgery, the surgeon removes the tissue expander and places a permanent implant, autologous tissue, or a combination of the two. The transverse rectus abdominis myocutaneous (TRAM) flap is the most common form of autologous tissue reconstruction, and it may be performed as a pedicle (a pedicled TRAM) or free flap (muscle-sparing free TRAM; Fig. 9.48). Finally, a latissimus dorsi myocutaneous flap may be used when additional skin is needed to close the wound or additional soft tissue is required in an implant-based reconstruction. The reconstructive method selected depends on the patient's goals, medical history, body habitus, physical examination, and potential need for adjuvant therapy.

In patients undergoing tissue expansion after mastectomy, very little, if any, breast tissue has been left in the mastectomy site, and the breast is left with little or no glandular tissue to image on mammography. Usually, a saline expander is left in the mastectomy site and gradually enlarged until the space is adequate to hold an appropriately sized implant. Patients with mastectomies with implant placement may undergo mammography if there is enough breast tissue to compress around the implant, but frequently, too little tissue is left to compress for an adequate view. Breast cancer recurrences can appear as suspicious calcifications or masses when breast tissue is adequately seen.

In the case of TRAM, latissimus dorsi, and other free flap reconstructions, skin, fat, and muscle are transferred to the mastectomy site with attachments to vascular structures and are shaped to form a breast. Traditionally, autologous flaps are not imaged by mammography, but mammography can be helpful in evaluating these structures when there are suspicious physical findings postoperatively. Autologous flaps appear radiographically as fat centrally, with (Fig. 9.49) or without (Fig. 9.50) muscle fibers around the edges of the flaps. Common mammographic findings in TRAM flaps are calcifications from fat necrosis (Fig. 9.51), benign dermal calcifications, calcified hematoma, and clustered microcalcifications. Areas of increased or decreased density without calcifications are also common and appear to be related to postsurgical changes and fat necrosis (Fig. 9.52). A nipple can be reconstructed out of skin and tattooed to provide color similar to the contralateral side. Rarely, the tattoo can be seen on mammography (Fig. 9.53).

Mammography can be a useful diagnostic tool for cancer recurrence in patients who have undergone autologous breast reconstruction. In a 2001 article by Shaikh et al., breast cancer recurrence in TRAM flaps appeared as masses with a differential diagnosis of granulomas or fat necrosis. In another study, Helvie et al. (1998) found six breast cancers in women undergoing TRAM flap reconstruction; they appeared as four suspicious masses and two suspicious microcalcification clusters. In a series by Casey et al. (2013), 66 breasts (18%) of 365 flaps in 272 patients developed breast masses, of which 54 were from fat necrosis seen within 3 months, 1 cancer at 24 months, and 11 other recurrent cancers, all suggested by diagnostic breast

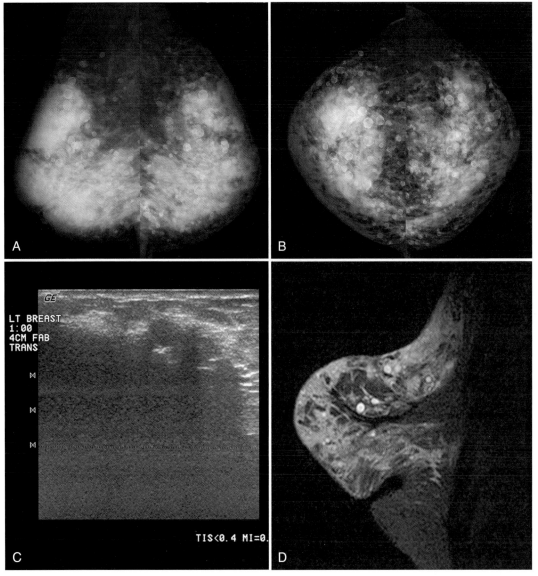

FIG. 9.44 Direct silicone injections. Mediolateral oblique (A) and craniocaudal (B) mammograms show dense tissue and multiple rim calcifications representing calcification around silicone injection granulomas. Ultrasound (C) of the left breast shows echogenic noise (snowstorm) that obscures all findings beneath it. Silicone-specific magnetic resonance image (D) shows multiple round masses of high signal intensity, characteristically representing silicone globules. Low-signal band in the center of breast is fibrosis (see Video 9.3).

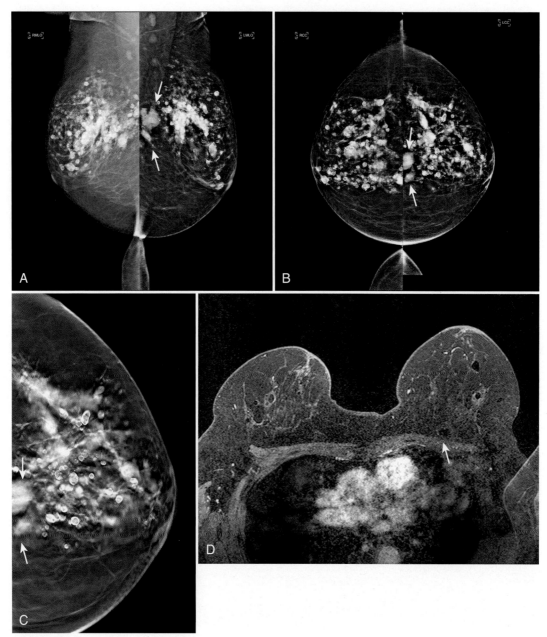

FIG. 9.45 Direct paraffin injections. Bilateral mediolateral oblique (A) and craniocaudal (CC; B) mammograms show multiple nodular shadows and multiple rim calcifications. There are 16-mm and 10-mm noncalcified masses in the upper central aspect of the left breast (*arrows*). They are suspicious for noncalcified granulomas but breast cancers could not be excluded. CC tomosynthesis key slice (C) of the left breast shows noncalcified masses (*arrows*) at the deep edge of the image (see Video 9.4). Axial contrast-enhanced fat-suppressed T1-wighted image (D) shows multiple nonenhanced nodules with slight rim enhancement, consisting of both calcified masses and noncalcified masses (*arrow*) on mammograms. They all were diagnosed as paraffin globules and paraffin injection granulomas without evidence of malignancy.

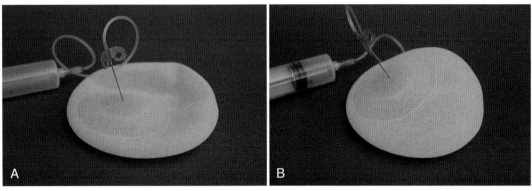

FIG. 9.46 Single-lumen expander. Before (A) and after (B) expansion. A tissue expander is a temporary device placed to expand the breast skin and muscle. Volume of the expander can be changed after surgery by injecting saline though the injection dome. Later adjustability allows the surgeon to shape the breast and achieve the size and symmetry the patient desires.

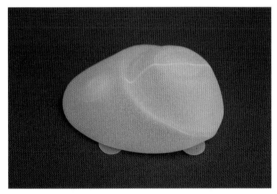

FIG. 9.47 Double-lumen expander. There is a variety in types, shapes, and sizes of breast expanders. The double-lumen breast expander shown here offers flexibility for optimal expansion results with inferior and superior fill chambers.

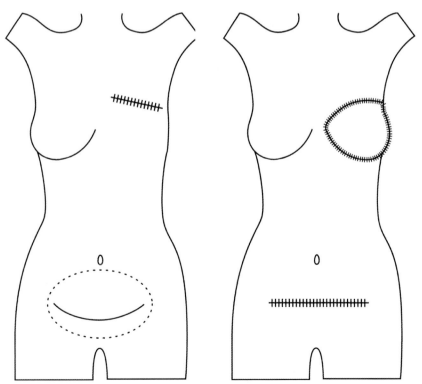

FIG. 9.48 Schematic of transverse rectus abdominis myocutaneous (TRAM) reconstruction showing the abdominal pedicle removed from the lower portion of the abdomen and tunneled under the skin to the mastectomy site where the breast is reconstructed. The TRAM surgery can also be done as a free flap.

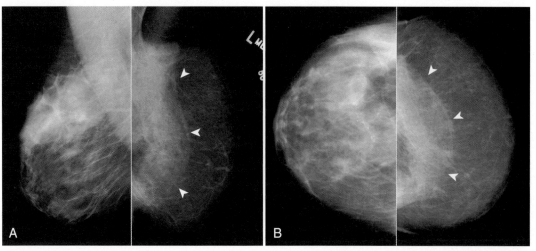

FIG. 9.49 Normal mammographic appearance of a transverse rectus abdominis musculocutaneous (TRAM) flap in the reconstructed left breast. The right breast is normal. Mediolateral oblique (A) and craniocaudal (B) mammograms show the anterior fatty portion and the muscular posterior portion (*arrowheads*) in the TRAM flap in the left breast. Heterogeneously dense fibroglandular tissue is seen in the normal right breast.

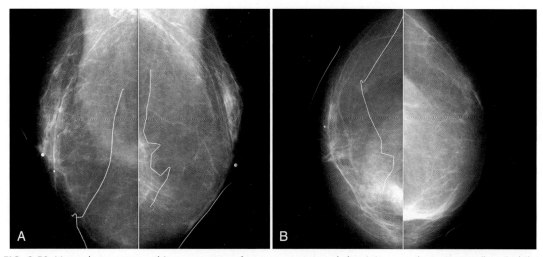

FIG. 9.50 Normal mammographic appearance of transverse rectus abdominis musculocutaneous flaps in bilateral reconstructed breasts. Mediolateral oblique (A) and craniocaudal (B) mammograms show fatty tissue and focal density in the breasts reconstructed from abdominal tissue. Note the relative fatty composition of the reconstructed breast and lack of normal glandular elements. Linear metallic scar markers show the location of the scars.

imaging of the palpable mass. The authors report that cancer was more likely to occur if the margins were close at less than 1 cm or if there was prior lymphovascular invasion. It is noted that most of these series of TRAM mammography investigations were performed because of palpable masses. Lee et al. (2008) showed that in asymptomatic women there were 265 TRAM reconstructions in 554 mammograms with 8 (1.4%) positive results and no cancers on biopsy. Because of the low probability of detecting nonpalpable breast cancer and decision analysis results showing "an additional 1.6 days of life expectancy for the screened cohort," they concluded that mammographic screening of asymptomatic women with TRAM flap reconstructions is "less effective than screening asymptomatic women in their 40s for primary breast cancer."

Two studies have looked at the efficacy of MRI of the breast after breast-conserving surgery and autogenous tissue reconstruction in patients with breast cancer for the detection of recurrent disease. Rieber et al. (2003) showed that on MRI in eight TRAM cases, the flap appeared to have fat signal intensity and the pedicle was isointense to pectoralis muscle, with easily seen fat necrosis. Kang et al. (2005) evaluated MRIs in 20 patients undergoing modified radical mastectomy and TRAM flap, and the opposite breast, showing that MRI depicted an enhancing TRAM flap/mastectomy site and with commonly seen postoperative skin thickenings, and less commonly, edema, fluid collection, hematoma, fat necrosis (Fig. 9.54), or lipofilling changes. The postoperative findings decreased on subsequent MRI studies. In the opposite breast, enhancing findings were seen in seven patients, and DCIS was seen in one. These two studies show that MRI may be helpful in showing postoperative findings in TRAM flap reconstructions and in finding cancer in the opposite breast; however, radiologists must be aware of the normal postoperative appearances of the breast after TRAM flap reconstructions to avoid misdiagnosis.

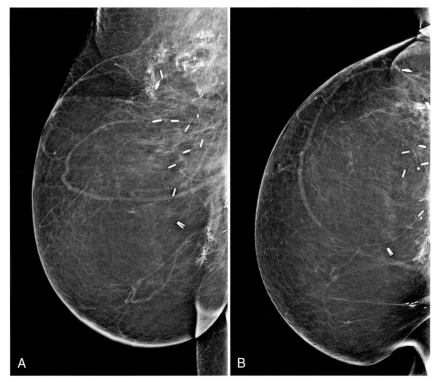

FIG. 9.51 Calcification in a transverse rectus abdominis musculocutaneous flap caused by fat necrosis. Mediolateral oblique (A) and craniocaudal (B) mammograms show dystrophic calcification caused by fat necrosis in the deep portion of the right breast. Note the relative fatty composition of the reconstructed breast and multiple metallic clips at flap pedicle.

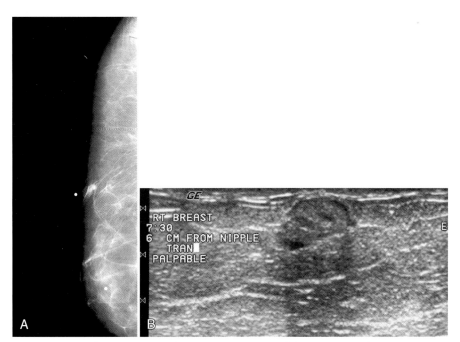

FIG. 9.52 Fat necrosis producing a mass after transverse rectus abdominis musculocutaneous (TRAM) reconstruction. A lateral mammogram (A) shows fatty tissue from a TRAM reconstruction with a skin marker over an upper oval equal-density palpable mass. The second skin marker in the lower portion of the breast shows the location of the reconstructed nipple. Ultrasound (B) shows a hypoechoic mass near the skin surface. The differential diagnosis includes recurrence of cancer, an epidermal inclusion cyst, and fat necrosis. Biopsy showed fat necrosis.

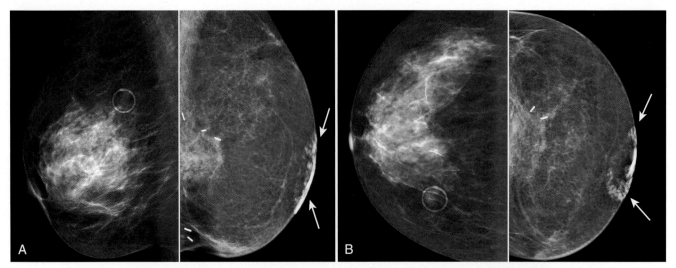

FIG. 9.53 Tattoo on transverse rectus abdominis musculocutaneous (TRAM) flap reconstruction. TRAM flap reconstruction in the left breast and a normal mammogram on the right breast. Mediolateral oblique (A) and craniocaudal (B) mammograms shows the fatty left TRAM reconstructed breast, clips at TRAM flap pedicle, and tattooed nipple–areolar complex (*arrows*) on the left.

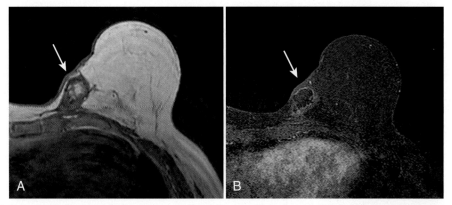

FIG. 9.54 Fat necrosis in a transverse rectus abdominis musculocutaneous (TRAM) flap on magnetic resonance image (MRI). (A) T1-weighted image. (B) T1-weighted contrast-enhanced differential subsampling with Cartesian ordering (DISCO) image. Left breast was reconstructed with a TRAM flap. Fat necrosis (*arrows*) in the TRAM flap appears as low signal intensity with central high intensity representing fat on T1-weighted image (A), and is contrast-enhanced with gadolinium on the edge around the low signal fat necrosis (B, *arrow*).

Another form of breast reconstruction involves autologous fat graft injection with or without the use of a vacuum-based external tissue expansion device called BRAVA to augment the volume of the reconstructed breast. In cases with autologous fat graft injection, findings caused by lipofilling are rarely identified on mammography (Fig. 9.55) but may appear as oil cysts on ultrasound and MRI. Fiaschetti et al. (2013) showed that in 15 patients with 20 breasts undergoing lipofilling there were many lipid cysts within the breasts on ultrasound, which is not surprising given the method by which the breasts are augmented. The most frequent complication in fat grafting is fat necrosis, which can be identified easily on mammography if it calcifies. Noncalcified fat necrosis can be identified on ultrasound, MRI, and, less commonly on mammography. Rubin et al. (2012) evaluated mammograms in 27 women treated with fat grafting to the breast for augmentation who had normal preaugmentation mammograms and compared them to postsurgical mammograms from 23 women who received reduction mammoplasty. They showed that there

was no significant difference in radiographic abnormality rates for oil cysts, benign calcifications, and calcifications warranting biopsy, and scarring and masses needing biopsy were more common in the reduction cohort. Further follow-up studies of this technique will yield further information in the future regarding the degree of calcification of the grafted fat and its appearance on imaging. In patients undergoing BRAVA, the enlarged vessels can be observed on mammography, because BRAVA increases the vascularity of the recipient site.

REDUCTION MAMMOPLASTY

Reduction mammoplasty and mastopexy are performed to reduce the breast size or to lift the breast, respectively. Reduction mammoplasty is most often performed for macromastia. After cancer surgery, patients often undergo breast reduction or mastopexy (breast lift) of the contralateral breast to achieve breast symmetry (Fig. 9.56). This surgery matches the "normal"

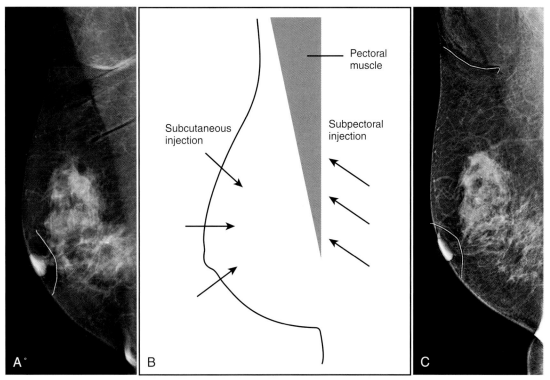

FIG. 9.55 Autologous fat graft injection. (A) Mediolateral oblique (MLO) mammogram before fat grafting. (B) Schema of fat injection. (C) MLO mammogram after fat grafting. This patient previously received lumpectomy with radiation therapy for breast cancer in the left breast (A). Subsequently, the patient received fat graft injection into subpectoral and subcutaneous spaces (B). The change related to fat injection is very subtle on mammography and is difficult to identify (C).

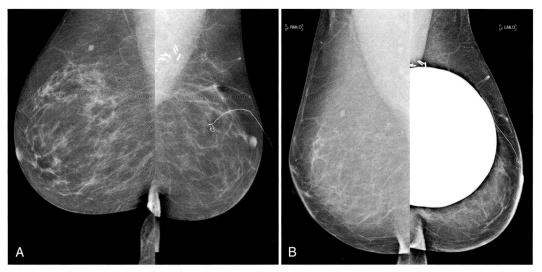

FIG. 9.56 Reduction mammoplasty for contralateral breast in a patient who received lumpectomy and subsequent breast reconstruction in left breast. Mediolateral oblique (MLO) mammograms before (A) and after (B) surgery. Preoperative MLO mammograms (A) show asymmetric breasts in size; the left breast is smaller than the right breast after lumpectomy for left breast cancer. Then, the patient received left breast reconstruction with implant placement and fat graft and right breast reduction mammoplasty. Postoperative MLO mammograms (B) show almost symmetric breasts.

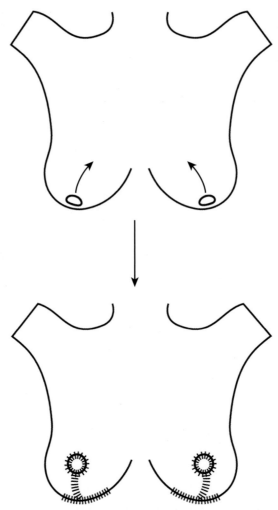

FIG. 9.57 Reduction mammoplasty. Schematic of reduction mammoplasty. Breast tissue is removed from the lower portion of the breast. The nipple is elevated and moved cranially to the upper part of the breast, but usually the nipple remains attached to the breast ducts. Typical reduction mammoplasty scars are shown in the bottom figure.

breast to the conserved breast. To perform a reduction mammoplasty, the surgeon removes skin and breast parenchyma from the lower portion and relocates the nipple superiorly (Fig. 9.57). The resulting scar runs around the areola, vertically down to the inframammary fold, and often within the inframammary fold. The resulting surgery leaves a smaller breast with normal visible skin in the region of the cleavage. The nipple is elevated and moved cranially to the upper part of the breast, but, usually, the nipple is kept attached to the breast ducts. In some instances in which the breast is very ptotic or very large (this increases the risk of nipple necrosis after breast reduction), the surgeon may choose to remove the nipple and then graft it back on to the breast.

Mammograms after reduction mammoplasty show characteristic skin thickening over the lower breast in the region of the scars. This is most evident on the mediolateral oblique or mediolateral view (Fig. 9.58; Video 9.5). The lower breast shows architectural distortion, and the overall pattern of the lower breast is distorted from scarring. Depending on the amount of tissue removed from various areas of the breast, the breast parenchymal pattern can be patchy and much different from the prereduction mammogram. The nipple is elevated cranially to the upper part of the breast, and the breast ducts attaching to the nipple may sometimes be seen on imaging. In some cases in which the surgeon removes the nipple and then grafts it back on to the breast, the breast ducts terminating to the nipples are not seen terminating to the nipple on the mammogram.

Reduction mammoplasty or any breast surgery can result in focal fat necrosis or oil cysts that have a characteristic appearance, or they may be atypical and form a palpable mass. Epidermal inclusion cysts can also form in biopsy scars and produce a dense smooth round or oval mass near the skin surface but not be connected to it. These masses represent epidermal cells that are displaced into breast tissue during biopsy. The epithelial cells can grow and form a round benign-appearing mass. In the case of fat necrosis, breast ultrasound may be helpful, but biopsy may be needed. Skin calcifications along the skin incisions may also develop but can be distinguished from intraparenchymal calcifications or cancer because of their typical skin location (Fig. 9.59; Video 9.6).

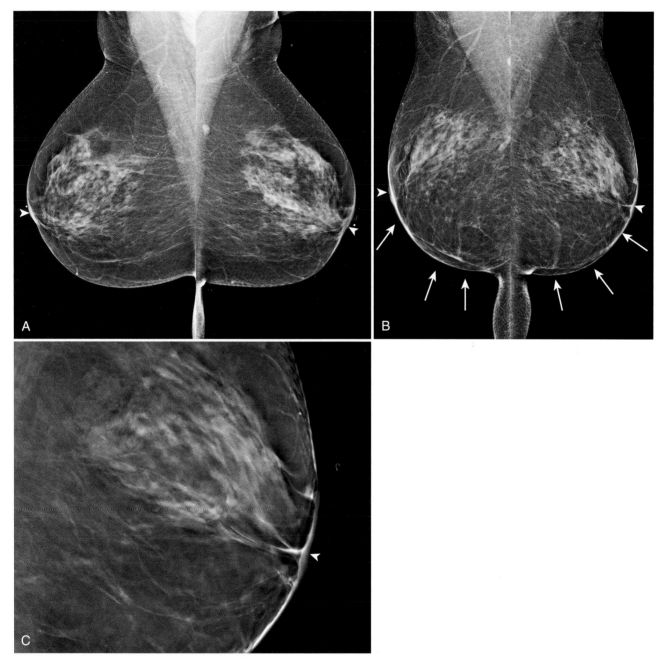

FIG. 9.58 Mammograms of a woman with bilateral reduction mammoplasty. (A) Bilateral mediolateral oblique (MLO) views before reduction. (B) Bilateral MLO views after reduction. (C) Cropped magnified tomosynthesis slice of left MLO projection after reduction. Compared with the presurgical mammograms (A), postsurgical mammograms (B) show smaller breasts with mildly distorted scattered fibroglandular tissue. Characteristic skin thickening (*arrows* in B) are apparent in the lower portions of the breast on MLO. The nipples (*arrowheads*) were moved cranially, but were kept attached to the breast ducts. Architectural distortion and the connection of ducts to the relocated nipple are more evident on tomosynthesis (C; see Video 9.5)

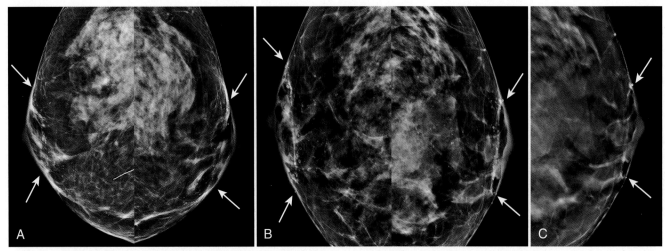

FIG. 9.59 Skin calcifications around the replaced nipple after reduction mammoplasty. (A and B) Photography-magnified mediolateral oblique (MLO; A) and craniocaudal (CC; B) digital mammograms. (C) Photography-magnified CC view of tomosynthesis of left breast. There are multiple dense tiny calcifications (*arrows*) around the replaced nipple along the incision (see Video 9.6).

Key Elements

No scientific evidence has shown a definite association between silicone breast implants and connective tissue disorders or breast cancer.

In the United States there was a moratorium on the use of silicone breast implants in 1992, but the ban was lifted and now silicone breast implants are approved for breast reconstruction and breast augmentation.

There is rare but reported primary breast anaplastic large cell lymphoma seen in patients with implants. This is a disease of the fibrous capsule surrounding the implant and not of the breast tissue around the implant, and is usually shown by an effusion and rarely a mass.

Breast implants may have single or multiple lumens, each containing silicone or other materials in the different shells.

Implants are placed in subpectoral or subglandular (above the pectoral muscle) locations.

Mammograms of breasts with implants use a limited-compression view that includes the implant and the tissue around it but does not use much compression (to not rupture the implant) and "implant-displaced views."

Even with the implant-displaced views, the radiologist sees only about 80% of the breast tissue.

Fibrous capsules form around all implants, sometimes becoming hard or calcified and impairing the implant's look and feel.

Implant complications include contracture of the fibrous capsule, calcification of the fibrous capsule, implant rippling, seroma, malposition, hematoma, infection, breast pain, and implant rupture.

Closed capsulotomy, or manual breaking of a hardened fibrous capsule, can result in implant rupture.

Implant rupture is classified as intracapsular (silicone contained in the fibrous capsule) or extracapsular (silicone outside the fibrous capsule).

Symptoms associated with silicone implant rupture are nonspecific and include axillary, breast, or chest wall masses; pain; and changes in breast size, shape, or texture.

The older generation implant models (first, second, or third generation) have not been manufactured for many decades; many of the initial implant rupture reports from the 1990s were of these older implants.

Newer generation silicone implants (fourth and fifth generation) have very small rupture rates in primary breast augmentation patients.

In 2012 the Poly Implant Prothèse silicone implant marketed in Europe was found to contain nonmedical industrial grade silicone and has a high rupture rate (14.4%; Wazir, 2015).

Extracapsular ruptures appear on mammography as silicone outside the implant in breast tissue, lymph nodes, or ducts or as a deformity in implant contour.

Intracapsular rupture of a silicone implant is almost impossible to detect on mammography, because the silicone gel is still contained within an intact fibrous capsule.

On mammography a bulging contour suggests, but is not definitive of, intracapsular rupture, because a lobulated contour can be also seen in capsular contracture or herniation of an intact implant envelope

Direct silicone or paraffin injections are used outside the United States for augmentation and cause eggshell-type calcifications or dense masses on mammography, snowstorm or echodense noise on ultrasound, and hard palpable silicone granuloma masses on physical examination.

A normal implant ultrasound shows radial folds and reverberations in the near field.

Ultrasound of extracapsular rupture shows the snowstorm sign, or echodense noise.

Ultrasound of intracapsular rupture shows the stepladder sign.

A false-positive ultrasound of intracapsular rupture is caused by a double-lumen or multilumen implant mimicking the stepladder sign.

Magnetic resonance imaging (MRI) of extracapsular rupture shows blobs of silicone outside the implant and signs of intracapsular rupture.

MRI of intracapsular rupture shows the linguine sign, subcapsular lines, teardrops, or the keyhole sign.

Nonspecific findings on MRI are water droplets, reactive fluid, and implant contour abnormalities.

False-positive findings of rupture on MRI are caused by intact multilumen implants simulating the linguine sign.

False-positive findings of rupture on all imaging methods include previous rupture with implant replacement but without removal of all intraparenchymal silicone.

To avoid false-positive diagnoses of rupture, know the implant type and whether previous rupture and removal of the implant have occurred.

After mastectomy, the breast may be reconstructed with a tissue expander followed by an implant, autologous tissue, or a combination of the two.

Autologous tissue reconstructions consist of transverse rectus abdominis or latissimus dorsi myocutaneous flaps performed as a pedicle or a free flap.

Mammographic findings of autologous tissue reconstruction include fat and muscle and, commonly, calcifications from fat necrosis and densities from postsurgical changes.

Cancer in reconstructed breasts is often detected by physical examination, with occasional mammographic findings of suspicious masses or calcifications.

Reduction mammoplasty produces a characteristic distortion of the lower portion of the breast and scarring, with relocation of the nipple higher on the breast.

Less common breast augmentation techniques include autologous fat graft injection and a vacuum-based external tissue expansion using lipofilling equipment.

Lipid cysts and fat necrosis can be seen on ultrasound or MRI with autologous fat graft injection; mammographic changes are difficult to see in the first few months.

SUGGESTED READINGS

Adrada BE, Miranda RN, Rauch GM, et al.: Breast implant-associated anaplastic large cell lymphoma: sensitivity, specificity, and findings of imaging studies in 44 patients, *Breast Cancer Res Treat* 147:1–14, 2014.

Ahn CY, DeBruhl ND, Gorczyca DP, et al.: Comparative silicone breast implant evaluation using mammography, sonography, and magnetic resonance imaging: experience with 59 implants, *Plast Reconstr Surg* 94:620–627, 1994.

Ahn CY, Shaw WW, Narayanan K, et al.: Residual silicone detection using MRI following previous breast implant removal: case reports, *Aesthetic Plast Surg* 19:361–367, 1995.

ALLERGAN®: Product labeling and safety information of NATRELLE® silicone-filled breast implants. http://www.allergan.com/assets/pdf/L034-03_Silicone_DFU.pdf. Accessed February 25, 2015.

From Baker Jr JL: Augmentation mammaplasty. In Owsley Jr JQ, Peterson RA, editors: *Symposium on esthetic surgery of the breast*, St. Louis, 1978, CV Mosby.

Beekman WH, Hage JJ, Taets van Amerongen AH, Mulder JW: Accuracy of ultrasonography and magnetic resonance imaging in detecting failure of breast implants filled with silicone gel, *Scand J Plast Reconstr Surg Hand Surg* 33:415–418, 1999.

Bengtson BP, Eaves 3rd FF: High-resolution ultrasound in the detection of silicone gel breast implant shell failure: background, in vitro studies, and early clinical results, *Aesthet Surg J* 32:157–174, 2012.

Berg WA, Caskey CI, Hamper UM, et al.: Diagnosing breast implant rupture with MR imaging, US, and mammography, *Radiographics* 13:1323–1336, 1993.

Berg WA, Caskey CI, Hamper UM, et al.: Single- and double-lumen silicone breast implant integrity: prospective evaluation of MR and US criteria, *Radiology* 197:45–52, 1995.

Breiting VB, Holmich LR, Brandt B, et al.: Long-term health status of Danish women with silicone breast implants, *Plast Reconstr Surg* 114:217–228, 2004.

Brown SL, Middleton MS, Berg WA, et al.: Prevalence of rupture of silicone gel breast implants revealed on MR imaging in a population of women in Birmingham, Alabama, *AJR Am J Roentgenol* 175:1057–1064, 2000.

Carlson GW, Moore B, Thornton JF, et al.: Breast cancer after augmentation mammaplasty: treatment by skin-sparing mastectomy and immediate reconstruction, *Plast Reconstr Surg* 107:687–692, 2001.

Carlson GW, Styblo TM, Lyles RH, et al.: Local recurrence after skin-sparing mastectomy: tumor biology or surgical conservatism? *Ann Surg Oncol* 10:108–112, 2003.

Casey 3rd WJ, Rebecca AM, Silverman A, et al.: Etiology of breast masses after autologous breast reconstruction, *Ann Surg Oncol* 20:607–614, 2013.

Center for Devices and Radiological Health/US Food and Drug Administration: *FDA update on the safety of silicone gel-filled breast implants*, http://www.fda.gov/downloads/MedicalDevices/ProductsandMedicalProcedures/ImplantsandProsthetics/Breast-Implants/UCM260090.pdf, June 2011. Accessed February 6, 2015.

Cher DJ, Conwell JA, Mandel JS: MRI for detecting silicone breast implant rupture: meta-analysis and implications, *Ann Plast Surg* 47:367–380, 2001.

Chung KC, Wilkins EG, Beil Jr RJ, et al.: Diagnosis of silicone gel breast implant rupture by ultrasonography, *Plast Reconstr Surg* 97:104–109, 1996.

Cicchetti S, Leone MS, Franchelli S, Santi PL: Evaluation of the tolerability of Hydrogel breast implants: a pilot study, *Minerva Chir* 57:53–57, 2002.

Collis N, Coleman D, Foo IT, Sharpe DT: Ten-year review of a prospective randomized controlled trial of textured versus smooth subglandular silicone gel breast implants, *Plast Reconstr Surg* 106:786–791, 2000a.

Collis N, Litherland J, Enion D, Sharpe DT: Magnetic resonance imaging and explantation investigation of long-term silicone gel implant integrity, *Plast Reconstr Surg* 120:1401–1406, 2007.

Collis N, Sharpe DT: Silicone gel-filled breast implant integrity: a retrospective review of 478 consecutively explanted implants, *Plast Reconstr Surg* 105:1979–1985, 2000b.

Cunningham B: The Mentor Core Study on silicone MemoryGel breast implants, *Plast Reconstr Surg* 120(7 Suppl 1):19S–32S, 2007a.

Cunningham B: The Mentor Study on contour profile gel silicone MemoryGel breast implants, *Plast Reconstr Surg* 120(7 Suppl 1):33S–39S, 2007b.

DeBruhl ND, Gorczyca DP, Ahn CY, Shaw WW, Bassett LW: Silicone breast implants: US evaluation, *Radiology* 189:95–98, 1993.

Destouet JM, Monsees BS, Oser RF, et al.: Screening mammography in 350 women with breast implants: prevalence and findings of implant complications, *AJR Am J Roentgenol* 159:973–981, 1992.

Derby BM, Codner MA: Textured silicone breast implant use in primary augmentation: core data update and review, *Plast Reconstr Surg* 135:113–124, 2015.

Di Benedetto G, Cecchini S, Grassetti L, et al.: Comparative study of breast implant rupture using mammography, sonography, and magnetic resonance imaging: correlation with surgical findings, *Breast J* 14:532–537, 2008.

Eidelman Y, Liebling RW, Buchbinder S, et al.: Mammography in the evaluation of masses in breasts reconstructed with TRAM flaps, *Ann Plast Surg* 41:229–233, 1998.

Eklund GW, Busby RC, Miller SH, Job JS: Improved imaging of the augmented breast, *AJR Am J Roentgenol* 151:469–473, 1988.

Fajardo LL, Harvey JA, McAleese KA, et al.: Breast cancer diagnosis in women with subglandular silicone gel-filled augmentation implants, *Radiology* 194:859–862, 1995.

Fajardo LL, Roberts CC, Hunt KR: Mammographic surveillance of breast cancer patients: should the mastectomy site be imaged? *AJR Am J Roentgenol* 161:953–955, 1993.

Feng LJ, Amini SB: Analysis of risk factors associated with rupture of silicone gel breast implants, *Plast Reconstr Surg* 104:955–963, 1999.

Fiaschetti V, Pistolese CA, Fornari M, et al.: Magnetic resonance imaging and ultrasound evaluation after breast autologous fat grafting combined with platelet-rich plasma, *Plast Reconstr Surg* 132:498–509, 2013.

Foster RD, Esserman LJ, Anthony JP, Hwang ES, Do H: Skin-sparing mastectomy and immediate breast reconstruction: a prospective cohort study for the treatment of advanced stages of breast carcinoma, *Ann Surg Oncol* 9:462–466, 2002.

Ganott MA, Harris KM, Ilkhanipour ZS, Costa-Greco MA: Augmentation mammoplasty: normal and abnormal findings with mammography and US, *Radiographics* 12:281–295, 1992.

Gorczyca DP: MR imaging of breast implants, *Magn Reson Imaging Clin North Am* 2:659–672, 1994.

Gorczyca DP, Schneider E, DeBruhl ND, et al.: Silicone breast implant rupture: comparison between three-point Dixon and fast spin-echo MR imaging, *AJR Am J Roentgenol* 162:305–310, 1994.

Gui GP, Kadayaprath G, Tan SM, et al.: Long-term quality-of-life assessment following one-stage immediate breast reconstruction using biodimensional expander implants: the patient's perspective, *Plast Reconstr Surg* 121:17–24, 2008.

Hammond DC, Migliori MM, Caplin DA, Garcia ME, Phillips CA: Mentor Contour Profile Gel implants: clinical outcomes at 6 years, *Plast Reconstr Surg* 129:1381–1391, 2012.

Handel N, Garcia ME, Wixtrom R: Breast implant rupture: causes, incidence, clinical impact, and management, *Plast Reconstr Surg* 132:1128–1137, 2013.

Harris KM, Ganott MA, Shestak KC, et al.: Silicone implant rupture: detection with US, *Radiology* 187:761–768, 1993.

Hayes MK, Gold RH, Bassett LW: Mammographic findings after the removal of breast implants, *AJR Am J Roentgenol* 160:487–490, 1993.

Heden P, Bone B, Murphy DK, et al.: Style 410 cohesive silicone breast implants: safety and effectiveness at 5 to 9 years after implantation, *Plast Reconstr Surg* 118:1281–1287, 2006a.

Heden P, Bronz G, Elberg JJ, et al.: Long-term safety and effectiveness of style 410 highly cohesive silicone breast implants, *Aesthetic Plast Surg* 33:430–436, 2009.

Heden P, Nava MB, van Tetering JP, et al.: Prevalence of rupture in Inamed silicone breast implants, *Plast Reconstr Surg* 118:303–312, 2006b.

Helvie MA, Bailey JE, Roubidoux MA, et al.: Mammographic screening of TRAM flap breast reconstructions for detection of nonpalpable recurrent cancer, *Radiology* 224:211–216, 2002.

Helvie MA, Wilson TE, Roubidoux MA, et al.: Mammographic appearance of recurrent breast carcinoma in six patients with TRAM flap breast reconstructions, *Radiology* 209:711–715, 1998.

Henriksen TF, Holmich LR, Fryzek JP, et al.: Incidence and severity of short-term complications after breast augmentation: results from a nationwide breast implant registry, *Ann Plast Surg* 51:531–539, 2003.

Herborn CU, Marincek B, Erfmann D, et al.: Breast augmentation and reconstructive surgery: MR imaging of implant rupture and malignancy, *Eur Radiol* 12:2198–2206, 2002.

Hogge JP, Zuurbier RA, de Paredes ES: Mammography of autologous myocutaneous flaps, *Radiographics* 19(Spec No):S63–S72, 1999.

Holmich LR, Friis S, Fryzek JP, Vejborg IM, et al.: Incidence of silicone breast implant rupture, *Arch Surg* 138:801–806, 2003.

Holmich LR, Fryzek JP, Kjoller K, et al.: The diagnosis of silicone breast-implant rupture: clinical findings compared with findings at magnetic resonance imaging, *Ann Plast Surg* 54:583–589, 2005a.

Holmich LR, Vejborg I, Conrad C, et al.: The diagnosis of breast implant rupture: MRI findings compared with findings at explantation, *Eur J Radiol* 53:213–225, 2005b.

Hsu W, Sheen-Chen SM, Eng HL, Ko SF: Mammographic microcalcification in an autogenously reconstructed breast simulating recurrent carcinoma, *Tumori* 94:574–576, 2008.

Hulka BS, Kerkvliet NL, Tugwell P: Experience of a scientific panel formed to advise the federal judiciary on silicone breast implants, *N Engl J Med* 342:812–815, 2000.

Ikeda DM, Borofsky HB, Herfkens RJ, et al.: Silicone breast implant rupture: pitfalls of magnetic resonance imaging and relative efficacies of magnetic resonance, mammography, and ultrasound, *Plast Reconstr Surg* 104:2054–2062, 1999.

Janowsky EC, Kupper LL, Hulka BS: Meta-analyses of the relation between silicone breast implants and the risk of connective-tissue diseases, *N Engl J Med* 342:781–790, 2000.

Kang BJ, Jung JI, Park C, et al.: Breast MRI findings after modified radical mastectomy and transverse rectus abdominis myocutaneous flap in patients with breast cancer, *J Magn Reson Imaging* 21:784–791, 2005.

Kessler DA: The basis of the FDA's decision on breast implants, *N Engl J Med* 326:1713–1715, 1992.

Khouri RK, Eisenmann-Klein M, Cardoso E, et al.: Brava and autologous fat transfer is a safe and effective breast augmentation alternative: results of a 6-year, 81-patient, prospective multicenter study, *Plast Reconstr Surg* 129:1173–1187, 2012.

Kim SH, Lipson JA, Moran CJ, et al.: Image quality and diagnostic performance of silicone-specific breast MRI, *Magn Reson Imaging* 31:1472–1478, 2013.

Kirkpatrick WN, Jones BM: The history of Trilucent implants, and a chemical analysis of the triglyceride filler in 51 consecutively removed Trilucent breast prostheses, *Br J Plast Surg* 55:479–489, 2002.

Kreymerman P, Patrick RJ, Rim A, et al.: Guidelines for using breast magnetic resonance imaging to evaluate implant integrity, *Ann Plast Surg* 62:355–357, 2009.

Kroll SS, Khoo A, Singletary SE, et al.: Local recurrence risk after skin-sparing and conventional mastectomy: a 6-year follow-up, *Plast Reconstr Surg* 104:421–425, 1999.

Kwek JW, Choi H, Ma J, Miller MJ: Gel-gel double-lumen silicone breast implant: mimic of intracapsular implant rupture, *AJR Am J Roentgenol* 187:W436–W437, 2006.

Lee JM, Georgian-Smith D, Gazelle GS, et al.: Detecting nonpalpable recurrent breast cancer: the role of routine mammographic screening of transverse rectus abdominis myocutaneous flap reconstructions, *Radiology* 248:398–405, 2008.

Leibman AJ, Kossoff MB, Kruse BD: Intraductal extension of silicone from a ruptured breast implant, *Plast Reconstr Surg* 89:546–547, 1992.

Lipworth L, Holmich LR, McLaughlin JK: Silicone breast implants and connective tissue disease: no association, *Semin Immunopathol* 33:287–294, 2011.

Maijers MC, Niessen FB: The clinical and diagnostic consequences of Poly Implant Prothèse silicone breast implants, recalled from the European market in 2010, *Plast Reconstr Surg* 131:394–402, 2013.

Marotta JS, Widenhouse CW, Habal MB, Goldberg EP: Silicone gel breast implant failure and frequency of additional surgeries: analysis of 35 studies reporting examination of more than 8,000 explants, *J Biomed Mater Res* 48:354–364, 1999.

Mason AC, White CS, McAvoy MA, Goldberg N: MR imaging of slipped stacked breast implants: a potential pitfall in the diagnosis of intracapsular rupture, *Magn Reson Imaging* 13:339–342, 1995.

Maxwell GP, Van Natta BW, Murphy DK, Slicton A, Bengtson BP: Natrelle style 410 form-stable silicone breast implants: core study results at 6 years, *Aesthet Surg J* 32:709–717, 2012.

McKeown DJ, Hogg FJ, Brown IM, et al.: The timing of autologous latissimus dorsi breast reconstruction and effect of radiotherapy on outcome, *J Plast Reconstr Aesthet Surg* 62:488–493, 2009.

McLaughlin JK, Lipworth L, Murphy DK, Walker PS: The safety of silicone gel-filled breast implants: a review of the epidemiologic evidence, *Ann Plast Surg* 59:569–580, 2007.

Medina-Franco H, Vasconez LO, Fix RJ, et al.: Factors associated with local recurrence after skin-sparing mastectomy and immediate breast reconstruction for invasive breast cancer, *Ann Surg* 235:814–819, 2002.

MENTOR®: Product information of MemoryShape™ breast implants. http://www.mentorwwllc.com/Documents/102942-001RevBPIDSFinal.pdf?v=2. Accessed February 25, 2015.

Middleton MS: Magnetic resonance evaluation of breast implants and soft-tissue silicone, *Top Magn Reson Imaging* 9:92–137, 1998.

Miranda RN, Aladily TN, Prince HM, et al.: Breast implant-associated anaplastic large-cell lymphoma: long-term follow-up of 60 patients, *J Clin Oncol* 32:114–120, 2014.

Mitnick JS, Vazquez MF, Plesser K, Colen SR: "Ductogram" associated with extravasation of silicone from a breast implant, *AJR Am J Roentgenol* 159:1126–1127, 1992.

Mitnick JS, Vazquez MF, Plesser K, et al.: Fine needle aspiration biopsy in patients with augmentation prostheses and a palpable mass, *Ann Plast Surg* 31:241–244, 1993.

Monticciolo DL, Nelson RC, Dixon WT, et al.: MR detection of leakage from silicone breast implants: value of a silicone-selective pulse sequence, *AJR Am J Roentgenol* 163:51–56, 1994.

Monticciolo DL, Ross D, Bostwick 3rd J, et al.: Autologous breast reconstruction with endoscopic latissimus dorsi musculosubcutaneous flaps in patients choosing breast-conserving therapy: mammographic appearance, *AJR Am J Roentgenol* 167:385–389, 1996.

Morris EA, Comstock CE, Lee CH, et al.: *ACR BI-RADS® magnetic resonance imaging. ACR BI-RADS® atlas, breast imaging reporting and data system*, Reston, VA, 2013, American College of Radiology.

Mund DF, Wolfson P, Gorczyca DP, et al.: Mammographically detected recurrent nonpalpable carcinoma developing in a transverse rectus abdominis myocutaneous flap. A case report, *Cancer* 74:2804–2807, 1994.

Munker R, Zorner C, McKiernan D, Opitz J: Prospective study of clinical findings and changes in 56 Trilucent implant explanations, *Aesthetic Plast Surg* 25:421–426, 2001.

Muzaffar AR, Rohrich RJ: The silicone gel-filled breast implant controversy: an update, *Plast Reconstr Surg* 109:742–748, 2002.

Noels EC, Lapid O, Lideman JH, Bastiaanner E: Breast implants and the risk of breast cancer: a meta-analysis of cohort studies, *Aesthet Surg J* 35:55–62, 2015.

Palmon LU, Foshager MC, Parantainen H, et al.: Ruptured or intact: what can linear echoes within silicone breast implants tell us? *AJR Am J Roentgenol* 168:1595–1598, 1997.

Patani N, Devalia H, Anderson A, Mokbel K: Oncological safety and patient satisfaction with skin-sparing mastectomy and immediate breast reconstruction, *Surg Oncol* 17:97–105, 2008.

Piza-Katzer H, Pulzl P, Balogh B, Wechselberger G: Long-term results of MISTI gold breast implants: a retrospective study, *Plast Reconstr Surg* 110:1425–1465, 2002.

Quaba O, Quaba A: PIP silicone breast implants: rupture rates based on the explantation of 676 implants in a single surgeon series, *J Plast Reconstr Aesthet Surg* 66:1182–1187, 2013.

Rieber A, Schramm K, Helms G, et al.: Breast-conserving surgery and autogenous tissue reconstruction in patients with breast cancer: efficacy of MRI of the breast in the detection of recurrent disease, *Eur Radiol* 13:780–787, 2003.

Rietjens M, Villa G, Toesca A, et al.: Appropriate use of magnetic resonance imaging and ultrasound to detect early silicone gel breast implant rupture in postmastectomy reconstruction, *Plast Reconstr Surg* 134:13e–20e, 2014.

Rivero MA, Schwartz DS, Mies C: Silicone lymphadenopathy involving intramammary lymph nodes: a new complication of silicone mammaplasty, *AJR Am J Roentgenol* 162:1089–1090, 1994.

Rizkalla M, Duncan C, Matthews RN: Trilucent breast implants: a 3-year series, *Br J Plast Surg* 54:125–127, 2001.

Rizkalla M, Webb J, Chuo CB, Matthews RN: Experience of explanation of Trilucent breast implants, *Br J Plast Surg* 55:117–119, 2002.

Rosculet KA, Ikeda DM, Forrest ME, et al.: Ruptured gel-filled silicone breast implants: sonographic findings in 19 cases, *AJR Am J Roentgenol* 159:711–716, 1992.

Rubin JP, Coon D, Zuley M, et al.: Mammographic changes after fat transfer to the breast compared with changes after breast reduction: a blinded study, *Plast Reconstr Surg* 129:1029–1038, 2012.

Saint-Cyr M, Nagarkar P, Schaverien M, et al.: The pedicled descending branch muscle-sparing latissimus dorsi flap for breast reconstruction, *Plast Reconstr Surg* 123:13–24, 2009.

Shah M, Tanna N, Margolies L: Magnetic resonance imaging of breast implants, *Top Magn Reson Imaging* 23:345–353, 2014.

Shaikh N, LaTrenta G, Swistel A, Osborne FM: Detection of recurrent breast cancer after TRAM flap reconstruction, *Ann Plast Surg* 47:602–607, 2001.

Silverstein MJ, Handel N, Gamagami P: The effect of silicone-gel-filled implants on mammography, *Cancer* 68(Suppl):1159–1163, 1991.

Silverstein MJ, Handel N, Gamagami P, et al.: Mammographic measurements before and after augmentation mammaplasty, *Plast Reconstr Surg* 86:1126–1130, 1990.

Slavin SA, Schnitt SJ, Duda RB, et al.: Skin-sparing mastectomy and immediate reconstruction: oncologic risks and aesthetic results in patients with early-stage breast cancer, *Plast Reconstr Surg* 102:49–62, 1998.

Soo MS, Kornguth PJ, Walsh R, et al.: Intracapsular implant rupture: MR findings of incomplete shell collapse, *J Magn Reson Imaging* 7:724–730, 1997.

Spear SL, Mardini S: Alternative filler materials and new implant designs: what's available and what's on the horizon? *Clin Plast Surg* 28:435–443, 2001.

Spear SL, Murphy DK: Allergan Silicone Breast Implant U.S. Core Clinical Study Group. Core Clinical Study Group. Natrelle round silicone breast implants: Core Study results at 10 years, *Plast Reconstr Surg* 133:1354–1361, 2014.

Stevens WG, Pacella SJ, Gear AJ, et al.: Clinical experience with a fourth-generation textured silicone gel breast implant: a review of 1012 Mentor MemoryGel breast implants, *Aesthet Surg J* 28:642–647, 2008.

Stewart NR, Monsees BS, Destouet JM, Rudloff MA: Mammographic appearance following implant removal, *Radiology* 185:83–85, 1992.

Stralman K, Mollerup CL, Kristoffersen US, Elberg JJ: Long-term outcome after mastectomy with immediate breast reconstruction, *Acta Oncol* 47:704–708, 2008.

Tugwell P, Wells G, Peterson J, et al.: Do silicone breast implants cause rheumatologic disorders? A systematic review for a court-appointed national science panel, *Arthritis Rheum* 44:2477–2484, 2001.

U.S. Food and Drug Administration: Guidance for Industry and FDA Staff—Saline, Silicone Gel and Alternative Breast Implants. http://www.fda.gov/medicaldevices/deviceregulationandguidance/guidancedocuments/ucm071228.htm. Accessed February 19, 2015a.

U.S. Food and Drug Administration: Regulatory history of implants in the US. http://www.fda.gov/MedicalDevices/ProductsandMedicalProcedures/ImplantsandProsthetics/BreastImplants/ucm064461.htm. Accessed February 6, 2015b.

Wazir U, Kasem A, Mokbel K: The clinical implications of Poly Implant Prothèse breast implants: an overview, *Arch Plast Surg* 42:4–10, 2015.

Wong JS, Ho AY, Kaelin CM, et al.: Incidence of major corrective surgery after post-mastectomy breast reconstruction and radiation therapy, *Breast J* 14:49–54, 2008.

Xu J, Wei S: Breast implant-associated anaplastic large cell lymphoma: review of a distinct clinicopathologic entity, *Arch Pathol Lab Med* 138:842–846, 2014.

Yoo H, Kim BH, Kim HH, Cha JH, Shin HJ, Lee TJ: Local recurrence of breast cancer in reconstructed breasts using TRAM flap after skin-sparing mastectomy: clinical and imaging features, *Eur Radiol* 24:2220–2226, 2014.

Young V, Watson M: Breast implant research: where we have been, where we are, where we need to go, *Clin Plast Surg* 28:451–483, 2001.

Young VL, Bartell T, Destouet JM, et al.: Calcification of breast implant capsule, *South Med J* 82:1171–1173, 1989.

Yueh JH, Slavin SA, Adesiyun T, et al.: Patient satisfaction in postmastectomy breast reconstruction: a comparative evaluation of DIEP, TRAM, latissimus flap, and implant techniques, *Plast Reconstr Surg* 125:1585–1595, 2010.

Chapter 10
Clinical Breast Problems and Unusual Breast Conditions

Debra M. Ikeda and Kanae K. Miyake

CHAPTER OUTLINE

Various breast symptoms and clinical problems are encountered in both benign breast conditions and breast cancer. This chapter briefly describes these conditions and elucidates how to distinguish them from malignancy.

THE MALE BREAST: GYNECOMASTIA AND MALE BREAST CANCER

The incidence of breast cancer in males is rare, constituting less than 1% of all breast cancers in the United States, so usually the symptoms for which men seek clinical attention are from benign disease. Men commonly present for breast imaging because of unilateral or bilateral breast enlargement, breast pain, or a palpable breast lump. Benign gynecomastia, an abnormal proliferation of benign ducts and supporting tissue that causes breast enlargement or a subareolar mass, with or without associated breast pain, is often the cause of many of these complaints in men.

Broad categories of conditions causing gynecomastia include high serum estrogen levels from endogenous or exogenous sources, low serum testosterone levels, endocrine disorders (hyperthyroidism or hypothyroidism), systemic disorders (cirrhosis, chronic renal failure with maintenance by dialysis, and chronic obstructive pulmonary disease), drug-induced (cimetidine, spironolactone, ergotamine, marijuana, anabolic steroids, and estrogen for prostate cancer), tumors (adrenal carcinoma, testicular tumors, and pituitary adenoma), or idiopathic (Box 10.1). Gynecomastia can occur at any age, but it may be seen in particular in neonates as a result of maternal estrogens circulating to the fetus through the placenta, in healthy adolescent boys 1 year after the onset of puberty because of high estradiol levels, or in older men as a result of decreasing serum testosterone levels.

Breast imaging in men is done in the same fashion as in women. The normal male breast is comprised of scant fatty tissue and a few major breast ducts. On the mammogram, the normal male breast consists of fat without obvious fibroglandular tissue, and the pectoralis muscles are usually larger than in women. In some men, there are faint strands of retroareolar tissue (Fig. 10.1); however, there is never as much tissue as in a woman in the normal male.

Pseudogynecomastia is a fatty proliferation of the breasts without proliferation of glandular tissue that simulates gynecomastia clinically, but unlike true gynecomastia, proliferation of glandular breast tissue does not occur.

In both pseudogynecomastia and in women with Turner syndrome, mammograms consist mostly of fat, similar to the normal male breast (Fig. 10.2).

Under a stimulus producing gynecomastia, ductal proliferation and stromal hyperplasia occurs with occasional ductal multiplication and elongation that produces breast enlargement, which may be reversible in the active phase if the stimulus is removed. If the stimulus persists, irreversible stromal fibrosis and ductal epithelial atrophy develop, and the breast enlargement may decrease but not completely resolve.

On the mammogram, gynecomastia in men is shown as glandular tissue in the subareolar region that is symmetric or asymmetric, unilateral or bilateral (Table 10.1). In a large series by Gunhan-Bilgen et al. (2002a), gynecomastia was unilateral in 45% and bilateral in 55% of 206 cases with mammograms. In the early phases of gynecomastia, the glandular tissue is flamelike, consisting of thin strands of glandular tissue extending from the nipple, like fingers extending posteriorly toward the chest wall (Fig. 10.3). With continued proliferation of breast ducts, the glandular tissue may take on a subareolar triangular nodular shape behind the nipple that can be symmetric (Figs. 10.4 and 10.5) or asymmetric (Fig. 10.6). When gynecomastia progresses to its later irreversible, stromal fibrotic phase it may take on the appearance of diffuse dense tissue (Fig. 10.7).

BOX 10.1 Causes of Gynecomastia

PHYSIOLOGIC

Liver disease
Renal failure
Chronic obstructive pulmonary disease
Diabetes
Hyperthyroidism
Hypothyroidism
Starvation/refeeding

DRUG RELATED

Sertraline (Zoloft)
Marijuana
Tricyclic antidepressants
Cimetidine
Spironolactone
Reserpine
Digitalis

HORMONAL

Neonates
Adolescence
Older men
Estrogen therapy
Testicular failure
Klinefelter syndrome
Hypogonadism

TUMORS

Lung
Pituitary
Adrenal
Hepatoma
Testicular

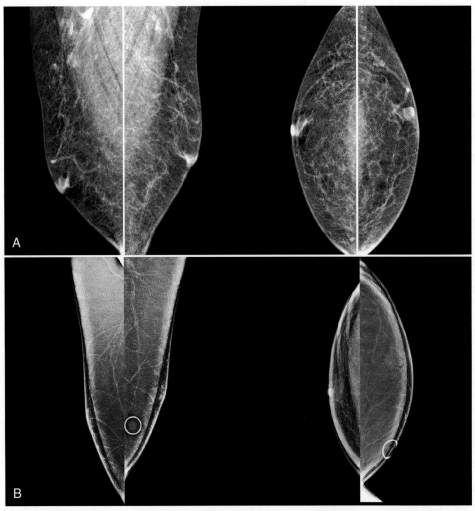

FIG. 10.1 Examples of male mammograms showing normal findings. (A) Mediolateral oblique (MLO; *left*) and craniocaudal (CC) mammograms (*right*) show mostly fatty tissue and normal, scant, flamelike strands of glandular tissue in the subareolar regions. (B) MLO (*left*) and CC (*right*) mammograms show thin subcutaneous fat on the thick pectoral muscles and tiny strands of retroareolar tissue that are much smaller than those in A. Note a ring marker placed on a mole.

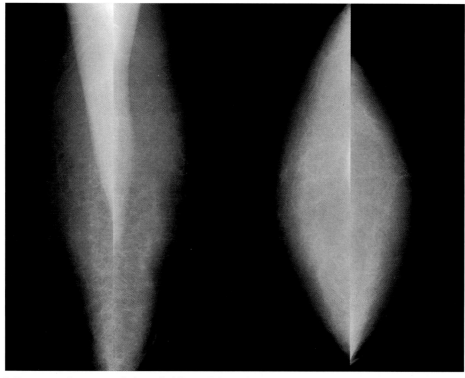

FIG. 10.2 Turner syndrome. Mediolateral oblique (*left*) and craniocaudal (*right*) mammograms show mostly fatty tissue, similar to the normal male breast, in this female patient with Turner syndrome.

TABLE 10.1   Mammographic Appearance of Gynecomastia

Type	Mammography	Gynecomastia
Normal	Fatty breast	N/A
Pseudogynecomastia	Fatty breast	N/A
Dendritic	Prominent radiating extensions	Epithelial hyperplasia
Nodular	Fan-shaped triangular density	Later phase
Diffuse	Diffuse density	Dense fibrotic phase

N/A, nonapplicable.

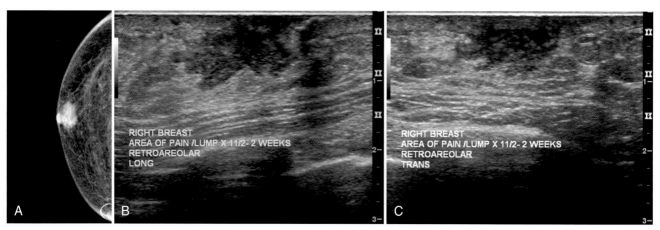

RIGHT BREAST
AREA OF PAIN /LUMP X 11/2- 2 WEEKS
RETROAREOLAR
LONG

RIGHT BREAST
AREA OF PAIN /LUMP X 11/2- 2 WEEKS
RETROAREOLAR
TRANS

A   B   C

FIG. 10.3 Gynecomastia in a male patient with a painful lump. Right mediolateral oblique view (A) shows a focal glandular tissue in the right subareolar region. Longitudinal (B) and transverse (C) ultrasounds show flamelike dendritic hypoechoic glandular tissue in a right retroareolar region that contains a painful lump.

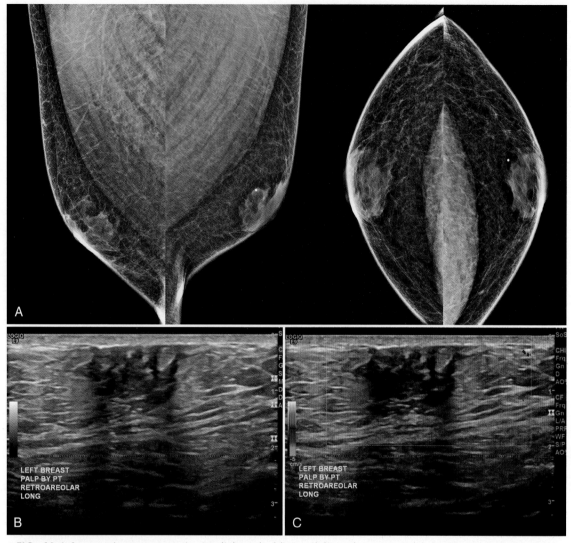

FIG. 10.4 Symmetric gynecomastia. Mediolateral oblique (*left*) and craniocaudal (*right*) mammograms (A) show triangular, focally dense breast tissue behind the nipple. Gray scale ultrasound (B) of the left breast shows hypoechoic dark strands of tissue extending from the nipple in a fingerlike triangular distribution. Doppler image (C) shows no abnormal vascularity in this hypoechoic tissue.

On ultrasound, gynecomastia is hypoechoic and consists of dark flamelike, fingerlike, or triangular structures extending posteriorly toward the chest wall from the nipple (see Figs. 10.3 to 10.7). Ultrasound is found to be of limited value when the mammogram clearly shows gynecomastia in symptomatic men but is clearly helpful when the mammogram is abnormal and suggesting cancer.

Male breast cancer accounts for less than 1% of all cancers found in men and is usually diagnosed at or around age 60 years old, which is older than the mean age for the diagnosis of breast cancer in women (Box 10.2). Male breast cancer has the same prognosis as breast cancer in women, but it is often detected at a higher stage than in women because of delay in diagnosis. Up to 50% of men have axillary adenopathy at initial evaluation. Risk factors include Klinefelter syndrome, high estrogen levels such as from prostate cancer treatment, and the development of mumps orchitis at an older age. Male breast cancer is generally manifested as a hard, painless, subareolar mass eccentric to the nipple. When the cancer is not subareolar, cancers in men are usually found in the upper outer quadrant. Clinical symptoms of nipple discharge or ulceration are not rare in association with male breast cancer.

On mammography, male breast cancers are generally dense noncalcified masses in the subareolar region (Figs. 10.8 and 10.9). Calcifications as the only indicator of cancers are less common in men than women, although calcifications may be present (Figs. 10.10 and 10.11). On ultrasound, male breast cancers are usually well circumscribed or irregularly marginated masses. Skin thickening, adenopathy (see Fig. 10.11), or skin ulceration are associated with a poor prognosis. Breast cancers in men are usually invasive ductal cancer in 85% of cases, and most of the remaining tumors are medullary, papillary, and intracystic papillary types. An associated component of ductal carcinoma in situ (DCIS) may be present. Invasive lobular carcinoma is rare. Treatment of breast cancer is the same for men as for women and consists of surgery, axillary node dissection, chemotherapy, and radiation therapy for invasive tumors; the prognosis is identical to women undergoing these treatments.

PREGNANT AND LACTATING PATIENTS AND PREGNANCY-ASSOCIATED BREAST CANCER

Pregnancy produces a proliferation of glandular breast tissue that results in breast enlargement and nodularity in response

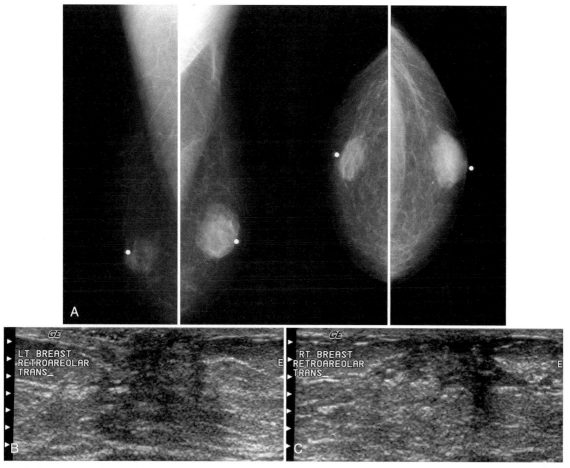

FIG. 10.5 Triangular nodular gynecomastia. Mediolateral oblique (*left*) and craniocaudal (*right*) mammograms (A) show triangular, focally dense breast tissue behind the nipple. Ultrasound of the left (B) and right (C) breast shows hypoechoic dark strands of tissue extending from the nipple in a fingerlike triangular distribution in this male with gynecomastia.

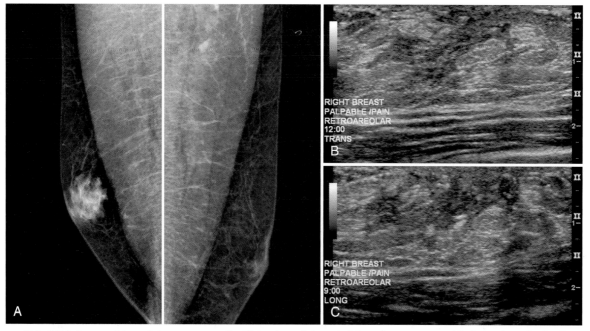

FIG. 10.6 Asymmetric nodular gynecomastia. Bilateral mediolateral oblique mammograms (A) show triangular focal asymmetric subareolar glandular breast tissue behind the right nipple, representing right gynecomastia, and a left normal mammogram. Ultrasound of the right retroareolar region on transverse (B) and longitudinal (C) scans show the typical, normal "fingerlike" hypoechoic dark strands of tissue from gynecomastia extending from the right nipple.

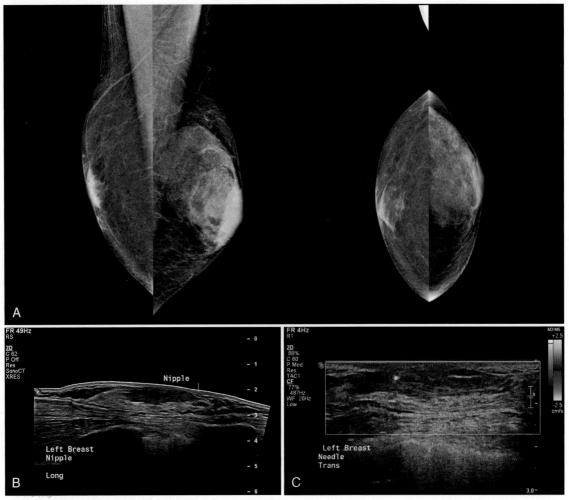

FIG. 10.7 Diffuse gynecomastia in left breast. Mediolateral oblique (*left*) and craniocaudal (*right*) mammograms (A) show asymmetric density behind the nipple. Density in the left breast is almost diffuse. Gray scale ultrasound (B) of the left breast shows hypoechoic dark tissue in the retroareolar area. Doppler image (C) shows no abnormal vascularity in this hypoechoic tissue.

BOX 10.2   Male Breast Cancer

Average age: 60 years
Hard, painless subareolar mass
Mass eccentric to the nipple or upper outer quadrant
Nipple discharge or ulceration not uncommon
Noncalcified round mass, variable border
Cancer usually ductal in origin
Treatment and prognosis identical to women's cancers

---

to female hormones. Fibroadenomas or adenomas of pregnancy respond to pregnancy hormones and may enlarge in this period. Breast masses are difficult to manage in a pregnant patient because surrounding breast nodularity and breast size increases over time. Most masses occurring in pregnancy are benign and include benign lactational adenomas, fibroadenomas, galactoceles, and abscesses (Box 10.3), but the diagnosis of exclusion is pregnancy-associated breast cancer.

Pregnancy-associated breast cancer is defined as breast cancer discovered during pregnancy or within 1 year of delivery (Box 10.4). The incidence of breast cancer in pregnant women is 0.2% to 3.8% of all breast cancers, or 1 in every 3000 to 10,000 pregnancies. Most pregnancy-associated breast cancers are usually invasive ductal cancer, and are usually estrogen receptor negative, similar to nonpregnant, premenopausal women of a similar age. The cancers generally present as a hard mass, but may be associated with bloody nipple discharge or breast edema.

Usually pregnant women are first imaged with breast ultrasound targeted to the area of concern. Pregnant patients often are reluctant to undergo mammography because they are worried about the effect of radiation on the fetus. If the doctor suspects cancer, and even though the breast tissue is dense from pregnancy, it is important to do the mammogram because it might show spiculated masses or suspicious calcifications. Furthermore, scattered radiation delivered by mammography to the fetus is low, and can be further reduced with lead shielding, with the dose about 0.004 Gy (Cardonick, 2014). Swinford et al. (1998) showed that the breast density is not always dense in pregnant and lactating women and varied from scattered fibroglandular density in pregnant patients to heterogeneously dense or dense in lactating women. In their series, mammography was as useful as it is in nonpregnant women who have clinical signs and symptoms of breast disease. In addition, imaging the breasts can be aided in lactating patients by pumping milk from the breasts before the study, thus reducing the breast density on the mammogram.

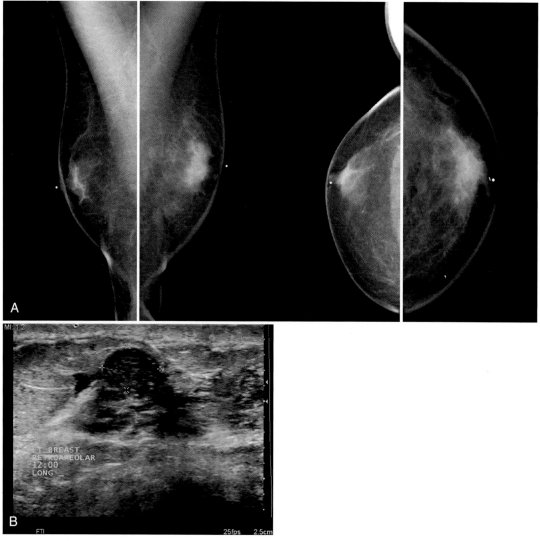

FIG. 10.8 Male breast cancer. In a patient with bilateral gynecomastia and a palpable mass in the left breast, bilateral mediolateral oblique (*left*) and craniocaudal (*right*) mammograms (A) show bilateral benign-appearing gynecomastia, with a marker on the right nipple and on an invisible palpable left breast mass obscured by the glandular tissue. Longitudinal ultrasound (B) shows a round, homogeneous, hypoechoic mass corresponding to the palpable finding within the gynecomastia. Biopsy showed invasive ductal cancer.

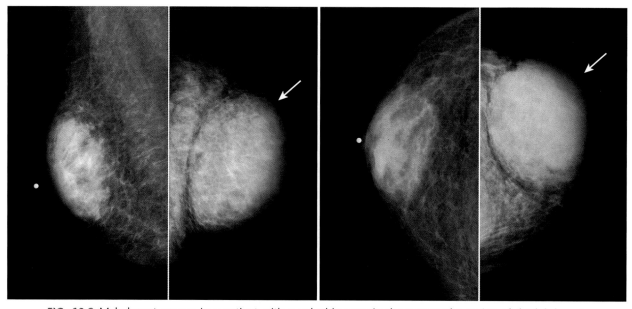

FIG. 10.9 Male breast cancer. In a patient with a palpable mass in the retroareolar region of the left breast, mediolateral oblique (*left*) and craniocaudal (*right*) mammograms show diffuse bilateral gynecomastia with a large oval retroareolar mass (*arrows*) on the left. Contrast the gynecomastia on the right, which shows indistinct breast tissue interfacing with fat, with the sharp smooth-bordered mass of the left breast cancer. Ultrasound-guided fine-needle aspiration of a portion of the mass showed invasive ductal cancer.

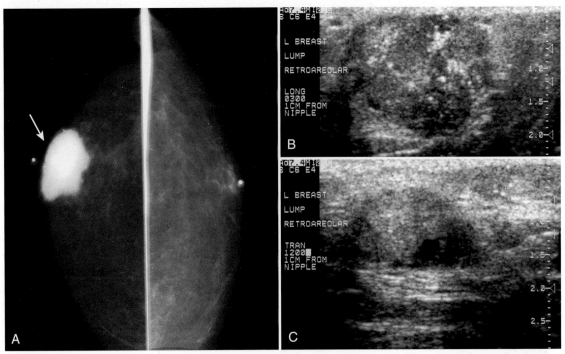

FIG. 10.10 Male breast cancer. Mediolateral oblique mammograms (A) show a round, irregular mass (*arrow*) with faint calcifications in the left breast. Longitudinal (B) and transverse (C) ultrasounds of a palpable mass in a man shows a suspicious hypoechoic oval mass with calcifications. Biopsy showed invasive ductal cancer.

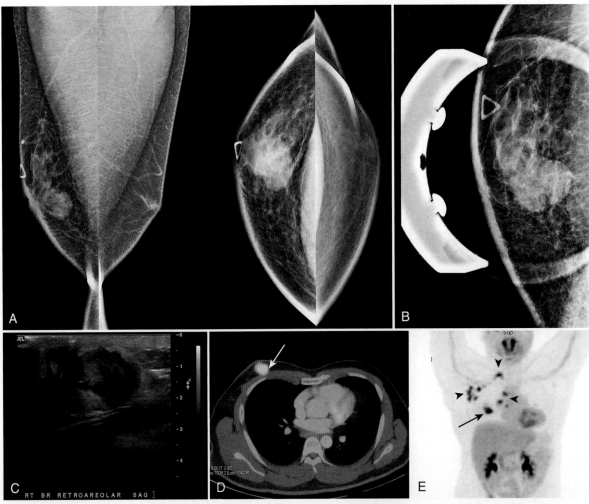

FIG. 10.11 Advanced male breast cancer. Mediolateral oblique (*left*) and craniocaudal (*right*) mammograms (A) show an asymmetric density with focally dense opacity in the right breast. Spot magnification lateral view (B) of right breast shows the mass accompanied with multiple faint calcifications. Ultrasound (C) of the palpable mass in the right breast shows a suspicious hypoechoic oval mass with irregular margins. Axial ^{18}F-fluorodeoxyglucose positron emission tomography (PET)/computed tomography image (D) and maximum intensity projection of the PET (E) show intense uptake (*arrows*) corresponding to the right breast mass. Biopsy showed invasive ductal cancer. Multiple lymph nodes metastases were present (E).

BOX 10.3 Pregnancy and Lactational Breast Problems

Growing fibroadenoma (rare)
Lactational adenoma (rare)
Cancer (rare)
Mastitis/abscess (common)
Galactocele (uncommon)
Benign bloody nipple discharge (uncommon)

BOX 10.4 Pregnancy-Associated Breast Cancer

Cancer diagnosed during pregnancy or within 1 year postpartum
Stage for stage, same prognosis as for nonpregnant patients
Mammography and ultrasound are indicated
Chemotherapy possible after the second trimester
Radiation therapy absolutely contraindicated

Mammography showed pregnancy-associated breast cancer in 78% of 23 pregnant women (Liberman et al., 1994) and in 86% of 15 cases (Ahn et al., 2003), as masses, pleomorphic calcifications, both masses and calcifications, asymmetries, and breast edema, or were negative because of dense breast tissue. Axillary lymphadenopathy, asymmetries, and skin or trabecular thickening were either primary findings or were associated findings of cancer. In both series, ultrasound was positive in all cases in which it was performed, usually showing irregular solid masses with irregular margins. In the series by Ahn et al. (2003), four masses also contained complex echo patterns or cystic components, and most showed acoustic enhancement.

Magnetic resonance imaging (MRI) contrast is generally contraindicated in the pregnant patient because gadolinium can cross the placenta and enter fetal circulation. There is experimental evidence showing the potential of the gadolinium ion to be freed from its chelate molecule and potentially enter the amniotic fluid (Expert Panel on MR Safety, 2013). Its effect on the fetus is unknown, and because of the association with nephrogenic systemic fibrosis in adults with impaired kidney function this consideration has led to a relative contraindication for the use of gadolinium in pregnant women. Other consensus groups have suggested that less toxic contrast media might be considered for use in MRI in pregnant women. In any case, there should be a strong, well-documented, thoughtful risk-benefit analysis supporting the benefits of a contrast-enhanced MRI study compared with theoretical but possible effects of free gadolinium ions on a developing fetus.

In a normal lactating breast, studies have shown that MRI can find breast cancer. A normal lactating breast will show dense, enhancing, diffuse glandular tissue and widespread high signal throughout the tissue on T2-weighted images. Breast cancer in a lactating breast on MRI shows higher signal intensity in the initial enhancement phase compared with normal surrounding lactational breast tissue (allowing the cancer to be detected), with that cancer showing a washout or plateau pattern in the late phases in the rare reported cases in the radiology literature.

A multidisciplinary approach to the pregnant patient is the cornerstone of care. Women with stages I and IIA breast cancer diagnosed during pregnancy have similar survival rates compared with nonpregnant women. However, a 2012 meta-analysis by Azim of 30 studies suggests pregnancy-associated breast cancers (cancers diagnosed postpartum) have a poorer prognosis compared with that of nonpregnant women. In pregnancy, diagnostic delays may cause breast cancer to be detected at a later stage, leading to a worse prognosis.

Treatment goals for pregnancy-associated breast cancer are the same as for nonpregnant women, which is to obtain both local and systemic control of the cancer, with the additional goal of minimizing fetal harm. Studies have shown that termination of the pregnancy does not usually improve patient survival, and the decision to terminate or continue the pregnancy is a personal one. However, the pregnancy gestational age can affect the treatment course since chemotherapy cannot be given in the first 12 weeks of gestation (the period of fetal organogenesis). Chemotherapy has been used safely in women after the first trimester. On the other hand, local control of the cancer by surgery can be performed at any gestational age with minimal risk to the fetus. Modified radical mastectomy was the usual treatment for pregnant women, who discuss breast-conserving surgery with their team just like nonpregnant patients. If women choose breast conservation, and radiation therapy is needed, radiation treatments would need to be postponed until they are postpartum. Pregnancy is an absolute contraindication for radiation therapy because of high fetal radiation dosages.

Benign conditions are the most frequent cause of breast masses in pregnant or lactating patients. Lactational mastitis is a common complication of breast feeding in which the breast becomes painful, indurated, and tender, usually as a result of *Staphylococcus aureus* infection. A cracked nipple may be the port of entry for the infecting bacteria, but it can be prevented by good nipple hygiene and care, along with frequent nursing to avoid breast engorgement. Treatment is administration of antibiotics and continuation of breast feeding. On occasion, antibiotic therapy is not sufficient to treat mastitis. If a hot, swollen, painful breast does not respond to antibiotics, ultrasound may identify an abscess and guide percutaneous drainage. On mammography, an abscess is a developing asymmetry or mass in a background of breast edema; it does not usually contain gas and is frequently located in the subareolar region (Fig. 10.12). On ultrasound, abscesses are fluid-filled structures with irregular margins in the early phase, but circumscribed margins develop in the later phase as the walls of the abscess form. The abscess may contain debris or multiple septations, which may be drained under ultrasound guidance, but some residua may remain because of thick debris. Ultrasound-guided percutaneous drainage may be curative in small abscesses <2.5 cm (Hook and Ikeda, 1999). Drainage may be palliative or curative in larger abscesses (Giess, 2014), but repeated drainages may be needed. If the abscess does not resolve or is refractory to either aspiration alone or catheter drainage placement, surgical incision and drainage may be needed. Some investigators report using ultrasound-guided aspiration for abscess irrigation and instilling antibiotics directly into the abscess cavity. This aids in resolution of the abscess and is done sometimes with percutaneous drain placement.

Both fibroadenomas and lactating adenomas are solid benign tumors diagnosed during pregnancy. Growth of preexisting fibroadenomas may be stimulated by elevated hormone levels of pregnancy, and the fibroadenoma may become clinically apparent. Infarction of fibroadenomas has been reported in the literature during pregnancy as well. On the other hand, the lactating adenoma is a firm, painless palpable mass occurring late in pregnancy or during lactation. The lactating adenoma is a circumscribed, lobulated mass containing distended tubules with an epithelial lining. The mass can enlarge rapidly during pregnancy and regress after cessation of lactation. Ultrasound typically shows an oval, well-defined hypoechoic mass that may contain echogenic bands representing the fibrotic bands seen on pathology (Fig. 10.13). It is not clear whether lactating adenomas arise from change stimulated by hormonal alterations in a fibroadenoma or tubular adenoma or if these tumors arise de novo.

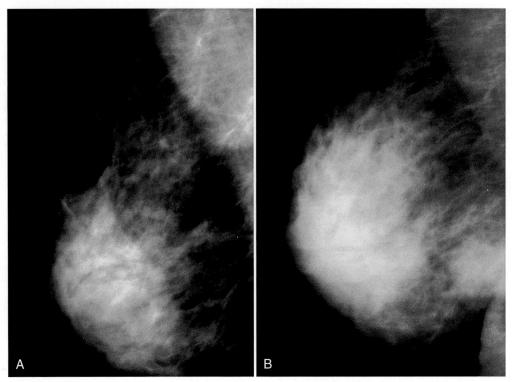

FIG. 10.12 Pregnancy-associated findings: abscess and mastitis. Mediolateral oblique mammogram (A) in a lactating patient shows dense tissue. After the development of mastitis and a lump near the chest wall, the mammogram (B) shows a developing density representing an abscess near the chest wall.

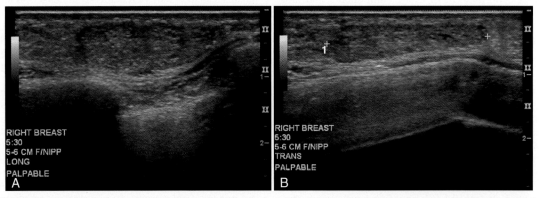

FIG. 10.13 Pregnancy-associated findings: lactating adenoma. Longitudinal (A) and transverse (B) ultrasounds in a patient with a palpable mass during pregnancy show an oval, homogeneous, well-circumscribed, palpable mass in the right breast that was larger during pregnancy and smaller after pregnancy. The differential diagnosis included fibroadenoma, adenoma of pregnancy, and well-circumscribed cancer. Biopsy showed lactating adenoma.

Sampling of solid masses for histologic examination in a pregnant or lactating patient can be accomplished safely by either percutaneous core biopsy or surgery. Milk fistula produced by damage to the breast ducts is an established, but uncommon complication of these biopsy procedures in women who are in the third trimester of pregnancy or who are lactating.

A galactocele produces a fluid-filled breast mass that can mimic a benign or malignant solid breast mass. On mammography, a galactocele is a round or oval, circumscribed mass of equal or low density (Fig. 10.14). Because a galactocele is filled with milk, the creamy portions of the milk may rise to the nondependent part of the galactocele and produce a rare, but pathognomonic fluid-fluid or fat-fluid appearance on the horizontal beam image (lateromedial view) at mammography. Ultrasound shows a fluid-filled mass that can have a wide range of sonographic appearances, depending on the relative amount of fluid and solid milk components within it. Galactoceles containing mostly fluid have well-defined margins with thin echogenic walls (Fig. 10.15). Galactoceles containing more solid milk components show variable findings, ranging from homogeneous medium-level echoes to heterogeneous contents with fluid clefts. Both distal acoustic enhancement and acoustic shadowing may be seen. A galactocele diagnosis

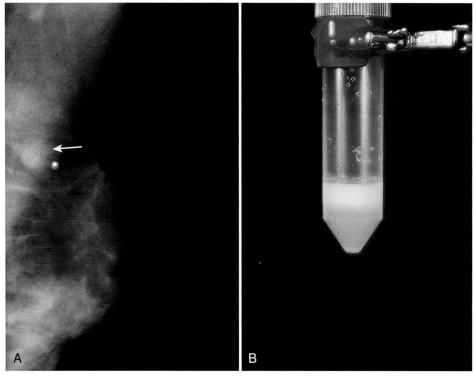

FIG. 10.14 Lactation-associated findings: galactocele. Mediolateral oblique mammogram (A) in a lactating patient with a marker over a palpable mass shows a low-density mass (*arrow*) in the upper portion of the left breast. Aspiration produced milky fluid with a fat-fluid level (B).

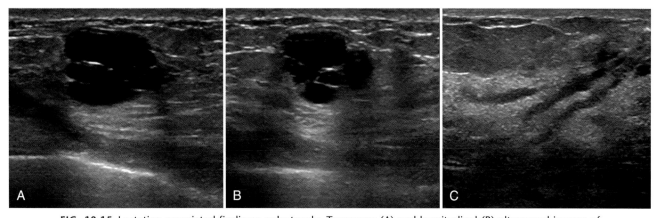

FIG. 10.15 Lactation-associated findings: galactocele. Transverse (A) and longitudinal (B) ultrasound images of galactocele show septated fluid-filled structure with enhanced through-sound. This galactocele had very little solid material in it. Prominent fluid-filled ducts during lactation are seen on ultrasound (C), showing the milk in the ducts before galactocele formation.

is made by an appropriate history of childbirth and lactation, with aspiration yielding milky fluid and leading to resolution of the mass. Aspiration is usually therapeutic.

PROBABLY BENIGN FINDINGS (BREAST IMAGING REPORTING AND DATA SYSTEM CATEGORY 3)

The Breast Imaging Reporting and Data System (BI-RADS) category 3, or Probably Benign, spectrum of findings (Box 10.5) include three entities: nonpalpable, noncalcified, round or lobulated, circumscribed solid masses (Fig. 10.16); nonpalpable focal asymmetries containing interspersed fat and concave scalloped margins that resemble fibroglandular tissue at diagnostic evaluation (Fig. 10.17); and solitary grouped punctate calcifications (Fig. 10.18). The Probably Benign category arose because mammography screening detects cancer but also uncovers indeterminate but benign-appearing lesions requiring recall. Fine-detail diagnostic mammographic views and ultrasound show that some indeterminate findings are typically benign and are dismissed, others are cancer, and yet others are most likely benign but do not fulfill all criteria for a typically benign finding (probably benign). Findings that qualify for the probably benign BI-RADS category 3 have a low probability (<2%) of malignancy and are followed with short-term mammography, so the diagnostic workup serves as a baseline for short-term, interval follow-up studies. In screening mammography series Sickles (1991), Varas et al. (1992, 2002), and Yasmeen et al. (2003) showed that probably benign findings have a small chance of malignancy. Probably

From Rosen EL, Baker JA, Soo MS: Malignant lesions initially subjected to short-term mammographic follow-up, *Radiology* 223:221–228, 2002; from ACR BI-RADS®–Mammography. *ACR BI-RADS® atlas, breast imaging reporting and data system.* Reston, Reston, VA, 2013, American College of Radiology.

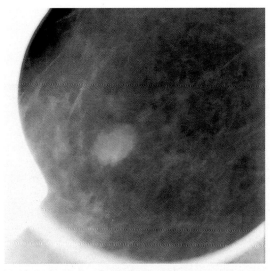

FIG. 10.16 Probably benign finding on mammography: noncalcified circumscribed mass. Spot mammogram shows a nonpalpable, round, well-circumscribed solid mass.

benign BI-RADS category 3 lesions were present in 5, 3, and 5% of all screening studies in their series, respectively.

Probably benign findings usually are found on baseline screening mammograms (no prior mammograms). These findings are designated as BI-RADS category 3 only after a full diagnostic mammographic evaluation and (in some cases) ultrasound. Probably benign findings have 6-month interval imaging only after the workup. BI-RADS 2013 emphasizes that a BI-RADS category 3 assignment is not allowed directly from screening. The reasoning for a full diagnostic workup before a category 3 assignment is that the workup (1) shows that some findings are truly benign such as cysts, skin calcifications, and lymph nodes, which may be returned to screening immediately or (2) shows cancer incompletely evaluated at screening, prompting biopsy.

For a single nonpalpable mass to be probably benign, the margin must be circumscribed around 75% of its edge; the remaining 25% may be obscured but must not show any signs of malignancy, such as ill-defined or spiculated borders. Multiple bilateral similar-appearing circumscribed or partially circumscribed masses may be considered BI-RADS category 2 (benign), because it has been shown that the rate of malignancy among multiple masses is 0.14%, which was lower than the age-matched U.S. incident breast cancer rate of 0.24%. For a focal asymmetry to be considered probably benign, it should not be associated with any mass, suspicious calcifications, or architectural distortion. Other inclusion criteria for the probably benign lesions are that they are nonpalpable, identifiable at imaging, and that the patients are likely to be compliant with follow-up imaging. Criteria that may exclude patients from short-term follow-up include extreme anxiety affecting the patient's quality of life, pregnancy or planned pregnancy, or a likelihood of noncompliance with follow-up.

Short-term 6-month mammographic unilateral follow-up for category 3 is an alternative to percutaneous core or surgical biopsy. Because the average breast cancer has a tumor volume doubling time of 100 days, growth should be detectable in 2 to 3 years. In the United States probably benign findings are usually followed for 2 to 3 years for this reason.

The usual follow-up for probably benign lesions is a 6-month unilateral mammogram, 12-month bilateral mammogram, and 24-month bilateral mammogram (with optional 36-month bilateral mammogram). If a category 3 finding is stable on the initial 6-month unilateral mammogram, the finding is assigned a category 3 again and recommended for another 6-month follow-up. At the next 6-month follow-up (or 1 year from initial detection) both breasts are imaged (because the opposite breast will be ready for a 12-month screening). If the finding is stable at this first 12-month follow-up, the BI-RADS code is changed to category 2 benign and recommended for a second 1-year follow-up. If the finding is stable at the 24-month follow-up, the B-IRADS code is still category 2 benign, and the patient is returned to screening

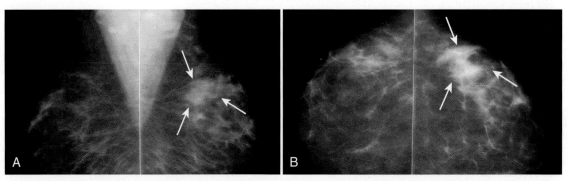

FIG. 10.17 Probably benign finding on mammography: focal asymmetry. Mediolateral oblique (A) and craniocaudal (B) mammograms show focal asymmetry (*arrows*) consisting of a nonpalpable greater volume of tissue in the upper outer portion of the left breast than in the right.

(with some facilities opting for a 36-month follow-up at this point). Probably benign breast lesions are selected on the basis that they will most likely not change in the time interval. Lesions in which growth is anticipated should undergo biopsy.

Rosen et al. (2002) reviewed the findings of cancers initially subjected to short-term follow-up to identify imaging criteria that should exclude initial assessment as BI-RADS category 3. They showed that cancers mistakenly classified as category 3 did not qualify as a probably benign finding and included palpable lesions, developing densities, architectural distortion, irregular spiculated masses, growing masses, pleomorphic calcifications, workups showing motion blur on magnification, and lesion progression of any type on mammograms. Their results emphasize that lesions should only be assessed as probably benign and assigned to short-term follow-up (instead of immediate biopsy) after optimal diagnostic workup. Data from the Breast Cancer Surveillance Consortium show that the few cancers that were initially assessed as probably benign are of early-stage and favorable prognosis, but only if full diagnostic imaging evaluation was initially performed. In contrast, cancers that were initially assessed as probably benign based on screening mammographic views and which were not recalled for diagnostic evaluation, were later stage (and of less favorable prognosis).

It is expected that a small number of cancers develop within BI-RADS category 3 lesions, with a probability of malignancy of less than 2%. Varas et al. (2002) showed that in their series of probably benign lesions, 0.4% of cases were cancer at follow-up, mostly stage 1 or less, as in the series by Sickles (1991).

Category 3 was based on longitudinal data derived from mammography, which is a well-established imaging modality. In clinical practice category 3 has been used with ultrasound and MRI but without the longitudinal data available for mammographic studies, specifically because mammography has been used for a longer period of time. However, data indicate that short-term follow-up may be indicated for palpable or nonpalpable circumscribed round, oval, or gently lobulated masses on mammography and ultrasound.

There is emerging data on MRI category 3 findings with carcinoma probability in MRI ranging from 0.6% to 10% (Liberman et al., 2003; Sadowski et al., 2005; Eby et al., 2007; Weinstein et al., 2010; Spick et al., 2014; Grimm et al., 2015). Data-supported recommendations for possible MRI category 3 lesions from BI-RADS 2013 indicate that short-term follow-up may be appropriate of a "1) new unique focus separate from background parenchymal enhancement (BPE) but has benign morphologic and kinetic features and 2) a mass on an initial examination with benign morphologic and kinetic features" (Morris et al., 2013). Normal background BPE is seen on almost all MRI examinations, and published data suggest that BPE should not be followed as a category 3 finding (Hambly, 2011). There should be caution regarding inappropriate overuse of the probably benign category in MRI. Among three single-institutional studies a high number, 8.5% (Spick et al., 2014), 17% (Sadowski et al., 2005), and 24% (Liberman et al. 2003), of the MRI cases were assessed as probably benign with a recommendation for short-term follow-up MRI. These numbers are substantially higher than those reported for mammographic lesions.

NIPPLE DISCHARGE AND GALACTOGRAPHY

Nipple discharge is a common reason for women to seek medical advice. Benign nipple discharge usually arises from multiple ducts, whereas nipple discharge from a papilloma or DCIS usually occurs from a single duct. Nipple discharge is of particular concern if it is spontaneous and from a single duct or if the discharge is bloody. Women may describe intermittent discharge producing tiny stains on their brassiere or nightgown, or they may be able to elicit the discharge themselves. Some women present for imaging evaluation after positive findings from ductal lavage in conjunction with an abnormal cytologic evaluation.

The most frequent causes of both nonbloody and bloody nipple discharge are benign conditions. The most common mass producing a bloody nipple discharge is a benign intraductal papilloma, with only approximately 5% of women found to have malignancy at biopsy. The bloody nipple discharge associated with papillomas is caused by twisting of the papilloma on its fibrovascular stalk with subsequent infarction and bleeding. Other causes of bloody discharge are cancer, benign findings such as duct hyperplasia/ectasia, and pregnancy as a result of rapidly proliferating breast tissue. Causes of nonbloody nipple discharge are fibrocystic change, medications acting as dopamine receptor blockers or dopamine-depleting drugs, rapid breast growth during adolescence, chronic nipple squeezing, or tumors producing prolactin or prolactin-like substances (Table 10.2).

Papillomas are benign masses consisting of a fibrovascular stalk with an attachment to the wall and breast duct epithelium; they have a variable cellular pattern and can produce nipple discharge. Papillomas may be single or multiple and may extend along the ducts for quite a distance. When large, papillomas can appear to be encysted and multilobulated. Some pathologists support the theory that peripheral papillomas have an increased risk for the subsequent development

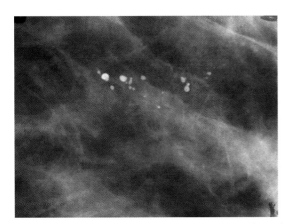

FIG. 10.18 Probably benign findings on mammography: solitary group of punctate calcifications. Photography-magnified mammographic view shows grouped punctate calcifications, including several round calcifications.

TABLE 10.2 Nipple Discharge

Color	Cause
Clear or creamy	Duct ectasia
Green, white, blue, black	Cysts, duct ectasia
Milky	Physiologic (neonatal)
	Endocrine (lactation/postlactation and pregnancy)
	Tumor (prolactinoma or other prolactin-producing tumor)
	Mechanical
	Drugs (dopamine receptor blockers/ dopamine-depleting drugs)
Bloody or blood related	Hyperplasia
	Papilloma
	Ductal carcinoma in situ or invasive cancer
	Pregnancy

of carcinoma, whereas solitary or central papillomas do not. Peripheral papillomas are associated with epithelial proliferation, which may have atypical features, raising the possibility that atypia within a peripheral papilloma increases the risk of malignancy rather than the location of the papilloma itself.

The mammogram is frequently negative in the setting of nipple discharge (Table 10.3). Mammographic findings described in association with nipple discharge include a negative mammogram, a single dilated duct in isolation (Fig. 10.19), and a small mass with or without calcifications in either a papilloma or papillary carcinoma. Ultrasound is frequently done in women with nipple discharge, usually done in the retroareolar region, and is often negative, but occasionally shows fluid-filled dilated ducts with or without an intraductal mass (Fig. 10.20; see 10.19B). Solid masses in a fluid-filled duct may represent debris, a papilloma, or cancer.

Papillomas on MRI deserve special mention because they mimic cancer by producing a round enhancing mass that frequently has rapid initial early enhancement and a late plateau or washout on kinetic curve analysis, which is indistinguishable from invasive cancer (Fig. 10.21). For this reason, papillomas are a common cause of false-positive MRI-guided breast biopsies. On MRI, intraductal papillomas can have three patterns. The first pattern is a small circumscribed enhancing mass at the terminus of a dilated breast duct, corresponding to the filling defect seen on galactography. The second pattern is an irregular, rapidly enhancing mass with occasional spiculation or rim enhancement in women without nipple discharge; this is the pattern that cannot be distinguished from invasive breast cancer. In some cases, blood or debris in the duct may cause precontrast high duct signal and is a cause of false-negative MRI studies because an enhancing mass cannot be detected against the high signal in the duct. Finally, despite the presence of a papilloma, the MRI may be negative, and the papilloma is undetected on contrast-enhanced fat-suppressed T1-weighted studies. Studies are mixed when recommending MRI for nipple discharge, with some studies showing good results detecting papillomas (Lubina, 2015), whereas others show the value of MRI is limited (van Gelder, 2015). Still others have used MRI galactography to show the ducts in an attempt to display pathology or intraductal masses with only limited success. We recommend that if the mammogram and ultrasound are negative, and there is no precontrast high duct signal to obscure enhancing intraductal masses, a negatvie MRI supports follow-up rather than surgery.

Galactography or ductography is a study that investigates single-duct nipple discharge by injecting radiopaque contrast into the discharging duct. When it shows filling defects in the ducts it helps subsequent surgical planning by identifying their location and distance from the nipple. Galactography may also show normal duct anatomy, duct ectasia, or fibrocystic change. To perform galactography, the radiologist wears magnifying glasses and expresses the nipple discharge to pinpoint the discharging duct in the nipple. The radiologist cleans the nipple, may use a topical anesthetic, and with sterile technique, cannulates the discharging duct with a 30-gauge blunt-tipped sialogram needle connected to tubing and a syringe filled with contrast. Usually, the needle will fall painlessly into the duct,

TABLE 10.3 Imaging of Nipple Discharge

Modality	Finding
Mammography	Negative (common) Dilated duct Mass with or without calcifications (papilloma or cancer)
Ultrasound	Negative (common) Fluid-filled ducts (normal or pathologic) Intraductal mass (papilloma, cancer, and debris)
Galactogram	Filling defect (papilloma, cancer, air bubble, and debris) Duct ectasia or cysts
Magnetic resonance imaging	Negative Fluid in dilated ducts Enhancing mass (cancer and papilloma)

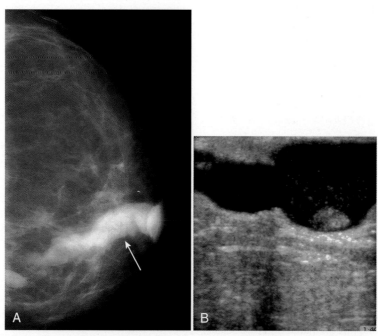

FIG. 10.19 Papilloma in a dilated duct on mammography. Left craniocaudal mammogram (A) shows a markedly dilated duct (without contrast) extending into the breast from the nipple. Ultrasound (B) revealed a fluid-filled dilated duct containing a mass, which was found to be a papilloma on biopsy.

but on occasion, warm compresses are needed to relax the duct opening. The radiologist injects 0.2 to 1 mL of contrast into the duct until they feel resistance or the patient feels a sense of fullness in the breast. Because the ducts are quite fragile, pain or burning may indicate duct perforation or contrast extravasation. The cannulation and/or the injection should not be painful. Either symptom is an indication to stop the procedure and reevaluate the situation.

After the injection, the radiologist either tapes the needle in place or withdraws the needle and the contrast-filled duct

is sealed with collodion for subsequent craniocaudal and mediolateral mammograms to see the contrast-filled ducts. Magnification views may help to evaluate the ducts for filling defects. After the mammogram, the radiologist expresses the contrast from the ducts by gentle massage. If duct filling is incomplete, if the contrast is diluted by retained secretions, or if an air bubble is simulating an intraductal filling defect, the contrast can be expressed from the nipple and then the duct can be reinjected immediately for a second, better, contrast-filled study.

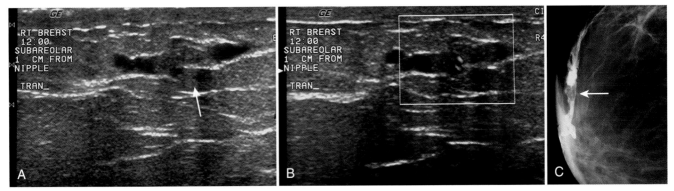

FIG. 10.20 Papilloma in a dilated duct on ultrasound. Gray scale ultrasound (A) shows the papilloma as a solid mass (*arrow*) surrounded by the distended, contrast-filled duct. On color Doppler ultrasound (B), a blood vessel is seen in its fibrovascular component. On galactography (C), this papilloma is depicted as a filling defect (*arrow*) in a dilated contrast-filled duct.

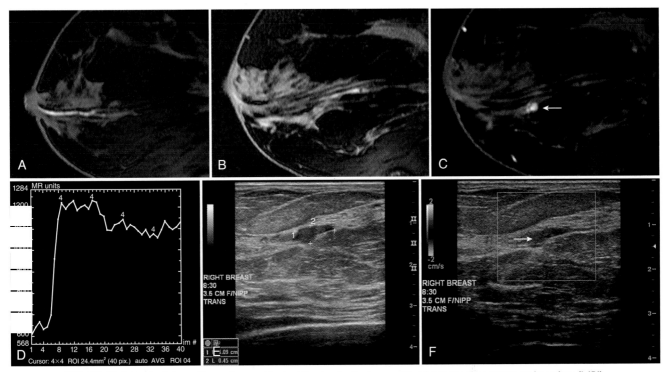

FIG. 10.21 Intraductal papilloma in a patient with nipple discharge. (A–D) Magnetic resonance imaging (MRI). Noncontrast T2-weighted sagittal MRI (A) shows a bright fluid-filled duct extending from the nipple into the midbreast. Noncontrast sagittal 3D spectral-spatial excitation magnetization transfer (3DSSMT) MRI (B) shows high signal fluid within the lower breast ducts before contrast enhancement. Postcontrast sagittal 3DSSMT MRI (C) shows a round enhancing mass in a duct (*arrow*), which previously had a slight high signal fluid within it on B. The kinetic curve of the round mass in C show fast initial enhancement and late washout, identical to kinetic curves in invasive cancer. (E and F) Breast ultrasound. B-mode image (E) shows a mass within a fluid-filled duct. Doppler ultrasound (F) shows a pulsating blood vessel (*arrow*) within the mass, accounting for the fast enhancement and washout. Biopsy showed intraductal papilloma.

A normal duct arborizes from a single entry point on the nipple into smaller ducts extending over almost an entire quadrant of the breast. Normal ducts are thin and smooth walled and have no filling defects or wall irregularities (Fig. 10.22A). Ductal ectasia is not uncommon; occasionally normal cysts or lobules fill from the dilated ducts (Fig. 10.22B). Ectatic ducts without a filling defect are usually normal. However, despite a normal galactogram, surgical excision of the discharging duct may still reveal papillomas or cancer on histology (ie, false-negative study; Fig. 10.22C).

Ducts containing malignancy or papillomas are typically dilated between the tumor and the nipple. Positive galactograms show a filling defect, an abrupt duct cutoff, or luminal irregularity and distortion (Figs. 10.23–10.25). Tumors causing the abnormal findings may be located inside a fluid-filled dilated duct or may compress the duct from outside the duct walls. On occasion, masses, either papilloma or intracystic cancer, may become encysted (Fig. 10.26). Air bubbles produce filling defects that mimic papilloma or cancer, but they are usually sharply defined and round and change position inside the duct on repeat injection, unlike fixed intraductal tumors. On the galactogram, extravasation is seen as contrast extending outside the duct lumen into the breast tissue and obscuring the underlying breast tissue and ducts (Fig. 10.27). In the rare instance of lymphatic or venous uptake of extravasated contrast, a draining tubular structure leading away from the extravasation site can be seen.

A positive galactogram usually leads to biopsy, either by preoperative needle localization or by ductoscopy. Preoperative needle localization of filling defects after galactography under x-ray guidance may be helpful for surgical planning, especially if the intraductal mass is deep in the breast. Negative

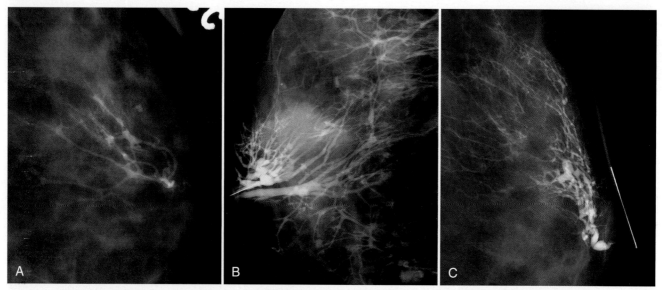

FIG. 10.22 Examples of normal galactograms. (A) Normal galactogram showing contrast filling nondilated ducts without an abrupt cutoff or intraductal filling defects to suggest cancer or a papilloma. (B) Normal galactogram demonstrating acinar filling. The galactogram shows two normally filling ducts, thin in diameter and without filling defects, and rounded acini filling in the periphery. (C) Normal galactogram showing nondilated contrast-filled ducts in a patient with nipple discharge. Ductoscopy revealed two microscopic papillomas (false-negative galactogram).

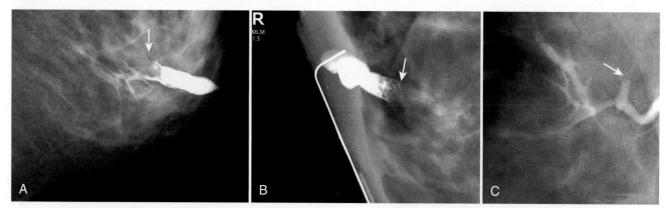

FIG. 10.23 Abnormal galactograms: examples of papilloma. (A) A filling defect (*arrow*) on the galactogram corresponded to a retroareolar papilloma at surgery. (B) Magnified right lateral mammogram after contrast injection into the duct shows the papillary filling defect (*arrow*), representing a papilloma. (C) Galactogram with an abrupt cutoff (*arrow*) in a proximal duct. Biopsy showed papilloma.

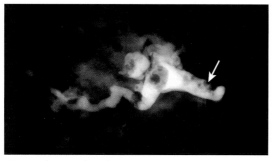

FIG. 10.24 Abnormal galactogram: ductal carcinoma in situ (DCIS). Galactogram showing cancer. A magnification view of a galactogram reveals an irregular filling defect (*arrow*) in the retroareolar region. Biopsy showed DCIS.

galactograms, despite the presence of a papilloma on biopsy, have been reported. Galactography has a sensitivity ranging from 69% to 78% for tumors.

In the early 1990s, surgeons reported using a tiny ductoscope to cannulate a discharging duct for identification of papillomas or other intraductal masses intraoperatively to guide surgery. Dooley (2003) reported that 16% of women undergoing ductoscopy at surgery had lesions detected by ductoscopy that were not seen on either ductograms or mammograms before surgery.

NIPPLE AND SKIN RETRACTION

Long-standing nipple inversion is not uncommon and is benign if it is present at birth. On the other hand, new nipple inversion is worrisome because retroareolar breast cancers can pull in the

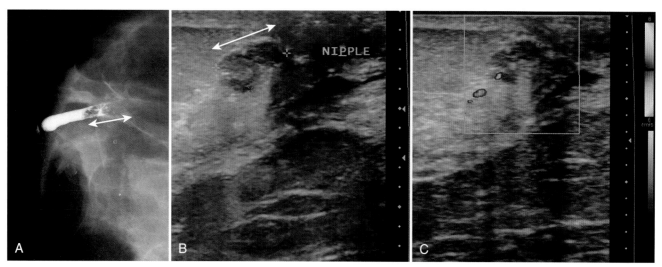

FIG. 10.25 Abnormal galactogram: ductal carcinoma in situ (DCIS) arising within an intraductal papilloma. Galactogram (A) shows a complex-appearing filling defect, which measures at least 10 to 15 mm in size (*double-headed arrow*) in a patient with 5-month history of spontaneous nipple discharge that started initially as brown nipple discharge. Gray scale ultrasound (B) shows a lobulated hypoechoic nodule just deep to the skin surface that measures 8.8 mm in size (*double-headed arrow*). The mass demonstrates vascularity with Doppler interrogation (C). Ultrasound-guided wire localization and lumpectomy were performed. The mass was proven as DCIS and atypical ductal hyperplasia arising within an intraductal papilloma.

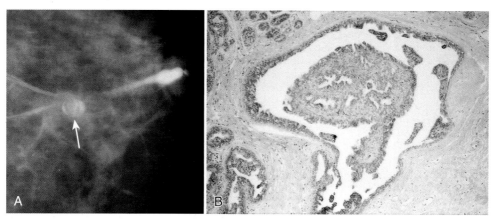

FIG. 10.26 Encysted papilloma. Galactogram (A) show a filling defect (*arrow*) in a cyst. Photomicrograph (B) of the encysted papilloma.

nipple by productive fibrosis or invasion, causing the nipple to retract or invert (Figs. 10.28 and 10.29).

Skin retraction or skin dimpling is not uncommon after surgical excisional biopsy. However, in the absence of biopsy, skin or nipple retraction may be a sign of breast cancer caused by superficial cancers tethering or invading the skin and pulling the skin in toward the breast. On physical examination, skin retraction or tethering might become evident when the woman raises her arms as she inspects her breasts in the mirror. Raising her arms or placing her hands on her hips pulls in the pectoralis muscle, which pulls on the cancer, which pulls on the skin, and dimples the skin in toward the cancer. On mammography with a BB marker placement on the site of skin dimpling, a suspicious mass sometimes may be identified under the BB marker (Fig. 10.30).

BREAST EDEMA

On clinical examination, breast edema may be evident as *peau d'orange* (a term signifying thickening and elevation of the skin around tethered hair follicles, making the skin's appearance similar to an orange peel). The edematous breast may be larger than the contralateral side. The differential diagnosis for breast edema depends on whether the edema is unilateral or bilateral (Box 10.6). Unilateral breast edema is caused by mastitis, inflammatory cancer (Figs. 10.31–10.33), local obstruction of lymph nodes (Fig. 10.34), trauma (Fig. 10.35), radiation therapy, or coumarin necrosis. Bilateral breast edema is caused by systemic etiologies, such as congestive heart failure, liver disease, anasarca, renal failure (Fig. 10.36), or other conditions that can cause edema elsewhere in the body. Alternatively, bilateral lymphadenopathy or superior vena cava obstruction for any reason may cause bilateral breast edema (Fig. 10.37). The key to diagnosis is to obtain an accurate clinical history and evaluate the breast for any signs of cancer.

The mammogram shows breast edema as skin thickening greater than 2 to 3 mm, coarsening of trabeculae in subcutaneous fat because of fluid within subdermal lymphatics, producing thick white lines in subdermal fat that have an appearance similar to Kerley B lines at the periphery of the lung on chest radiographs in congestive heart failure. An edematous breast is much denser and whiter than the contralateral side because of fluid in the breast tissue.

The differential diagnosis for increased bilateral breast density on mammography includes breast edema, exogenous hormone therapy, and weight loss. Increased breast density from edema is caused by breast tissue fluid overload. Increased breast density from exogenous hormone therapy is caused by hormonally

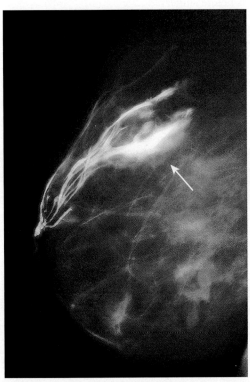

FIG. 10.27 Extravasation on galactography. The mammogram shows extravasation (*arrow*) of contrast outside the normal thin ducts.

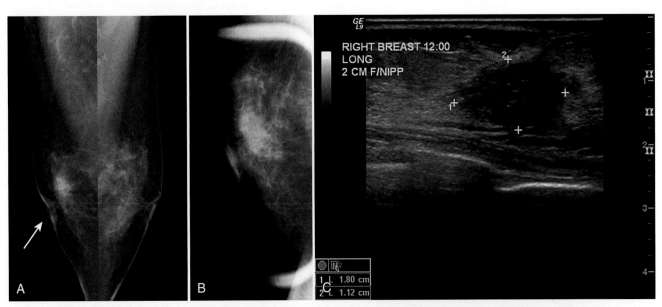

FIG. 10.28 Nipple retraction caused by cancer. Mediolateral oblique (MLO) mammograms (A) show a retroareolar mass under the right nipple. Note the slightly retracted position of right nipple (*arrow*) compared with the left nipple. Spot-magnified MLO view (B) shows a spiculated mass below the nipple. Ultrasound (C) shows a hypoechoic mass with irregular margin behind the nipple. Biopsy showed ductal carcinoma in situ.

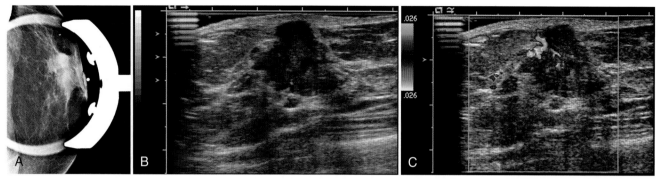

FIG. 10.29 Nipple retraction and inversion caused by cancer. Spot-magnified mammogram (A) shows a mass involving the nipple. Gray scale ultrasound (B) shows a hypoechoic mass with irregular margin, extending to the nipple, corresponding the mass in A. Color Doppler image (C) shows hypervascularity within the tumor. Pathology was invasive breast cancer.

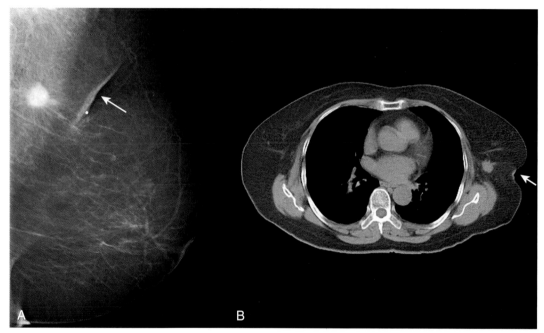

FIG. 10.30 Skin retraction and skin thickening. Left mediolateral oblique mammogram (A) shows an axillary spiculated mass, proven to be invasive ductal cancer, accompanied with a secondary sign of indrawing of the skin (*arrow*), marked by a metallic BB skin marker. The dark air is seen adjacent to the skin fold. An axial plane of computed tomography (B) shows the skin thickening (*arrow*) at the site of skin retraction caused by the spiculated mass.

BOX 10.6 Causes of Breast Edema

UNILATERAL

Mastitis
Staphylococcus aureus (common)
Tuberculosis (rare)
Syphilis (rare)
Hydatid disease (rare)
Molluscum contagiosum
Abscess complicating mastitis
Recurrent subareolar abscess
Inflammatory cancer
Trauma

Coumarin necrosis
Unilateral lymph node obstruction
Radiation therapy

BILATERAL

Congestive heart failure
Anasarca
Renal failure
Lymphadenopathy
Superior vena cava syndrome
Liver disease

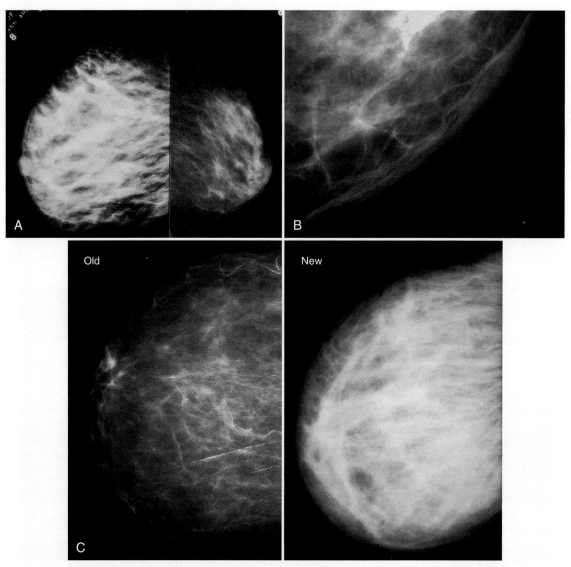

FIG. 10.31 Unilateral breast edema: three examples with inflammatory breast cancer. (A) Unilateral breast edema on the right breast secondary to inflammatory cancer. Note the larger and whiter appearance of the right breast compared with the left, as well as marked coarsening of the trabeculae. (B) Breast edema. A cropped, magnified mammogram shows skin thickening and atypical engorgement of the subdermal lymphatics in subcutaneous fat causing a trabecular pattern similar to Kerley B lines on a chest radiograph. Inflammatory cancer was the diagnosis. (C) Normal mammogram before the development of inflammatory cancer (*left*) and mammogram with breast edema 8 months later (*right*).

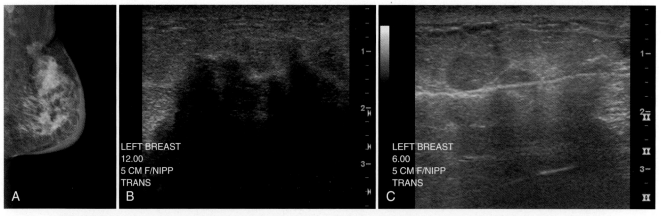

FIG. 10.32 Unilateral breast edema: mammographic and ultrasonographic appearance of inflammatory breast cancer. Left mediolateral oblique mammogram (A) shows marked skin thickening and an extensive breast cancer and axillary adenopathy. Note the marked skin thickening and breast edema. Left breast ultrasound (B) shows the marked skin thickening in the near field and a markedly shadowing spiculated invasive ductal cancer. Ultrasound image during a core biopsy of a lower invasive ductal cancer in the same patient (C) shows the skin thickening in the near field to greater advantage. The fat is gray, compatible with breast edema.

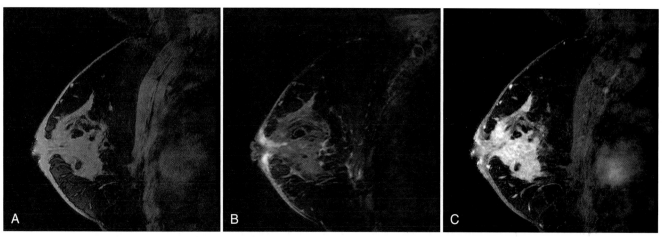

FIG. 10.33 Unilateral breast edema: magnetic resonance imaging (MRI) appearance of inflammatory breast cancer. In a patient with a large retroareolar breast cancer, precontrast sagittal 3D spectral-spatial excitation magnetization transfer (3DSSMT) MRI (A) shows skin thickening, nipple retraction, and dense tissue behind the nipple. Sagittal precontrast T2-weighted fat-suppressed MRI (B) shows breast edema with fluid in the periareolar region and within thickened skin. Postcontrast sagittal 3DSSMT MRI (C) shows marked enhancement of a large cancer in the retroareolar region, skin thickening, and enhancement of the areola and skin, which is abnormal. Biopsy showed inflammatory cancer.

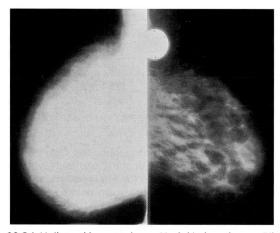

FIG. 10.34 Unilateral breast edema: Hodgkin lymphoma. Bilateral mediolateral oblique mammograms show unilateral breast edema from lymphoma and obstruction of the right axillary lymphatics. Note the chemotherapy port on the left.

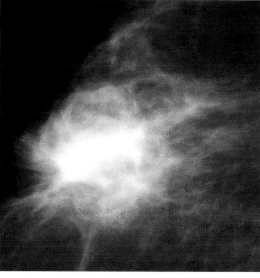

FIG. 10.35 Unilateral breast edema: trauma. Mammogram shows focal edema and hematoma from trauma.

driven proliferation of stromal and epithelial breast tissue (Fig. 10.38). Increased breast density caused by weight loss is not due to any increase in breast tissue, but to loss of fat (Fig. 10.39). A history of recent weight loss should lead to the correct diagnosis in the latter case.

To distinguish between breast edema and exogenous hormone therapy or weight loss, the radiologist looks for skin thickening, which is found with breast edema only (Box 10.7). Increased breast density from breast edema can occur anywhere; skin thickening in dependent portions of the breast is common. Increased breast density from exogenous hormone therapy is usually bilateral but without skin thickening, and occurs in regions where breast tissue was previously present.

On ultrasound, breast edema is characterized by skin thickening, loss of the normal sharp margins of Cooper's ligaments, increased echogenicity of surrounding tissues, graying of the normally dark subcutaneous fat and, in severe cases, fluid in dilated subdermal lymphatics, which are seen as tubular fluid-filled structures just under the skin line. Breast ultrasound may show invasive ductal cancer hidden on the mammogram

by overlying breast edema, should inflammatory cancer be suspected.

On MRI, breast edema is manifested as skin thickening and coarsening of breast trabeculae and Cooper's ligaments. Locally advanced cancer is usually seen as an irregular mass with rapid initial enhancement and a late plateau or washout phase. The breast skin does not usually enhance, and if there is enhancement within the skin, skin invasion by cancer should be suspected (see Fig. 10.33).

Inflammatory cancer is a rare (1% of all cancers) aggressive breast cancer with a poor prognosis. It is the most important differential diagnosis for unilateral breast edema. The definition of inflammatory cancer varies, but it usually has the clinical signs of an enlarging erythematous breast with *peau d'orange*, with focal, red, raised skin invaded by tumor. Inflammatory cancer is often mistaken for mastitis because of its clinical features, but it does not respond to antibiotics. On mammography, inflammatory cancer shows breast edema

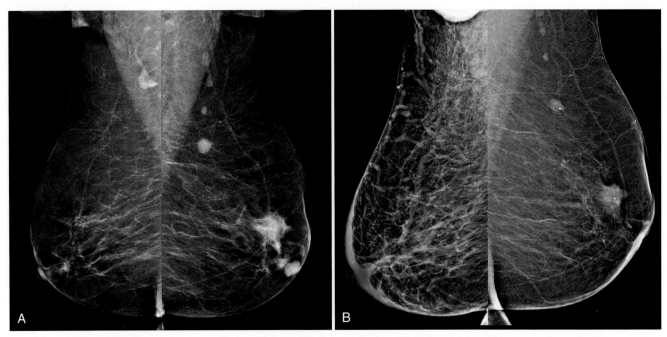

FIG. 10.36 Bilateral breast edema: renal failure. Previous mediolateral (MLO) mammograms (A) show multiple breast cancers in the left breast. No edema is observed. This patient received chemotherapy and suffered from secondary renal failure associated with the chemotherapy. Current MLO mammograms (B) show the skin thickening and coarsening of trabeculae in the bilateral breasts (more on the right side).

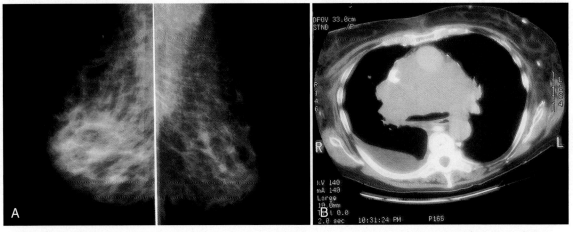

FIG. 10.37 Bilateral breast edema: superior vena cava (SVC) compression secondary to granulomatous disease. A bilateral mammogram (A) shows bilateral breast edema, worse on the right because the patient preferentially lies on her right side. Contrast-enhanced computed tomography (B) shows SVC syndrome from mediastinal adenopathy, collateral vessels in the left chest, and right pleural effusion

(see Figs. 10.31 and 10.32), occasionally displaying the underlying cancer as a breast mass, focal or global asymmetry, suspicious calcifications, nipple retraction, or axillary adenopathy. Ultrasound shows breast edema in 96% of cases, masses in 80% (see Fig. 10.32), and dilated lymphatic channels in 68%. On MRI, one report of inflammatory cancer described a "patch enhancement" pattern with some "areas of focal enhancement" and washout on the late phase of the dynamic curve. The enhancement rate on MRI for inflammatory cancer is reported to be quite rapid in the initial postcontrast phase and slightly less rapid in mastitis. The MRI shows breast edema, skin thickening, and skin enhancement (see Fig. 10.33). On biopsy, breast cancer is present in the dermal lymphatics in 80% of cases. The usual management is biopsy to make the

diagnosis of inflammatory cancer, neoadjuvant chemotherapy with or without subsequent surgery, and radiation therapy, depending on tumor response, or any combination of these treatments.

Mastitis is a common cause of unilateral breast edema, and clinical findings of pain, erythema, and *peau d'orange* are typical. The most common bacterial cause of mastitis is *S. aureus*. Rare causes of breast infection include tuberculosis, syphilis, hydatid disease, and molluscum contagiosum. Clinically, mastitis produces breast cellulitis, which if untreated, may progress to small focal microabscesses or a larger abscess collection that may become walled off. On mammography, mastitis appears as unilateral breast edema. When mastitis progresses to abscess, abscesses are tender palpable masses, usually in the retroareolar

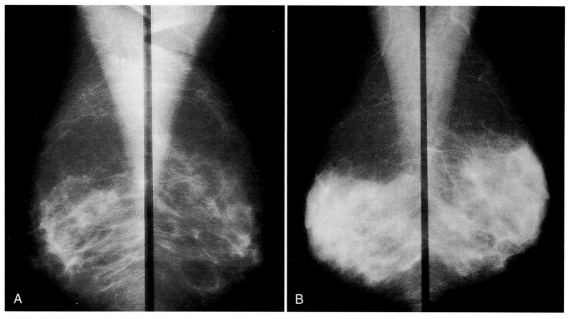

FIG. 10.38 Exogenous hormone replacement therapy. Bilateral mediolateral oblique mammograms before (A) and after (B) hormone replacement therapy show increased glandular tissue bilaterally in locations where glandular tissue previously existed. Unlike breast edema, there is no skin thickening or coarsening of trabeculae in subcutaneous fat.

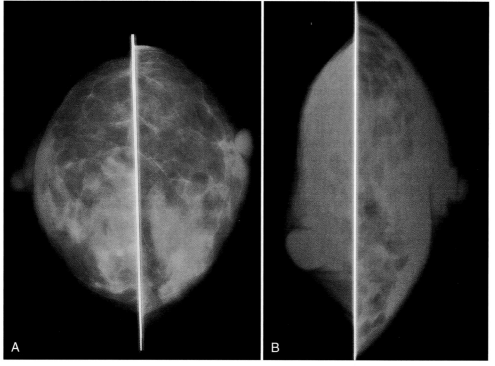

FIG. 10.39 Weight loss. Bilateral craniocaudal mammograms before (A) and after (B) weight loss show increased breast density on the mammogram because of loss of fat.

BOX 10.7	Hormone Changes versus Breast Edema on Mammography

HORMONE CHANGES	**BREAST EDEMA**
Increased breast density	Increased breast density
Breast density increased at sites with glandular tissue	Diffuse or focal; may develop where no glandular tissue occurred previously
Normal skin	Skin thickening
Normal subcutaneous fat	Subcutaneous trabecular thickening
Normal skin on physical examination	*Peau d'orange* on physical examination

region. On mammography the abscess is an ill-defined or irregular mass without calcifications and usually, without gas. Rarely, an abscess contains gas, but most often only after aspiration has been attempted. On ultrasound, the abscess is an irregular, ill-defined hypoechoic mass, sometimes containing septations or debris, with enhanced through-transmission of sound, not usually containing gas. Because antibiotics cannot cross abscess walls, larger abscesses require either percutaneous or operative drainage. For this reason, ultrasound is particularly helpful in the setting of mastitis to detect and define abscesses requiring drainage.

Recurrent subareolar abscesses are special entities caused by plugging of the major retroareolar breast ducts with subsequent infection. They are commonly associated with a fistulous tract that forms from the abscess that drains to the skin. The resulting abscess is chronic and may be drained percutaneously or operatively many times without resolution or with frequent recurrence unless the abscess is excised with its the fistulous tract.

An extremely rare cause of unilateral breast edema is breast necrosis from coumarin (warfarin [Coumadin]) therapy. On this therapy necrosis is more common in the abdomen,

---

BOX 10.8 Coumarin Necrosis

Rare cause of breast edema
Exact mechanism unknown
Associated protein C or S deficiency
Painful swelling and petechiae
Hemorrhagic bullae
Full-thickness skin necrosis
Discontinue coumarin or change anticoagulants

---

buttocks, and thighs, rather than in the breast, in 0.01% to 1% of coumarin-treated patients (Box 10.8). Although it has been associated with protein C or protein S deficiency, the exact mechanism of coumarin-induced necrosis is unknown. Painful lesions, swelling, and petechiae from thrombosis of small vessels and inflammation occur after initiation of coumarin treatment; large hemorrhagic bullae result and develop to full-thickness fat and skin necrosis. Discontinuing the use of coumarin is recommended to stop the necrosis. Heparin or other anticoagulants may be necessary in patients who require sustained anticoagulation in the short term. Heparin-induced skin necrosis has also been reported in association with type II heparin-induced thrombocytopenia, but heparin is often used in the setting of coumarin necrosis. In some cases, the skin lesions heal spontaneously after shallow tissue sloughing. In other cases, skin grafts are required, and in extreme cases, mastectomy is required.

HORMONE CHANGES

Normal young women have extremely dense breast tissue, gradually replaced by fat during the aging process. On mammography, the breasts usually appear very white in younger patients and become darker and darker as glandular tissue is replaced by fatty tissue with age (Fig. 10.40). The overall breast density at any time in the patient's life depends on the patient's age, her genetic predisposition for retaining glandular tissue, and her hormonal status.

Exogenous hormone replacement therapy, pregnancy, and lactation reverse the trend toward fatty breast tissue by causing a proliferation of the glandular elements and periductal stroma of the breast, resulting in a denser mammogram (Fig. 10.41; see also Fig. 10.38). Unlike in breast edema, hormone

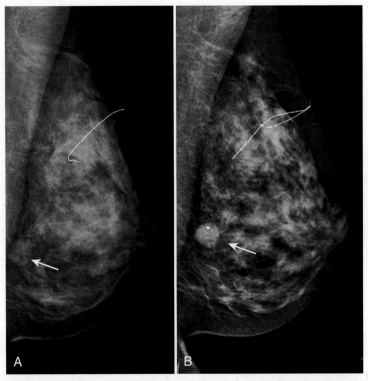

FIG. 10.40 Breast tissue density before and after menopause. Left mediolateral oblique (MLO) mammogram before menopause (A) shows extremely dense breast and a suspicious mass (*arrow*) in the lower breast. Left MLO mammogram obtained 6 years after menopause (B) shows decreased glandular tissue. The mass (*arrow*) in the lower breast is visualized more clearly and calcification is observed. This mass was an involuting fibroadenoma. Note linear markers placed in scars from previous biopsy.

changes make the breast tissue denser and the skin does not become thickened. With breast edema, the entire breast becomes denser and the skin thickens to more than the normal 2 to 3 mm, and the subdermal lymphatics become engorged. This does not happen with exogenous hormone replacement therapy.

Some women report breast tenderness, pain, fullness, and lumpiness with exogenous hormone replacement therapy. The frequency of increased breast density on mammography in women undergoing exogenous hormone therapy varies from 23% to 34%. The highest percentage of women with increased density were receiving continuous-combined hormone therapy consisting of conjugated equine estrogen, 0.625 mg/day; plus medroxyprogesterone acetate, 2.5 mg/day; or other combinations, with the progestin component most affecting increased breast density. In another report, continuous-combined hormone therapy produced increased breast density on mammography, but estrogen-only therapy did not.

Other medications also change breast density. Raloxifene hydrochloride, a drug used for bone mineral density, has been reported to produce increased breast density on mammography in a very small number of women. Case studies of two women undergoing injections of medroxyprogesterone (Depo-Provera) for contraception reported a decrease in breast density on mammograms during the injections and an increase in breast density when the injections were discontinued. Tamoxifen used for adjuvant or prophylactic treatment of breast cancer has been reported to decrease mammographic tissue density in some women, with one case report describing a return to baseline breast density after termination of drug therapy. Isoflavones are phytoestrogens contained in soy foods and have been reported to have both estrogenic and antiestrogenic effects. A double-blind, randomized trial of women undergoing mammography after isoflavone supplements showed no significant decrease in breast density or change in dense tissue over a 12-month period.

Because breast density changes with hormone therapy, new or focal asymmetries on mammograms in women undergoing hormone therapy may be cancer or may be benign developing asymmetries caused by hormone treatment. Tomosynthesis, spot compression fine-detail views, and ultrasound help to exclude a mass. Discontinuing exogenous hormone therapy for 3 months and reimaging may exclude a mass. Similarly, increased BPE on contrast-enhanced breast MRI in women receiving exogenous hormone replacement therapy is reversible when the therapy is discontinued for 1 month.

BREAST PAIN

Breast pain is an extremely common complaint. However, in the absence of an associated palpable lump, it is a very infrequent sign of breast cancer. Nevertheless, because both breast pain and breast cancer are common, the purpose of workup is to reassure the patient and exclude a coexistent cancer. Breast pain may be focal or diffuse and may vary with the menstrual cycle (ie, cyclic) or not (ie, noncyclic). Generally, both diffuse and cyclic breast pain are benign breast symptoms that do not warrant imaging evaluation and generally need only patient reassurance.

Although *focal* breast pain, pain that can be identified by the patient with one finger, is worrisome to the patient, studies have shown that it is most often not caused by cancer. On the other hand, because both focal breast pain and cancer are common, mammography is reasonable to exclude cancer and reassure the patient. Consideration should be given to ultrasound in women with focal pain to exclude a breast cyst that may be causing the pain.

Cyclic mastalgia has many causes, including cyclic enlargement as a result of menses or multiple cysts. Relief from breast pain may be achieved in some cases by aspiration of the cyst, decrease in caffeine intake, or analgesics. Home remedies for breast pain have included 400 U of vitamin E per day, vitamin

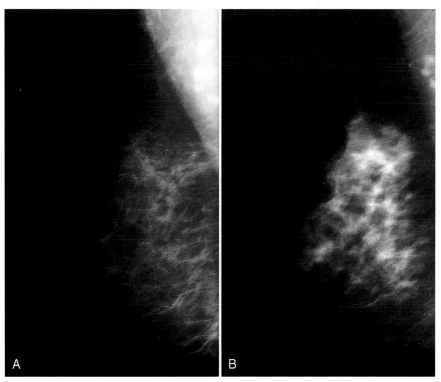

FIG. 10.41 Exogenous hormone replacement therapy. Mediolateral oblique mammograms before (A) and after (B) hormone replacement therapy show a denser breast where breast tissue previously existed.

B6, analgesics, decrease in fat and salt intake, use of sports bras, and evening primrose oil. In extreme cases, progestins, danazol, tamoxifen, or bromocriptine is used to relieve mastodynia.

AXILLARY LYMPHADENOPATHY

Normal axillary lymph nodes on the mammogram are reniform and have a thin, smooth, sharply marginated white cortex that surrounds a fatty hilum. With lymphadenopathy, the normal lymph nodes become denser, rounder, with loss of their normal fatty hila, with or without lymph node enlargement (Figs. 10.42–10.44). Abnormal lymph nodes may also contain calcifications, gold deposits mimicking calcifications from treatment of rheumatoid arthritis, or silicone from a previously ruptured breast implant. The differential diagnosis for axillary adenopathy without a definite breast mass varies for unilateral versus bilateral findings (Box 10.9). Causes of unilateral axillary adenopathy include metastatic breast cancer and mastitis. Bilateral axillary adenopathy is usually caused by systemic etiologies, such as infection, collagen vascular diseases like rheumatoid arthritis, lymphoma, leukemia, or metastatic tumor.

Calcific particles in abnormal axillary lymph nodes may represent calcified metastasis from breast cancer (Fig. 10.45) or calcifying infections such as tuberculosis (Box 10.10). In the case of tuberculous mastitis, patients have axillary swelling and breast enlargement without a breast mass, enlarged dense or matted axillary lymph nodes, or breast edema with or without findings of pulmonary tuberculosis. The finding of macrocalcifications rather than pleomorphic microcalcifications in the lymph nodes may suggest tuberculous mastitis, but biopsy is necessary to exclude metastatic breast cancer. Migration of silicone into axillary lymph nodes from ruptured silicone breast implants or migration of gold particles from therapy for rheumatoid arthritis

may mimic calcifications in lymph nodes, but the clinical history should provide clues to the correct diagnosis.

Lymphadenopathy on mammography without underlying clinical reasons for the abnormal lymph nodes should prompt a critical review for breast cancer. In a series of 21 women with lymphadenopathy found at screening mammography, 50% had malignancy (lymphoma, metastatic carcinoma, and leukemia), and the other 50% were caused by benign causes (reactive changes, healed granulomatous disease, rheumatoid arthritis, amyloid, and infection).

Primary breast cancer presenting as isolated lymph node metastasis in the setting of normal mammographic and physical examination findings is an uncommon clinical problem that accounts for less than 1% of all breast cancers. Both breast ultrasound and contrast-enhanced breast MRI are useful in this scenario. Once the primary tumor is found, breast conservation rather than mastectomy is a potential option (see Fig. 10.45). A breast cancer diagnosis is helpful for the patient who otherwise would be treated for metastatic lymphadenopathy of unknown primary. In some cases the primary breast cancer is never identified (see Fig. 10.44B). In a pathology series by Haupt et al. (1985), 43 women with lymph nodes showing metastases suggestive of breast cancer origin were reviewed. The primary breast tumor was found in 31 (72%) women but never identified in the remaining 12. Survival rates between the two groups were similar, and the 12 women that never had a tumor discovered never had another primary malignancy detected in the follow-up period.

PAGET DISEASE OF THE NIPPLE

Paget disease of the nipple is a distinct clinical entity that heralds an underlying breast cancer. Ductal carcinoma almost always coexists with Paget disease, either in the ducts

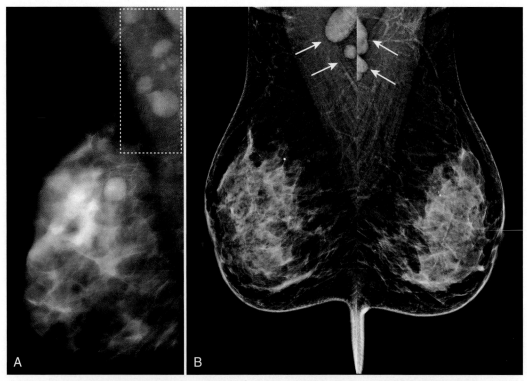

FIG. 10.42 Axillary lymphadenopathy: examples of benign conditions. (A) Abnormal dense round lymph nodes (*box*) in the axilla have lost their fatty hila and are rounder and bigger than normal lymph nodes as a result of lupus and rheumatoid arthritis. (B) Bilateral axillary lymphadenopathy (*arrows*) was diagnosed as reactive lymphoid hyperplasia.

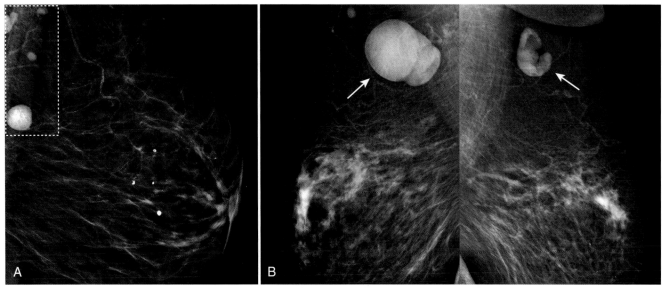

FIG. 10.43 Axillary lymphadenopathy: examples of lymphoma. (A) Abnormal round lymph nodes (*box*) in a patient with lymphoma on left mediolateral oblique (MLO) mammography. (B) Bilateral MLO views show bilateral axillary lymphadenopathy (*arrows*) in another patient with lymphoma.

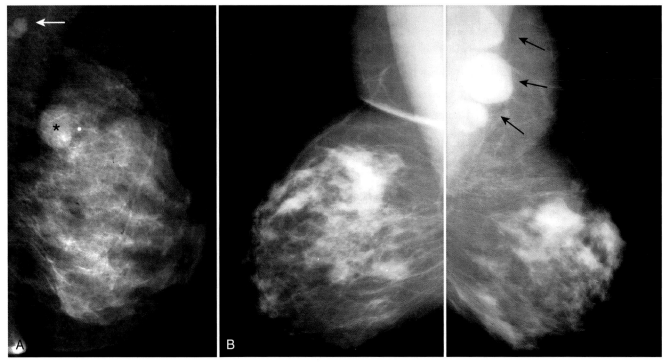

FIG. 10.44 Axillary lymphadenopathy: examples of metastasis from breast cancer. (A) Left mediolateral oblique (MLO) view shows a mass (*) in the upper breast representing an invasive ductal cancer with an abnormal lymph node (*arrow*) in the left axilla. Even though the lymph node still has its fatty hilum, it is worrisome for cancer metastases because it is rounder, denser, and has a thicker cortex than a normal lymph node. Metastatic disease was found in the lymph node at sentinel lymph node biopsy. (B) Breast cancer presenting as axillary lymphadenopathy. Bilateral MLO mammograms show adenopathy in the left axilla, which was consistent with the diagnosis of breast cancer. Additional views of the left breast by mammography and ultrasound did not demonstrate any masses. Examination after mastectomy showed no primary breast cancer. The patient was treated for breast cancer empirically. No breast cancer in the opposite breast and no additional tumors were found elsewhere in 5 years of follow-up.

BOX 10.9   Axillary Lymphadenopathy

UNILATERAL
Mastitis
Cancer

BILATERAL
Widespread infection
Rheumatoid arthritis
Collagen vascular disease
Lymphoma
Leukemia
Metastatic cancer

beneath the nipple or elsewhere in the breast, and it has a high rate of overexpression of the c-erb-B2 oncogene. The underlying pathology is almost always high-grade DCIS, but an invasive component may also be present. Affected women have a bright, reddened nipple that progresses to eczematous changes that may extend to the areola, with subsequent ulceration and nipple destruction if the process is unchecked. A delay of several months often occurs before women seek advice, unless there is associated nipple discharge. Paget disease of the nipple may mimic dermatitis of the nipple, resulting in delayed diagnosis. If the patient's symptoms do not respond to a trial of topical steroids, the diagnosis of Paget disease should be considered.

The nipple and mammogram are normal in almost 50% of cases (Fig. 10.46) despite clinical signs of Paget disease and/or

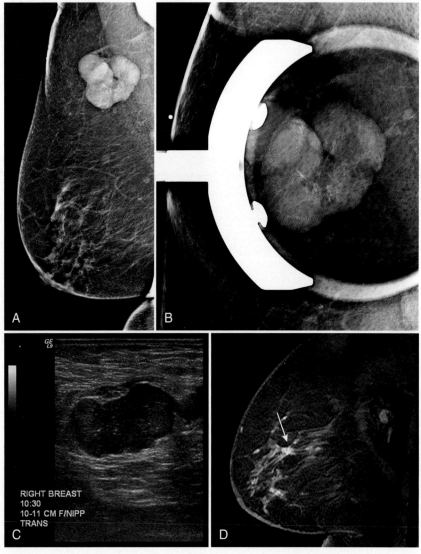

FIG. 10.45 Calcified axillary lymphadenopathy: metastasis from breast cancer. Right mediolateral oblique (MLO) mammogram (A) shows markedly enlarged axillary lymph node. Spot compression mammogram (B) visualizes calcified particles with in the enlarged lymph node. Ultrasound (C) shows hypoechoic mass with tiny high spots, corresponding to the enlarged lymph node with calcification. Pathology was metastatic adenocarcinoma from right breast cancer. Sagittal contrast-enhanced magnetic resonance image (MRI; D) of the right breast shows an irregular mass (*arrow*), 13 mm in diameter, which was occult on mammography. This right breast mass was diagnosed as primary invasive ductal cancer by MRI-guided biopsy.

an underlying breast cancer (Box 10.11). On abnormal mammograms, the underlying cancer has suspicious microcalcifications, a spiculated mass, or both (Fig. 10.47), often in the subareolar region; but it does not necessarily lie directly adjacent to the nipple or areola. In women with Paget disease, skin or areolar thickening, nipple retraction, subareolar masses, or calcifications leading to the nipple should be viewed with suspicion

on mammography. Spot compression magnification mammography of the nipple and retroareolar region is often helpful for identifying subtle abnormalities. Conversely, nipple–areolar abnormalities or thickening detected at mammography should be correlated with the physical examination to exclude clinical findings of Paget disease. MRI may be helpful in detecting the underlying breast cancer. Although mastectomy has been the mainstay of treatment, women without a palpable mass and a normal mammogram and MRI have been successfully treated with breast conservation.

SARCOMAS

Sarcomas are rare tumors of the breast or the underlying chest wall, and their classification depends on the cell type involved (Fig. 10.48). Ultrasound shows a hypoechoic mass and may be

---

BOX 10.10   Lymphadenopathy with Calcifications

Metastatic calcifying cancer
Granulomatous disease
Gold particles from rheumatoid arthritis therapy
Migrated silicone from implant rupture

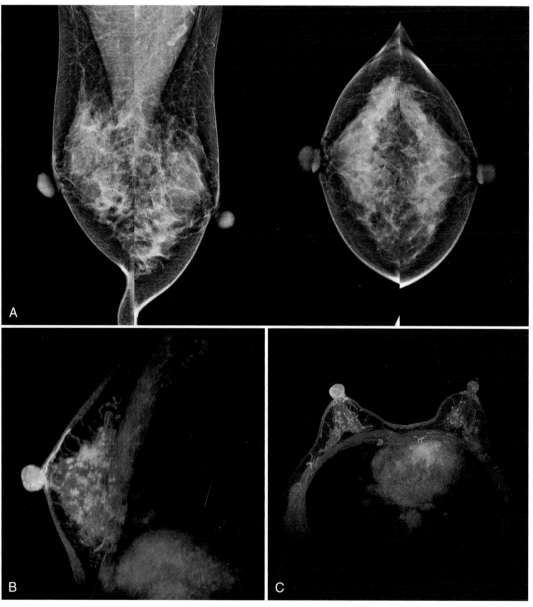

FIG. 10.46 Pagetoid involvement of invasive breast cancer. This patient had persistent right nipple rash for 6 months, which at times had associated bleeding. Mediolateral oblique (*left*) and craniocaudal (*right*) mammograms (A) show no apparent abnormality. Targeted ultrasound of the periareolar portion of the right breast was also negative for suspicious findings. However, sagittal (B) and axial (C) magnetic resonance images show abnormal enhancement in the slightly swelling right nipple, and multiple small masses and clumped nonmass enhancement in the right breast. Biopsy-proved invasive carcinoma with pagetoid involvement of the nipple.

BOX 10.11 Paget Disease of the Nipple

Heralds underlying ductal cancer
Bright red nipple
Eczematous nipple–areolar changes
Ulceration
Cancer location often subareolar, but may be anywhere in the breast
Normal mammogram in 50%
Nipple change, skin/areolar thickening in 30%
Subareolar mass/calcifications are suspicious

helpful in determining whether the origin of the sarcoma is from the breast or chest wall (Fig. 10.49). Mammography shows high-density masses without calcifications or spiculation, unless the tumor has osseous elements (Fig. 10.50). MRI is useful for demonstrating pectoralis muscle or chest wall involvement, because sarcomas tend to be large and locally invasive. On ultrasound, angiosarcoma is an echogenic mass because of the large number of small vessels within it.

On MRI, angiosarcoma shows low signal intensity on T1-weighted images, higher signal intensity on T2-weighted images, and enhancement of the mass with a low-intensity central region.

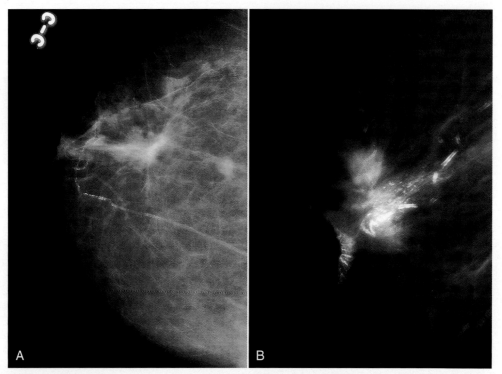

FIG. 10.47 Examples of Paget disease. (A) Craniocaudal mammogram shows nipple retraction and a second invasive ductal cancer deep in the breast in a patient with Paget disease. (B) Mediolateral oblique mammogram in a patient with Paget disease shows destruction of the nipple covered with a radiopaque salve and a retroareolar dense mass producing retraction.

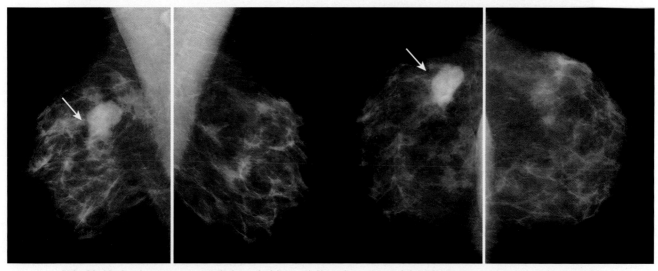

FIG. 10.48 Carcinosarcoma. Mediolateral oblique (*left*) and craniocaudal (*right*) mammograms in a 37-year-old woman with a palpable mass show a dense lobulated mass (*arrows*) in the right breast with an obscured lower border. Pathologic examination demonstrated the epithelial and mesenchymal differentiation required to make the diagnosis. (From Smathers RL: *Mammography: diagnosis and intervention,* Medical Interactive [compact disc]. Copyright Mammography Specialists Medical Group, Inc. Contribution from Ralph Smathers, M.D.)

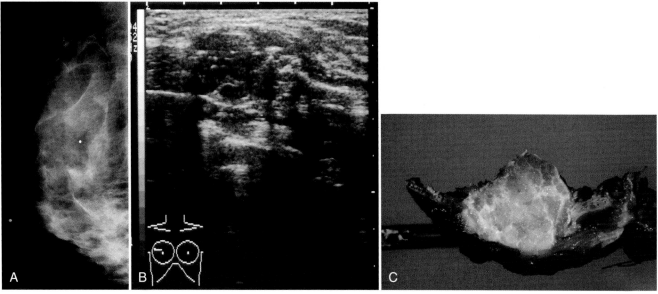

FIG. 10.49 Chondrosarcoma of the rib. Mediolateral oblique mammogram (A) shows a marker over a slowly growing mass, which proved to be only dense tissue. Ultrasound (B) reveals a complex heterogeneous mass invading the chest wall, predominantly posterior to the pectoralis muscle and measuring 6 cm. Pathologic examination (C) showed a grade I chondrosarcoma containing mature hyaline cartilage and reactive bone in continuity with the rib. (From Smathers RL: *Mammography: diagnosis and intervention,* Medical Interactive [compact disc]. Copyright Mammography Specialists Medical Group, Inc. Contribution from Ralph Smathers, M.D.)

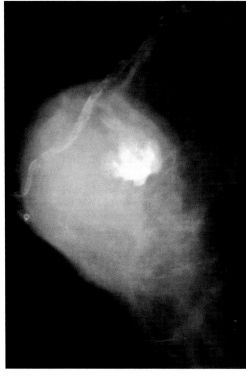

FIG. 10.50 Fibrosarcoma of the breast with osseous trabeculae. Craniocaudal mammogram shows a dense mass containing dense calcification resembling bone. (From Elson BC, Ikeda DM, Andersson I, Wattsgard C: Fibrosarcoma of the breast: mammographic findings in 5 cases, *AJR Am J Roentgenol* 158:994, 1992.)

At pathology, sinusoids containing red blood cells are present. Angiosarcoma of the breast may be primary or secondary to radiation, usually received as adjunctive therapy after breast conservation surgery (ie, lumpectomy). Secondary angiosarcoma usually occurs approximately 10 years after the initial radiation therapy.

BOX 10.12 Mondor Disease

Thrombophlebitis of the superficial veins of the breast
Painful, ropelike, palpable cord
Thrombosed vein causes a furrow/dimpling
Self-limited
Related to trauma or surgery
Mammography is negative, or long tubular density is noted
Ultrasound: hypoechoic tube or cord with or without flow

MONDOR DISEASE

Mondor disease is acute thrombophlebitis of the superficial veins of the breast (Box 10.12). It is rare, is often associated with trauma or recent surgery, and has been reported after sonography-guided or stereotactic core biopsy, but it may be idiopathic in origin. Patients report acute pain, discomfort, and tenderness along the lateral aspect of the breast, the chest wall, or the region of the thrombosed vein; they may also report a cordlike, painful elongated mass just below the skin, which represents the thrombosed, hardened vein. Extension of the arm may produce a long narrow furrow in the skin as a result of retraction from the thrombosed vein, similar to skin dimpling from breast cancer.

Physical examination shows a tender palpable cord extending toward the outer portion of the breast that is produced by fibrosis and obliteration of the superficial vein; in the acute phase, it is occasionally accompanied by discoloration of the overlying skin. Thereafter, the vein diminishes in painfulness over a period of 3 to 4 weeks as a result of either recanalization or complete obliteration of the vein by phlebosclerosis and hyalinization. Because Mondor disease is self-limited and the palpable finding resolves over a 2- to 12-week period, supportive care is the appropriate treatment.

Case reports describe negative mammographic findings in women with Mondor disease or, rarely, a long linear or tubular density on the mammogram corresponding to the thrombosed vein (Fig. 10.51). Case reports of ultrasound in Mondor disease

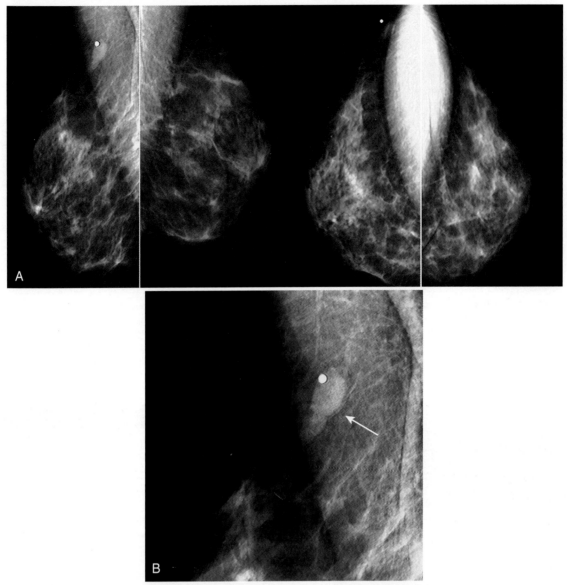

FIG. 10.51 Mondor disease. Mediolateral oblique (MLO; *left*) and craniocaudal (*right*) mammograms (A) of a marker over a tender, elongated, dilated ductlike structure in the right axilla of a young woman. Spot compression on the MLO view (B) shows a tubular mass (*arrow*) representing the superficial thrombophlebitis that results in the nodular, superficial tender vein typical of Mondor disease.

show a noncompressible hypoechoic tubular cord in the subcutaneous tissue, with or without flow on color Doppler imaging, depending on the degree of recanalization.

GRANULOMATOUS MASTITIS

Granulomatous mastitis is a rare disease, occurring in young premenopausal women after their last childbirth. It has been correlated with breast feeding and oral contraceptive use, and a possible autoimmune component has been implicated in its etiology. Affected patients may have galactorrhea, pain, inflammation, a breast mass, induration, and skin ulcerations.

Women undergoing mammography are found to have asymmetries (former asymmetric densities), focal asymmetries, or ill-defined breast masses (Fig. 10.52), or negative mammograms. Calcifications were not usually a feature of granulomatous mastitis but were reported in 11% (2/19) of a series in which mammograms were done (Handa, 2014). On ultrasound, findings

include irregular masses, focal regions of inhomogeneous patterns associated with hypoechoic tubular/nodular structures, or decreased parenchymal echogenicity with acoustic shadowing, all suggestive of malignancy (see Fig. 10.52; Fig. 10.53). In one 2013 series by Gautier, MRI showed masses or nodules with rapid enhancement with a late-phase washout seen and adjacent non-mass enhancement, sometimes with fistulous tracts thought to represent the inflammatory response.

Because the mammographic, sonographic, and MRI features suggest breast cancer, biopsy is frequently performed on women with granulomatous mastitis, often by percutaneous needle biopsy. Biopsy shows a chronic noncaseating granulomatous inflammation of the breast composed of giant cells, leukocytes, epithelioid cells, macrophages, and abscesses. There is usually no infection and the etiology of the granulomas is unknown. Treatment consists of surgical excision, oral steroid therapy, antiinflammatory drugs or colchicines, or methotrexate, as well as antibiotic treatment of any associated

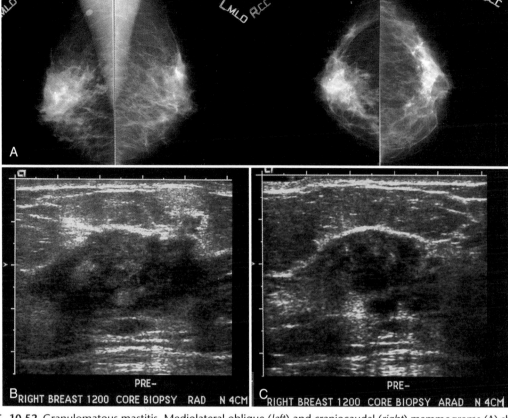

FIG. 10.52 Granulomatous mastitis. Mediolateral oblique (*left*) and craniocaudal (*right*) mammograms (A) show a marker over a palpable right breast mass shown as a focal asymmetry. Radial (B) and antiradial (C) ultrasounds show a complex irregular heterogeneous mass corresponding to the palpable finding and the mammographic mass. Biopsy showed granulomatous mastitis.

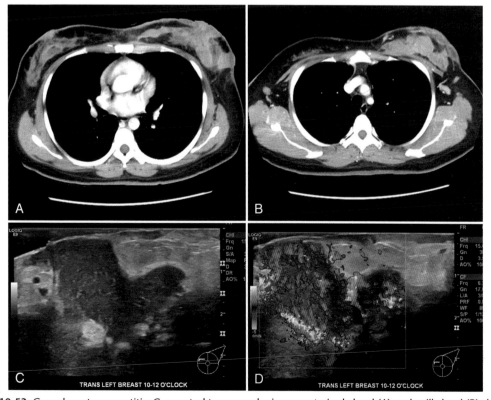

FIG. 10.53 Granulomatous mastitis. Computed tomography images at nipple level (A) and axilla level (B) show a large, heterogeneous, fungating mass in the left breast measuring approximately 11 × 11 × 3 cm associated with skin thickening and areas of necrosis and ipsilateral enlarged axillary lymph nodes. A smaller heterogeneous, enhancing mass in the right breast measuring 3 × 1 cm also extends to the skin with smaller adjacent nodules. Gray scale (C) and color Doppler (D) ultrasounds show solid, hypervascular bilateral breast masses without evidence of a drainable fluid collection as clinically queried. Differential considerations included inflammatory breast cancer versus infectious or granulomatous mastitis. Final diagnosis was granulomatous mastitis.

abscesses. Recurrence rates of up to 50% have been reported, but they can be reduced by immunosuppressive treatment until complete remission.

DIABETIC MASTOPATHY

Diabetic mastopathy produces hard, irregular, sometimes painful mobile breast masses that may be recurrent or bilateral in patients with a history of long-term insulin-dependent type 1 diabetes, in younger premenopausal diabetic women, or in rare patients with thyroid disease (Box 10.13). Diabetic mastopathy is caused by an autoimmune reaction to the accumulation of abnormal matrix proteins caused by hyperglycemia. It leads to atrophy and obliteration of glandular breast tissue and the production of fibrosis, which forms a hard mass simulating breast cancer. Because of the hardness of the mass, needle biopsy is often performed, but it may be insufficient for diagnosis necessitating histologic sampling. Pathologic examination reveals fibrosis with a dense lymphocytic infiltration around breast lobules and ducts.

Mammography shows a regional asymmetric density with ill-defined margins but no microcalcifications. Ultrasound demonstrates a hypoechoic mass or region displaying marked acoustic shadowing in most cases, which can be suggestive of scirrhous breast cancer (Fig. 10.54).

Case reports of diabetic mastopathy on MRI describe a decreased area of signal intensity with "poor" or "heterogeneous" enhancement or "nonspecific" enhancement in the initial postcontrast phase. Heterogeneous "spotting enhancement" or a "benign gradual-type dynamic curve" is reported in the late enhancement phase.

On biopsy, fibrosis with perivascular, periductal, or perilobular lymphocytic infiltrates is seen. Frequently, patients will undergo

---

BOX 10.13   Diabetic Mastopathy

Long-term insulin-dependent diabetics
Thyroid disease (rare)
Autoimmune reaction causing fibrosis
Periductal and perilobular lymphocytic infiltration
May result in a hard mass
Surgery can result in recurrent masses

---

surgical excisional biopsy to exclude cancer. Unfortunately, surgery may exacerbate the disease, with recurrences developing in the same location. Therefore surgery is usually not recommended if the finding is proven to be diabetic mastopathy by core biopsy, because the entity is benign.

DESMOID TUMOR

Desmoid tumor, or extraabdominal desmoid, is also known as desmoid type fibromatosis, and aggressive fibromatosis. Desmoid tumor in the breast is a rare entity, accounting for less than 0.2% of all breast tumors. Desmoid tumor is an infiltrative, locally aggressive fibroblastic/myofibroblastic process that may recur locally, may be multicentric, has been associated with previous trauma or surgery, and has been reported in women with breast implants. In the breast, desmoid tumor is manifested as a solitary, hard painless mass, occasionally fixed to the skin or pectoral fascia. Because treatment involves wide surgical excision, the primary tumor is evaluated for its origin within either the breast or the underlying musculoaponeurotic structures. The extent of invasion into surrounding structures is also evaluated to facilitate surgical planning. It is important to remove the entire tumor because of its predilection to recur again and again.

On mammography, desmoid tumors appear as irregular-shaped, high-density spiculated or indistinct masses with rare associated calcifications Ultrasound typically shows an irregular hypoechoic solid mass with or without posterior acoustic shadowing (Fig. 5.55). On MRI, T1- and T2-weighted signal intensity and gadolinium contrast enhancement of desmoid tumors varies depending on their histopathologic features. Reports of chest wall desmoid tumors on computed tomography show variable tumor composition, caused by collagen content and amount of solid or necrotic tissue (Fig. 10.56). Because it is difficult to differentiate between desmoid tumors and breast cancers, biopsy is required.

Treatment of desmoid tumors is complete local surgical excision. Recurrence of desmoid tumor is less likely with wide excision and clear histologic margins. Tumor recurrence usually occurs within 3 years of excision and for this reason breast reconstruction is generally delayed for 3 years. Because surgical trauma has been associated with recurrence, informed consent is necessary before breast reconstruction. Recurrences are treated by radical excision. Radiation therapy is used as an alternative to surgery for tumors if complete excision would

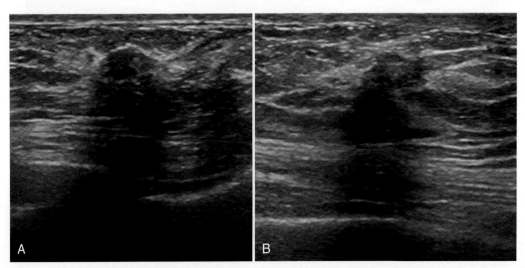

FIG. 10.54 Diabetic mastopathy. Ultrasound scans of diabetic mastopathy in longitudinal (A) and transverse (B) images show an ill-defined shadowing mass mimicking breast cancer. Biopsy showed diabetic mastopathy.

result in a poor functional outcome or if tumors have positive margins (Box 10.14). Because of its variable clinical course and behavior, a team approach and individualized treatment is recommended.

TRICHINOSIS

Trichinosis is caused by the ingestion of raw or undercooked meat containing encysted larvae of the Trichinella genus. Diarrhea is produced during the intestinal phase of adult development, and then myositis, fever, and periorbital edema develop during larval migration (Box 10.15). After gastric digestion releases the encysted larvae, the larvae migrate into the intestinal mucosa, mature, and mate. The adult female releases new larvae into mucosal blood vessels, and the larvae are distributed throughout the body over a period of 4 to 6 weeks. The larvae enter skeletal muscles, most commonly the diaphragm, tongue, periorbital muscles, deltoid, pectoralis, gastrocnemius, and intercostal muscles, in which they encyst and calcify in 6 to 18 months, with a further life span of 5 to 10 years in the encysted form. During migration, larvae may also produce myocarditis, pneumonitis, or central nervous system symptoms

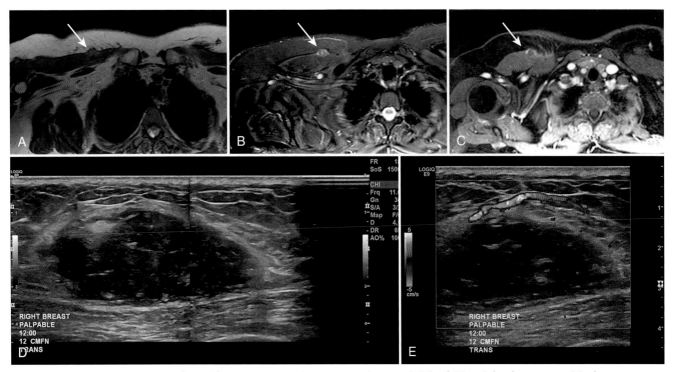

FIG. 10.55 Recurrent desmoid tumor. Magnetic resonance images (MRI) of T1-weighted sequence (A), fat-suppressed T2-weighted sequence (B), and contrast-enhanced fat-suppressed T1-weighted sequence (C) show a 13-mm enhancing nodule (*arrow*) with slightly higher signal intensity compared with the muscle on T1- and T2-wighted images within the anterior aspect of the right pectoralis muscle. Gray scale (D) ultrasound obtained 1 year later than MRI study (A–C) shows interval growth of a palpable 4.5 × 4.6 × 2.2-cm hypoechoic ovoid solid mass with irregular margins, without apparent posterior acoustic shadowing. Although prominent vascularity is seen within the breast tissue, the mass itself is not particularly vascular by color Doppler assessment (E). This patient has a history of desmoid fibromatosis of the chest with prior resection. Diagnosis was recurrent desmoid tumor.

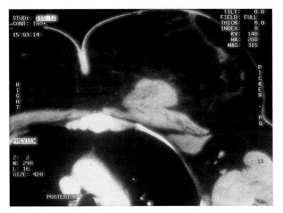

FIG. 10.56 Desmoid. Computed tomography scan shows a soft-tissue mass adjacent to the pectoralis muscle in the left breast. Biopsy revealed a desmoid tumor.

BOX 10.14   Desmoid Tumor

Synonyms: extraabdominal desmoid/fibromatosis
Recurrent unless widely resected
Associated with previous trauma or surgery, implants
Solitary spiculated hard painless mass, occasionally fixed
If recurrent, recurs within 3 years

BOX 10.15   Trichinosis

Ingestion of encysted worm larvae in undercooked meat
Tiny linear calcified encysted larvae in the pectoralis muscle
No calcifications in breast tissue

---

from vasculitis of small arteries or capillaries, but encystment does not usually occur in these locations. Ingestion of the encysted larvae by a new host perpetuates the life cycle of the organism. In the United States most Trichinella infections are asymptomatic and are acquired by ingesting undercooked pork, feral meat, wild boar, bear, or walrus.

On mammography, the calcified encysted larvae are seen as tiny linear calcifications smaller than 1 mm that are aligned along the long axis of the pectoralis muscle, parallel to the muscular fibers (Fig. 10.57). Because the calcifications are within the

muscle, they should not be mistaken for breast cancer. At this point patients are asymptomatic.

Parasitic diseases that have been reported to calcify in breast tissue include hydatid disease, paragonimiasis, Dirofilaria repens infection, schistosomiasis, myiasis, and loiasis.

DERMATOMYOSITIS

Dermatomyositis and some collagen vascular diseases can rarely produce calcifications within the soft tissues of the arms and legs. In the breast, bizarre sheetlike calcifications form in a configuration similar to that of fat necrosis; the calcifications align along the breast tissues and generally point at the nipple (Fig. 10.58). Dermatomyositis is not a specific indicator of breast cancer. However, mammography is often performed because of an association of dermatomyositis with malignancies.

FOREIGN BODIES

Foreign bodies can be seen within the breast on mammography. Some acupuncture practitioners break acupuncture needle tips off in the breast tissue after placement, and the tiny sheared-off metallic needle tip fragments can be seen inside the breast tissue.

The most common foreign bodies seen in the breast on mammography are metallic markers placed percutaneously after core needle biopsy guided by stereotaxis, ultrasound, or MRI (Fig. 10.59). The markers have different shapes, depending on the manufacturer, and may contain a pellet or pellets that are visible by ultrasound. For patients who desire removal of the markers, case reports describe the use of an 11-gauge stereotactic vacuum-assisted probe technique that can remove the markers percutaneously. Percutaneous breast biopsy devices may produce tiny residual metallic shavings or fragments from the biopsy probe or needle itself and are usually not seen on the mammogram. These fragments are ferromagnetic and can occasionally cause signal voids on MRI.

Fragments of preoperatively placed hookwires have been reported in the breast after preoperative needle localization; these fragments may have been transected at surgery or may be caused by breakage of the wire at the hooked end. Specimen radiography shows if the target, hookwire, and hookwire tip

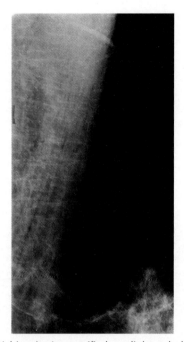

FIG. 10.57 Trichinosis. A magnified mediolateral oblique view of the upper part of the breast shows innumerable tiny calcifications aligned along the pectoralis muscle that represent the calcified encysted larvae of *Trichinella*.

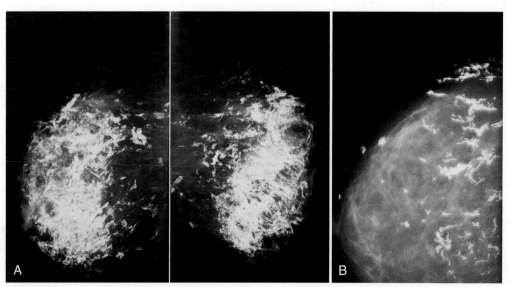

FIG. 10.58 Dystrophic calcifications: examples of collagen vascular disease. (A) Bilateral mediolateral oblique mammograms show extensive dystrophic calcifications in both breasts. (B) Dystrophic calcifications seen in another patient on craniocaudal mammogram. Dermatomyositis with calcifications was the diagnosis.

were removed, and this information is conveyed to the surgeon in the operating room. Although some hookwire fragments were reported as stable within the breast 1.5 to 11 years after surgery, other fragments become symptomatic as a result of migration within and through the breast into the soft tissues of other parts of the body.

Round Dacron Hickman catheter cuffs may be left inside the breast after removal of a Hickman catheter. The rounded, short tubelike Dacron structure has a characteristic appearance in the upper part of the breast on mammography (Fig. 10.60A–B). A needle may also be retained in the breast, which can be visualized on mammography (Fig. 10.60C).

Suture material may calcify after lumpectomy and radiation therapy. The result is a linear or curvilinear calcified suture. The diagnosis can be made if the suture still contains a knot (Fig. 10.60D).

Surgeons occasionally place metallic surgical clips in breast cancer biopsy cavities for radiation oncologists to plan electron beam boosts. This practice is becoming less common, as

discussed in Chapter 8. Other materials may lodge in the breast, and the clinical history may help in the diagnosis (Fig. 10.61).

HIDRADENITIS SUPPURATIVA

This condition involves hidradenitis of the apocrine sweat glands, which are usually located in the axilla and the inguinal region. In the breast, these glands are also found in the inframammary folds, between the breasts, and around the areola. Hidradenitis suppurativa has been reported in obese patients in regions where the skin surfaces of the breasts or chest wall rub together. Severe hidradenitis causes masses with local inflammation. Severe cases are treated by excision of local disease, but local recurrence is common after treatment.

NEUROFIBROMATOSIS

This autosomal dominant disease is composed of two main types, the most common of which is also known as von Recklinghausen

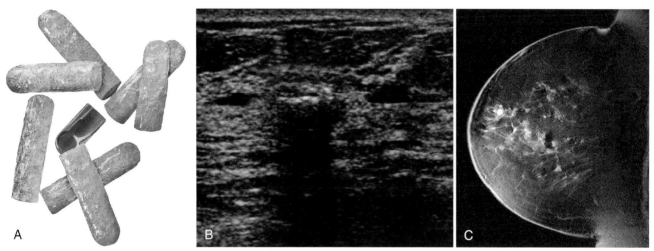

FIG. 10.59 Examples of foreign bodies: metallic clips and pellets. Metallic clips and pellets are often placed for marking the biopsy site after percutaneous needle biopsy. (A) Pellets and a metallic marker. (B) Echogenic ultrasound appearance after a gel marker is placed. (C) Magnetic resonance imaging signal void from a metallic marker.

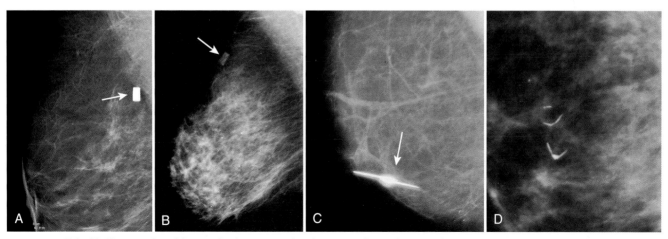

FIG. 10.60 Examples of foreign bodies: retained catheter, needle, and suture after procedure. (A) Cropped digital mammogram shows an opaque tubelike structure (*arrow*) in the upper right breast representing a retained cuff from a prior catheter. (B) Another retained Dacron Hickman catheter cuff (*arrow*) in the upper part of the right breast is seen as a radiopaque tube. (C) A needle (*arrow*) was iatrogenically placed by this patient into her own breast, and it subsequently broke and calcified. (D) Mammography shows sutures containing knots and a small calcified suture fragment.

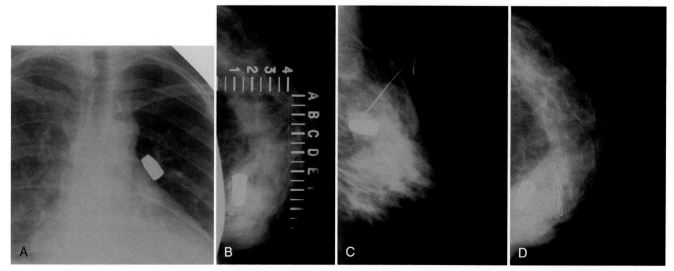

FIG. 10.61 Foreign bodies: bullet. Cropped chest radiograph (A) shows a bullet projected over the left breast. To remove the bullet, the patient underwent needle localization, shown here in the alphanumeric grid (B). Mediolateral oblique (C) and craniocaudal (D) mammograms of the left breast show the bullet at the end of the hookwire.

disease (type 1) and is found in 90% of patients. Affected patients may have café au lait skin lesions, neurofibromas of the neural plexus or peripheral nerve sheaths, and neurilemmomas.

The skin lesions of neurofibroma can mimic a deep breast tissue mass and limit evaluation of the breast. However, like any skin lesion, neurofibromas may be outlined with air, and correlation with the breast history form is advisable. Furthermore, the description of cutaneous findings on the technologist's sheet should enable the radiologist to distinguish neurofibromas on the skin from masses of ductal origin inside the breast (Fig. 10.62).

LYMPHANGIOMA

Lymphangioma or lymphangiomatosis is a rare benign malformation characterized by fibrous tissue containing thin-walled ectatic vascular channels lined with endothelial cells filled with lymph fluid. Lymphangiomas are classified as capillary lymphangioma, cavernous lymphangioma, cystic lymphangioma (cystic hygroma), and hemolymphangioma (vascular lymphatic malformation) based on the size of lymphatic spaces and the presence of vascular elements. The cystic lymphangioma is the most common type and is believed to result from lymph sac sequestration with failure to join central lymphatic channels. Clinically, lymphangioma typically presents as a fairly well circumscribed, soft, cystic mass, and is usually first diagnosed in childhood. Lymphangioma can arise at any part of the body except for the central nervous system, and is most common in the neck and axillary region. Involvement of the breast is extremely rare. In the breast, the distribution of lymphangioma is mainly toward the tail and the axilla, because it occurs along lymphatic drainage routes.

Because this disease basically occurs in children, mammography is not usually obtained because of the radiation exposure. Few reports show nonspecific appearance of breast cystic lymphangioma on mammography. Calcifications were not a common feature of lymphangioma but have been reported in adult lymphangiomas outside of the breast (Fig. 10.63). On ultrasonography, cystic lymphangioma is typically shown as a multiloculated, hypoechoic, cystic mass with linear septa. The tumor has well-defined margins, but the margins may not be observed, especially if it extends to the surrounding tissues. On computed tomography, lymphangioma usually appears as a homogeneous,

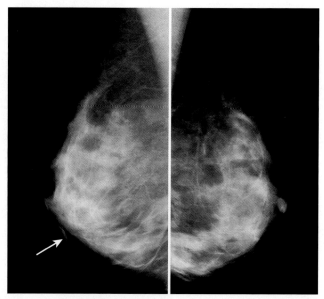

FIG. 10.62 Neurofibromatosis simulating breast masses. Bilateral lateral mammograms show a neurofibroma simulating a retroareolar mass on the left and a long neurofibroma extending from inferior to the nipple on the right (*arrow*).

low-attenuation mass, but may present as a higher attenuation or be comprised of a combination of fluid, solid tissue, and fat. On MRI, lymphangioma is typically seen as a septated mass that has heterogeneous T1- and high T2-weighted signal intensity, reflecting its fluid content. The mass demonstrates peripheral and septal enhancement after administration of gadolinium. Signal intensity may be altered because of complications such as spontaneous or traumatic hemorrhage. Other complications include rupture and infection.

POLAND SYNDROME

Poland syndrome is an absence of the pectoralis muscle on x-ray. It is usually unilateral. The mammogram shows absence of the pectoralis muscle on one side (Fig. 10.64).

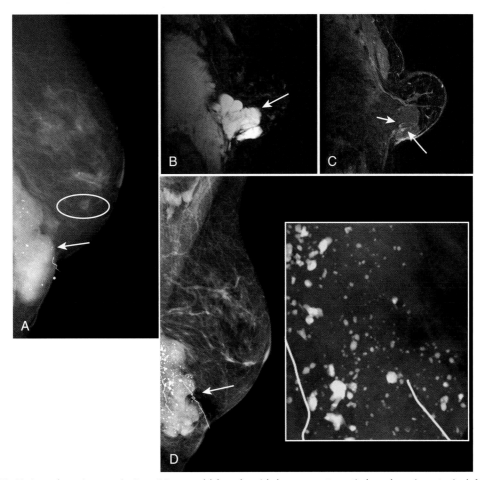

FIG. 10.63 Lymphangiomatosis. In a 55-year-old female with known systematic lymphangiomatosis, left lateral mammogram (A) shows a lobulated mass (*arrow*) with multiple, mostly round calcifications (*circle*) in the lower left breast. Sagittal T2-weighted image (B) of the left breast shows that the lobulated mass (*arrow*) has a high signal intensity, and extends from the thorax into the left lower breast. Sagittal contrast-enhanced T1-weighted image (C) demonstrates septal enhancement within the mass (*arrows*) with a low signal intensity. This was diagnosed as lymphangiomatosis involving the breast. Eight years later, left mediolateral oblique mammogram with its photographically magnified view (*right*; D) demonstrates that the mass is stable in size, but more calcifications developed with time (*arrow*). Generally, calcification is rare in lymphangioma, but can be seen in older patients. Note grouped pleomorphic microcalcifications (*circle*) in the central left breast in A, representing ductal carcinoma in situ diagnosed by partial resection. There is a linear scar marker on the lower left breast in A and D.

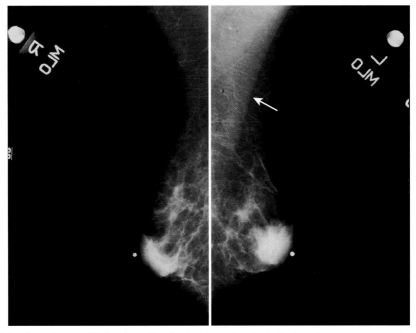

FIG. 10.64 Poland syndrome. Bilateral mediolateral oblique implant-displaced mammograms show a pectoralis muscle (*arrow*) on the left and absence of the pectoralis muscle on the right.

Key Elements

The normal male breast shows only fat on mammography.

Gynecomastia is unilateral or bilateral, symmetric or asymmetric, and is shown as glandular tissue in a retroareolar flamelike dendritic, triangular nodular, or diffuse appearance on mammography.

Gynecomastia causes breast lumps and pain and has physiologic, drug-related, and medical-related etiologies.

Breast cancer in men is rare, is manifested as a mass eccentric to the nipple or in the upper outer quadrant, and has the same prognosis as breast cancer in women.

Breast cancer in men develops at 1% the rate in women, occurs in older men, and on mammography is usually a noncalcified spiculated or circumscribed retroareolar or periareolar mass.

Pregnancy-related conditions include mastitis, lactational adenoma, enlarging fibroadenoma, galactocele, and pregnancy-associated breast cancer.

Pregnancy-associated breast cancer is defined as cancer diagnosed during pregnancy or within 1 year of delivery.

Stage for stage, the prognosis for pregnancy-associated breast cancer is the same as for nonpregnant women.

On mammography, pregnancy-associated breast cancer is detected as masses or pleomorphic calcifications.

Probably benign findings (Breast Imaging Reporting and Data System [BI-RADS] category 3) include single or multiple groups of small, round, or oval calcifications; circumscribed masses; and nonpalpable focal asymmetries that resemble fibroglandular tissue at diagnostic evaluation.

To identify subtle signs of malignancy and definitively benign entities, screen-detected findings should be recalled for full diagnostic imaging evaluation (including fine-detail diagnostic mammographic views and often ultrasound) before rendering a BI-RADS category 3 assessment and assigning short-term imaging follow-up.

Nipple discharge characteristics that should be investigated are new, bloody, or spontaneously occurring copious serous discharge.

Mammograms and ultrasound are frequently negative in the setting of nipple discharge.

A positive galactogram shows a filling defect, an abrupt duct cutoff, or luminal irregularity.

The differential diagnosis of intraductal masses on galactography includes papilloma, cancer, debris, and an air bubble.

Unilateral breast edema may be caused by mastitis, inflammatory cancer, local obstruction of lymph nodes, trauma, radiation therapy, or coumarin necrosis.

Bilateral breast edema is caused by systemic etiologies, such as congestive heart failure, liver disease, anasarca, renal failure, bilateral lymphadenopathy, or superior vena cava syndrome.

Although breast edema, exogenous hormone therapy, and weight loss all result in increased breast density, distinction between these causes is made by the presence of skin thickening, which is seen only with breast edema.

Inflammatory cancer is the most important differential diagnosis for unilateral breast edema and is a rare (1% of all cancers) aggressive breast cancer with a poor prognosis.

The most common cause of mastitis is *Staphylococcus aureus*; rare causes include tuberculosis, syphilis, hydatid disease, and molluscum contagiosum.

An extremely rare cause of unilateral breast edema is coumarin (warfarin [Coumadin]) therapy, producing necrosis of the breast.

Axillary lymphadenopathy on mammography is shown as replacement of the fatty hilum of lymph nodes by dense tissue, a rounded lymph node shape, and overall generalized increased density with or without lymph node enlargement.

The differential for abnormal lymph nodes containing calcifications includes calcifying metastatic disease, granulomatous disease, gold deposits from therapy for rheumatoid arthritis mimicking calcifications, or silicone from a previously ruptured breast implant.

The differential for unilateral axillary adenopathy includes metastatic breast cancer or mastitis.

The differential for bilateral axillary adenopathy is systemic conditions such as infection, collagen vascular diseases like rheumatoid arthritis, lymphoma, leukemia, and metastatic tumor.

Primary breast cancer manifested as isolated lymph node metastasis in women with normal mammographic findings and normal physical examinations is uncommon and accounts for less than 1% of all breast cancers.

Paget disease of the nipple heralds an underlying breast cancer with a high rate of overexpression of the c-erb-B2 oncogene.

Women with Paget disease of the nipple have a bright red nipple, eczematous nipple changes that may extend to the areola, and subsequent ulceration or nipple destruction.

Sarcomas are rare malignant tumors of the breast or underlying chest wall. Their classification depends on the cell type; mammography shows high-density masses without calcifications or spiculation.

Mondor disease is a rare benign and self-limited acute thrombophlebitis of the superficial veins of the breast. It is often associated with trauma or recent surgery and produces a tender palpable cord extending toward the outer portion of the breast.

Mammography is usually negative in women with Mondor disease or rarely shows a long linear or tubular density corresponding to the thrombosed vein.

Granulomatous mastitis is a rare benign cause of a breast mass in young premenopausal women after their last childbirth; it has been correlated with breast feeding and oral contraceptive use, and a possible autoimmune component has been implicated in its etiology.

Patients with granulomatous mastitis may have galactorrhea, inflammation, a breast mass, induration, and skin ulcerations. Treatment is surgery, but the recurrence rate is high.

Diabetic mastopathy is a benign cause of hard, irregular, sometimes painful mobile breast masses in long-term insulin-dependent diabetes, younger premenopausal diabetic women, or rare patients with thyroid disease.

Diabetic mastopathy is caused by an autoimmune reaction to the accumulation of abnormal matrix proteins caused by hyperglycemia. It produces a hard fibrotic mass with a lymphocytic reaction; treatment is surgery, but the recurrence rate is high.

Desmoid tumor is also known as an extraabdominal desmoid or fibromatosis.

Desmoid tumor is an infiltrative, locally aggressive fibroblastic/myofibroblastic process that is treated by surgery, may recur locally, may be multicentric, is associated with previous trauma or surgery, and has been reported in women with breast implants.

Trichinosis is caused by ingesting raw or undercooked meat containing encysted larvae of the Trichinella genus. The larvae give rise to tiny linear calcifications in the pectoralis muscles and not in the breast.

Dermatomyositis and some collagen vascular diseases can rarely produce bizarre sheetlike calcifications that are found to align along the breast tissues on mammography.

Foreign bodies in the breast seen on mammography include percutaneous metallic markers, acupuncture needle tips, hookwire fragments, calcifying sutures, vascular clips to mark breast cancer cavities for radiation therapy, Dacron Hickman catheter cuffs, and other foreign objects.

Hidradenitis suppurativa is a benign condition that produces breast lumps representing hidradenitis of the apocrine sweat glands in the axilla, between the breasts, and in the inframammary folds.

Neurofibromatosis is an autosomal dominant disease also known as von Recklinghausen disease (type 1); affected patients may have café au lait skin lesions and neurofibromas of the neural plexus or peripheral nerve sheaths. The skin lesions can cause apparent breast masses on mammography.

SUGGESTED READINGS

Ad-El DD, Meirovitz A, Weinberg A, et al.: Warfarin skin necrosis: local and systemic factors, *Br J Plast Surg* 53:624-626, 2000.

Ahn BY, Kim HH, Moon WK, et al.: Pregnancy- and lactation-associated breast cancer: mammographic and sonographic findings, *J Ultrasound Med* 22:491-499, 2003.

Al-Kkawari HAT, Al-Manfouhi HA, Madda JP, et al.: Radiologic features of granulomatous mastitis, *Breast J* 17:645-650, 2011.

Armant F, Deckers S, Van Calsteren K, et al.: Breast cancer in pregnancy: recommendations of an international consensus meeting, *Eur J Cancer* 46:3158-3368, 2010.

Azim HA, Santoro L, Russell-Edu W, et al.: Prognosis of pregnancy-associated breast cancer: a meta-analysis of 30 studies, *Cancer Treat Rev* 38(7):834-842, 2012.

Bayer U, Horn LC, Schulz HG: Bilateral, tumorlike diabetic mastopathy—progression and regression of the disease during 5-year follow up, *Eur J Radiol* 26:248-253, 1998.

Bejanga BI: Mondor's disease: analysis of 30 cases, *J R Coll Surg Edinb* 37:322-324, 1992.

Bergkvist L, Frodis E, Hedborg-Mellander C, Hansen J: Management of accidentally found pathological lymph nodes on routine screening mammography, *Eur J Surg Oncol* 22:250-253, 1996.

Berkowitz JE, Gatewood OM, Goldblum LE, Gayler BW: Hormonal replacement therapy: mammographic manifestations, *Radiology* 174:199-201, 1990.

Birdwell RL, Ikeda DM, O'Shaughnessy KF, Sickles EA: Mammographic characteristics of 115 missed cancers later detected with screening mammography and the potential utility of computer-aided detection, *Radiology* 219:192-202, 2001.

Brenner RJ: Follow-up as an alternative to biopsy for probably benign mammographically detected abnormalities, *Curr Opin Radiol* 3:588-592, 1991.

Brenner RJ: Percutaneous removal of postbiopsy marking clip in the breast using stereotactic technique, *AJR Am J Roentgenol* 176:417-419, 2001.

Bruwer A, Nelson GW, Spark RP: Punctate intranodal gold deposits simulating microcalcifications on mammograms, *Radiology* 163:87-88, 1987.

Camuto PM, Zetrenne E, Ponn T: Diabetic mastopathy: a report of 5 cases and a review of the literature, *Arch Surg* 135:1190-1193, 2000.

Cardonick E: Pregnancy-associated breast cancer: optimal treatment options, *Int J Womens Health* 6:935-943, 2014.

Chow JS, Smith DN, Kaelin CM, Meyer JE: Case report: galactography-guided wire localization of an intraductal papilloma, *Clin Radiol* 56:72-73, 2001.

Crowe DJ, Helvie MA, Wilson TE: Breast infection. Mammographic and sonographic findings with clinical correlation, *Invest Radiol* 30:582-587, 1995.

Cyrlak D, Wong CH: Mammographic changes in postmenopausal women undergoing hormonal replacement therapy, *AJR Am J Roentgenol* 161:1177-1183, 1993.

Dale PS, Wardlaw JC, Wootton DG, et al.: Desmoid tumor occurring after reconstruction mammaplasty for breast carcinoma, *Ann Plast Surg* 35:515-518, 1995.

Daniel BL, Gardner RW, Birdwell RL, et al.: Magnetic resonance imaging of intraductal papilloma of the breast, *Magn Reson Imaging* 21:887-892, 2003.

Dershaw DD, Moore MP, Liberman L, Deutch BM: Inflammatory breast carcinoma: mammographic findings, *Radiology* 190:831-834, 1994.

Diesing D, Axt-Fliedner R, Hornung D, et al.: Granulomatous mastitis, *Arch Gynecol Obstet* 269(4):233-236, 2004.

Doberl A, Tobiassen T, Rasmussen T: Treatment of recurrent cyclical mastodynia in patients with fibrocystic breast disease. A double-blind placebo-controlled study—the Hjorring project, *Acta Obstet Gynecol Scand* (Suppl 123)177-184, 1984.

Dominici LS, Lester S, Liao GS, et al.: Current surgical approach to Paget's disease, *Am J Surg* 204:18-22, 2012.

Dooley WC: Ductal lavage, nipple aspiration, and ductoscopy for breast cancer diagnosis, *Curr Oncol Rep* 5:63-65, 2003.

D'Orsi CJ, Sickles EA, Mendelson EB, Morris EA, et al.: *ACR BI-RADS® atlas, breast imaging reporting and data system*, Reston, VA, 2013, American College of Radiology.

Duijm LE, Guit GL, Hendriks JH, et al.: Value of breast imaging in women with painful breasts: observational follow up study, *BMJ* 317:1492-1495, 1998.

Dursun M, Yilmaz S, Yahyayev A, et al.: Multimodality imaging features of idiopathic granulomatous mastitis: outcome of 12 years of experience, *Radiol Med* 117:529-538, 2012.

Eby PR, DeMartini WB, Peacock S, et al.: Cancer yield of probably benign breast MR examinations, *J Magn Reson Imaging* 26:950-955, 2007.

Elson BC, Ikeda DM, Andersson I, Wattsgard C: Fibrosarcoma of the breast: mammographic findings in five cases, *AJR Am J Roentgenol* 158:993-995, 1992.

Evans GF, Anthony T, Turnage RH, et al.: The diagnostic accuracy of mammography in the evaluation of male breast disease, *Am J Surg* 181:96-100, 2001.

Expert Panel on MR Safety Kanal E, Barkovich AJ, Bell C, et al.: ACR Guidance Document on MR Safe Practices, *J. Magn Reson Imaging* 37:501-530, 2013.

Fields EC, DeWitt P, Fisher CM, et al.: Management of male breast cancer in the United States: a surveillance, epidemiology and end results analysis, *Int J Radiat Oncol Biol Physics* 87:747-752, 2013.

Finder CA, Kisielewski RW, Kedas AM: Residual metal shavings and fragments associated with large-core biopsy needles: a follow-up, *Radiology* 208:833-834, 1998.

Garstin WI, Kaufman Z, Michell MJ, Baum M: Fibrous mastopathy in insulin dependent diabetics, *Clin Radiol* 44:89-91, 1991.

Gautier N, Lalonde L, Tran-Thanh D, et al.: Chronic granulomatous mastitis: imaging, pathology and management, *Eur J Radiol* 82:165-175, 2013.

Giess CS, Golshan M, Flaherty K, Birdwell RL: Clinical experience with aspiration of breast abscesses based on size and etiology at an academic medical center, *J Clin Ultrasound* 42:513-521, 2014.

Godwin Y, McCulloch TA, Sully L: Extra-abdominal desmoid tumour of the breast: review of the primary management and the implications for breast reconstruction, *Br J Plast Surg* 54:268-271, 2001.

Graf O, Helbich TH, Hopf G, et al.: Probably benign breast masses at US: is follow-up an acceptable alternative to biopsy? *Radiology* 244:87-93, 2007.

Grimm IJ, Anderson AL, Baker JA, et al.: Frequency of malignancy and imaging characteristics of probably benign lesions seen at breast MRI, *AJR Am J Roentgenol* 205:442-447, 2015.

Gunhan-Bilgen I, Bozkaya H, Ustun EE, Memis A: Male breast disease: clinical, mammographic, and ultrasonographic features, *Eur J Radiol* 43:246-255, 2002a.

Gunhan-Bilgen I, Ustun EE, Memis A: Inflammatory breast carcinoma: mammographic, ultrasonographic, clinical, and pathologic findings in 142 cases, *Radiology* 223:829-838, 2002b.

Hambly NM, Liberman L, Dershaw DD, et al.: Background parenchymal enhancement on baseline screening breast MRI: impact on biopsy rate and short term follow up, *AJR* 196:218-224, 2011.

Handa P, Leibman AJ, Sun D, et al.: Granulomatous mastitis: changing clinical and imaging features with image-guided biopsy correlation, *Eur Radiol* 24:2404-2411, 2014.

Harenberg J, Hoffmann U, Huhle G, et al.: Cutaneous reactions to anticoagulants. Recognition and management, *Am J Clin Dermatol* 2(2):69-75, 2001.

Harvey JA, Nicholson BT, Cohen MA: Finding early invasive breast cancers: a practical approach, *Radiology* 248:61-76, 2008.

Haupt HM, Rosen PP, Kinne DW: Breast carcinoma presenting with axillary lymph node metastases. An analysis of specific histopathologic features, *Am J Surg Pathol* 9:165-175, 1985.

Homer MJ, Smith TJ: Asymmetric breast tissue, *Radiology* 173:577-578, 1989.

Hook GW, Ikeda DM: Treatment of breast abscesses with US-guided percutaneous needle drainage without indwelling catheter placement, *Radiology* 213:579-582, 1999.

Ikeda DM, Birdwell RL, O'Shaughnessy KF, et al.: Analysis of 172 subtle findings on prior normal mammograms in women with breast cancer detected at follow-up screening, *Radiology* 226:494-503, 2003.

Ikeda DM, Helvie MA, Frank TS, et al.: Paget disease of the nipple: radiologic-pathologic correlation, *Radiology* 189:89-94, 1993.

Ikeda DM, Sickles EA: Mammographic demonstration of pectoral muscle microcalcifications, *AJR Am J Roentgenol* 151:475-476, 1988.

Ingram AD, Mahoney MC: An overview of breast emergencies and guide to management by interventional radiologists, *Tech Vasc Interv Radiol* 17(1):55-63, 2014.

Joshi S, Dialani V, Marotti J, et al.: Breast disease in the pregnant and lactating patient: radiological-pathological correlation, *Insights Imaging* 4(5):527-538, 2013.

Kasper V, Baumgarten C, Bonvalot S, et al.: Management of sporadic desmoid-type fibromatosis: A European consensus approach based on patients' and professionals' expertise—A Sarcoma Patients EuroNet and European Organisation for Research and Treatment of Cancer/Soft Tissue and Bone Sarcoma Group initiative, *Eur J Cancer* 51(2):127-136, 2015.

Kedas AM, Byrd LJ, Kisielewski RW: Residual metal shavings and fragments associated with large-core breast biopsy, *Radiology* 200:585, 1996.

Kerlikowske K, Smith-Bindman R, Abraham LA, et al.: Breast cancer yield for screening mammographic examinations with recommendation for short-interval follow-up, *Radiology* 234:684-692, 2005.

Kim MJ, Wapnir IL, Ikeda DM, et al.: MRI enhancement correlates with high grade desmoid tumor of breast, *Breast J* 18(4):374-376, 2012.

Kopans DB, Swann CA, White G, et al.: Asymmetric breast tissue, *Radiology* 171:639-643, 1989.

Kushwaha AC, Whitman GJ, Stelling CB, et al.: Primary inflammatory carcinoma of the breast: retrospective review of mammographic findings, *AJR Am J Roentgenol* 174:535-538, 2000.

Leibman AJ, Kossoff MB: Mammography in women with axillary lymphadenopathy and normal breasts on physical examination: value in detecting occult breast carcinoma, *AJR Am J Roentgenol* 159:493-495, 1992.

Leroux-Stewart J, Rabasa-Lhoret R: Diabetic mastopathy: case report and summary of literature, *Can J Diabetes* 38:305-306, 2014.

Leung JWT, Kornguth PJ, Gotway MB: Utility of targeted sonography in the evaluation of focal breast pain, *J Ultrasound Med* 21:521-526, 2002.

Leung JWT, Sickles EA: Multiple bilateral masses detected on screening mammography: assessment of need for recall imaging, *AJR Am J Roentgenol* 175:23-29, 2000.

Leung JWT, Sickles EA: Developing asymmetry identified on mammography: correlation with imaging outcome and pathologic findings, *AJR Am J Roentgenol* 188:667-675, 2007a.

Leung JWT, Sickles EA: The probably benign assessment, *Radiol Clin North Am* 23:773-789, 2007b.

Liberman L, Giess CS, Dershaw DD, et al.: Imaging of pregnancy-associated breast cancer, *Radiology* 191:245-248, 1994.

Liberman L, Morris EA, Benton CL, et al.: Probably benign lesions at breast magnetic resonance imaging: preliminary experience in high-risk women, *Cancer* 98:377-388, 2003.

Lim HS, Jeong SJ, Lee JS, et al.: Paget disease of the breast: mammographic, US, and MR imaging findings with pathologic correlation, *Radiographics* 31:1973-1987, 2011.

Liu GJ, Chen WG, Duan G, et al.: Mammographic findings of gynecomastia, *Di Yi Jun Yi Da Xue Xue Bao* 22:839-840, 2002.

Lubina N, Schedelbeck U, Roth A, et al.: 3.0 Tesla breast magnetic resonance imaging in patients with nipple discharge when mammography and ultrasound fail, *Eur Radiol* 25:1285-1293, 2015.

Mahoney MC, Ingram AD: Breast emergencies: types, imaging features, and management, *AJR Am J Roentgenol* 202:W390-W399, 2014.

Matsuoka K, Ohsumi S, Takashima S, et al.: Occult breast carcinoma presenting with axillary lymph node metastases: follow-up of 11 patients, *Breast Cancer* 10:330-334, 2003.

Memis A, Bilgen I, Ustun EE, et al.: Granulomatous mastitis: imaging findings with histopathologic correlation, *Clin Radiol* 57:1001-1006, 2002.

Montrey JS, Levy JA, Brenner RJ: Wire fragments after needle localization, *AJR Am J Roentgenol* 167:1267-1269, 1996.

Morris EA, Comstock CE, Lee CH, et al.: ACR BI-RADS magnetic resonance imaging. In *ACR BI-RADS atlas, breast imaging reporting and data system*, Reston, VA, 2013, American College of Radiology.

Murakami R, Kumita S, Yamaguchi K, Ueda T: Diabetic mastopathy mimicking breast cancer, *Clin Imaging* 33:234-236, 2009.

Murray ME, Given-Wilson RM: The clinical importance of axillary lymphadenopathy detected on screening mammography, *Clin Radiol* 52:458-461, 1997.

Nicholson BT, Harvey JA, Cohen MA: Nipple-areolar complex: normal anatomy and benign and malignant processes, *Radiographics* 29(2):509-523, 2009.

Orel SG, Dougherty CS, Reynolds C, et al.: MR imaging in patients with nipple discharge: initial experience, *Radiology* 216:248-254, 2000.

Park YM, Kim EK, Lee JH, et al.: Palpable breast masses with probably benign morphology at sonography: can biopsy be deferred? *Acta Radiol* 49:1104-1111, 2008.

Parsi K, Younger I, Gallo J: Warfarin-induced skin necrosis associated with acquired protein C deficiency, *Australas J Dermatol* 44:57-61, 2003.

Raza S, Chikarmane SA, Neilsen SS, et al.: BI-RADS 3, 4, and 5 lesions: value of US in management—follow-up and outcome, *Radiology* 248:773-781, 2008.

Rieber A, Tomczak RJ, Mergo PJ, et al.: MRI of the breast in the differential diagnosis of mastitis versus inflammatory carcinoma and follow-up, *J Comput Assist Tomogr* 21:128-132, 1997.

Rosen EL, Baker JA, Soo MS: Malignant lesions initially subjected to short-term mammographic follow-up, *Radiology* 223:221-228, 2002.

Sachs DD, Gordon AT: Hidradenitis suppurativa of glands of Moll, *Arch Ophthalmol* 77:635-636, 1967.

Sadowski EA, Kelcz F: Frequency of malignancy in lesions classified as probably benign after dynamic contrast-enhanced breast MRI examination, *J Magn Reson Imaging* 21:556-564, 2005.

Sardanelli F, Boetes C, Borisch B, et al.: Magnetic resonance imaging of the breast: recommendations from the EUSOMA working group, *Eur J Cancer* 46(8):1296-1316, 2010.

Sawhney S, Petkovska L, Ramadan S, et al.: Sonographic appearances of galactoceles, *J Clin Ultrasound* 30:18-22, 2002.

Schnarkowski P, Kessler M, Arnholdt H, Helmberger T: Angiosarcoma of the breast: mammographic, sonographic, and pathological findings, *Eur J Radiol* 24:54-56, 1997.

Serels S, Melman A: Tamoxifen as treatment for gynecomastia and mastodynia resulting from hormonal deprivation, *J Urol* 159:1309, 1998.

Shin JH, Han BK, Ko EY, et al.: Probably benign breast masses diagnosed by sonography: is there a difference in the cancer rate according to palpability? *AJR Am J Roentgenol* 192:187-191, 2009.

Sickles EA: Mammographic features of 300 consecutive nonpalpable breast cancers, *AJR Am J Roentgenol* 146:661-663, 1986.

Sickles EA: Nonpalpable, circumscribed, noncalcified solid breast masses: likelihood of malignancy based on lesion size and age of patient, *Radiology* 192:439-442, 1994.

Sickles EA: Periodic mammographic follow-up of probably benign lesions: results in 3,184 consecutive cases, *Radiology* 179:463-468, 1991.

Sickles EA: Probably benign breast lesions: when should follow-up be recommended and what is the optimal follow-up protocol? *Radiology* 213:11-14, 1999.

Sickles EA: The spectrum of breast asymmetries: imaging features, work-up, management, *Radiol Clin North Am* 45:765-771, 2007.

Sonnenblick EB, Margolies LR, Szabo JR, Jacobs LM, Patel N, Lee KA: Digital breast tomosynthesis of gynecomastia and associated findings—a pictorial review, *Clin Imaging* 38:565-570, 2014.

Spick C, Szolar DH, Baltzer PA, et al.: Rate of malignancy in MRI-detected probably benign (BI-RADS 3) lesions, *AJR Am J Roentgenol* 202:684-689, 2014.

Stomper PC, Waddell BE, Edge SB, Klippenstein DL: Breast MRI in the evaluation of patients with occult primary breast carcinoma, *Breast J* 5:230-234, 1999.

Swinford AE, Adler DD, Garver KA: Mammographic appearance of the breasts during pregnancy and lactation: false assumptions, *Acad Radiol* 5:467-472, 1998.

Talele AC, Slanetz PJ, Edmister WB, et al.: The lactating breast: MRI findings and literature review, *Breast J* 9:237-240, 2003.

Tilanus-Linthorst MM, Obdeijn AI, Bontenbal M, Oudkerk M: MRI in patients with axillary metastases of occult breast carcinoma, *Breast Cancer Res Treat* 44:179-182, 1997.

Trop I, Dugas A, David J, et al.: Breast abscesses: evidence-based algorithms for diagnosis, management, and follow-up, *Radiographics* 31:1683-1699, 2011.

van Gelder L, Bisschops RH, Menke-Pluymers MB, Westenend PJ, Plaisier PW: Magnetic resonance imaging in patients with unilateral bloody nipple discharge; useful when conventional diagnostics are negative? *World J Surg* 39:184-186, 2015.

Varas X, Leborgne F, Leborgne JH: Nonpalpable, probably benign lesions: the role of follow up mammograpy, *Radiology* 184(2):409-414, 1992.

Varas X, Leborgne JH, Leborgne F, Mezzera J, Jaumandreu S, Leborgne F: Revisiting the mammographic follow-up of BI-RADS category 3 lesions, *AJR Am J Roentgenol* 179:691-695, 2002.

Vashi R, Hooley R, Butler R, Geisel J, Philpotts L: Breast imaging of the pregnant and lactating patient: physiologic changes and common benign entities, *AJR Am J Roentgenol* 200:329-336, 2013.

Weinstein SP, Hanna LG, Gatsonis C, Schnall MD, Rosen MA, Lehman CD: Frequency of malignancy seen in probably benign lesions at contrast-enhanced breast MR imaging: findings from ACRIN 6667, *Radiology* 255:731-737, 2010.

Woo JC, Yu T, Hurd TC: Breast cancer in pregnancy: a literature review, *Arch Surg* 138:91-99, 2003.

Yasmeen S, Romano PS, Pettinger M, et al.: Frequency and predictive value of a mammographic recommendation for short-interval follow-up, *J Natl Cancer Inst* 95:429-436, 2003.

Youk JH, Kim EK, Ko KH, Kim MJ: Asymmetric mammographic findings based on the fourth edition of BI-RADS: types, evaluation, and management, *Radiographics* 29:e33, 2009.

Chapter 11

^{18}F-FDG PET/CT and Nuclear Medicine for the Evaluation of Breast Cancer

Camila Mosci, Kanae K. Miyake, and Andrew Quon

CHAPTER OUTLINE

Since its introduction in the early 1990s as a promising functional imaging technique, positron emission tomography (PET) and subsequently PET combined with computed tomography (PET/CT), has gained widespread acceptance in several oncologic procedures such as tumor staging and restaging, treatment efficacy assessment during or after treatment, and radiotherapy planning. PET is a sensitive and specific noninvasive technology used to depict the whole-body distribution of positron-emitting biomarkers. The fundamental strength of PET over conventional imaging is the ability to convey functional information that even the most exquisitely detailed anatomic image cannot provide. The primary radiotracer used in PET/CT imaging is ^{18}F-fluorodeoxyglucose (^{18}F-FDG), a glucose analog taken up by cells in proportion to their rate of glucose metabolism. The increased glycolytic rate and glucose avidity of malignant cells in comparison to normal tissue is the basis of the ability of ^{18}F-FDG PET/CT imaging to accurately differentiate cancer from benign tissue regardless of morphology (Gambhir, 2002). This ability to sensitively detect malignancy within the entire body in one scan as well as the ability to differentiate benign from cancerous structures has allowed PET/CT imaging to positively impact the care of cancer patients, particularly those with breast cancer, over the last 10 years.

This chapter reviews ^{18}F-FDG PET and PET/CT imaging of breast cancer. In addition, it outlines conventional nuclear medicine techniques, including lymphoscintigraphy and bone scintigraphy, which are often used in the assessment of breast cancer.

PET/CT SCANNING PRINCIPLES

PET and PET/CT Scanners

In positron decay, a nuclide transforms one of its core protons into a neutron and emits a positron (β^+). The β^+ will annihilate with an atomic electron and they will convert their mass into energy and produce a pair of photons (called annihilation photons) that travels in opposite directions exactly 180 degrees apart from each other. The radiotracers used in this imaging technique, such as ^{18}F-FDG, are positron emitters. The equipment measures the two annihilation photons that are produced after positron emission. This is the key difference from the conventional radiotracers used in nuclear medicine that only emit single photons in any direction at each decay event. Accordingly, PET scanners are designed as a ring of multiple pairs of photon detectors arranged 180 degrees apart from each other with the patient lying in the middle of this ring. These pairs of photon detectors, which are made of either bismuth germanium oxide, gadolinium orthosilicate, or lutetium orthosilicate crystals, are electronically linked such that they accept only pairs of photons that arrive at both detectors at exactly the same time point and reject scattered photons that arrive at incongruent time points (Fig. 11.1; Box 11.1). This design allows for superior photon sensitivity and spatial resolution, because a lead-based collimator, such as those used in conventional nuclear medicine scanners, is no longer needed to reduce scattered photons that hit the camera face at tangential angles.

PET/CT scanners are integrated units with the individual PET and CT components nearly identical to their stand-alone counterparts. Integrated PET/CT has the added advantage of using the CT data for attenuation correction (see Box 11.1) and anatomic localization and, additionally, more sophisticated PET/CT fusion software can be used for interpretation. CT-based attenuation correction, however, may introduce artifacts on PET when imaging high-density materials such as bowel contrast and metallic prostheses. The field of view of a modern PET/CT scanner is approximately 16 to 18 cm wide (see Box 11.1). The bed is advanced into the scanner in six to seven increments

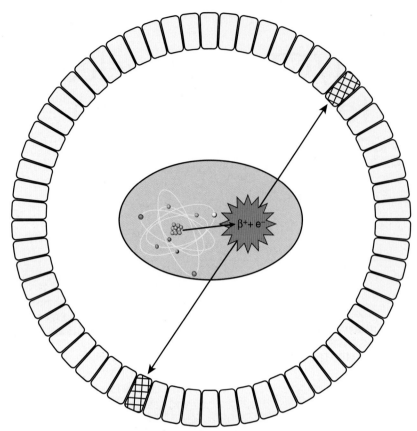

FIG. 11.1 Schematic of a positron emission tomography (PET) scanner. Inside a PET scanner: a positron is emitted and annihilated after interaction with an electron. Two gamma rays are emitted 180 degrees apart and detected by paired detectors. (Courtesy Andrei Iagaru, M.D., Andrew Quon, M.D., Stanford University School of Medicine.)

BOX 11.1   Essentials of Positron Emission Tomography and Positron Emission Tomography/Computed Tomography Instrumentation

Scintillation crystal types:
Bismuth germanium oxide
Gadolinium orthosilicate
Lutetium orthosilicate
Scanner field of view: 16–18 cm in the axial dimension, 68–72 cm gantry diameter
Attenuation correction:
Computed tomography (CT)-based (integrated positron emission tomography [PET]/CT)
Germanium 68 rod source (stand-alone PET)

---

for a patient to be scanned from the base of the skull to the midthigh. An additional six to seven increments are required for scanning the extremities. Typically, each increment, termed a *bed position*, requires 1 to 5 minutes of acquisition time before moving on to the next section of the body. The acquisition time is dependent on a variety of factors including patient weight and girth, scanner sensitivity, and amount of injected radiotracer. In contrast to conventional cross-sectional imaging, scanning starts at the pelvis and moves cranially to minimize the amount of urine accumulation in the bladder.

¹⁸F-Fluorodeoxyglocose

¹⁸F-FDG is the primary radiotracer in clinical use for oncologic PET and PET/CT scanning, including breast cancer. Once injected, ¹⁸F-FDG is transported into cells via the glucose transporter system (GLUT) and quickly phosphorylated by hexokinase II. After phosphorylation, it is trapped within the cell where it decays with a physical half-life of 110 minutes. Typically, imaging commences at 45 to 90 minutes after injection of tracer to allow for adequate time for tumor accumulation and background washout from renal clearance (Box 11.2).

Patient preparation before and after ¹⁸F-FDG injection is critical for high-quality scanning (see Box 11.2). Because ¹⁸F-FDG is a glucose analog, increased serum levels of insulin and/or glucose may alter the biodistribution of ¹⁸F-FDG. High levels of either endogenous or injected insulin cause significant uptake of FDG in muscle and greatly decrease the sensitivity of the scan. For this reason, diabetic patients who have used regular insulin within 4 hours of FDG injection usually require rescheduling, as do patients who have eaten a meal within 8 hours. A less significant and somewhat controversial factor is that high levels of circulating glucose may potentially compete with FDG at tumor sites, decreasing sensitivity of the scan as well. Patients should be instructed to fast for at least 4 to 6 hours before the intravenous administration of ¹⁸F-FDG so that PET images are not affected by circulating glucose as well as endogenous insulin. Most institutions reschedule the study if a patient's blood glucose level is greater than 150 to 200 mg/dL. Detailed procedure guidelines for tumor imaging with ¹⁸F-FDG PET/CT are provided by the Society of Nuclear Medicine and Molecular Imaging (SNMMI) (Delbeke et al., 2006).

Accurate interpretation requires knowledge of the physiology of ¹⁸F-FDG as well as the limitations of PET scanning. Box 11.3 summarizes the pearls in the interpretation of ¹⁸F-FDG PET/CT for breast cancer assessment. Greater ¹⁸F-FDG uptake levels suggest a greater likelihood of malignancy; however, it is not reliable when used alone. Equally important is learning to differentiate

PATIENT PREPARATION

BEFORE ^{18}F-FLUORODEOXYGLUCOSE (FDG) INJECTION

Overnight fast (recommend 4- to 6-h fast)

Insulin-dependent diabetics:

　　Morning scan: Skip morning breakfast and insulin dose

　　Afternoon scan: Have morning meal and insulin dose, fast thereafter

Noninsulin-dependent diabetics:

　　Fast overnight and skip morning oral hypoglycemic medication

After FDG Injection

Minimize physical activity and talking

Minimize visual stimulation

Drink three to four glasses of water

Urinate immediately before scan

RADIOTRACER

^{18}F-FDG

Intravenous dose

5–7 mCi (3D acquisition)

10–15 mCi (2D acquisition)

INSTRUMENTATION

Begin scanning at 45 to 90 min after injection of tracer

Start at pelvis and scan toward head

Field of view per bed position: 16–18 cm

Length of acquisition: 3–7 min per bed position

BOX 11.3 Breast Cancer Interpretation Pearls

PRIMARY BREAST LESIONS

Focal lesions are more suspicious

Malignancies have standardized uptake value beyond background tissue

Lesions <1 cm difficult to characterize

Invasive ductal carcinoma is ^{18}F-fluorodeoxyglucose (FDG)-avid

Lobular carcinoma is poorly FDG-avid

Fibrous or dense breasts have greater background FDG activity and hamper lesion detection

DISTANT LESIONS

Axillary metastasis <1 cm difficult to characterize

Sentinel lymph node dissection superior to positron emission tomography for staging axilla

Osteolytic bone metastases: high sensitivity

Osteoblastic bone metastases: moderate sensitivity

focal from nonfocal lesions through experience (there is no clinically used quantitative parameter for focality), with focal lesions more likely to be malignant than benign.

Physiologic tracer uptake of considerable intensity is typically seen in the brain, liver, bowel, mediastinal blood pool, myocardium, and lymphoid tissue. Additionally, marked tracer uptake is seen in the kidneys, ureters, and bladder where ^{18}F-FDG is excreted. A multitude of common physiologic variants can also occur. These include marked fat activity, particularly in the head and neck (termed *brown fat* uptake; Fig. 11.2), skeletal muscle uptake caused by physical activity after the injection of ^{18}F-FDG, and increased areolar and ovarian activity dependent on lactation

and hormonal cycles. Even with abnormal ^{18}F-FDG uptake beyond these physiologic variants, a host of benign processes may cause abnormal findings on PET scanning. These include infection and inflammation, certain benign or adenomatous lesions (including fibroadenomas and phyllodes tumor), and granulomatous disease. Physiologic or benign tracer uptake of considerable intensity may mimic or mask tumor uptake. Causes of false-positives and false-negatives are summarized in Boxes 11.4 and 11.5, respectively. Common benign breast lesions that have no elevated ^{18}F-FDG activity are listed in Box 11.6.

Quantitative Values

Quantitative analysis plays an important role in oncology PET studies for various settings, particularly in the assessment of treatment effect. Standardized uptake value (SUV) is a quantitative value that is measurable on ^{18}F-FDG PET and PET/CT. It represents the image-derived radioactivity concentration in a target at a certain time point, normalized on the basis of the radioactivity concentration in the hypothetical case of an even distribution of the injected radioactivity across the entire body. The SUV is calculated according to the following formula: $SUV = C/(ID/W)$, where C represents the decay-corrected tissue activity concentration in megabecquerels per kilogram measured with PET, ID is the injected dose in megabecquerels, and W is patient weight in kilograms. A metric similar to SUV, called the standardized uptake value lean body mass (SUL) is the SUV corrected with the lean body mass index. This value accounts for variability in SUV secondary to body fat composition. Thinner patients tend to have a lower SUV compared with obese patients.

Several parameters have been developed to determine the single representative value of the SUV (or SULs) of a target (Table 11.1). The most common parameter in clinical practice (the de facto standard) is SUVmax. The "max" designation infers the single-voxel value of the hottest point within a region of interest or volume of interest (VOI). SUVmax or SULmax may be highly variable because of the voxel-to-voxel noise in a PET image. For this reason, other metrics may be used. For example, in the PET Response Criteria in Solid Tumors, Wahl et al. (2009) recommend the use of SULpeak for therapeutic monitoring, because SUVpeak (the average value of SULs within a 1 cm³-volume VOI that includes the hottest voxel) is less susceptible to noise compared with SULmax.

Recently there has been an increasing interest in the use of volumetric parameters of metabolism, such as metabolic tumor volume (MTV) and total lesion glycolysis (TLG), particularly for the estimation of prognosis. MTV is the volume of tumor tissues with increased ^{18}F-FDG uptake that meets a predefined minimum SUV threshold (a common threshold standard is 40% of SUVmax within a VOI). TLG can be calculated by multiplying MTV by SUVmean (or SULmean), which weights the volumetric burden and metabolic activity of tumors. Other quantitative parameters that require more complex data-collection procedures are being used as well.

CLINICAL UTILITY OF ^{18}F-FLUORODEOXYGLUCOSE POSITION EMISSION TOMOGRAPHY AND POSITION EMISSION TOMOGRAPHY/COMPUTED TOMOGRAPHY FOR BREAST CANCER

Breast cancer is the second most common cancer in the world and, by far, the most frequent cancer among women with an estimated 1.67 million new cancer cases diagnosed in 2012 (World Health Organization, 2015). In 2014 an estimated 232,670 new cases and 40,430 deaths from breast cancer were expected in the United States (Siegel et al., 2014). The incidence of breast cancer has increased over the past few decades, but mortality appears to be declining, suggesting a benefit from the combination of early diagnosis and effective treatment.

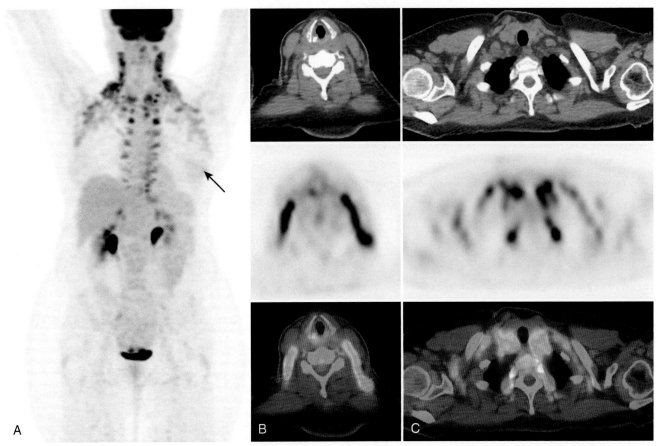

FIG. 11.2 Physiologic uptake in brown fat on ¹⁸F-fluorodeoxyglucose positron emission tomography (PET)/computed tomography (CT). A 63-year-old female with a left breast cancer. (A) Maximal intensity projection PET image. (B and C) Axial views (CT, *top*; PET, *middle*; and PET/CT, *bottom*) of the same patient at the level of the neck (B) and the supraclavicular region (C). Moderate to intense uptake, corresponding to the lucent fat tissue on CT, is observed in the neck, axilla, and paraspinal regions, bilaterally, representing physiologic uptake in brown fat. Pretreatment with a β-blocker or diazepam can be helpful to reduce the physiologic uptake in brown fat. Note physiologic uptake in the brain, mediastinal blood pool, myocardium, and liver, as well as in the kidneys, ureters, and bladder, where ¹⁸F-FDG is excreted. Mild uptake (A, *arrow*) in the left breast represents the primary infiltrating lobular carcinoma.

BOX 11.4   False-Positive Breast Lesions on Positron Emission Tomography/Computed Tomography

WITHIN BREAST TISSUE

Fibroadenoma (10% of lesions)
Granuloma
Infection/inflammation
Proliferative dysplasia
Ductal ectasia
Phyllodes tumor
Lactating breast
Areolar activity
Postsurgical changes
Dense fibrous tissue

DISTANT SITES

Brown fat in the head and neck
Infection
Fractures
Bowel
Bladder/ureter

BOX 11.5   False-Negative Breast Lesions on PET/CT

Lobular carcinoma
Carcinoma in situ
Small lesion size (<1 cm)

BOX 11.6   Benign Breast Lesions with no ¹⁸F-Fluorodeoxyglucose Activity

Cysts
Normal fibroglandular tissue
Fibroadenomas (10%)
Implants

If at the time of diagnosis only local disease is confirmed, the patient undergoes curative-intended surgery followed by adjuvant local and systemic treatment depending on the extent of surgery and nodal stage. If distant metastases are diagnosed, the disease is considered incurable and palliative treatment such as systemic chemotherapy and radiation should be considered. The detection of disseminated disease has a considerable influence on treatment management clarifying the importance for accurate

TABLE 11.1 Definition of Quantitative Values Used in Positron Emission Tomography Imaging

Quantitative Values	Definition
SUVmax (SULmax)	Single-voxel value of the hottest point within a target
SUVmean (SULmean)	Average value of the whole single-voxel SUVs (or SULs) within a delineated target
$SUV_{70\%}$ ($SUL_{70\%}$)	Average value of the single-voxel SUVs (or SULs) within a VOI that is defined as the 3D isocontour at 70% of the maximum voxel value
SUVpeak (SULpeak)	Average value of SUVs (or SULs) within a $1cm^3$–volume VOI that includes the hottest voxel
MTV	Volume of tumor tissues with increased ^{18}F-FDG uptake
TLG	Calculated by multiplying MTV by SUVmean (or SULmean)

^{18}F-FDG, ^{18}F-fluorodeoxyglucose; *MTV*, metabolic tumor volume; *SUL*, standard uptake value normalized with lean body mass index; *SUV*, standard uptake value; *TLG*, total lesion glycolysis; *VOI*, volume of interest.

TABLE 11.2 National Comprehensive Cancer Network® (NCCN®) Recommendations in Patients with Breast Cancer: ^{18}F-Fluorodeoxyglucose Positron Emission Tomography/ Computed Tomography versus Bone Scintigraphy

	^{18}F-FDG PET/CT	Bone Scintigraphy
DCIS		
Clinical stage 0	Not recommended	Not recommended
LOCALIZED INVASIVE BREAST CANCER		
Clinical stages IA, IIA, and IIB	Not recommended	Indicated for patients with localized bone pain or elevated alkaline phosphatase (2A)
Clinical stage IIIA (T3-N1M0)	Optional (2B)	Considered[a] (2A)
Preoperative systemic therapy for stage IIA (T2-N01M0), IIB, and IIIA (T3-N1M0)	Optional (2B)	Considered[a] (2A)
After lumpectomy with surgical axillary staging; Four or more positive axillary lymph nodes	Optional (2B)	Considered (2A)
LOCALLY ADVANCED INVASIVE BREAST CANCER (NONINFLAMMATORY)		
Clinical stage IIIA (T0-3N2M0), IIIB. and IIIC	Optional[b,c] (2B)	Considered[a] (2A)
INFLAMMATORY BREAST CANCER		
Clinical stage T4d, N0-3, M0	Recommended as workup (2B); particularly when standard staging studies are equivocal or suspicious	Recommended as workup (2A)
PATIENTS WITH METASTATIC DISEASE		
Clinical stage IV metastatic cancer (baseline)	Optional workup (2B)	Recommended as workup[a] (2A)
Monitoring metastatic disease	Optional (2B)	Recommended (2A)
AFTER TREATMENT		
No clinical signs and symptoms suggestive of recurrence (initially stage I to III)	Not recommended	Not recommended
Recurrent cancer	Optional (2B)	Recommended[a] (2A)

[a]^{18}F-fluoride (^{18}F-NaF) positron emission tomography (PET)/computed tomography (CT) (2B) is also indicated.
[b]FDG PET/CT can be performed at the same time as diagnostic CT. The use of PET or PET/CT scanning is not indicated in the staging of clinical stage I, II, or operable III breast cancer. FDG PET/CT is most helpful in situations where standard staging studies are equivocal or suspicious, especially in the setting of locally advanced or metastatic disease.
[c]FDG PET/CT may also be helpful in identifying unsuspected regional nodal disease and/or distant metastases in locally advanced breast cancer when used in addition to standard staging studies.
Number in parenthesis indicates category of evidence; *category 1*, high-level evidence; *category 2A*, lower level evidence, uniform NCCN consensus that the intervention is appropriate; *category 2B*, lower level evidence, NCCN consensus that the intervention is appropriate; *category 3*, any level of evidence, major NCCN disagreement that the intervention is appropriate.
From National Comprehensive Cancer Network (NCCN): NCCN clinical practice guidelines in oncology, breast cancer. Version 2.2016. Panel chair, et al., NCCN Clinical Practice Guidelines in Oncology (NCCN Guidelines®) Breast Cancer. Version 2.2016. © 2014 National Comprehensive Cancer Network, Inc. Available at NCCN.org. Accessed: 2016.

staging. Prediction of treatment response to avoid unnecessary toxicity and change to a potentially effective treatment is also very important.

The National Comprehensive Cancer Network® NCCN Clinical Practice Guidelines in Oncology (NCCN Guidelines®) (2015) suggest that ^{18}F-FDG PET/CT may be used in staging, restaging, and treatment monitoring in breast cancer (Table 11.2). Additionally, ^{18}F-FDG PET/CT has a higher diagnostic performance than radionuclide bone scintigraphy for detection of osseous metastases, but the relative costs of the two examinations should be considered depending on local practice and reimbursement patterns. Overall, the role of PET/CT in clinical diagnosis and management of breast cancer patients is increasing and evolving and include the advent of newer tracers such as ^{18}F-fluoride (^{18}F-NaF) PET/CT bone scanning.

Detection of Breast Cancer

Noninvasive breast cancer has been previously shown to be poorly imaged by ^{18}F-FDG PET (Avril et al., 2000; Fig. 11.3); thus the majority of ^{18}F-FDG PET research studies in the literature have been performed on patients with invasive breast cancer. Earlier small studies in selected patient groups reported 100% sensitivity and accuracy. However, larger and more recent series (Avril et al., 2000; Garami et al., 2012; Schirrmeister et al., 2001) showed ^{18}F-FDG PET sensitivity varying in the range from 84% to 93%. The overall specificity of ^{18}F-FDG PET is relatively high but false-positives do occur in some benign inflammatory lesions and fibroadenomas (Jones et al., 1999; Palmedo et al., 1997).

The two major contributing factors that explain the varied statistical results between studies are histopathology and size of the lesion (see Box 11.3). Invasive breast cancer includes multiple histologic types comprising infiltrating ductal, infiltrating lobular, and combined infiltrating carcinoma. Infiltrating ductal carcinoma has a higher level of ^{18}F-FDG uptake; therefore it is detected at a significantly higher sensitivity than infiltrating lobular breast cancer (Avril et al., 2000; Crippa et al., 1998). This difference in ^{18}F-FDG uptake between the two histologic types suggests that tumor aggressiveness is not the sole determinant of ^{18}F-FDG uptake. The mechanism of the variable ^{18}F-FDG uptake by breast cancer cells is likely modulated by multiple factors, such as GLUT-1 expression, hexokinase I activity, tumor microvessel density, amount of necrosis, number of lymphocytes, tumor cell density, and mitotic activity (Bos et al., 2002).

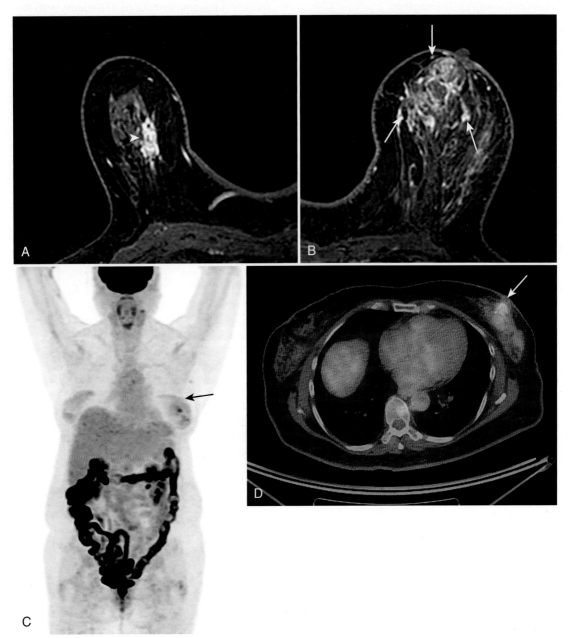

FIG. 11.3 Ductal carcinoma in situ (DCIS) on ^{18}F-fluorodeoxyglucose (FDG) positron emission tomography (PET)/computed tomography (CT). A 62-year-old female with bilateral DCIS. (A and B) Contrast-enhanced magnetic resonance imaging. Axial image of the right breast (A) shows 2.1-cm mass enhancement (*arrowhead*) accompanied with nonmass enhancement below it, representing DCIS. Axial image of the left breast (B) shows clumped nonmass enhancement (*arrows*) extending 5.2 × 3.5 × 3.5 cm, representing another DCIS with postbiopsy hematoma. (C and D) ^{18}F-FDG PET/CT. Maximal intensity projection PET image (D) and axial PET/CT image (C) show moderate uptake (SUVmax 3.9; *arrows*) in the left breast, corresponding to the DCIS or postprocedure change; however, no apparent uptake is detected in the DCIS in the right breast. Note intense physiologic bowel uptake.

Studies have shown that breast tumor size significantly affects ^{18}F-FDG PET/CT results (Fig. 11.4). Many studies have shown that sensitivity of PET is substantially low in the detection of breast cancers smaller than 1 cm (Avril et al., 1996; Kumar et al., 2006). Garami et al. (2012) described that PET/CT sensitivity varies in the different T (size) groups: 42.8% in T1a, b malignancies, and 93.9% and 98.0% in stages T1c and T2, respectively. Small lesions are at the limit of the resolution of modern PET systems, which is approximately 6 mm (with the newest PET/CT systems possibly having a spatial resolution of 4 mm). Lesions in this size range and smaller will be below the threshold of detectability. Quantitative values in small lesions are also affected by partial volume effects.

In summary, the results of ^{18}F-FDG PET for the initial detection and diagnosis of primary breast cancer vary largely because of heterogeneity of the disease and tumor size (see Boxes 11.4–11.6). Improvements in spatial resolution and scanner sensitivity as well as the advent of dual modality PET/CT scanning may lead to ^{18}F-FDG PET being more useful for breast cancer diagnosis (Fueger et al., 2005). ^{18}F-FDG PET may also play an important adjunctive role in selected patients with dense breasts in which mammography has a much poorer sensitivity (Vranjesevic et al., 2003). Indeed, to increase diagnostic accuracy in detecting breast tumors dedicated breast-PET scanners such as positron emission mammography (PEM) as well as PET/magnetic resonance imaging (MRI) has been applied.

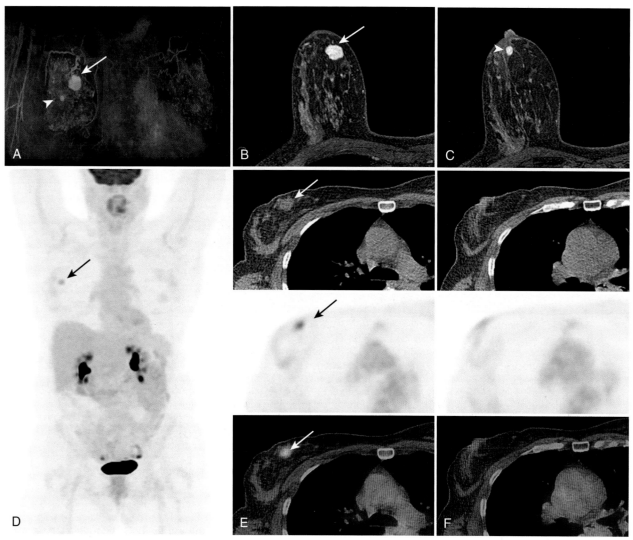

FIG. 11-4 Difference of uptake between larger and smaller breast cancers on ¹⁸F-fluorodeoxyglucose (FDG) positron emission tomography (PET)/computed tomography (CT). A 48-year-old female with two invasive ductal carcinomas in the right breast. (A–C) Contrast-enhanced magnetic resonance images. Frontal view of maximal intensity projection (MIP) image (A) and two axial images (B and C) show a 1.9-cm index tumor (*arrow* in A and B) and a 7.5-mm additional tumor (*arrowhead* in A and C). (D–F) ¹⁸F-FDG PET/CT. MIP PET images (D) show a focal moderate uptake (SUVmax 3.6) corresponding to the index tumor (*arrow*); however, there is no apparent uptake for the additional tumor. Axial views (CT, *top*; PET, *middle*; and PET/CT, *bottom*) of the patient show the details of the index tumor (E) and the additional tumor (F). It is often difficult to detect subcentimeter breast cancer on whole-body PET/CT.

Initial Staging

The TNM staging system is used for classification, prognostication, and treatment planning in breast cancer patients. The 5-year relative survival rate decreases according to stage at presentation from 99% in localized disease, to 84% in node-positive disease, and 24% in distant disease.

The performance of ¹⁸F-FDG PET imaging in initial staging of primary breast cancer can be separated into two general categories: (1) staging of axillary lymph nodes in which PET or PET/CT has presented mixed results and (2) staging of mediastinal and internal mammary lymph nodes (IMLs) and distant metastatic disease in which ¹⁸F-FDG PET or PET/CT has consistently performed well.

Axillary lymph node involvement in breast cancer patients is an indicator of prognosis and an important factor in determining medical management and therapy. An increase in the number of tumor-positive axillary nodes is related to a worsened prognosis

irrespective of primary tumor size. Because conventional anatomic imaging cannot reliably detect axillary nodal metastasis, patients with invasive breast cancer routinely undergo sentinel lymph node biopsy (SLNB) and axillary lymph node dissection (ALND) for accurate staging. This practice is under debate, because the identification of axillary nodal involvement may not improve overall survival rate, and because ALND is associated with a high incidence of morbidities, such as lymphedema and decreased range of motion of the ipsilateral arm and shoulder girdle. Therefore ¹⁸F-FDG PET has been extensively studied for noninvasive staging of axilla. These results have been mixed (Fig. 11.5). Early results were quite encouraging with high sensitivities and specificities reported. However, a larger prospective multicenter study involving 360 women with 308 assessable axillary lymph nodes by Wahl et al. (2004) reported lower sensitivity for ¹⁸F-FDG PET in detecting axillary nodal disease; the overall sensitivity, specificity, and positive and negative predictive values were 61%, 80%, 62%, and 79%, respectively, using

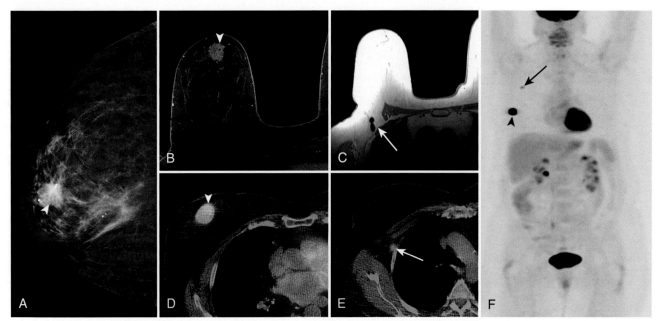

FIG. 11.5 ¹⁸F-fluorodeoxyglucose (FDG) positron emission tomography (PET)/computed tomography (CT) for nodal staging. A 68-year-old female with a newly diagnosed right breast cancer. (A) Craniocaudal mammogram of the right breast shows a 2.2-cm retroareolar irregular mass (*arrowhead*) with a metallic biopsy marker, representing an invasive ductal cancer. Note the architectural distortion in the breast parenchyma caused by previous surgery. (B and C) Magnetic resonance (MR) images. Contrast-enhanced fat suppressed T1-weighter (B) shows an enhanced mass corresponding to the primary cancer (*arrowhead*). T1-weighted MR image (C) shows axillary lymph nodes (*arrow*) measuring up to a 7-mm short axis. Although not enlarged, the lack of fatty hilum makes them suspicious for possible metastatic involvement. (D and E) ¹⁸F-FDG PET/CT. Axial PET/CT fusion images of primary cancer (D) and of right axillary lymph nodes (E) and maximal intensity projection PET image (F). Intense focal uptake is observed corresponding to the primary tumor (*arrowheads* in D and F). Axillary lymph nodes are also hypermetabolic (*arrows* in E and F), consistent with metastatic lymph nodes. Pathologically, the lymph nodes were positive for metastatic disease. ¹⁸F-FDG PET/CT contributed to an increase the confidentiality of axillary lymph node metastasis in this case.

pathologic results obtained by ALND as the gold standard. They stated that ¹⁸F-FDG PET may fail to detect tumor in the axilla when few and small nodal metastases are present, whereas it may be highly predictive for nodal involvement when multiple intense foci of tracer uptake are identified. A prospective study involving 250 patients by Cermik et al. (2008) demonstrated that ¹⁸F-FDG PET had different sensitivities depending on the axillary lymph node pathologic stages. PET can detect axillary lymph node involvement with higher sensitivity in patients with higher nodal stages: 41% in pN1, 67% in pN2, and 100% in pN3. The specificity was 89% for the pN0 stage. Koolen et al. (2012) analyzed dual-modality PET/CTs in 311 patients who presented with primary invasive breast cancer >3 cm and/or proven axillary node metastasis and were scheduled for neoadjuvant chemotherapy (NAC), using cytology or histopathology obtained with ultrasound-guided fine-needle aspiration or SLNB before NAC as gold standards. Sensitivity, specificity, positive predictive value, negative predictive value, and accuracy of FDG-avid nodes for the detection of axillary metastases were 82%, 92%, 98%, 53%, and 84%, respectively. On the other hand, Choi et al. (2012) evaluated 154 subjects with invasive breast cancer using histopathological results and imaging follow-up as gold standards and found a PET/CT sensitivity of 37.3% and specificity of 95.8% to detect metastatic axilla, whereas the U.S. corresponding estimates were 41.2% and 93.7%.

Earlier studies suggesting a high sensitivity of ¹⁸F-FDG PET for the detection of axillary metastases did not use the more sensitive methods of serial sectioning and cytokeratin immunohistochemistry currently used in the assessment of SLNs. With increasing numbers of trials and larger sample sizes, more recent studies have consistently suggested that ¹⁸F-FDG PET and PET/CT may

not have a sufficient negative predictive value to justify foregoing ALND. Although the sensitivity is suboptimal, the specificity of ¹⁸F-FDG PET and PET/CT appears to be relatively high, ranging from 89% to 96%. FDG-avid lymph nodes may be highly predictive for nodal involvement. Koolen et al. (2012) suggested that patients with FDG-avid nodes can skip SLNB to exclude the axillary metastasis and may undergo ALND without SLNB.

Another current issue found in axially nodal staging is an inherent sampling error of core needle biopsy that leads to underestimation of invasive breast cancer in patients with carcinoma in situ. Omission of axillary node staging is recommended in subjects with pure ductal carcinoma in situ (DCIS) to avoid procedure morbidity. However, approximately one-quarter of these patients are subject to underestimation of invasive breast carcinoma; consequently, additional axillary lymph node staging is performed. There are still no established factors with which to identify patients who truly need axillary lymph node staging at the same time as breast surgery and those who can safely forego it. Shigematsu et al. (2014) evaluated cases of DCIS at primary needle biopsy who underwent curative surgery, and the association between the SUVmax on ¹⁸F-FDG PET/CT before excision and the underestimation of invasive breast cancer was examined. Their findings showed that SUVmax on ¹⁸F-FDG PET/CT was a strong independent predictive factor of underestimation of invasive breast cancer in cases of DCIS diagnosed at needle biopsy.

In contrast to the mixed results and indeterminable roles of ¹⁸F-FDG PET in axillary lymph node staging, many studies have consistently demonstrated that ¹⁸F-FDG PET is superior to conventional imaging in the detection of nodal metastasis in extraaxillary lymph nodes, such as internal mammary, periclavicular, or mediastinal lymph nodes (Figs. 11.6 and 11.7). The

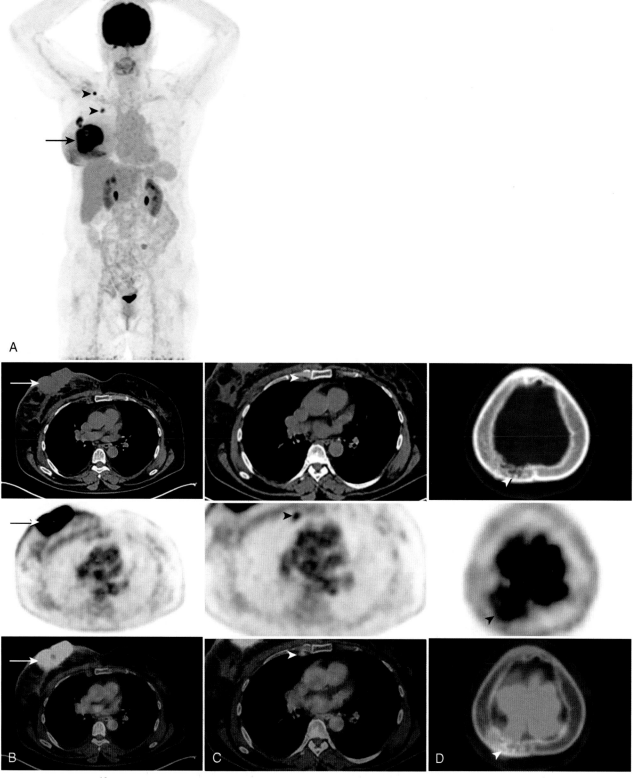

FIG. 11.6 ¹⁸F-fluorodeoxyglucose positron emission tomography (PET)/computed tomography (CT) for initial staging. A 56-year-old woman with diagnosis of infiltrative ductal carcinoma of the right breast. (A) Maximal intensity projection PET image shows increased uptake in the primary tumor (*arrow*) and lymph nodes (*arrowheads*). (B–D) Axial views in detail of the same patient: CT (*top*), PET (*middle*), and PET/CT (*bottom*) of the primary tumor (B, *arrows*), internal mammary lymph node (C, *arrowheads*), and lytic bone lesion on the scalp (D, *arrowheads*).

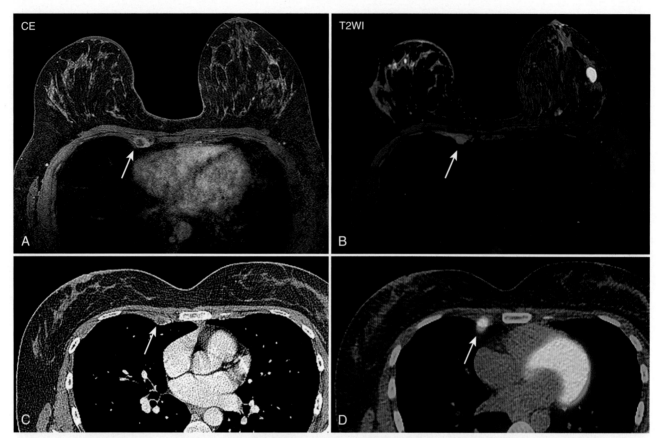

FIG. 11.7 ¹⁸F-fluorodeoxyglucose (FDG) positron emission tomography (PET)/computed tomography (CT) for initial staging. A 34-year-old female with a newly diagnosed right invasive breast cancer. (A and B) Magnetic resonance imaging. Axial contrast-enhanced fat-suppressed T1-weighted image (A) shows a small oval mass with heterogeneous enhancement (*arrow*), measuring 10 x 24 x 20 mm, in the right middle to lower internal mammary chain. This mass appears as a high signal on axial fat-suppressed T2-weighted image (B, *arrow*). The differential diagnosis includes a vascular varix, a schwannoma, and an enlarged lymph node. (C) Axial contrast-enhanced CT image. Heterogeneous enhancement is seen within the mass (*arrow*). (D) Axial ¹⁸F-FDG PET/CT fusion image. The mass has intense FDG uptake (SUVmax 6.2), and nodal metastasis was diagnosed. PET/CT contributed to the diagnosis of metastatic internal mammary lymph node.

presence of a tumor-positive extraaxillary lymph node results in a further decrease in survival (Carter et al., 1989; Sugg et al., 2000; Brito et al., 2001). Koolen et al. (2012) reported that occult lymph node metastases in the internal mammary chain and periclavicular area were detected in 8% and 10% of 311 patients scheduled for NAC, respectively, resulting in changed regional radiotherapy planning in 16% of the patients. Another study (Aukema et al., 2010) involving stage II and III breast cancer patients demonstrated that ¹⁸F-FDG PET/CT detected extraaxillary lymph nodes in 28% of the patients. Moreover, it showed suspicious uptake in extraaxillary lymph nodes that were not detected by conventional imaging (ultrasound and SLNB) in 17% of the patients, impacting the TNM staging.¹⁸F-FDG PET is also effective in detecting distant lesions and provides staging information even at the time of initial diagnosis (Fig. 11.8). PET/CT scans are always performed as whole-body scans, which is beneficial because spread of cancer to organs not primarily suspected of disease can be demonstrated. Also, PET/CT allows for simultaneous acquisition of a diagnostic-quality contrast-enhanced CT; therefore it is considered a better diagnostic strategy in unknown disease stage, compared with conventional methods that are restricted to examining the location or organ of interest. A second primary cancer can also be detected on PET/CT (Fig. 11.9). Several investigators (Dose et al., 2002; Moon et al., 1998) have shown that ¹⁸F-FDG PET is relatively sensitive (86%–93%) in the evaluation of metastases

from breast cancers. A recent study of dual modality PET/CT showed that the sensitivity and specificity in the detection of distant metastases is approximately 97.4% and 91.2%, respectively, compared with 85.9% and 67.3%, respectively, in conventional images (Niikura et al., 2011). Alberini et al. (2009) found that PET/CT detected distant metastases in 31% of patients with inflammatory breast cancer but these metastases were recognized in only 33% of them with conventional imaging. In patients who were not suspected of having distant metastases, distant metastases were also found in a nonnegligible percentage of patients with noninflammatory, but large (>3 cm) breast cancers (Fuster et al., 2008), as well as in two series of patients in whom PET/CT was used in the workup of patients with stage II or III breast cancer (Groheux et al., 2008; Segaert et al., 2010). ¹⁸F-FDG PET/CT has also been demonstrated to be superior to bone scintigraphy for depicting bone metastases from breast cancer (Liu et al., 2011). Details about the comparison of PET, PET/CT, and bone scintigraphy will be discussed later in this chapter.

The staging of distant metastasis is one of the most important parts of ¹⁸F-FDG PET and PET/CT in patients with breast cancer. Since 2004, the Centers of Medicare Services has approved of coverage for ¹⁸F-FDG PET scanning for the staging patients with distant metastasis. Additionally, NCCN guidelines consider ¹⁸F-FDG PET/CT may be used for clinical stage III and IV breast cancer patients (as an optional examination) or for those with inflammatory breast cancer.

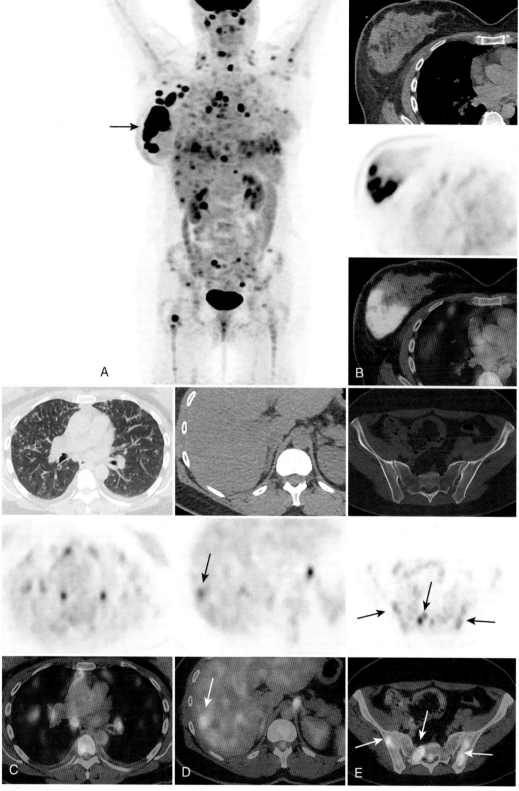

FIG. 11.8 ¹⁸F-fluorodeoxyglucose (FDG) positron emission tomography (PET)/computed tomography (CT) for initial staging. A 48-year-old female with a history of recently diagnosed stage IIIA T3N1 infiltrating ductal carcinoma of the right breast. (A) Maximal intensity projection PET image shows a large intense uptake (*arrow*), representing the newly diagnosed primary breast cancer. In addition, PET demonstrates multiple foci of increased uptake, suggesting multiple nodal and distant metastases. (B–E) Axial views (CT, *top*; PET, *middle*; and PET/CT, *bottom*) of the breast (B), the lung (C), the liver (D), and the pelvis (E). The primary cancer is shown to occupy a hypermetabolic area in the outer right breast (B). In the lung, nodular interlobular septal thickening, with diffuse FDG uptake, is considered to represent lymphangitic spread of tumor (C). Hepatic (D, *arrow*) and osseous metastases (E, *arrows*) are also present. Hypermetabolic lymph nodes are seen not only in the right axilla, but also in the mediastinum, at the bilateral hilum, and in the upper abdomen. FDG PET/CT contributed to detect additional metastatic lymph nodes and distant metastases, resulting in upstaging the patient to stage IV.

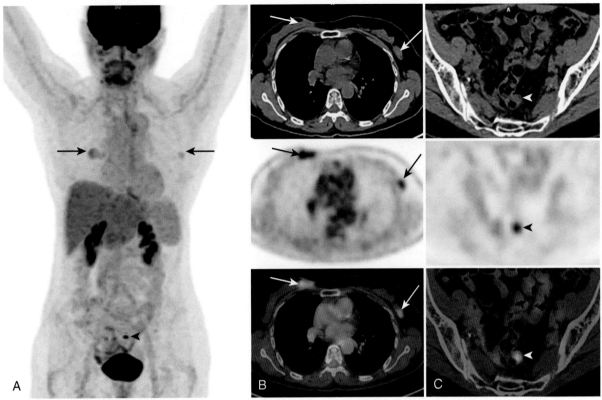

FIG. 11.9 Second cancer detected on ¹⁸F-fluorodeoxyglucose positron emission tomography (PET)/computed tomography (CT) for initial staging. A 62-year-old female with bilateral breast cancer submitted to four cycles of chemotherapy. (A) Maximal intensity projection PET image shows primary breast tumor bilaterally (*arrows*) and second primary tumor on the colon (*arrowhead*). (B and C) Axial views in detail of the primary tumor (B, *arrows*) on CT (*top*), PET (*middle*), and PET/CT (bottom) and the colon cancer (C, *arrowheads*) on CT (*top*), PET (*middle*), and PET/CT (*bottom*).

It is particularly helpful when standard staging studies are equivocal or suspicious. Riedl et al. (2014) suggested that PET/CT also might be valuable for stage IIB disease in younger patients, because it revealed distant metastases in 17% of asymptomatic stage IIB breast cancer patients younger than 40 years old in their study.

Cost-effectiveness of ¹⁸F-FDG PET/CT in breast cancer was analyzed in a meta-analysis (Sloka et al., 2005). In this study, the representative population was a 55-year-old woman presenting with stage I or II breast cancer. Authors compared PET and ALND in selected patients with ALND in all patients. A cost savings of $695 per person is expected for the PET strategy, with an increase in life expectancy (7.4 days), compared with the non-PET strategy. This cost savings remained in favor of the PET strategy when subjected to a sensitivity analysis.

Prognostic Estimation

Several reports have shown that SUV and MTV obtained with PET/CT are useful for predicting survival (Ueda et al., 2008; Oshida et al., 1998; Inoue et al., 2004).

Intratumoral metabolic heterogeneity can be demonstrated by analyzing ¹⁸F-FDG distribution within tumors (Kubota et al., 1992). The heterogeneity is an important feature of malignant tumors. It is caused by haphazard cellular proliferation, necrosis, and accumulation of extracellular material and appears as cellular morphologic characteristics, gene expression, metabolism, and motility, and as variations in behavioral characteristics such as angiogenesis and changes in proliferative, immunogenic, and metastatic potential (Son et al., 2014). Son et al. (2014) evaluated the prognostic implication of findings of intratumoral metabolic heterogeneity on pretreatment ¹⁸F-FDG PET/CT scans in patients with invasive ductal breast carcinoma and found that

intratumoral metabolic heterogeneity significantly affected the overall survival in these patients. The heterogeneity factor may act as a robust surrogate marker for the prediction of overall survival in these patients.

Another cohort involving 253 subjects studied the prognostic SUV, MTV, and TLG in patients with newly diagnosed metastatic breast cancer. They found that FDG avidity is a prognostic biomarker. SUVmax and TLG were both predictors of survival in breast cancer patients with bone metastases. They also found that TLG may be a more informative biomarker of overall survival than SUVmax for patients with lymph node and liver metastases (Ulaner et al., 2013).

Treatment Monitoring

¹⁸F-FDG PET is a metabolic imaging modality that has high sensitivity in the detection of therapy-induced glucose metabolic rate changes, which may not be evident in anatomic images after treatment. This concept has naturally led to the evaluation of PET for treatment monitoring. Two different clinical situations may be considered in treatment monitoring: (1) patients undergoing NAC for locally advanced, operable tumor and (2) patients undergoing chemotherapy for metastatic tumor.

Many recent publications have reported encouraging results for a role of ¹⁸F-FDG PET/CT in early evaluation of the response to NAC (Duch et al., 2009; Groheux et al., 2014; Lee et al., 2014; Ogino et al., 2014; Schelling et al., 2000). NAC has been used largely for controlling locally advanced breast cancer or large tumors. It results in significant tumor shrinkage, enabling breast conservation surgery and predicting response to postoperative adjuvant chemotherapy. Early prediction of response offers an opportunity to change chemotherapy strategy in case of ineffectiveness and to avoid unwarranted side effects. Anatomic imaging with mammography, ultrasonography, and MRI are used to assess how tumors respond. However, these methods are dependent on tumor size, have limited reproducibility, and cannot distinguish fibrosis from viable tumor. The delay between the treatment and tumor shrinkage limits the accuracy of these methods, such as when several cycles of chemotherapy are necessary to significantly change lesion size. Although the optimal interpretation criteria and, specifically, an optimum cutoff value for the SUV reduction rate is still not clearly defined, Duch et al. (2009) recommended a cutoff value of >40% of SUVmax decrease in the primary tumor to appropriately detect therapeutic response. They also stated that low baseline SUVmax can underestimate response to treatment. Groheux et al. (2014) described a cutoff value of 42% to predict response and found that the change in tumor uptake after two cycles of NAC can predict early the inefficacy in triple negative breast cancer. Using a cutoff of 50% another group found sensitivity, specificity, and accuracy of PET/CT in detecting responders of 93%, 75%, and 87%, respectively (Kumar et al., 2009).

There are few studies regarding the utility of PET/CT in monitoring patients with metastatic breast disease (Figs. 11.10 and 11.11). Moreover, in most studies, PET is performed without CT (Jansson et al., 1995; Gennari et al., 2000; Couturier et al., 2006). There is some evidence that hybrid ¹⁸F-FDG PET/CT provides useful information for assessing the efficacy of chemotherapy. The presence of persistently FDG-avid lesions after chemotherapy has been reported to correlate with poorer prognosis in patients with bone metastasis (Du et al., 2007). A decrease in SUV and an increase in CT-based attenuation in bone metastases are potential predictors of response duration. Furthermore PET/CT allows evaluation of response in many different metastases, enabling the identification of a heterogeneous response (Groheux et al., 2013).

NCCN guidelines suggest ¹⁸F-FDG PET/CT as an optional study for monitoring the therapeutic effect of preoperative systemic therapy as well as systemic therapy for metastatic disease. However, they also state that PET imaging may be challenging in monitoring metastatic breast cancer, because of the absence of a reproducible, validated, and widely accepted set of standards for disease activity assessment. Further studies are warranted to clarify the utility of ¹⁸F-FDG PET/CT in this situation.

PET image interpretation in breast cancer includes notable pitfalls in interpretation. In estrogen receptor-positive tumors, metastases may actually show *increased* ¹⁸F-FDG intensity after therapy as a predictive response to successful antiestrogen treatment, which is described as "metabolic flare." This transient increase in ¹⁸F-FDG activity after hormone therapy initiation may be the result of an initial stimulation of tumor growth by estrogen-like agonist effects induced by increased levels of the hormone (Mortimer et al., 2001). The metabolic flare occurs as early as 7 to 10 days after treatment initiation and may be the earliest and most accurate predictor of hormonal therapy response. Another phenomenon seen after the initiation of chemotherapy is diffuse bone marrow uptake of the axial skeleton (Fig. 11.12). Diffusely and homogeneously increased bone marrow uptake represents rebound hyperactive bone marrow or hematopoiesis caused by chemotherapy and can be accompanied with increased uptake in the spleen. The other causes of diffuse bone marrow uptake include the administration of granulocyte colony-stimulating factor or erythropoietin, severe anemia, cytokines from tumors, leukemia, and myelodysplastic syndrome. Diffuse bone marrow uptake can also represent diffuse bone marrow metastases or malignant bone marrow infiltration (although this is more common in patients with lymphoma). Diffuse bone or bone marrow metastases from breast cancer tends to be shown as heterogeneous, nodular multiple uptake foci rather than uniform diffuse uptake.

Recurrence Evaluation

Up to 30% of breast cancer patients will have recurrent disease within 10 years of initial treatment, and restaging is critical for therapeutic management of the patient (Kruse et al., 2013). ¹⁸F-FDG PET can be very helpful in evaluating asymptomatic, already treated breast cancer patients who may pose a diagnostic challenge for detecting occult recurrences (Fig. 11.13). In a large series of 132 patients evaluated for disease recurrence, Pecking et al. (2001) reported that ¹⁸F-FDG PET detected lesions in 106 patients, with an overall sensitivity of 94% and a positive predictive value of 96%. A meta-analysis by Isasi et al. (2005) of the diagnostic performance of ¹⁸F-FDG PET in detecting breast cancer recurrence and metastasis found a median sensitivity of 92.7% and median specificity of 81.6%. Published data consistently demonstrate that ¹⁸F-FDG PET has a similar or superior diagnostic accuracy compared with other conventional imaging modalities in the detection of recurrent breast cancer. Hybrid PET/CT also seems to perform better than conventional imaging modalities. Groheux et al. (2013) reviewed publications investigating the role of ¹⁸F-FDG PEC/CT in the detection of recurrent disease and found a sensitivity between 85% and 97%, specificity between 52% and 100%, and an accuracy between 60% and 98%. The 2012 meta-analysis by Evangelist et al. of 13 articles that evaluated the role of PET and PET/CT in breast cancer recurrence detection in the presence of elevated tumor markers provided pooled sensitivity of 87.8%, pooled specificity of 69.3%, and pooled accuracy of 82.8%. ¹⁸F-FDG PET and PET/CT may have an important role, particularly in the setting of asymptomatic patients with rising tumor markers levels and negative conventional imaging results.

PET appears to lead to a change in management in a significant number of patients. A recent publication by Manohar et al. (2012) described that ¹⁸F-FDG PET/CT had a major impact on management in 41% of the patients analyzed for a major change in treatment. Another group, Cochet et al. (2014), found that the management impact of PET/CT was high (change of treatment modality or intent) in 48% patients and medium (change in radiation treatment volume or dose fractionation) in 9% of the patients.

Radiation Planning

An ever-growing application of PET/CT is radiation treatment planning. Fused PET and CT images provide radiation oncologists with critical information with a single study including (1) the volume and extent of viable tumor and (2) the presence of unexpected regional disease to be included in the radiation field. Studies showed that ¹⁸F-FDG PET/CT improved the accuracy of target definition and PET/CT reduced the interobserver variability compared with CT alone (Nestle et al., 2006; MacManus et al., 2009; Tejwani et al., 2012).

Initial studies in patients with varied tumor types have confirmed that using PET/CT both in pretreatment planning and in follow-up evaluations have a significant impact on radiotherapy management in up to 56% of patients (Ciernik et al., 2003; Giraud et al., 2001).

DEVELOPING POSITRON EMISSION TOMOGRAPHY TECHNOLOGIES

Current efforts to improve PET resolution and sensitivity include the development of time-of-flight calculation techniques that account for the slight difference in time that the pairs of photons arrive at the detectors to further localize the origin of positron decay within the patient (Surti et al., 2006). Integrated PET/MRI and dedicated high-resolution breast PET systems are being developed and evaluated at several institutions worldwide.

Dedicated Breast Position Emission Tomography Systems

The PET systems dedicated for breast are high-resolution PET imaging systems with a limited field of view. These systems have sophisticated detectors that consist of small detector elements and are placed close to the breast, increasing photon reception and yielding higher photon sensitivity and improved spatial resolution compared with whole-body PET systems. Dedicated breast PET systems can be classified into two types (Bowen

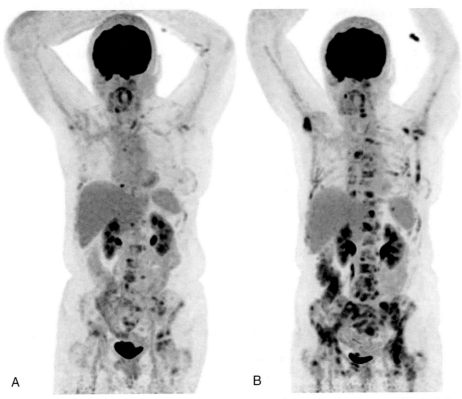

FIG. 11.10 ^{18}F-fluorodeoxyglucose positron emission tomography (PET)/computed tomography (CT) for treatment monitoring. A 66-year-old female with metastatic breast cancer. (A) Maximal intensity projection (MIP) PET image shows an uptake in osteoblastic lesions in the axial and appendicular skeleton. (B) MIP PET image of the study performed after six cycles of chemotherapy demonstrates multiple new bone lesions, suggesting progressive metabolic disease.

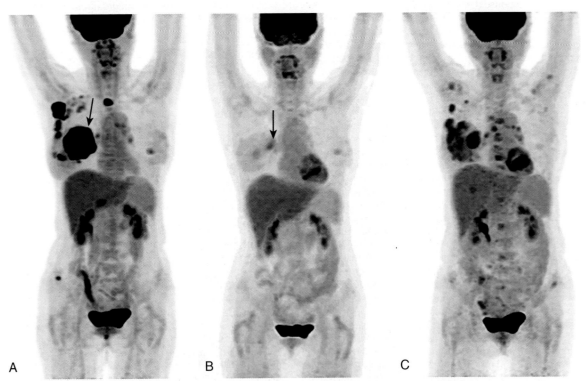

FIG. 11.11 ^{18}F-fluorodeoxyglucose (FDG) positron emission tomography (PET)/computed tomography (CT) for treatment monitoring. A 52-year-old female with a locally advanced infiltrating ductal carcinoma of the right breast. Maximal intensity projection (MIP) PET images obtained at initial diagnosis (A), 8 months (B), and 20 months (C) after the initiation of chemotherapy. At the initial diagnosis (A), PET shows hypermetabolic right breast cancer (*arrow*); hypermetabolic right axillary, subpectoral, and supraclavicular lymph nodes; and several hypermetabolic osseous foci involving the fourth cervical and second thoracic spine and the right iliac wing suspicious for metastases, suggesting stage IV breast cancer. After the initiation of chemotherapy (B), FDG activity of all the abnormal uptake foci remarkably decreased, suggesting interval partial metabolic response. An arrow indicates the residual faint uptake at the primary site. On CT (not shown), there were multiple new sclerotic foci throughout the axial skeleton, but non–FDG-avid, likely representing sequelae of treatment. However, the third PET (C) shows increased uptake in right breast mass, right breast subcutaneous nodules, mediastinal lymph nodes, a right hepatic lobe lesion, and several sclerotic osseous lesions, representing progression of metabolic disease.

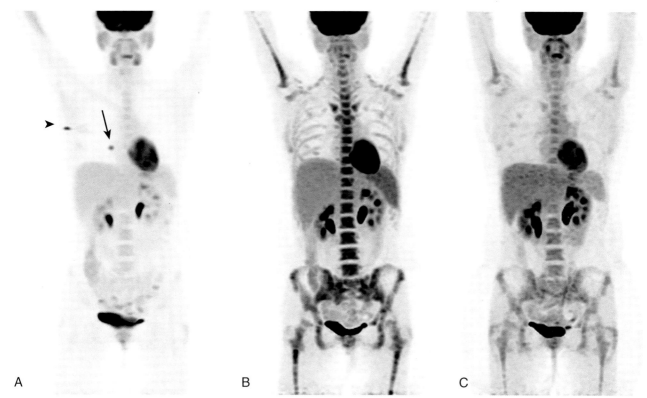

FIG. 11.12 Diffuse bone marrow uptake on ¹⁸F-Fluorodeoxyglucose positron emission tomography (PET)/computed tomography (CT) during chemotherapy. A 34-year-old woman with a recent history of right lumpectomy for infiltrating ductal carcinoma. Maximum intensity projection (MIP) PET images before (A), during (B), and after (C) eight cycles of adjuvant chemotherapy. Diffuse increased uptake of bone marrow not seen in the first study (A) is observed in the axial and proximal appendicular skeleton in the second study (B) performed 2 months after the start of chemotherapy. This uptake decreased in the third study (C) obtained 2 weeks after the completion of chemotherapy. No suspicious lytic or sclerotic osseous lesions were visualized on the CT (not shown). The diffuse bone marrow uptake is considered to reflect rebound hyperfunction of bone marrow induced by chemotherapy. Note that focal uptake in the medial and lateral right chest on the first PET represents a metastatic internal mammary lymph node (*arrow* in A) and a postoperative change in the right breast (*arrowhead* in A), respectively, which have resolved in B.

et al., 2009): PEM and fully tomographic dedicated PET systems (Fig. 11.14). PEM has two planar or curved detector heads that are integrated with breast compression paddles and provides planner and limited-angle tomography images. A PEM scanner was cleared for marketing by the U.S. Food and Drug Administration (FDA) in the 2000s and is currently the most common, commercially available dedicated breast PET system in the United States. The fully tomographic dedicated PET system is a newer generation of dedicated breast PET systems, and acquires fully tomographic three-dimensional (3D) images without breast compression by rotating two or more detector heads around the breast or by completely encircling the breast with detectors. The clinical utility of the dedicated breast PET systems is under investigation. Potential advantages of dedicated scanners over the conventional whole-body PET scanners include the visualization of small breast cancers, possibly leading to improvement of cancer detection with PET techniques (Fig. 11.15). A study that directly compared PEM and whole-body PET (not including PET/CT) in 69 patients with known breast cancers demonstrated that ¹⁸F-FDG PEM had significantly higher sensitivities for breast cancers, either for known index cancers and additional ipsilateral unsuspected cancers, than whole-body PET with ¹⁸F-FDG (Kalinyak et al., 2014). A meta-analysis of studies published between 2000 and 2012 (Caldarella et al., 2014) showed that pooled sensitivity and specificity of PEM using ¹⁸F-FDG are 85% (95% confidence interval [CI], 83%–88%) and 79% (95% CI, 74%–83%), respectively, on a per lesion-based analysis in the early detection of breast malignancy in women with known breast cancers or suspicious breast lesions.

CONVENTIONAL NUCLEAR MEDICINE TECHNIQUES FOR THE DIAGNOSIS OF BREAST CANCER

Lymphoscintigraphy

The SLN is defined as the first lymph node to drain the area under investigation. Thus SLNs are the first nodes to receive metastatic cells. Lymphoscintigraphy is a nuclear medicine technique that labels the SLN using a radiocolloid, such as ⁹⁹ᵐTc-sulfur colloid, ⁹⁹ᵐTc-nanocoloid, and ⁹⁹ᵐTc-antimony trisulfide (Buscombe et al., 2007). After peritumoral, subdermal, or periareolar injections of a radioactive tracer within the breast, serial gamma-camera images (planner images with or without single-photon emission computed tomography [SPECT]) are obtained to visualize lymphatic drainage status and sentinel nodes (Fig. 11.16). This technique allows a surgeon to identify and resect one or more SLNs using a gamma ray detector and precludes the need for an extensive and potentially morbid resection of multiple axillary lymph nodes. The SNMMI and the European Association of Nuclear Medicine provide practice guidelines for lymphoscintigraphy and sentinel node localization in patients with breast cancer (Giammarile et al., 2013).

SLNB has been applied to the management of several malignancies, including breast carcinoma, where it has had a profound impact on decreasing postoperative morbidity. Since the 1990s, SLNB has become the standard staging procedure for patients with invasive breast cancer, replacing ALND (Fisher et al., 1983). Before the adoption of SLNB in breast carcinoma, widespread performance of ALND carried the risk of decreased shoulder range

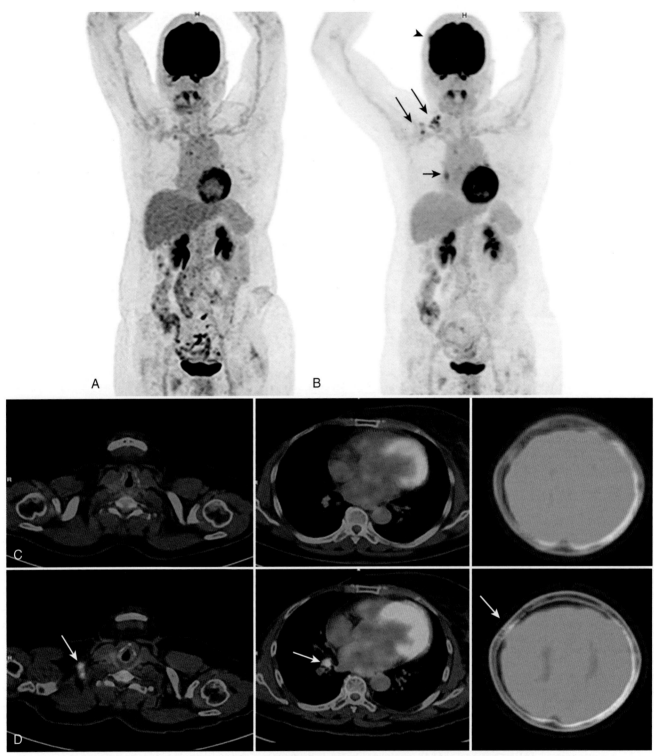

FIG. 11.13 Detecting of recurrence with on ¹⁸F-Fluorodeoxyglucose positron emission tomography (PET)/computed tomography (CT). A 67-year-old woman with breast cancer submitted to surgery and chemoradiation therapy 4 years ago. (A) Maximum intensity projection (MIP) PET image of the first PET/CT study does not demonstrate any abnormality. (B) An MIP PET image of the second study, performed 10 months later, shows hypermetabolic metastatic lesions in cervical, supraclavicular, right axillary, and mediastinal lymph nodes (*arrows*) and on the skull (*arrowhead*). (C and D) Axial PET/CT views in details of the same patient. In the first scan (C), no abnormalities are detected, but the second scan (D) demonstrates elevated uptake (*arrows*) in supraclavicular lymph nodes (*left*), right hilar lymph node (*middle*), and lytic lesion on the right frontal bone (*right*).

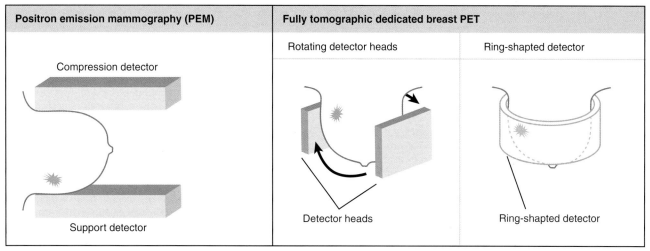

FIG. 11.14 Dedicated breast scanners. Dedicated breast position emission tomography (PET) scanners can be generalized into two types: positron emission mammography (PEM) and fully tomographic dedicated PET systems. PEM (*left*) has two planar or curved detector heads that are integrated with breast compression paddles and provides planar and limited-angle tomography images. The fully tomographic dedicated PET system acquires fully tomographic 3D images by rotating two or more planar heads (*middle*) or by completely encircling the breast with a ring-shaped detector (*right*).

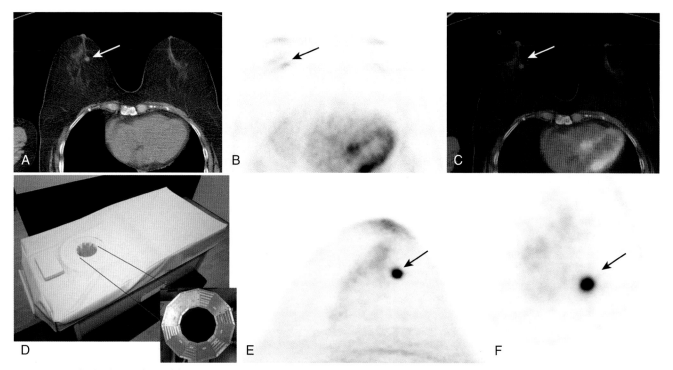

FIG. 11.15 Dedicated breast positron emission tomography (PET). A 74-year-old female with a 7-mm invasive breast cancer in the right breast. (A–C) Conventional whole-body 18F-fluorodeoxyglucose (FDG) PET/computed tomography (CT) obtained in the prone position. Axial views of CT (A), PET (B), and PET/CT fusion (C) demonstrate faint uptake in the 7-mm primary tumor (*arrows*, SUVmax 1.0). (D–F) 18F-FDG dedicated breast PET. Picture of the system (D), maximal intensity projection image (E), and coronal slice (F). The patient's right breast was then examined with dedicated breast PET equipped with a ring-shaped detector in prone position (D). In contrast to the whole-body PET/CT, the tumor is clearly visualized as intense focal uptake (*arrows*) on dedicated breast PET (E and F). Uptake to the normal structures, such as the breast tissue, nipple, and skin, is also more obvious. (From Miyake KK, et al. Performance evaluation of a new dedicated breast pet scanner using NEMA NU4-2008 standards, *J Nucl Med* 55:1198–1203, 2014.)

of motion and lymphedema, with a significant impact on patients' quality of life. This surgical approach conserves the regional lymphatic chain for axillary staging because it restricts lymphatic dissection only to patients whose biopsies show metastasis in at least one lymph node. Indications for SLNB are established for, but are not limited to, T1 or T2 tumors, DCIS with mastectomy, older age, obesity, male breast cancer, and tumors treated with preoperative systemic therapy (Giammarile et al., 2013).

No imaging modality is accurate enough to detect lymph node metastases when a primary breast cancer is at an early stage (I or II), but SLNB is a highly reliable method for screening axillary nodes and for identifying metastatic and micrometastatic disease in regional lymphatic nodes (Benson et al., 2007; Veronesi et al., 2003, 2006). The IMLs represent a second regional basin of lymph drainage from the breast and are considered a major prognostic factor since they are associated with a less favorable prognosis. The SLNB technique is able to visualize lymph nodes in the internal mammary basin, making its resection feasible. The literature is controversial regarding the indication for an IML-SLNB procedure when there is evidence of IML drainage on lymphoscintigraphy. However, recent studies with large cohorts demonstrated that IML biopsy is predictable and safe and has the potential to alter the stage and adjuvant therapy of breast cancer patients (see Gnerlich et al., 2014; Caudle et al., 2014; Veronesi et al., 2008).

Bone Scintigraphy

The skeleton is the most frequent site of distant metastases from breast cancer. Bone represents the first site of distant metastasis for 26% to 50% of patients with metastatic breast cancer (Coleman et al., 1987; Hortobagyi, 1991). Breast cancer preferably metastasizes in vertebrae (especially thoracolumbar), followed by ribs, sternum, pelvis, femur, and skull (Kakhki et al., 2013). Bone metastases are classified as osteolytic, osteoblastic, or mixed-pattern on the basis of radiographic appearance (Nielsen et al., 1991). Osteolytic pattern is the predominant type of metastases from breast cancer, as seen in up to half of them, and has

been reported to be associated with poorer prognosis compared with the other patterns (Cook et al., 1998). A sclerotic appearance is seen in about 15% to 20% (Roodman, 2004).

Bone scanning using ⁹⁹ᵐTc-methylene diphosphonate (MDP) is the most commonly used radiotracer for the evaluation of bone metastases. It is incorporated in hydroxyapatite crystals in bone and is excreted in urine. Routine scanning is usually performed 2 to 5 hours after injection of ⁹⁹ᵐTc-MDP. SNMMI provides procedure guidelines for bone scintigraphy (Donohoe, 2003). Hot spots on bone scanning therefore are present wherever there is osteoblastic activity and increased skeletal vascularity (Hamaoka et al., 2004). The advantage of bone scanning is that it is a widely available examination obtained at reasonable cost.

Detection of Bone Metastases

Published sensitivity and specificity rates of bone scintigraphy in the detection of bone metastases have been varied, with sensitivity ranging from 76% to 96% and specificity from 81% to 100% on the patient basis (Niikura et al., 2011; Balci et al., 2012; Groheux, 2013). False-negatives are occasionally encountered in rapidly growing osteolytic metastases or in lesions at sites with slow bone turnover or avascular sites. False-positives are caused by degenerative joint disease, trauma (bone fracture and bruise), inflammation, and benign bone tumors (such as fibrous dysplasia and enchondroma). Because of this lack of specificity, foci noted on bone scanning should often be further assessed by using x-ray, CT, or MRI for correlation and confirmation. Histologic confirmation may also be required for the final diagnosis of suspicious lesions.

There have been debates on which imaging modality is reliable and practical enough to assess bone metastases among various techniques, such as bone scintigraphy (either with planar imaging or SPECT and SPECT/CT), ¹⁸F-FDG PET and PET/CT, MRI, x-ray, and CT. Each modality represents different aspects of bone metastases and has different features and diagnostic performance (Tables 11.3 and 11.4). Generally, the sensitivity for detecting bone metastasis tends to be constantly high for ¹⁸F-FDG PET/CT

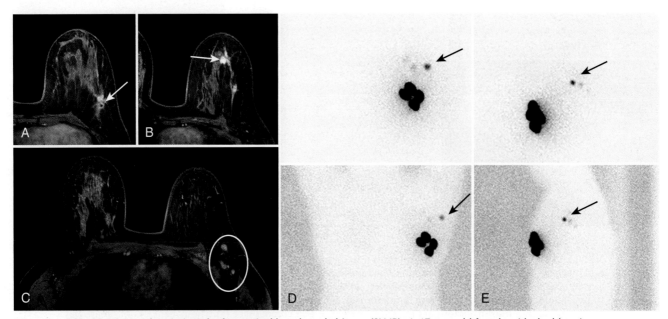

FIG. 11.16 Lymphoscintigraphy for sentinel lymph node biopsy (SLNB). A 47-year-old female with double primary breast cancers (invasive ductal carcinomas) in the right breast, scheduled for SLNB for initial staging. (A–C) Axial contrast-enhanced fat-suppressed T1-weighted magnetic resonance images at different levels show an 18-mm enhanced mass with a biopsy marker (A, *arrow*) and a 6-mm enhanced mass (B, *arrow*), associated with slightly enlarged lymph nodes in the right axilla (C, *circle*). (D and E) Anterior (D) and lateral (E) planar images of lymphoscintigraphy obtained after the four-point injection of ⁹⁹ᵐTc-filtered sulfur colloid around the areola. One hot SLN (D and E, *arrows*) is depicted in the right axilla. Surgery was performed the next day. Two SLNs were resected under the guidance of a gamma detector, and one of the two, with higher radioactivity, was pathologically proven to have metastasis.

TABLE 11.3 **Visualized Structure, Cost and Availability, and Technical Disadvantage of Imaging Modalities**

Imaging Modality	Visualized Structure	Cost and Availability	Technical Advantages and Disadvantage
Bone scan (planar image with/without SPECT)	Osteoblastic metabolism	Low cost Widely available	Whole-body scanning
Bone SPECT/CT	Osteoblastic metabolism	Not commonly available	Whole-body scanning, radiation exposure
FDG PET	Tumor glucose metabolism	High cost	Whole-body scanning
FDG PET/CT	Tumor glucose metabolism, bone structure, bone marrow, tumors	High cost	Radiation exposure
MRI	Bone marrow, tumors	High to moderately high cost	Artifacts caused by field inhomogeneity, no radiation exposure
X-ray	Bone structure	Low cost Widely available	Radiation exposure
CT	Bone structure, bone marrow, tumors	Moderately high cost Widely available	Radiation exposure

CT, computed tomography; *FDG,* ¹⁸F-fluorodeoxyglucose; *MRI,* magnetic resonance imaging; *PET,* positron emission tomography; *SPECT,* single-photon emission computed tomography.
Modified from Hamaoka et al: Bone imaging in metastatic breast cancer, *J Clin Oncol* 22:2942-2953, 2004.

TABLE 11.4 **Diagnostic Performance in the Detection of Bone Metastases from Breast Cancer in Imaging Modalities**

Imaging Modality	Reported Sensitivity[a]	Reported Specificity[a]	FN causes[b]	FP Causes[b]
Bone scan, planar image	76%–96%[c-f]; meta-analysis, 78%–87%[g-i]	81%–100%[c-f]; meta-analysis 79%–96%[g-i]	Osteolytic metastases	Degeneration Trauma, compression fracture Inflammation Benign tumor
Bone SPECT	85%[j]	99%[j]	Osteolytic metastases	Degeneration Trauma, compression fracture Inflammation Benign tumor
FDG PET	78%[c]; meta-analysis 81%–83%[g,h]	98%[c]; meta-analysis 93%–94%[g,h]	Cortex only lesion Osteoblastic metastases	Trauma, compression fracture Inflammation Benign tumor
FDG PET/CT	98%–100[d-f,k]; meta-analysis 93%[i]	85%–98%[d-f,k]; meta-analysis 99%[i]		Trauma, compression fracture Inflammation Benign tumor
Whole-body MRI	92%[l]; meta-analysis 97%[h]	90%[l]; meta-analysis 97%[h]	Cortex only lesion	Edema Trauma, compression fracture Inflammation
X-ray	50%–54%[m,n]	n.a.	BM-only lesion Mineral density change under threshold Osteopenia	Trauma, compression fracture Inflammation Benign tumor
CT	93%[n]	n.a.	Mineral density change under threshold	Trauma, compression fracture Inflammation Benign tumor

[a]Sensitivities and specificities on the patient basis are shown.
[b]Modified from Hamaoka et al: Bone imaging in metastatic breast cancer, *J Clin Oncol* 22:2942-2953, 2004.
[c]Ohta et al: Whole body PET for the evaluation of bony metastases in patients with breast cancer: comparison with 99Tcm-MDP bone scintigraphy, *Nucl Med Commun* 22:875-879, 2001.
[d]Niikura N, Costelloe CM, Madewell JE, et al: FDG-PET/CT compared with conventional imaging in the detection of distant metastases of primary breast cancer, *Oncologist* 16:1111-1119, 2011.
[e]Balci TA, Koc ZP, Komek H: Bone scan or (18)f-fluorodeoxyglucose positron emission tomography/computed tomography; which modality better shows bone metastases of breast cancer? *Breast Care (Basel)* 7:389-393, 2012.
[f]Groheux et al. 2013.
[g]Shie P, Cardarelli R, Brandon D, Erdman W, Abdulrahim N: Meta-analysis: comparison of F-18 Fluorodeoxyglucose-positron emission tomography and bone scintigraphy in the detection of bone metastases in patients with breast cancer, *Clin Nucl Med* 33:97-101, 2008.
[h]Liu T, Cheng T, Xu X, Yan WL, Liu J, Yang HL: A meta-analysis of 18FDG-PET, MRI and bone scintigraphy for diagnosis of bone metastases in patients with breast cancer, *Skeletal Radiol* 40:523-531, 2011.
[i]Rong, et al: Comparison of 18 FDG PET-CT and bone scintigraphy for detection of bone metastases in breast cancer patients, a meta-analysis, *Surg Oncol* 22:86-91, 2013.
[j]Uematsu T, Yuen S, Yukisawa S, et al: Comparison of FDG PET and SPECT for detection of bone metastases in breast cancer, *AJR Am J Roentgenol* 184:1266-1273, 2005.
[k]Manohar K, Mittal BR, Senthil R, Kashyap R, Bhattacharya A, Singh G: Clinical utility of F-18 FDG PET/CT in recurrent breast carcinoma, *Nucl Med Commun* 33:591-596, 2012.
[l]Engelhard, et al: Comparison of whole-body MRI with automatic moving table technique and bone scintigraphy for screening for bone metastases in patients with breast cancer, *Eur Radiol* 14:99-105, 2004.
[m]Galasko CS, et al: Skeletal metastases and mammary cancer, *Ann R Coll Surg Engl* 50:3-28, 1972.
[n]Kido DK, Gould R, Taati F, Duncan A, Schnur J: Comparative sensitivity of CT scans, radiographs and radionuclide bone scans in detecting metastatic calvarial lesions, *Radiology* 128:371-375, 1978.
BM, bone marrow; *CT,* computed tomography; *FDG,* ¹⁸F-fluorodeoxyglucose; *FN,* false-negative; *FP,* false-positive; *MRI,* magnetic resonance imaging; *n.a.,* nonapplicable; *PET,* positron emission tomography; *SPECT,* single-photon emission computed tomography.

and MRI, low for x-ray, and varies in bone scintigraphy and ^{18}F-FDG PET (utilized without integrated CT). The specificity tends to be high in PET, PET/CT, and MRI, and varies in bone scan. Liu et al. (2011) performed a meta-analysis of 13 articles to compare the diagnostic value of bone scintigraphy, ^{18}F-FDG PET, and MRI. They found that the pooled sensitivity estimates for MRI (97.1%) were significantly higher than for bone scintigraphy (87.0%) and ^{18}F-FDG PET (83.3%), and that the pooled specificity estimates for PET (94.5%) and MRI (97.0%) were both significantly higher than for bone scintigraphy (88.1%) on a per patient basis. In another meta-analysis (Shie et al., 2008) the pooled patient-based sensitivity and specificity for bone scintigraphy versus ^{18}F-FDG PET were 78% versus 81% and 79% versus 93%, respectively. The authors stated that ^{18}F-FDG PET may better serve to detect bone metastases than bone scintigraphy because of its superior specificity. Rong et al. (2013) investigated the diagnostic performance of the dual modality, ^{18}F-FDG PET/CT, compared with bone scintigraphy in a meta-analysis. The pooled patient-based sensitivity, specificity, and area under the curve for bone scintigraphy versus ^{18}F-FDG PET/CT were 81% versus 93%, 96% versus 99%, and 0.94 (95% CI, 0.92–0.96) versus 0.98 (95% CI, 0.98–1.00), respectively, suggesting a higher diagnostic performance of PET/CT for detection of bone metastases from breast cancer compared with bone scintigraphy. These studies may suggest that ^{18}F-FDG PET/CT and MRI are currently the most powerful imaging modalities in the detection of bone metastases.

^{18}F-FDG PET visualizes hyperactive glucose metabolism of tumor cells and potentially depicts metastatic foci that are not visualized on bone scintigraphy because of the absence of sufficient bone remodeling reaction (thus, osteolytic metastases; Fig.

11.17). However, a limitation has been reported in the detection of osteoblastic metastasis (Fig. 11.18). Cook et al. (1998) found that ^{18}F-FDG-PET was superior to bone scan in the detection of osteolytic metastases; however, it was less sensitive in the detection of osteoblastic metastases. Because osteoblastic lesions can be detected as sclerotic lesions on CT, dual-modality PET/CT has the improved sensitivity compared with PET. It is important to assess not only ^{18}F-FDG uptake but also bone density on CT images when ^{18}F-FDG PET/CT is interpreted for the presence of bone metastases.

Bone SPECT using the same radioactive tracer as conventional bone scintigraphy provides tomographic image slices through the body. Available data on the diagnostic performance of bone SPECT are limited, but its ability to provide precise anatomic localization of radioactive tracer may be helpful in improving the diagnostic performance of the conventional bone scintigraphy. Uematsu et al. (2005) reported that ^{99m}Tc-MDP SPECT was significantly superior to ^{18}F-FDG PET for its sensitivity (85% versus 17%) and accuracy (96% versus 85%) on a per lesion basis in 900 bone lesions of 15 patients with breast cancer.

Although ^{18}F-FDG PET/CT and MRI seem to perform better than bone scintigraphy, bone scintigraphy is still currently recommended as the first imaging study for detecting bone metastasis in asymptomatic patients with breast cancer by the NCCN because of it low cost (Costelloe et al., 2009). NCCN guideline 20015 recommends considering the use of bone scintigraphy for patients with increased risk of bone metastases, whereas they place ^{18}F-FDG PET/CT as an optional test (see Table 11.2). Indications include patients with stage III, stage IV, or recurrent invasive breast cancer; those with inflammatory breast cancer; those

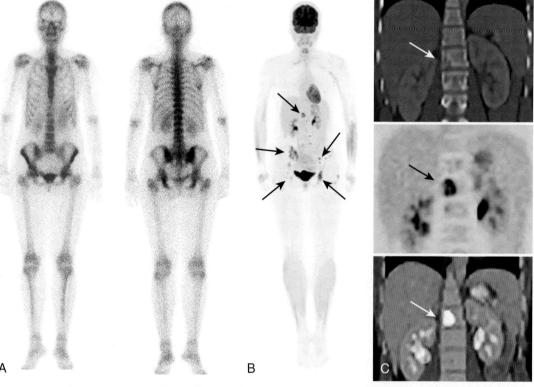

FIG. 11.17 Detection of bone metastasis: ^{99m}Tc-methylene diphosphonate (MDP) bone scintigraphy versus ^{18}F-fluorodeoxyglucose (FDG) positron emission tomography (PET)/computed tomography (CT). A 32-year-old female with a previous history of mastectomy for right breast cancer. (A) Anterior (*left*) and posterior (*right*) planar images of bone scintigraphy for restaging show no apparent abnormal uptake. (B and C) ^{18}F-FDG PET/CT. Maximal intensity projection PET image shows multiple hypermetabolic osseous lesions in the lumbar spine, sacrum, and pelvic bones (*arrows* in B). Coronal slices of CT (C, *top*), PET (C, *middle*), and PET/CT (C, *bottom*) demonstrate focal intense uptake corresponding to an osteolytic lesion in the first lumbar vertebral body (*arrows*). In this case osteolytic metastases were better depicted on ^{18}F-PET/CT compared with bone scintigraphy.

who are scheduled for preoperative systemic therapy; those who are proved to have four or more positive axillary lymph nodes by surgical axillary staging; and for monitoring therapeutic effect. Bone scintigraphy is not indicated for patients with early stage (stage I–IIB) breast cancer, unless they have localized bone pain or elevated alkaline phosphatase, because bone scintigraphy has a low detection rate for bone metastasis in early-stage breast cancers and relatively high false-positive rates. Previous studies by Puglisi and Hamaoka have suggested the rates at which bone metastasis is detected by bone scan are 0.8% to 5.1% for stage I, 2.6% to 5.6% for stage II, 14.0% to 16.8% for stage III, and 40.3% for stage IV (Puglisi et al., 2005; Hamaoka et al., 2004).

Improvement of cost and availability and development in technology may change the diagram of the diagnostic strategy for bone metastases in the future. Some authors reported the utility of combined 18F-FDG PET/MRI (Catalano et al., 2015). Similarly, combined SPECT and CT (SPECT/CT) has been reported to have superior diagnostic accuracy than SPECT by allowing anatomic localization and morphologic characterization of bone (Zhang, 2013). Recently growing evidence has suggested that sodium 18F-NaF PET/CT has a good diagnostic performance in the detection of bone metastases (Bastawrous et al., 2014). 18F-NaF was approved for clinical use by the FDA in 1972, but had not been commonly used because older PET machines did not provide images with sufficient quality. However, recent developments

in technology and availability of hybrid PET/CT scanners have encouraged a renewed interest in 18F-NaF PET/CT for bone imaging. 18F-NaF can be easily produced in a cyclotron, and PET/CT is usually performed 0.5 to 1.5 hours after intravenous injection of 18F-NaF, which accumulates in bone as a result of ion exchange, physiologically similar to 99mTc-MDP. However, the effective radiation dose is twice as great compared with 99mTc-MDP. 18F-NaF has rapid blood clearance because of minimal binding to serum proteins and is excreted in urine. Abnormally increased uptake of 18F-NaF reflects increased bone remodeling (predominantly osteoblastic activity) and/or increased blood flow. With faster blood clearance and twofold higher skeletal uptake as well as advantages of PET/CT over conventional nuclear medicine scintigraphy (primarily higher spatial resolution), 18F-NaF PET/CT provides better images with higher bone-to-background ratio and is superior to visualize small bone metastases compared with bone scan (Figs. 11.19 and 11.20). In an early study by Schirrmeister et al. (1999) that investigated the accuracy of 18F-NaF PET compared with 99mTc-MDP bone scintigraphy in the detection of bone metastases in 34 patients with breast cancer, 18F-NaF PET provided a higher detection rate and a higher accuracy than planar bone scan. 18F-NaF accumulates sclerotic metastases very well. Osteolytic metastases may be NaF avid and often show as rim-shaped uptake (photopenic lesions with peripheral uptake). However, osteolytic lesions often exhibit little to no radiotracer

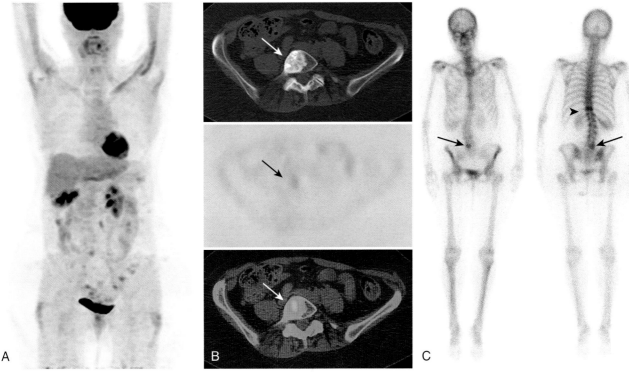

FIG. 11.18 Detection of bone metastasis: 99mTc-methylene diphosphonate (MDP) bone scintigraphy versus 18F-fluorodeoxyglucose (FDG) positron emission tomography (PET)/computed tomography (CT). A 65-year-old female with a history of bone metastasis after lumpectomy of breast cancer. Radiation therapy and chemotherapy were completed 10 months ago. (A and B) 18F-FDG PET/CT for restaging. Maximal intensity projection of PET (A) shows no abnormal 18F-FDG uptake. Axial slices of CT (B, *top*), PET (B, *middle*), and PET/CT (B, *bottom*) demonstrate a non–FDG-avid sclerotic lesion (*arrows*) in the fifth lumbar (L5) vertebral body, in which there had been a bone metastasis treated with radiation therapy. Because of no apparent 18F-FDG activity, it appeared to be posttreatment change. (C) Anterior (*left*) and posterior (*right*) planar images of bone scintigraphy obtained 2 weeks after A. However, on bone scintigraphy, there is increased radiopharmaceutical uptake at L5 (*arrow*), suspicious for residual disease versus posttreatment change. Linear uptake at the T11 vertebral body (*arrowhead*) is consistent with compression fracture. Later, bone metastasis progressed. In retrospect, positive bone scan may reflect residual disease in this case, although it is generally difficult to differentiate residual disease and posttreatment change for sclerotic lesions with positive bone scan.

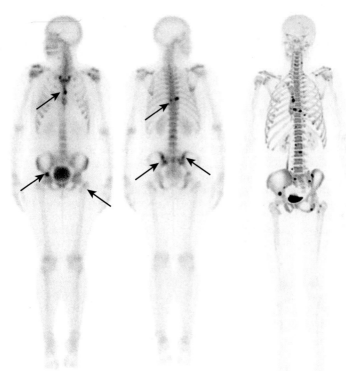

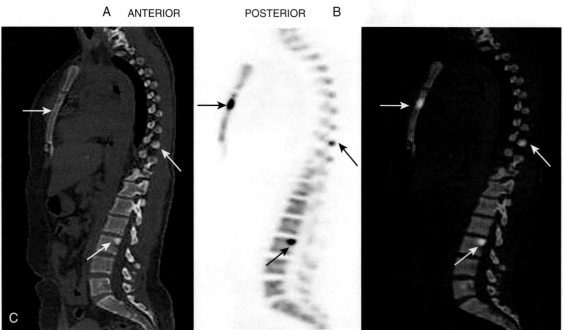

A   ANTERIOR   POSTERIOR   **B**

FIG. 11.19 Sodium ¹⁸F-fluoride (¹⁸F-NaF) positron emission tomography (PET)/computed tomography (CT) for investigation of bone metastases. A 29-year-old female with recently diagnosed stage III breast cancer. (A) Anterior (*left*) and posterior (*right*) planar images of bone scintigraphy show hot spots in the sternum, the T8 and T9 vertebrae, sacroiliac bilaterally, right acetabulum, and left femur (*arrows*). (B and C) ¹⁸F-NaF PET/CT of the same patient performed 3 days after A. Maximal intensity projection PET image (B) demonstrates a high contrast image with superior bone-to-background ratio to bone scan and visualizes more lesions with increased uptake in the sternum, vertebrae, pelvic bones, right parietal bone, left scapula, humerus, and femurs. Sagittal views (C) in detail of the same patient (CT, *left*; PET, *middle*; and PET/CT, *right*) show NaF-avid sclerotic lesions (*arrows*) in the sternum, T9 and L3.

activity leading to false-negatives. Conversely, because ¹⁸F-NaF is not a tumor-specific agent, benign conditions, such as degenerative disk disease, arthritis, trauma, fibrous dysplasia, and Paget's disease, can be shown as abnormal uptake, producing false-positives and resulting in low specificity of ¹⁸F-NaF PET studies. Careful combination reading of CT images may help in improving the specificity.

Monitoring the Response of Bone Metastases to Treatment

In the setting of monitoring disease before and after initiation of therapy, a positive but stable-appearing bone scan reflecting osteoblastic foci may be secondary to either ongoing malignant disease or a physiologic osseous reaction to treated disease and is therefore nonspecific (Fig. 11.21). On the other hand,

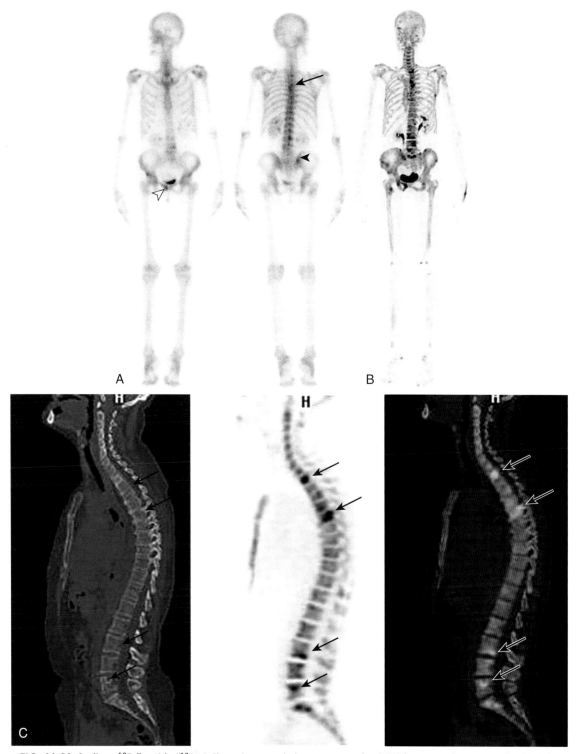

FIG. 11.20 Sodium 18F-fluoride (18F-NaF) positron emission tomography (PET)/computed tomography (CT) for investigation of bone metastases. A 53-year-old female with breast cancer. (A) Anterior (*left*) and posterior (*right*) planar images of bone scintigraphy show hot spots in thoracic vertebrae (*arrow*), right sacrum (*black arrowhead*), and right pubis (*white arrowhead*). (B and C) 18F-NaF PET/CT of the same patient performed 7 days after A. Maximal intensity projection PET image (B) depicts more metastatic lesions with clear increased uptake in the right orbit, vertebrae, sixth left costal arch, sacrum, pelvic bones, and right femur. Both osteoblastic and osteolytic lesions accumulated 18F-NaF. Sagittal views (C) of CT (*left*), PET (*middle*), and PET/CT (*right*) show multiple vertebrae lesions (*arrows*), some of them without anatomic correlation.

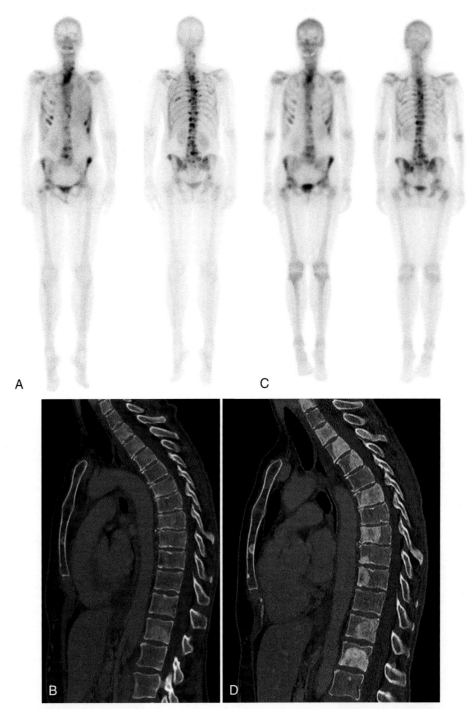

FIG. 11.21 ⁹⁹ᵐTc-methylene diphosphonate (MDP) bone scintigraphy for treatment monitoring. A 60-year-old female with newly diagnosed stage I invasive ductal carcinoma of the left breast. (A and B) Anterior (*left*) and posterior (*right*) planar images of bone scintigraphy (A) and sagittal computed tomography (CT; B) at the initial staging. On bone scintigraphy (A), diffuse osseous uptake is seen in the bilateral ribs; cervical, thoracic, and lumbar spine; left iliac crest; right sacroiliac joint; right greater trochanter; and right femoral neck. CT (B) on the same day shows diffuse sclerotic and mixed lytic and sclerotic osseous lesions. This patient was diagnosed to have diffuse bone metastasis and was upgraded to stage IV. (C and D) Anterior (*left*) and posterior (*right*) planar images of bone scintigraphy (C) and sagittal CT (D) after the initiation of chemotherapy. CT (D) shows increased osseous sclerotic metastasis, whereas bone scintigraphy (C) shows stable appearance of diffuse osseous uptake, suggesting residual disease or posttreatment bone change. Later, osseous metastasis progressed. In retrospect, positive bone scan may reflect residual disease in this case, although it is generally difficult to differentiate residual disease and posttreatment change for sclerotic lesions with positive bone scan.

TABLE 11.5 Diagnostic Performance in the Assessment of Therapeutic Response of Bone Metastases from Breast Cancer in Imaging Modalities

Imaging Modality	Time Course Appearance of Responded Lesions	Therapy-Related FN Causes	Therapy-Related FP Causes
Bone scan (planar image, SPECT)	Decrease of uptake		Flare phenomenon
FDG PET	Decrease of uptake		Diffuse bone marrow uptake Tam-induced flare phenomenon
FDG PET/CT	Decrease of uptake From lytic to sclerotic Regression of mass		Diffuse bone marrow uptake Tam-induced flare phenomenon
Whole-body MRI	Regression of mass		
X-ray	From lytic to sclerotic	Delayed appearance of response	
CT	From lytic to sclerotic Regression of mass	Delayed appearance of response	

CT, computed tomography; *FDG,* ¹⁸F-fluorodeoxyglucose; *FN,* false-negative; *FP,* false-positive; *MRI,* magnetic resonance imaging; *PET,* positron emission tomography; *SPECT,* single-photon emission computed tomography; *Tam,* tamoxifen. Modified from Hamaoka et al: Bone imaging in metastatic breast cancer, *J Clin Oncol* 22:2942–2953, 2004.

a negative scan is regarded as a sign of response in patients with an initial positive scan (Table 11.5). Responding disease can result in increased activity (aforementioned "flare" phenomenon) on the bone scintigraphy, especially on the first follow-up scan after initiating a new therapy. Citing these variable factors, Hamaoka et al. (2004) stated that the bone scan has poor specificity in assessing the treatment response of bone metastases.

Several groups have investigated a diagnostic utility of ¹⁸F-FDG PET or PET/CT specifically in monitoring bone metastases. Du et al. (2007) evaluated the change of functional and morphologic appearances of 146 bone metastases in 25 patients with breast cancer on serial ¹⁸F-FDG PET/CT studies. They demonstrated that the most common pattern of bone metastases was an FDG-avid osteolytic type (72/146, 49%), 81% of which became ¹⁸F-FDG negative and osteoblastic on CT after treatment. The study also showed the presence of persistently FDG-avid lesions correlated with poorer prognosis, likely suggesting that ¹⁸F-FDG uptake reflects the tumor activity. Teteishi et al. (2008) showed that a decrease in SUV and an increase in CT-based attenuation in bone metastases are potential predictors of response duration. However, PET imaging is still considered as challenging because of the absence of a reproducible, validated, and widely accepted set of standards for disease activity assessment. Similarly, the role of ¹⁸F-NaF PET/CT in monitoring therapeutic effect has not yet been firmly established.

No consensus has been reached as to the imaging modality for monitoring therapeutic effect. NCCN allows the use of bone scintigraphy and optional ¹⁸F-FDG PET/CT for monitoring; however, it also states that studies of functional imaging, such as bone scintigraphy and PET imaging, are particularly challenging when used to assess

response (see Table 11.2). The Response Evaluation Criteria in Solid Tumors system considers bone metastases to be "unmeasurable."

Although functional imaging such as bone scintigraphy, ¹⁸F-FDG PET, and PET/CT, are not always helpful, it is reasonable to monitor tumors with functional imaging if patients initially had a positive scan. In addition, functional imaging may detect the functional changes caused by therapy, which may not be evident in anatomic images particularly early after treatment.

CONCLUSIONS

Nuclear medicine has an important role in breast cancer imaging. ¹⁸F-FDG PET/CT has gained widespread acceptance in staging, restaging, treatment efficacy assessment during or after treatment, and radiotherapy planning. SLNB has become the standard staging procedure for patients with invasive breast cancer, whereas bone scintigraphy and, more recently, ¹⁸F-NaF PET/CT are the modalities of choice for bone metastases evaluation. Looking toward the future, PET/MRI and PEM are being evaluated and preliminary data show promising results.

Key Elements

Indications of ¹⁸F-fluorodeoxyglucose (¹⁸F-FDG) positron emission tomography (PET)/computed tomography (CT) in breast cancer include staging, restaging and treatment monitoring, and radiotherapy planning.

¹⁸F-FDG PET/CT is indicated in invasive breast cancer evaluation. Noninvasive breast cancer has been shown to be poorly imaged by this modality.

The overall specificity of ¹⁸F-FDG PET/CT in the detection of breast cancer is relatively high; however, false-positives do occur in some benign inflammatory lesions and fibroadenoma. FDG avidity is a prognostic biomarker in breast cancer.

¹⁸F-FDG PET/CT performs well in staging mediastinal and internal mammary lymph nodes and distant metastatic disease.

¹⁸F-FDG PET/CT can be helpful in evaluating asymptomatic, already treated breast cancer patients who may pose a diagnostic challenge for detecting occult recurrences.

¹⁸F-FDG PET/CT has an important role in the setting of asymptomatic patients with rising tumor markers levels and negative conventional imaging results.

The sentinel lymph node (SLN) is the hypothetical first lymph node to drain metastatic cancer cells. The sentinel node biopsy has become a standard staging procedure for patients with invasive breast cancer, and is replacing axillary lymph node dissection.

Lymphoscintigraphy is a nuclear medicine technique to label SLN using a radiocolloid, such as ⁹⁹ᵐTc-sulfur colloid, ⁹⁹ᵐTc-nanocoloid, and ⁹⁹ᵐTc-antimony trisulfide. Lymphoscintigraphy allows a surgeon to identify and resect one or more SLNs using a gamma ray detector and precludes the need for an extensive and potentially morbid resection of multiple axillary lymph nodes.

The skeleton is the most frequent site of distant metastases from breast cancer. Bone scintigraphy using radiotracers, such as ⁹⁹ᵐTc-methylene diphosphonates), is the most commonly used examination for the evaluation of bone metastases because of its low cost and wide availability.

¹⁸F-FDG PET/CT and ¹⁸F-fluoride (¹⁸F-NaF) PET/CT have been shown to have higher diagnostic performance than conventional bone scintigraphy for detection of bone metastases, but the relatively high costs should be considered depending on local practice and reimbursement patterns.

SUGGESTED READINGS

Alberini JL, Lerebours F, Wartski M, et al.: 18F-fluorodeoxyglucose positron emission tomography/computed tomography (FDG-PET/CT) imaging in the staging and prognosis of inflammatory breast cancer, *Cancer* 115:5038-5047, 2009.

Aukema TS, et al.: Detection of extra-axillary lymph node involvement with FDG PET/CT in patients with stage II-III breast cancer, *Eur J Cancer* 46:3205-3210, 2010.

Avril N, Dose J, Janicke F, et al.: Metabolic characterization of breast tumors with positron emission tomography using F-18 fluorodeoxyglucose, *J Clin Oncol* 14:1848-1857, 1996.

Avril N, Rose CA, Schelling M, et al.: Breast imaging with positron emission tomography and fluorine-18 fluorodeoxyglucose: use and limitations, *J Clin Oncol* 18:3495-3502, 2000.

Balci TA, Koc ZP, Komek H: Bone scan or (18)f-fluorodeoxyglucose positron emission tomography/computed tomography; which modality better shows bone metastases of breast cancer? *Breast Care (Basel)* 7:389-393, 2012.

Bastawrous SP, Bhargava P, Behnia F, Djang DS, Haseley DR: Newer PET application with an old tracer: role of 18F-NaF skeletal PET/CT in oncologic practice, *Radiographics* 34:1295-1316, 2014.

Benson JR, Della Rovere GQ, Axilla Group: Management Consensus: management of the axilla in women with breast cancer, *Lancet Oncol* 8:331-348, 2007.

Bos R, van Der Hoeven JJ, van Der Wall E, et al.: Biologic correlates of (18)fluorodeoxyglucose uptake in human breast cancer measured by positron emission tomography, *J Clin Oncol* 20:379-387, 2002.

Bowen SL, Wu Y, Chaudhari AJ, et al.: Initial characterization of a dedicated breast PET/CT scanner during human imaging, *J Nucl Med* 50:1401-1408, 2009.

Brito RA, Valero V, Buzdar AU, et al.: Long-term results of combined-modality therapy for locally advanced breast cancer with ipsilateral supraclavicular metastases: The University of Texas M.D. Anderson Cancer Center experience, *J Clin Oncol* 19:628-633, 2001.

Buscombe J, Paganelli G, Burak ZE, et al.: Sentinel node in breast cancer procedural guidelines, *Eur J Nucl Med Mol Imaging* 34: 2154-1259, 2007.

Caldarella C, Treglia G, Giordano A: Diagnostic performance of dedicated positron emission mammography using fluorine 18-fluorodeoxyglucose in women with suspicious breast lesions: a meta-analysis, *Clin Breast Cancer* 14:241-248, 2014.

Carter CL, Allen C, Henson DE, et al.: Relation of tumor size, lymph node status, and survival in 24,740 breast cancer cases, *Cancer* 63:181-187, 1989.

Catalano OA, Nicolai E, Rosen BR, et al.: Comparison of CE-FDG-PET/CT with CE-FDG-PET/MR in the evaluation of osseous metastases in breast cancer patients', *Br J Cancer* 112:1452-1460, 2015.

Caudle AS, Yi M, Hoffman KE, et al.: Impact of identification of internal mammary sentinel lymph node metastasis in breast cancer patients, *Ann Surg Oncol* 21:60-65, 2014.

Cermik TF, Mavi A, Basu S, Alavi A: Impact of FDG PET on the preoperative staging of newly diagnosed breast cancer, *Eur J Nucl Med Mol Imaging* 35:475-483, 2008.

Choi YJ, Shin YD, Kang YH, et al.: The effects of preoperative (18)F-FDG PET/CT in breast cancer patients in comparison to the conventional imaging study, *J Breast Cancer* 15:441-448, 2012.

Ciernik IF, Dizendorf E, Baumert BG, et al.: Radiation treatment planning with an integrated positron emission and computer tomography (PET/CT): a feasibility study, *Int J Radiat Oncol Biol Phys* 57:853-863, 2003.

Cochet A, David S, Moodie K, et al.: The utility of 18 F-FDG PET/CT for suspected recurrent breast cancer: impact and prognostic stratification, *Cancer Imaging* 14:1-9, 2014.

Coleman RE, Rubens RD: The clinical course of bone metastases from breast cancer, *Br J Cancer* 55:61-66, 1987.

Cook GJ, Houston S, Rubens R, Maisey MN, Fogelman I: Detection of bone metastases in breast cancer by 18FDG PET: differing metabolic activity in osteoblastic and osteolytic lesions, *J Clin Oncol* 16:3375-3379, 1998.

Costelloe CM, Rohren EM, Madewell JE, et al.: Imaging bone metastases in breast cancer: techniques and recommendations for diagnosis, *Lancet Oncol* 10:606-614, 2009.

Couturier O, Jerusalem G, N'Guyen JM, Hustinx R: Sequential positron emission tomography using [18F]fluorodeoxyglucose for monitoring response to chemotherapy in metastatic breast cancer, *Clin Cancer Res* 12:6437-6443, 2006.

Crippa F, Agresti R, Seregni E, et al.: Prospective evaluation of fluorine-18-FDG PET in presurgical staging of the axilla in breast cancer, *J Nucl Med* 39:4-8, 1998.

Delbeke D, Coleman RE, Guiberteau MJ, et al.: Procedure guideline for tumor imaging with 18F-FDG PET/CT 1.0, *J Nucl Med* 47:885-895, 2006.

Donohoe KJ: *Society of Nuclear Medicine procedure guideline for bone scintigraphy,* version 3, 2003. http://snmmi.files.cms-plus.com/docs/pg_ch34_0403.pdf. Accessed August 1, 2016.

Dose J, Bleckmann C, Bachmann S, et al.: Comparison of fluorodeoxyglucose positron emission tomography and "conventional diagnostic procedures" for the detection of distant metastases in breast cancer patients, *Nucl Med Commun* 23:857-864, 2002.

Du Y, Cullum I, Illidge TM, Ell PJ: Fusion of metabolic function and morphology: sequential [18F]fluorodeoxyglucose positron-emission tomography/computed tomography studies yield new insights into the natural history of bone metastases in breast cancer, *J Clin Oncol* 10(25):3440-3447, 2007.

Duch J, Fuster D, Munoz M, et al.: 18F-FDG PET/CT for early prediction of response to neoadjuvant chemotherapy in breast cancer, *Eur J Nucl Med Mol Imaging* 36:1551-1557, 2009.

Engelhard, et al.: Comparison of whole-body MRI with automatic moving table technique and bone scintigraphy for screening for bone metastases in patients with breast cancer, *Eur Radiol* 14:99-105, 2004.

Evangelista L, Cervino AR, Ghiotto C, Al-Nahhas A, Rubello D, Muzzio PC: Tumor marker-guided PET in breast cancer patients-a recipe for a perfect wedding: a systematic literature review and meta-analysis, *Clin Nucl Med* 37:467-474, 2012.

Fisher B, Bauer M, Wickerham DL, et al.: Relation of number of positive axillary nodes to the prognosis of patients with primary breast cancer. An NSABP update, *Cancer* 52:1551-1557, 1983.

Fueger BJ, Weber WA, Quon A, et al.: Performance of 2-deoxy-2-[F-18]fluoro-D-glucose positron emission tomography and integrated PET/CT in restaged breast cancer patients, *Mol Imaging Biol* 7:369-376, 2005.

Fuster D, Duch J, Paredes P, et al.: Preoperative staging of large primary breast cancer with [18F]fluorodeoxyglucose positron emission tomography/computed tomography compared with conventional imaging procedures, *J Clin Oncol* 26:4746-4751, 2008.

Galasko CS, et al.: Skeletal metastases and mammary cancer, *Ann R Coll Surg Engl* 50:3-28, 1972.

Gambhir SS: Molecular imaging of cancer with positron emission tomography, *Nat Rev Cancer* 2:683-693, 2002.

Garami Z, Hascsi Z, Varga J, et al.: The value of 18-FDG PET/CT in early-stage breast cancer compared to traditional diagnostic modalities with an emphasis on changes in disease stage designation and treatment plan, *Eur J Surg Oncol* 38:31-37, 2012.

Gennari A, Donati S, Salvadori B, et al.: Role of 2-[18F]-fluorodeoxyglucose (FDG) positron emission tomography (PET) in the early assessment of response to chemotherapy in metastatic breast cancer patients, *Clin Breast Cancer* 1:156-161, 2000. discussion 62-63.

Giammarile F, Alazraki N, Aarsvold JN, et al.: The EANM and SNMMI practice guideline for lymphoscintigraphy and sentinel node localization in breast cancer, *Eur J Nucl Med Mol Imaging* 40:1932-1947, 2013.

Giraud P, Grahek D, Montravers F: CT and (18)F-deoxyglucose (FDG) image fusion for optimization of conformal radiotherapy of lung cancers, *Int J Radiat Oncol Biol Phys* 49:1249-1257, 2001.

Gnerlich JL, Barreto-Andrade JC, Czechura T, et al.: Accurate staging with internal mammary chain sentinel node biopsy for breast cancer, *Ann Surg Oncol* 21:368-374, 2014.

Groheux D, Espie M, Giacchetti S, Hindie E: Performance of FDG PET/CT in the clinical management of breast cancer, *Radiology* 266:388-405, 2013a.

Groheux D, Giacchetti S, Delord M, et al.: 18F-FDG PET/CT in staging patients with locally advanced or inflammatory breast cancer: comparison to conventional staging, *J Nucl Med* 54:5-11, 2013b.

Groheux D, Hindie E, Giacchetti S, et al.: Early assessment with 18F-fluorodeoxyglucose positron emission tomography/computed tomography can help predict the outcome of neoadjuvant chemotherapy in triple negative breast cancer, *Eur J Cancer* 50:1864-1871, 2014.

Groheux D, Moretti JL, Baillet G, et al.: Effect of (18)F-FDG PET/CT imaging in patients with clinical Stage II and III breast cancer, *Int J Radiat Oncol Biol Phys* 71:695-704, 2008.

Hamaoka T, Madewell JE, Podoloff DA, Hortobagyi GN, Ueno NT: Bone imaging in metastatic breast cancer, *J Clin Oncol* 22:2942-2953, 2004.

Hortobagyi GN: Bone metastases in breast cancer patients, *Semin Oncol* 18:11-15, 1991.

Inoue T, Yutani K, Taguchi T, Tamaki Y, Shiba E, Noguchi S: Preoperative evaluation of prognosis in breast cancer patients by [(18)F]2-Deoxy-2-fluoro-D-glucose-positron emission tomography, *J Cancer Res Clin Oncol* 130:273-278, 2004.

Isasi CR, Moadel RM, Blaufox MD: A meta-analysis of FDG-PET for the evaluation of breast cancer recurrence and metastases, *Breast Cancer Res Treat* 90:105-112, 2005.

Jansson T, Westlin JE, Ahlstrom H, Lilja A, Langstrom B, Bergh J: Positron emission tomography studies in patients with locally advanced and/or metastatic breast cancer: a method for early therapy evaluation, *J Clin Oncol* 13:1470-1477, 1995.

Jones A, Bernstein, Davis, Bryce, Wilson, Mankoff: Pilot Feasibility Study to Assess the Utility of PET Scanning in the Pre-Operative Evaluation of Internal Mammary Nodes in Breast Cancer Patients Presenting with Medial Hemisphere Tumors, *Clin Positron Imaging* 2:331, 1999.

Kakhki VR, Anvari K, Sadeghi R, Mahmoudian AS, Torabian-Kakhki M: Pattern and distribution of bone metastases in common malignant tumors, *Nucl Med Rev Cent East Eur* 16:66-69, 2013.

Kalinyak JE, Berg WA, Schilling K, Madsen KS, Narayanan D, Tartar M: Breast cancer detection using high-resolution breast PET compared to whole-body PET or PET/CT, *Eur J Nucl Med Mol Imaging* 41:260-275, 2014.

Kido DK, Gould R, Taati F, Duncan A, Schnur J: Comparative sensitivity of CT scans, radiographs and radionuclide bone scans in detecting metastatic calvarial lesions, *Radiology* 128:371-375, 1978.

Koolen BB, Valdés Olmos RA, Elkhuizen PH, et al.: Locoregional lymph node involvement on 18F-FDG PET/CT in breast cancer patients scheduled for neoadjuvant chemotherapy, *Breast Cancer Res Treat* 135:231-240, 2012.

Kruse V, Cocquyt V, Borms M, Maes M, Van de Wiele C: Serum tumor markers and PET/CT imaging for tumor recurrence detection, *Ann Nucl Med* 27:97-104, 2013.

Kubota R, Yamada S, Kubota K, Ishiwata K, Tamahashi N, Ido T: Intratumoral distribution of fluorine-18-fluorodeoxyglucose in vivo: high accumulation in macrophages and granulation tissues studied by microautoradiography, *J Nucl Med* 33:1972-1980, 1992.

Kumar A, Kumar R, Seenu V, et al.: The role of 18F-FDG PET/CT in evaluation of early response to neoadjuvant chemotherapy in patients with locally advanced breast cancer, *Eur Radiol* 19:1347-1357, 2009.

Kumar R, Chauhan A, Zhuang H, Chandra P, Schnall M, Alavi A: Clinicopathologic factors associated with false negative FDG-PET in primary breast cancer, *Breast Cancer Res Treat* 98:267-274, 2006.

Lee SM, Bae SK, Kim TH, et al.: Value of 18F-FDG PET/CT for early prediction of pathologic response (by residual cancer burden criteria) of locally advanced breast cancer to neoadjuvant chemotherapy, *Clin Nucl Med* 39:882–886, 2014.

Liu T, Cheng T, Xu X, Yan WL, Liu J, Yang HL: A meta-analysis of 18FDG-PET, MRI and bone scintigraphy for diagnosis of bone metastases in patients with breast cancer, *Skeletal Radiol* 40:523–531, 2011.

MacManus M, Nestle U, Rosenzweig KE, et al.: Use of PET and PET/CT for radiation therapy planning: IAEA expert report 2006-2007, *Radiother Oncol* 91:85–94, 2009.

Manohar K, Mittal BR, Senthil R, Kashyap R, Bhattacharya A, Singh G: Clinical utility of F-18 FDG PET/CT in recurrent breast carcinoma, *Nucl Med Commun* 33:591–596, 2012.

Miyake KK, Matsumoto K, Inoue M, et al.: Performance evaluation of a new dedicated breast pet scanner using NEMA NU4-2008 standards, *J Nucl Med* 55:1198–1203, 2014.

Moon DH, Maddahi J, Silverman DH, Glaspy JA, Phelps ME, Hoh CK: Accuracy of whole-body fluorine-18-FDG PET for the detection of recurrent or metastatic breast carcinoma, *J Nucl Med* 39:431–435, 1998.

Mortimer JE, Dehdashti F, Siegel BA, Trinkaus K, Katzenellenbogen JA, Welch MJ: Metabolic flare: indicator of hormone responsiveness in advanced breast cancer, 2001 *J Clin Oncol* 19:2797–2803, 2001.

National Comprehensive Cancer Network (NCCN): NCCN Clinical Practice Guidelines in Oncology, *Breast Cancer*, 2015. Version 2.

Nestle U, Kremp S, Grosu AL: Practical integration of [18F]-FDG-PET and PET-CT in the planning of radiotherapy for non-small cell lung cancer (NSCLC): the technical basis, ICRU-target volumes, problems, perspectives, *Radiother Oncol* 81:209–225, 2006.

Nielsen OS, Munro AJ, Tannock IF: Bone metastases: pathophysiology and management policy, *J Clin Oncol* 9:509–524, 1991.

Niikura N, Costelloe CM, Madewell JE, et al.: FDG-PET/CT compared with conventional imaging in the detection of distant metastases of primary breast cancer, *Oncologist* 16:1111–1119, 2011.

Ogino K, Nakajima M, Kakuta M, et al.: Utility of FDG-PET/CT in the evaluation of the response of locally advanced breast cancer to neoadjuvant chemotherapy, *Int Surg* 99:309–318, 2014.

Ohta M, et al.: Whole body PET for the evaluation of bony metastases in patients with breast cancer: comparison with 99Tcm-MDP bone scintigraphy, *Nucl Med Commun* 22:875–879, 2001.

Oshida M, Uno K, Suzuki M, et al.: Predicting the prognoses of breast carcinoma patients with positron emission tomography using 2-deoxy-2-fluoro[18F]-D-glucose, *Cancer* 82:2227–2234, 1998.

Palmedo H, Bender H, Grunwald F, et al.: Comparison of fluorine-18 fluorodeoxyglucose positron emission tomography and technetium-99m methoxyisobutylisonitrile scintimammography in the detection of breast tumours, *Eur J Nucl Med* 24:1138–1145, 1997.

Pecking AP, Mechelany-Corone C, Bertrand-Kermorgant F, et al.: Detection of occult disease in breast cancer using fluorodeoxyglucose camera-based positron emission tomography, *Clin Breast Cancer* 2:229–234, 2001.

Puglisi F, Follador A, Minisini AM, et al.: Baseline staging tests after a new diagnosis of breast cancer: further evidence of their limited indications, *Ann Oncol* 16:263–266, 2005.

Riedl CC, Slobod E, Jochelson M, et al.: Retrospective analysis of 18F-FDG PET/CT for staging asymptomatic breast cancer patients younger than 40 years, *J Nucl Med* 55:1578–1583, 2014.

Rong, et al.: Comparison of 18 FDG PET-CT and bone scintigraphy for detection of bone metastases in breast cancer patients, a meta-analysis, *Surg Oncol* 22:86–91, 2013.

Roodman GD: Mechanisms of bone metastasis, *Discov Med* 4:144–148, 2004.

Schelling M, Avril M, Nahrig J, et al.: Positron emission tomography using [(18)F] Fluorodeoxyglucose for monitoring primary chemotherapy in breast cancer, *J Clin Oncol* 18:1689–1695, 2000.

Schirrmeister H, Guhlmann A, Kotzerke J, et al.: Early detection and accurate description of extent of metastatic bone disease in breast cancer with fluoride ion and positron emission tomography, *J Clin Oncol* 17:2381–2389, 1999.

Schirrmeister H, Kuhn T, Guhlmann A, et al.: Fluorine-18 2-deoxy-2-fluoro-D-glucose PET in the preoperative staging of breast cancer: comparison with the standard staging procedures, *Eur J Nucl Med* 28:351–358, 2001.

Segaert I, Mottaghy F, Ceyssens S, et al.: Additional value of PET-CT in staging of clinical stage IIB and III breast cancer, *Breast J* 16:617–624, 2010.

Segall G, Delbeke D, Stabin MG, et al.: SNM practice guideline for sodium 18F-fluoride PET/CT bone scans 1.0, *J Nucl Med* 51:1813–1820, 2010.

Shie P, Cardarelli R, Brandon D, Erdman W, Abdulrahim N: Meta-analysis: comparison of F-18 Fluorodeoxyglucose-positron emission tomography and bone scintigraphy in the detection of bone metastases in patients with breast cancer, *Clin Nucl Med* 33:97–101, 2008.

Shigematsu H, Kadoya T, Masumoto N, et al.: Role of FDG-PET/CT in prediction of underestimation of invasive breast cancer in cases of ductal carcinoma in situ diagnosed at needle biopsy, *Clin Breast Cancer* 14:358–364, 2014.

Siegel R, Ma J, Zou Z, Jemal A: Cancer statistics, *CA Cancer J Clin* 64:9–29, 2014.

Sloka JS, Hollett PD, Mathews M: Cost-effectiveness of positron emission tomography in breast cancer, *Mol Imaging Biol* 7:351–360, 2005.

Son SH, Kim DH, Hong CM, et al.: Prognostic implication of intratumoral metabolic heterogeneity in invasive ductal carcinoma of the breast, *BMC Cancer* 14:585, 2014.

Sugg SL, Ferguson DJ, Posner MC, Heimann R: Should internal mammary nodes be sampled in the sentinel lymph node era? *Ann Surg Oncol* 7:188–192, 2000.

Surti S, Karp JS, Popescu LM, Daube-Witherspoon ME, Werner M: Investigation of time-of-flight benefit for fully 3-D PET, *IEEE Trans Med Imaging* 25:529–538, 2006.

Tateishi U, Gamez C, Dawood S, Yeung HW, Cristofanilli M, Macapinlac HA: Bone metastases in patients with metastatic breast cancer: morphologic and metabolic monitoring of response to systemic therapy with integrated PET/CT, *Radiology* 247:189–196, 2008.

Tejwani A, Lavaf A, Parikh K, et al.: The role of PET/CT in decreasing inter-observer variability in treatment planning and evaluation of response for cervical cancer, *Am J Nucl Med Mol Imaging* 2:307–313, 2012.

Ueda S, Tsuda H, Asakawa H, et al.: Clinicopathological and prognostic relevance of uptake level using 18F-fluorodeoxyglucose positron emission tomography/computed tomography fusion imaging (18F-FDG PET/CT) in primary breast cancer, *Jpn J Clin Oncol* 38:250–258, 2008.

Uematsu T, Yuen S, Yukisawa S, et al.: Comparison of FDG PET and SPECT for detection of bone metastases in breast cancer, *AJR Am J Roentgenol* 184:1266–1273, 2005.

Ulaner GA, Eaton A, Morris PG, et al.: Prognostic value of quantitative fluorodeoxyglucose measurements in newly diagnosed metastatic breast cancer, *Cancer Med* 2:725–733, 2013.

Veronesi U, Arnone P, Veronesi P, et al.: The value of radiotherapy on metastatic internal mammary nodes in breast cancer. Results on a large series, *Ann Oncol* 19:1553–1560, 2008.

Veronesi U, Paganelli G, Viale G, et al.: A randomized comparison of sentinel-node biopsy with routine axillary dissection in breast cancer, *N Engl J Med* 349:546–553, 2003.

Veronesi U, Paganelli G, Viale G, et al.: Sentinel-lymph-node biopsy as a staging procedure in breast cancer: update of a randomised controlled study, *Lancet Oncol* 7:983–990, 2006.

Vranjesevic D, Schiepers C, Silverman DH, et al.: Relationship between 18F-FDG uptake and breast density in women with normal breast tissue, *J Nucl Med* 44:1238–1242, 2003.

Wahl RL, Jacene H, Kasamon K, Lodge MA: From RECIST to PERCIST: evolving Considerations for PET response criteria in solid tumors, *J Nucl Med* 50(Suppl 1):122S–150S, 2009.

Wahl RL, Siegel BA, Coleman RE, Gatsonis CG: P. E.T. Study Group: prospective multicenter study of axillary nodal staging by positron emission tomography in breast cancer: a report of the staging breast cancer with PET Study Group, *J Clin Oncol* 22:277–285, 2004.

World Health Organization (WHO): International Agency for Research on Cancer: GLOBOCAN 2012: Estimated cancer incidence, mortality and prevalence worldwide in 2012. http://globocan.iarc.fr/Pages/fact_sheets_cancer.aspx Accessed July 27, 2015.

Zhang Y, Shi H, Cheng D, et al.: Added value of SPECT/spiral CT versus SPECT in diagnosing solitary spinal lesions in patients with extraskeletal malignancies, *Nucl Med Commun* 34:451–458, 2013.

Index

Pages followed by b, t, or f refer to boxes, tables, or figures, respectively.

466